P9-DCZ-521

THE COMPLETE & UP-TO-DATE

FAT

BOOK

NEWLY REVISED AND EXPANDED

THE COMPLETE & UP-TO-DATE

FAT BOOK

*A guide to the fat, calories, and
fat percentages in your food*

4TH EDITION

Karen J. Bellerson

AVERY
a member of Penguin Putnam Inc.
NEW YORK

SOURCES OF NUTRITION INFORMATION

United States Department of Agriculture Handbook No. 8 (revised), "Composition of Foods Raw, Processed, Prepared," sections 8–1 through 8–22; Handbook No. 456, "Nutritive Value of American Foods in Common Units"; Home and Garden Bulletin No. 232, "Nutrition and Your Health: Dietary Guidelines for Americans."

Food manufacturers and processors, as well as their product labels.

Individual fast-food chains.

Every effort has been made to ensure that the information in this book is complete and accurate. However, neither the publisher nor the author is engaged in rendering professional advice or services to the individual reader. The ideas, procedures, and suggestions herein are not intended as a substitute for consulting with a physician. All matters regarding health require medical supervision. Calories, fat content, and fat percentages for processed foods are subject to change, and might in the future vary from listings in this book, which are based on research conducted in 2000. Neither the author nor the publisher shall be liable or responsible for any loss, injury, or damage allegedly arising from any information or suggestion in this book.

Most Avery books are available at special quantity discounts for bulk purchase for sales promotions, premiums, fundraising, and educational needs. Special books or book excerpts also can be created to fit specific needs. For details, write Putnam Special Markets, 375 Hudson Street, New York, NY 10014.

a member of
Penguin Putnam Inc.
375 Hudson Street
New York, NY 10014
www.penguinputnam.com

Copyright © 1991, 1993, 1997, 2001 by Karen J. Bellerson
All rights reserved. This book, or parts thereof, may not be
reproduced in any form without permission.
Published simultaneously in Canada

Library of Congress Cataloging-in-Publication Data

Bellerson, Karen J.
    The complete & up-to-date fat book : a guide to the fat, calories, and fat percentages in
your food / Karen J. Bellerson.—4th ed.
        p.   cm.
    ISBN 1-58333-099-2
    1. Food—Fat content—Tables.   I. Title: Complete and up-to-date fat book.   II. Title.
TX551.B39   2001   2001022137
613.2'84—dc21

Printed in the United States of America

10 9 8 7 6 5 4 3 2

To You, the Reader

In honor of a new millennium and the ten years of successful publication that this book has enjoyed, I dedicate this edition to you. For without you, none of it would have been possible. You have my gratitude and wishes for a lifetime of vibrantly good health.

Contents

Acknowledgments

My heartfelt gratitude to my editor, Laura Shepherd, for orchestrating yet another revision of *The Complete and Up-to-Date Fat Book*. A book of such complexity is not published and does not reach such a measure of success without the expertise of those who know what they are doing, and Laura's insight and enthusiasm to my ideas were invaluable. To judge from the continuing quality and precision of the editing, Chris Mariadason appears to have found his life's calling! Thank you, Chris!

As always, my appreciation goes also to those food manufacturers who make nutritional information about their products available and who have listened to consumers' requests for tastier healthful food choices.

For all of you who take the time to write me (whether to ask questions, make comments, or offer suggestions), I want you to know that your letters are of great help to me. Thank you very much for allowing me to play a small part in your endeavors to pursue a healthier, nutritionally sound lifestyle.

Preface

We who have no time for our health today
may have no health for our time tomorrow.

Hello, and thank you for joining me in our never-ending quest for healthy eating habits, this time at the beginning of a new millennium, with the fourth edition of The Complete & Up-to-Date Fat Book. *In my desire to bring you the most complete and up-to-date nutritional data available, I continue to educate not only you but myself as well. By this I mean that the constantly changing food industry keeps me on my toes with its ingenuity in manufacturing new food products. It is an endless challenge, which I gladly accept, to keep up with the extraordinary abundance of food products making their debut on our grocery shelves.*

Many food manufacturers, along with nutritional watchdogs such as the Center for Science in the Public Interest, the National Cancer Institute, the American Heart Association, and the publishers of numerous nutrition and health newsletters, take our nutritional habits very seriously. They persevere in proving the direct relationship between a high-fat diet (in which more than 30 percent of daily calories come from fat) and a higher risk of developing cancer, heart disease, stroke, diabetes, high blood pressure (hypertension), and other life-threatening diseases. Along these same lines, professionals throughout the health field promote the very real health benefits of a low-fat nutritional lifestyle.

In their endeavors to bring their findings to the public's attention, some of these groups publish dietary guidelines, which almost seem to be clones of one another in the close similarity of their content. I offer you the guidelines of one such group, the National Cancer Institute. These are geared to cancer prevention, but they are consistent with the Dietary Guidelines for Americans *(which you will find on pages 2–3).*

NATIONAL CANCER INSTITUTE DIETARY GUIDELINES

- *Reduce daily fat intake to 30 percent of calories or less.*
- *Increase fiber to 20–30 grams/day, with an upper limit of 35 grams.*

- *Include a variety of fruits and vegetables in the daily diet.*
- *Avoid obesity.*
- *Consume alcoholic beverages in moderation, if at all.*
- *Minimize consumption of salt-cured, salt-pickled, and smoked foods.*

As much as I agree with the above recommendations, there is one that is, sadly, missing from this list and others published in this country. I am referring to the proven fact that healthful eating habits encompass more than just sustained physical well-being, and involve more than just what you eat. The following recommendations, found in published dietary guidelines from some other countries, reinforce that fact.

- *Britain's number-one dietary guideline is: "Enjoy your food."*
- *Japanese dietary advice includes "Avoid too much salt," and furthermore: "Happy eating makes for happy family life. Sit down and eat together and talk. Treasure family taste and home cooking."*
- *The Norwegian government tells its people that "food and joy equal health."*
- *Vietnam advocates preparing "a healthy family meal that is delicious" and to serve it "with affection."*

As charming as the above advice is, it also makes perfect sense. Why? As you will find, following it often leads to a welcome bonus of more harmony within the family circle. And those of you who have teenagers may very well enjoy a double bonus by following any of these guidelines. Research strongly indicates that teenagers who eat with adult family members an average of five times a week tend to be more mentally alert, more motivated to do well in their school studies, and less likely to use drugs or experience depression than those who eat with their parent/parents only three times a week or less.

As you read this book and plan your meals, keep in mind that it is your total diet that counts, not the nutrient content of a single food. Educating yourself in how much and what kind of dietary fat is in the foods you eat will enable you to make wise choices and keep your eating habits balanced and in moderation to make room for all your favorite foods. Remember, too, that small, gradual changes can add up to lifelong eating habits. Choose those foods that fit in with your personal tastes and preferences, balancing good nutrition, variety, and great taste!

Let me leave you with the following proverb, hoping you will take it to heart: "The best physicians are Dr. Diet, Dr. Quiet, and Dr. Merryman!"

Until next time,

Introduction

Only saturated fats and dietary cholesterol raise blood cholesterol. A high level of cholesterol in the blood is a major risk factor for coronary heart disease, which leads to heart attack.

—American Heart Association

The single most influential dietary change one can make to lower the risk of these diseases [cardiovascular disease, diabetes, and certain forms of cancer] is to reduce intake of foods high in fats and to increase the intake of foods high in complex carbohydrates and fiber.

—The Surgeon General's Report on Nutrition and Health, 1988

More than half of all adults in the United States are overweight or obese, and the rates of obesity in children and teens have doubled since the late 1970s. Obesity increases the risk of diabetes, heart disease, stroke, and other health problems. Each year in this country, obesity causes tens or even hundreds of thousands of premature deaths, and *costs the public tens of billions of dollars.*

—Centers for Disease Control and Prevention

Health specialists are calling it a "fat epidemic," and no wonder, with the latest numbers showing that more than half of Americans are overweight and one out of three adults is obese. The fat-and-fatter trend has initiated more research into obesity than ever, focusing on its causes and effects. This is especially significant in light of findings that link higher fat intake to a myriad of serious health problems, including heart and respiratory disease, diabetes, osteoarthritis, and some forms of cancer.

For decades, studies have shown the influence of diet on the development of such diseases. Much of what we know today about the diet–disease relationship dates back to World War II, during which the incidence of death from heart attacks among Western Europeans declined greatly. The cause of this dramatic decline was found to lie in the wartime rationing of foods such as meat, dairy products, and eggs. Once the war was over and high-fat foods were once again available, the incidence of heart disease rose. In-depth studies were begun in earnest to investigate the negative effects of these foods.

Today we know that populations with low-fat diets tend to have a lower occurrence of heart disease, stroke, and diabetes, and countless studies prove that there is a very real relationship between diet and the risk of devel-

1

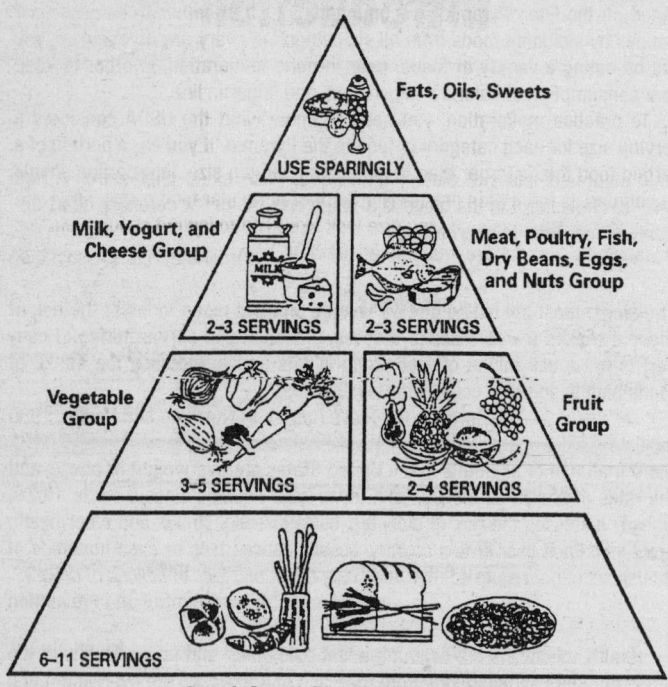

Fats, Oils, Sweets

USE SPARINGLY

Milk, Yogurt, and
Cheese Group

Meat, Poultry, Fish,
Dry Beans, Eggs,
and Nuts Group

2–3 SERVINGS

2–3 SERVINGS

Vegetable
Group

Fruit
Group

3–5 SERVINGS

2–4 SERVINGS

6–11 SERVINGS

Bread, Cereal, Rice, and Pasta Group

Figure 1.   Food Guide Pyramid

oping a life-threatening disease. In response to many of these findings, the
United States Department of Agriculture (USDA) replaced its Four Basic Food
Groups (milk; meat; vegetables and fruits; breads and cereals) with the Food
Guide Pyramid (released in January 1996; see Figure 1) as a formula for a
healthy diet.

Notice that fats, oils, and sweets are the smallest part of the Food Guide
Pyramid. This reflects advice from major health organizations recommending
a diet consisting of 55 to 60 percent carbohydrates, 15 percent protein, and
no more than 30 percent fat. Some experts feel that only 25 percent or less of
calories should come from fat, in order to lower the risk of heart disease and
certain kinds of cancer.

The Food Guide Pyramid can help you plan a healthy, balanced diet that
meets your individual nutritional needs and caloric intake, while taking into

consideration your particular food likes and dislikes. When making choices based on the Food Pyramid's recommendations, remember to balance your choices by including foods from all six categories every day. In doing so, you will be eating a variety of foods. Bear in mind moderation, in order to keep your consumption of calories, fat, sodium, and sugar in line.

To practice moderation, you need to know what the USDA considers a serving size for each category of food in the Pyramid. If you eat a portion of a certain food that is larger than the indicated serving size, that portion should be counted as more than one serving for that particular food group.

Exactly what does a serving size look like? The following should help you to visualize a standard recommended serving:

A golf ball   = 1-ounce meatball
A deck of cards   = 3 ounces cooked lean meat
A baseball   = 1 cup milk or other liquid dairy product
3 stacked dominoes = 1½ ounces cheese

Table 1 on page 4 shows the USDA's recommended serving sizes for the various types of foods in the Pyramid.

Other USDA dietary guidelines include these:

1. Eat a variety of foods.
2. Balance the food you eat with physical activity and maintain or improve your weight.
3. Choose a diet low in fat, saturated fat, and cholesterol.
4. Choose a diet with plenty of grain products, vegetables, and fruits.
5. Choose a diet moderate in sugars.
6. Choose a diet moderate in salt and sodium.
7. If you drink alcoholic beverages, do so in moderation. Children, adolescents, and pregnant women should abstain.

Okay, you're convinced that you need to get the fat out of your diet, but where do you begin? Before we go into some simple guidelines, let's look at a few basic facts about dietary fat.

FAT: A NECESSARY NUTRIENT

The fact is that we need some fat in our diets. *Adults need a minimum daily intake of 15 to 25 grams of dietary fat to meet the body's needs.* Children under age two should not have their dietary fat restricted, because that may interfere with their development.

Our bodies use fat in numerous ways—ways most of us are unaware of. We use fat in manufacturing antibodies to fight disease. Fat acts as carriers for the fat-soluble vitamins (A, D, E, and K). Fat is one of the body's three nutrient energy sources, and it aids in digestion by slowing down the stomach's secretions of hydrochloric acid. This is what produces that satisfying feeling of fullness after a meal. Fat deposits in the body cushion, protect, and hold in place vital organs such as the kidneys, heart, and liver, and also give the body its shape. Fat is the body's insulation against environmental temperature changes. As you can see, fat is a vital nutrient, and should not be totally eliminated from our diets.

All fats are composed of building blocks called fatty acids. There are two types of fatty acids: nonessential, which our body is able to manufacture, and essential, which we cannot make and must obtain through our diets. Essential fatty acids are necessary for normal growth; for healthy skin, blood, arteries, and nerves; and for a smoothly running metabolism.

Table 1.   Serving Sizes

Food Group	Amount
Bread, cereal, rice, and pasta (6–11 servings daily)	1 slice bread ½ hamburger roll, bagel, or English muffin 1 ounce ready-to-eat cereal (be sure to check labels, as 1 ounce may equal anywhere from ¼ cup to 2 cups, depending on the cereal) ½ cup cooked cereal, rice, or pasta 3 or 4 plain crackers (small)
Vegetables (3–5 servings daily)	1 cup raw leafy vegetables ½ cup other vegetables, cooked or chopped raw ¾ cup vegetable juice
Fruit (2–4 servings daily)	1 medium apple, banana, orange, nectarine, or peach ½ cup chopped raw, cooked, or canned fruit ¾ cup fruit juice
Milk, yogurt, and cheese (2–3 servings daily)	1 cup milk or yogurt 1½ ounces natural cheese 2 ounces processed cheese
Meat, poultry, fish, dry beans, eggs, and nuts (2–3 servings daily)	2–3 ounces cooked lean meat, poultry, or fish 1½ cups cooked dry beans 2–3 eggs 4–6 tablespoons peanut butter

CHOLESTEROL AND LIPOPROTEINS (LDL AND HDL)

The main reason to be concerned with the fat in your diet is that fat—both the amount and the type—affects blood cholesterol. Cholesterol is a white, waxy, fatty substance found in all foods that come from animal sources, particularly organ meats such as brains, kidney, and liver. Because plants do not manufacture cholesterol, there is no cholesterol in them; this applies as well to oils that come from vegetable sources. While cholesterol is not a fatty acid, it is a fatlike substance and is often referred to as a fat.

Cholesterol, too, is essential to our well-being. We need it to help build cell membranes, to produce hormones (estrogen, progesterone, and testosterone), and to manufacture bile acids needed for eliminating excess cholesterol from the body. If we have more cholesterol than we need in our blood, however, it clogs the arteries. For the average person, about 75 percent of the cholesterol found in the body—all the body needs—is manufactured in the liver, even if that person eats no animal products; the other 25 percent comes from the diet.

Cholesterol is carried through the bloodstream by molecules called lipoproteins. The cholesterol manufactured by the liver is carried to the cells that need it by low-density lipoproteins (LDLs). High levels of LDLs in the bloodstream can result in clogged arteries, causing high blood pressure, stroke, and heart disease. This is why LDL is referred to as "bad cholesterol"—or, as I call it, "lethal cholesterol." *LDL levels can be reduced through a proper diet.*

Now we come to the high-density lipoproteins (HDLs), or "good cholesterol," which I refer to a "healthy cholesterol." HDLs pick up excess cholesterol from various body tissues and carry it to the liver. It is then metabolized by the liver, processed through the intestines, and eliminated from the body. High levels of HDL are associated with a decreased risk of coronary heart disease. HDL levels can be raised through regular exercise. Total cholesterol, the sum of the total of LDL plus HDL, is also important, because it allows us to see the ratio of LDL to HDL.

TYPES OF DIETARY FATS IN INDIVIDUAL FOODS

Because of differences in their chemical structure, the fatty acids in the foods we eat fall in to three categories: polyunsaturated, monounsaturated, and saturated. Most foods contain a combination of all three kinds of dietary fat, usually with a higher content of one of them. The relative percentage of each type of fat in any one food is what makes it a healthier or less healthy choice than another.

Polyunsaturated Fats

Polyunsaturated fats are found in most foods. Omega-3 polyunsaturated fats are found primarily in certain fish, while omega-6 polyunsaturated fats are found mainly in nuts, plant oils, seeds, and soybeans. These fats are liquid at room temperature. Polyunsaturated fats reduce blood cholesterol, but if eaten in excess they may lower the level of protective "good cholesterol," or HDL. Some studies speculate a link between a high consumption of polyunsaturated fats and breast cancer.

Foods in which polyunsaturated fats are the main type of fat include those listed below. **Note that the foods listed here are not necessarily high in fat.** They are simply higher in polyunsaturated fats than in the other two types of fats.

Bagels
Barbecue sauce
Bluefish
Brazil nuts
Chickpeas (garbanzo beans)
Cod
Corn chips
Cornmeal
French bread
Haddock
Herring
Italian bread
Lentils
Mackerel
Mussels
Oysters
Oatmeal bread
Pine nuts
Popcorn (air-popped)
Potato chips
Potato salad (made with mayonnaise)
Pumpernickel
Pumpkin seeds
Rainbow trout
Raisin bread
Refried beans
Rye bread
Salad dressings (most types)
Salmon
Sardines
Scallops
Sesame seeds
Soybeans
Squash
Squash seeds
Sunflower seeds
Sweet potatoes
Tofu
Tuna salad (made with mayonnaise)
Vegetable and nut oils (see table, page 463)
Walnuts
Whitefish

Monounsaturated Fats

Monounsaturated fats are found in most foods, but mainly in vegetable and nut oils such as canola (rapeseed), olive, and peanut. These fats too are liquid at room temperature. They reduce total blood cholesterol while not lowering the protective "good cholesterol," HDL.

The following foods are higher in monounsaturated fats than in the other two types of fats. Those marked with an asterisk are also high in saturated fats.

Almonds
Animal fats* (most
    types)
Avocados
Beef* (leaner cuts)
Biscuits
Bread* (most
    types)
Brownies
Cake* (most types)
Cashews
Chestnuts
Chicken
Cookies* (most
    types)
Croissants*

Doughnuts* (most
    types)
Eggs*
Fruitcake
Gingerbread
Hazelnuts
Lard*
Macadamia nuts
Margarine (stick types)
Muffins*
Oatmeal
Ocean perch
Pastry (including pie
    crust)
Peanut butter
Peanuts

Pecans
Pies* (most types)
Pistachios
Popcorn (popped in
    vegetable oil)
Pork*
Sausage* (most types)
Spaghetti (with tomato
    sauce)
Taco*
Veal* (leaner cuts)
Vegetable and nut oils
    (see table, page 463)
Vegetable
    shortening

Saturated Fats

All meat and dairy products contain saturated fats. Coconut, palm, and palm kernel oils, although of plant origin, are also high in saturated fat, as is cocoa butter, which is used in making chocolate. (This is why I recommend substituting powdered cocoa in recipes that call for chocolate.) Saturated fats are generally solid at room temperature. *Saturated fats—even more than dietary cholesterol—raise total blood cholesterol.*

The following foods are higher in saturated fats than in the other two types of fats. Other foods high in saturated fats appear in the list of foods high in monounsaturated fat. Those foods are marked with an asterisk, and, while monounsaturated fats predominate, they contain significant amounts of saturated fats as well.

Beef (fattier cuts)
Beef tallow
Boston brown bread
    (canned)
Butter
Cheese (most types)
Cheesecake
Chili (with beef)
Chocolate

Cocoa butter
Cocoa mixes
Coconut
Coconut products
Cottage cheese (4% fat)
Cream
Cream soups (most
    types)
Custard (baked)

Duck
Eggnog
Fried foods (fried in
    saturated oils)
Garlic spread
Granola
Gravy (brown,
    packaged)
Hot dogs

Ice cream
Lamb
Luncheon meats
Malts
Milk (whole, 2%, and 1%)
Nondairy creamer
Nondairy whipped topping
Pies (cream types)
Pizza
Pompano

Popcorn (most microwave types)
Pork (fattier cuts)
Puddings
Quiche
Sauces (butter-, egg-, milk-based, such as béarnaise, hollandaise, white, or cheese sauce)
Seaweed
Shakes

Snack cakes (most types, those with chocolate frosting)
Sour cream
Turkey (dark meat or self-basting)
Veal (fattier cuts)
Vegetable and nut oils (especially coconut, palm, and palm kernel; see table, page 463)

Remember, the essential fatty acids—the ones that must be obtained through the diet—are unsaturated. This means we can get all the fat we need from unsaturated fats; there is no biological need for saturated fat.

The American Heart Association points out that the body can use all three types of fats, but it recommends, for the average person, that:

• Total daily fat intake (saturated, monounsaturated, polyunsaturated) should be limited to no more than 30 percent of total calories.

• Daily saturated fat intake should be limited to 7 to 10 percent of total calories.

• Daily polyunsaturated fat intake should be no more than 10 percent of total calories.

• Daily monounsaturated fat intake should be no more than 15 percent of total calories.

Recommended Daily Fat Gram Budget per Caloric Intake*

Total Daily Calories	Total Daily Fat (in grams†)	Daily Saturated Fat (in grams†)
1,200	40	9–12
1,500	50	11–15
1,800	60	13–18
2,000	67	14–20
2,200	73	15–22
2,500	83	18–25
3,000	100	21–30

*For healthy people over age two

†There are 9 calories in 1 gram of fat. To calculate your maximum allowable total daily fat, see the formula on page 14.

Hydrogenated Fats and Trans-Fatty Acids

The American Heart Association further recommends a total daily fat intake equivalent to between 5 and 8 teaspoons of fats and oils, to reduce the possibility of an excess of trans-fats.

You may have read of, and been confused by, the term "trans fatty acids." These are simply types of fats formed when liquid polyunsaturated or monounsaturated oils are subjected to a process called hydrogenation, in which hydrogen is added to an oil to convert it to a solid or semisolid at room temperature, so that it can be used in baked goods, nondairy creamers, whipped toppings, and other processed foods. The hydrogenation of unsaturated fats causes them to act like saturated fats in the bloodstream, raising blood cholesterol and LDL. On the labels of such products as margarine, shortening, chips, and baked goods, the amount of trans fatty acids is included in the amount of total fat, but not in the amount of saturated fat. Be aware that both polyunsaturated and monounsaturated fats can be hydrogenated. While some trans fats occur naturally in dairy products and other foods of animal origin, most are formed by hydrogenation. When you read product labels, watch for the words "hydrogenated" or "partially hydrogenated," which indicate the presence of trans fatty acids.

The Food and Drug Administration is currently proposing that trans fat be listed as part of the saturated fat content on food labels. Under this proposal, food products advertised as "low in saturated fat" could contain more than 0.5 grams of trans fat, aside from the current requirement of less than 1 gram of saturated fat per serving, and a food labeled as "low-cholesterol" could contain no more than 2 grams of saturated fat and trans fat combined per serving size. The American Heart Association recommends using liquid vegetable oil and liquid or soft margarines whenever possible. The harder and more solid a margarine is, the more trans fatty acids it contains.

"Fake Fats"

For years we have heard about ongoing research in the area of "fake fats," or fat substitutes. Manufacturers have been eager to develop low- or no-calorie substitutes for fat that would have the characteristics of fat: the texture, "mouth feel," and flavor, as well as the ability to stand up under a wide range of manufacturing processes.

Even the United States Department of Agriculture has scientists working on the development of an acceptable fat replacement. Dr. George Inglett, a research chemist at the department's Agricultural Research Service National Center for Agricultural Utilization Research in Peoria, Illinois (and developer of Oatrim-10, an earlier fat substitute), has developed a fat substitute known as

Z-Trim. This is a purified insoluble fiber made from seed hulls of oats, soybeans, peas, and rice, or corn or wheat bran and dried to a white powder. Since Z-Trim is made of natural dietary fiber, it does not upset the digestive system when consumed in ordinary amounts. Fantesk, which uses biopolymers and water to mimic fat in food products, is another fat substitute developed at the National Center for Agricultural Utilization Research. It has been licensed for use in ice cream and processed meat products.

Simplesse is one of the better-known fake fats. Made of egg whites and milk protein, it has been on the market for several years. Whereas fat has 9 calories per gram, Simplesse has only 1 to 2 calories per gram. Because it consists largely of protein and contains only the fat found in skim milk, its safety, like that of Z-Trim and Fantesk, has not been questioned by the FDA.

Procter & Gamble scientists have been working on their fake fat, Olestra, for twenty-five years or so. Finally, after P&G had spent more than $200 million in research and produced more than 150,000 pages of supporting data, the FDA gave the green light of Olestra (marketed under the trade name Olean) in January 1996.

Olestra is a chemically engineered variation of natural fat made from sugar and vegetable oil. It is reported to be virtually fat-free and can withstand cooking at high temperatures without breaking down. Although Olestra has the taste and consistency of fat, it cannot be digested or absorbed by the body like fat. Its ability to "pass through the body undigested" has made Olestra controversial among health care professionals and others within the public health community.

When the FDA cleared Olestra for use in the manufacture of salty, savory snack foods only (until studies of long-term effect can be done), there were both cheers and boos to be heard across the nation. Enthusiasm came from those who focused on new and improved low-fat and fat-free products they hoped to see on grocery shelves, while opposition came from nutritional watchdogs who focused on the possible side effects of consuming foods containing Olestra. Their very real concerns included the fact that since Olestra cannot be absorbed by the body, some of the fat-soluble vitamins (A, D, E, and K), when eaten at the same time as Olestra, will be dissolved in the Olestra and will also pass through the body. Vitamins eaten at least two hours before or after the Olestra should not be affected. Also, Olestra sharply decreases the levels of some carotenoids in the bloodstream. Carotenoids, a group of more than 500 related compounds found in fruits and vegetables (beta-carotene and lycopene are the best-known) are also fat-soluble. Large quantities of carotenoids from fruits and vegetables are associated with lower rates of cancer; lower levels of carotenoids in the bloodstream are associated with heart disease and stroke. Further, because Olestra is not digested or absorbed, it may have negative gastrointestinal side effects.

Because of the concerns suggested above, and so that consumers will know if any foods they purchase contain Olestra (Olean), the FDA is requiring

P&G to make sure that all foods containing Olestra are packaged in containers that carry the following statement: "This product contains Olestra. Olestra may cause abdominal cramping and loose stools. Olestra inhibits the absorption of some vitamins and other nutrients. Vitamins A, D, E, and K have been added."

The American Heart Association discourages the use of substitute (fake) fats or sugars, particularly in children's diets. In the absence of evidence for overall health benefits, it feels that people, especially children, are better off developing a taste for fruits, vegetables, and whole-grain foods instead of foods containing fat or sugar substitutes and, as is often the case, little nutritional value.

FOOD LABELS: "NUTRITION FACTS"

As you walk down the aisles of your supermarket, make it a practice to look at the array of foods offered. You will see hundreds of new food products flooding the market each year from our industrious food manufacturers. Before you buy, read nutrition labels to decide whether a particular food will fit in with your ultimate goal of a healthy eating lifestyle.

Although the standard food nutrition label offers a lot of information (see Figure 2), people often tell me they are confused by it. **The "% Daily Value" column especially causes confusion.** Some consumers make the mistake of assuming that the percentage across from "Total Fat" represents the percentage of calories that come from fat. Don't be misled; it has nothing to do with the percentage of calories from fat. Rather, "% Daily Value" indicates what part of a 2,000-calorie-a-day diet is constituted by the corresponding nutrient. Thus, in the label in Figure 2, the "5%" opposite "Total Fat" means that one serving of the product provides 5 percent of daily fat intake. Of course, if you eat more or less than 2,000 calories a day, the "% Daily Value" listed will not reflect the true percentage for you. However, you can still use these numbers to get a general idea of a particular food's nutritional values relative to an average daily diet and thus determine whether to include the food in your eating plans. *Remember that the guidelines shown on food labels are for healthy adults and children two years of age or older.* A low-fat diet may be harmful to children younger than two years of age.

Also potentially confusing are the many descriptive words that appear on food labels, words such as "lite," "reduced-calorie," "low-fat," and "no sodium." I offer the following definitions in hopes they will help clarify matters:

• *Cholesterol-free.* Containing less than 2 milligrams of cholesterol and 2 grams or less of saturated fat per serving. This in no way indicates that a product is fat-free.

• *Extra-lean.* Containing less than 5 grams of total fat, less than 2 grams of saturated fat, and less than 95 milligrams of cholesterol per serving.

- *Fat-free.* Containing less than 0.5 grams of fat per serving.
- *High-fiber.* Containing 5 grams or more of fiber per serving.
- *Lean.* Containing less than 10 grams of total fat, less than 4 grams of saturated fat, and less than 95 milligrams of cholesterol per serving (but not as little as extra-lean).
- *Less.* Referring to a food, altered or not, containing 25 percent less of a nutrient or of calories than other comparable foods.
- *Light* or *lite.* Containing one-third fewer calories or no more than half the fat of the higher-calorie, higher-fat version; or containing no more than half the sodium of the higher-sodium version.
- *Low-saturated-fat.* Containing 1 gram or less of saturated fat per serving.
- *Low-calorie.* Containing 40 or fewer calories per serving.
- *Low-fat.* Containing 3 grams of fat or less per serving.
- *Reduced-fat.* Referring to nutritionally altered product containing 25 percent less of a nutrient or of calories than the regular product.

Figure 2 offers a sample of the most widely used nutrition information label. Other, smaller styles of label are used when the larger ones do not fit on the packaging. The smaller labels show the same nutritional information as the larger version, but in a different format. If a package is too small for any type of readable label (as, for example, certain candy wrappers), the manufacturer must list an address or telephone number from which consumers may request nutritional information.

Another style of label is used for food products that are to have ingredients added to them by the consumer during preparation. Boxed pancake mix is an example of such a product. This type of label shows the nutritional information for one serving of the packaged contents "as packaged" and separate nutritional information for one serving of the finished product with the added ingredients included.

Recently, a bill was introduced in Washington mandating that the Department of Agriculture require, within one year, the same nutritional label on fresh meat and poultry that is now required for processed meat and poultry. This would be particularly beneficial to the consumer, as red meat is one of the largest sources of artery-clogging saturated fat.

CAUTION: "FAT-FREE" PRODUCTS CAN BE HAZARDOUS TO YOUR WEIGHT!

Grocery shelves carry more and more fat-free products, and average fat consumption in the United States decreased from 40 percent of daily calories in

Nutrition Facts

Serving Size ½ cup (114g)
Servings Per Container 4

Amount Per Serving

Calories 90   Calories from Fat 30

	% Daily Value*
Total Fat 3g	**5%**
Saturated Fat 0g	**0%**
Cholesterol 0mg	**0%**
Sodium 300mg	**13%**
Total Carbohydrate 13g	**4%**
Dietary Fiber 3g	**12%**
Sugars 3g	
Protein 3g	

Vitamin A	80%	Vitamin C	60%
Calcium	4%	Iron	4%

* Percent Daily Values are based on a 2,000 calorie diet. Your daily values may be higher or lower depending on your calorie needs:

	Calories	2,000	2,500
Total Fat	Less than	65g	80g
Sat Fat	Less than	20g	25g
Cholesterol	Less than	300mg	300mg
Sodium	Less than	2,400mg	2,400mg
Total Carbohydrate		300g	375g
Fiber		25g	30g

Calories per gram:
Fat 9 • Carbohydrate 4 • Protein 4

More nutrients may be listed on some labels.

Figure 2.   Sample Food Product Label

the 1960s to 34 percent in 1990. Yet these changes have not had the expected effect on people's weight. Why? A clue may lie in the following statistics: The percentage of Americans concerned about their fat intake climbed from 16 in 1987 to 65 in 1995, according to the Food Marketing Institute, while only 13 percent of us appeared to be concerned about calorie intake. Is it any wonder, then, that the National Center for Health Statistics reports that 33 percent more of us are obese (defined as 30 percent or more over healthy weight) than just fifteen years before?

Studies done by the Department of Nutrition and Food Studies at New York University indicate that while we Americans are consuming more calories than ever, we are not compensating with an increase in physical activity.

Along these same lines, Dr. Marion Nestle, a professor in and chair of the department, remarks: "The ubiquity of fast-food outlets and soda vending machines, the huge increase in portion sizes at restaurants, the decline in school physical education programs, and the many hours spent on the Internet and watching television are all contributing to the obesity epidemic."

Although the biggest culprit behind the obesity statistics seems to be lack of exercise, it is becoming increasingly evident that consumers see fat-free products as being totally healthful. They forget the fact that fat-free foods still contain calories—in some cases, as many as (if not more than) their higher-fat counterparts. (Sugar, it should be remembered, is sometimes used to make up for the flavor lost in cutting out fat.) Studies show that some people use the absence of fat as a license to binge on fat-free and low-fat foods. *Remember this: Both the amount of fat and the number of calories are important. Don't buy the myth that "calories don't count." If you eat more calories than you burn, regardless of the source, you will gain weight. Whether the extra calories come from fat, from carbohydrates, or from protein, you will store them as body fat.*

So while fat-free products may be of a higher quality than they were a few years ago, and while they will offer a viable way to cut the amount of fat we consume, portion control is still very much in order. You might try keeping things in perspective by reminding yourself that while a one-and-a-half-ounce serving of "fat-free" cake has less than 0.5 grams of fat, it still has almost the same number of calories as a tablespoon of butter.

GUIDELINES FOR REDUCING THE FAT IN YOUR DIET

As mentioned earlier, fat is needed for healthy body functions and should not be eliminated from the diet. According to a Surgeon General's Report on Nutrition and Health: "Adults need a minimum daily intake of 15 to 25 grams of fat to meet these necessities." The American Heart Association, the American Health Foundation, the American Cancer Society, the National Heart, Lung, and Blood Institute, the National Center for Nutrition and Dietetics, the American Diabetes Association, and the Surgeon General all recommend that no more than 30 percent of daily calories come from fat, and that no more than a third of those fats (or 10 percent of daily calories) be saturated fats. Below you will see how to calculate these percentages.

THE FAT GRAM BUDGET FORMULA

Fortunately, since you have decided to reduce your dietary fat, a simple formula will let you know the exact maximum number of fat grams you can allow yourself every day. To calculate your maximum daily allowance, multiply your daily calorie intake by .3, and divide that total by 9 (there are 9 calories in each gram of fat). For a daily intake of 1,500 calories, your calculation would be:

$$1,500 \times .3 = 450$$
$$450 \div 9 = 50$$

So you should have a maximum of 50 grams of fat per day.

To make things even easier, I have listed the fat gram budgets for specific daily calorie intakes in Table 2. It shows 10 percent, 20 percent, 30 percent maximum daily fat gram budgets for diets of 1,200 to 3,000 calories per day. (Note that the data are rounded; decimal fractions have been dropped.) The table opens with a daily intake of 1,200 calories; it is not recommended that anyone eat fewer than 1,200 calories (for women) or 1,500 calories (for men), in order to ensure that daily nutritional needs are met. In using your daily fat gram budget, remember that the fact that you have budgeted X amount of fat grams for the day doesn't mean you have to eat that entire amount. Just make sure not to go over budget!

Table 2.   Maximum Daily Fat Gram Budget

Daily Calorie Intake	Fat Grams Allowed			Daily Calorie Intake	Fat Grams Allowed		
	10%	20%	30%		10%	20%	30%
1,200	13	27	40	2,200	24	49	73
1,300	14	29	43	2,300	26	51	76
1,400	16	31	46	2,400	27	53	80
1,500	17	33	50	2,500	28	56	83
1,600	16	36	53	2,600	29	58	86
1,700	19	38	56	2,700	30	60	90
1,800	20	40	60	2,800	31	62	93
1,900	21	42	63	2,900	32	64	96
2,000	22	44	66	3,000	33	67	100
2,100	23	47	70				

Of course, to calculate your daily fat gram budget, you need to know your daily calorie intake. If you don't already know this, keep a diary for three or four days. Write down the calorie amounts for everything you eat and drink for these days, add the daily totals, then divide by the number of days you kept track.

People often wonder how many calories they should be consuming on a daily basis. Table 3 will give you a general idea of what your daily calorie consumption should be, making it easier for you to figure your fat gram budget. Keep in mind, though, that everyone has a different metabolism, so the appropriate amount of daily calories for you may vary slightly, above or below the amount listed.

Table 3.   Daily Calorie Requirements

Age / Sex / Activity Level	Calorie Requirements
Minimum calories for adequate nutrition (women)	1,200
Minimum calories for adequate nutrition (men)	1,500
Sedentary women	1,600
Moderately active women; children 4–6 years; women 51 and over	1,800
Active women; sedentary men; teen girls; children 7–10 years	2,000–2,200
Very active women; average men 50 and over; boys 11–14 years	2,200–2,600
Active men; teen boys	2,600–2,800
Active to very active men 25–50; athletes in training	3,000–4,000

Source: U.S. Department of Health and Human Services, Food and Drug Administration, FDA Special Report, May 1993.

MAKING SMARTER, HEALTHIER CHOICES

Here are some tips to follow as you take stock of your eating habits and improve your nutrition by reducing your intake of dietary fat:

• Beef and pork have become leaner than ever because the animals are fed a less fattening diet and are taken to market sooner, before they have a chance to build up a store of fat. You can now choose cuts of beef or pork that have little more fat than a skinless breast of chicken. Stay with the following cuts, boneless and trimmed of visible fat, and keep your cooked portions to 3 ounces (trimmed of all visible fat), prepared without added fat:

Beef (USDA Select)	*Pork*	*Veal*
Chuck arm pot roast	Cured ham (lean)	Cutlets
Eye of round	Loin Roast	Sirloin
Flank steak	Sirloin chops	Tenderloin
Top round	Tenderloin	
Top sirloin	Top loin	

• Familiarize yourself with the number of grams of fat and the percentage of calories from fat in the foods you eat most often, so that it becomes second nature to compute your fat consumption.

• Once you are familiar enough with where the fat is in the foods you eat, make your fat gram budget an average covering three to four days instead of focusing on each meal. This allows some flexibility, which is important for healthy lifelong habit changes.

• When putting together a macaroni, potato, tuna, or turkey salad, don't forget fat-free and reduced-fat mayonnaise on the market today.

• Use a reduced-fat or fat-free margarine or spread instead of butter or regular margarine or spread. Either comes in spreadable, squeezable, and sprayable forms.

• Use canned evaporated skim milk as a substitute for heavy cream, and low-fat or skim milk in place of whole milk or cream in your recipes.

• There is quite a selection of low-fat and fat-free salad dressings available now, in many flavors and styles. Try them until you find one or more to your taste. You can avoid as many as 6 to 10 grams of fat per tablespoon by not using regular salad dressings.

• For desserts, go ahead and splurge on occasion, but more often indulge in the wide range of frozen yogurt desserts in your grocery store's freezer section. Again, because of the wide range, you may have to try more than one or two to find a favorite or favorites. There are also "lighter" ice creams, even in such gourmet flavors as caramel nut fudge sundae and mocha almond fudge. Low-fat and fat-free bakery goods give almost unlimited choices for anyone's sweet tooth. *Remember, though: Moderation and portion control!*

• Substitute low-fat, reduced-fat, or fat-free cheeses for cheeses that are higher in fat. The fat avoided here is between 6 and 10 grams per ounce!

• Most breads are low in fat (1 gram per slice), but be careful when you reach for a croissant to make that sandwich. One butter croissant can have 20 or more grams of fat and 360 calories!

• Dry cereals make a great-tasting snack. Most of them have 0 to 3 grams of fat per serving. Read the labels on granola-type cereals, though, as most of them are higher in fat.

• Canadian bacon is a tasty lower-fat substitute for bacon. Bacon bits also have less fat, and can be used as a pizza topping too.

• When contemplating potato snacks, consider this: While ten French fries have 8 grams of fat, a 1.5-ounce package of potato chips has a whopping 15 grams!

• You can thicken sauces without fat by substituting puréed vegetables for cream or whole milk.

• Make your own bread coatings with plain bread crumbs and your choice of spices. Dip food into skim milk, buttermilk, or egg whites before coating in the bread crumbs and baking.

• Use powdered low-fat or skim milk instead of nondairy creamer.

• Reduce the amount of oil or melted butter in your recipes by a third to a half, and replace the subtracted amount with water, fruit juice, or yogurt. If you buy commercial mixes, buy only those to which you add the fat or oil, so you can control the amount.

• Instead of pan-frying or deep-frying, bake or broil meat, fish, or poultry and baste it with wine, lemon or tomato juice or another juice, broth, or low-fat or fat-free salad dressing to keep it from drying out.

• Instead of using whole eggs, replace each yolk with two egg whites, or use a low-fat egg substitute. Omelets can be made with one whole egg and an additional egg white or two.

• Use partly skimmed ricotta instead of full-fat cream cheese for a luscious cheesecake.

• When using oil, make sure it's the least saturated type available. Although an oil may be low in saturated fat, all oils have 14 grams of fat per tablespoon. (See Oil, pages 463–64.)

• Cocoa powder is an excellent low-fat substitute for baking chocolate, which is high in fat. Use a mixture of 3 tablespoons cocoa, 2 teaspoons sugar, and 1 tablespoon water or other liquid for each 1-ounce square baking chocolate. If the recipe *absolutely* requires baking chocolate, use a smaller amount than called for.

• Coconut-flavored extract and coconut milk (the liquid found inside the coconut, which has only 0.5 gram of fat per cup) are excellent substitutes for coconut when you want that taste. Add shredded carrots and you can have the texture of coconut without the fat.

• Instead of preparing a pan with cooking oil or shortening, use a nonstick pan sprayed with a small amount of cooking spray. Or spread a small amount of oil over the surface of the pan with a paper towel.

These changes can be made easily. Learn the low-fat substitutes to use in your home cooking, and stay away from high-fat store-bought products. Read your labels. Once you have learned from this book how to recognize the fat content of the foods available to you, making healthier eating choices will become a way of life.

LET'S GET STARTED!

By following the suggestions in this book, even just a little at a time, and educating yourself about the sources of dietary fat, you will be on your way to a healthy, low-fat lifestyle. Check the fat content of the foods you usually eat against your daily fat gram budget and see what foods you may need to change or replace with lower-fat choices. Then find appropriate low-fat substitutes for these higher-fat foods to bring you in line with your budget. Sound easy? With the variety of lower-fat foods available, it's easier than ever!

You may be startled by exactly how much dietary fat you have been eating. Moreover, you may find that if a favorite food takes a big enough bite (no pun intended) out of your daily fat gram budget, you will want that favorite food less often and will automatically begin to make more nutritionally sound food selections.

Food for Thought

According to the USDA, the following are America's top ten fat sources:

1. Margarine
2. Whole milk
3. Shortening
4. Mayonnaise and salad dressing
5. American cheese
6. Ground beef
7. Reduced-fat milk
8. Eggs
9. Butter
10. Vanilla ice cream

Write It Down

In the beginning, you will find that keeping a daily account of your food intake cannot be overrated. Keep track of *everything* you eat and drink, so you can accurately total the fat grams and calories for each day. This way, you will have a precise idea of what you are eating and where you need to make adjustments. Your diary will be invaluable also in keeping track of your eating habits and help you form new, healthier ones. It will, furthermore, help you:

- Recognize your eating patterns and reevaluate your food choices.
- Remember what you have eaten throughout the day.
- Gain control over what you eat.
- Budget your fat grams and calories more realistically.
- Think twice about straying from a healthy low-fat lifestyle.
- Take pride in seeing your progress in writing.

At the back of this book you will find a Personal Food Diary to help you start recording your new eating habits.

GET ACQUAINTED WITH *THE COMPLETE AND UP-TO-DATE FAT BOOK*

This is a well-researched, in-depth, and comprehensive nutritional guide. As you shop for and prepare low-fat foods, it will be a valuable source of information for your healthy eating lifestyle. Although extreme care has been taken in recording the data in this book, you may come across occasional discrepancies between the information here and the nutritional data on product labels or other sources of nutritional information. There are a number of possible reasons for this.

First, manufacturers are given a little flexibility, so they may round off their data and still be in accordance with governmental regulations on product labeling. If a certain product contains 2.3 grams of fat, for example, the manufacturer may list the fat content as 2 grams, dropping the .3. The same is done with data on calories. If a product serving has 134 calories, the manufacturer may list the calorie content as either 130 or 135. Wherever possible, I have kept nutritional data intact, rounding off neither fat nor calorie content.

Second, when I gathered data from product labels and compared this with data I received directly from manufacturers, there was at times a difference between the two because the labels listed the nutritional data of old product formulas while the manufacturer provided up-to-date information reflecting a change in the formulas. In these cases, the book gives the more recent data obtained directly from the manufacturer. Also, product serving sizes may change and in turn alter the nutritional data. Be sure, when comparing products, that you are comparing them in the same serving size—that is, a quarter-cup of one product against a quarter-cup of another.

Other discrepancies may be due to differences in the analytical methods and sampling techniques used by various food manufacturers.

As you can see, data in this book are listed in four columns. "Amount" means the serving size of food served or used in a recipe. Any deviation in serving size will mean a change in the data in all the other columns. The fat content of each food is expressed as the number of fat grams (the measurement used for dietary fat) per serving. The calorie column needs no explanation.

In the fourth column, under "% Fat Calories," I have given the percentage of calories from fat for all foods listed. To figure the percentage of fat in the rare food that is not listed:

1. Multiply the number of fat grams by 9 (calories per gram) to get total fat calories (TFC).
2. Divide TFC by the total calorie content of your chosen food.

EXAMPLE: 1 ounce cheddar cheese contains 9 grams and 110 calories
9 (fat grams) x 9 (calories per gram) = 81 (TFC)
81 (TFC) ÷ 110 (total calories) = 0.73, or 73 percent

Since a high-fat food is defined as any food in which 30 percent or more of the calories come from fat, this cheddar cheese would be considered high-fat.

Some of the figures in the "% Fat Calories" column have been rounded, as mentioned, and the percentage might be off slightly, but not so much that it matters. For example, 100 percent of the calories in oils and fats come from fat. But if you look at the listing for butter and calculate the percentage of calories from fat (11 fat grams x 9 calories per gram ÷ 100 calories = 99 percent), the result differs slightly from the "% Fat Calories" listed (100 percent). Because we know that all oils and fats contain 100 percent fat calories, I did not want to mislead you by listing the calculated 99 percent instead of the absolute 100 percent.

You will find both generic and brand-name products in these tables. The listing of a product by brand name is not an endorsement. If certain brand-name products are not listed, it means that there was no nutritional data available at the time the list was compiled, and they were not included for that reason only. Data are given for food products available in wholesale clubs and through wholesale distributors; these are identified as "food service products."

Serving size, fat grams, total calories, and percentage of calories from fat are provided for most products listed. In most cases, the entries are given alphabetically for easy reference. Where appropriate, some types of foods are presented in groups, such as "Frozen Entrée/Dinner," "Mexican Food," and "Asian Food." After the A-to-Z list is a separate section on fast foods, organized alphabetically by individual franchise name.

Since cereals and soups are frequently prepared with milk, quick-reference charts for adding milk can be found in the cereal and soup sections. And because it is important to choose the least saturated oil available when using oil in food preparation, charts on pages 463–64 show the percentages of saturated, polyunsaturated, and monounsaturated fats contained in the most commonly used fats and oils.

The book features main headings for foods in uppercase boldface letters. In some instances, subheadings (smaller and bold) with solid boxes before them have been added for clarity. Description of foods are in upper/lowercase, with brand names in parentheses.

If you are unable to find a particular food, look for the entry of a similar food. The nutritional data should be similar, if not exactly the same. When comparing foods, make sure you are comparing the same serving size, weight measure, and/or volume. The Table of Equivalent Measures (page 24) should help you not only in comparing serving sizes but in making exchanges as well. Finally, note that all servings of cooked vegetables are drained of liquid, unless otherwise specified.

Your copy of *The Complete and Up-to-Date Fat Book* will be a treasured companion as you take control of your eating habits. You will discover that by adopting a low-fat lifestyle you will reap many rewards—rewards such as more energy, better sleep, lower grocery bills, more control over your weight, and perhaps most important, vibrant health and a more satisfying quality of life as a whole!

Abbreviations and Symbols

~	=	approximately
<	=	less than
"	=	inch
–	=	trace amount or less
dia	=	diameter
lb	=	pound
oz	=	ounce
pkg	=	package
pkt	=	packet
sec	=	second
Tbs	=	tablespoon
tsp	=	teaspoon
w/	=	with
w/o	=	without

For dishes described as "homemade," the data assume the use of standard ingredients in preparation—no low-fat substitutes. The data given are guidelines for the dishes as you might make them in your own kitchen. Data on dishes made from packaged mixes assume that they are prepared according to package directions and, unless noted otherwise, without low-fat substitute ingredients.

Table of Equivalent Measures

VOLUME

1 tablespoon	=	½ fluid ounce
		3 teaspoons
1 fluid ounce	=	2 tablespoons
¼ cup	=	2 fluid ounces
		4 tablespoons
⅓ cup	=	5⅓ tablespoons
½ cup	=	4 fluid ounces
		8 tablespoons
⅔ cup	=	10⅔ tablespoons
¾ cup	=	6 fluid ounces
		12 tablespoons
1 cup	=	½ pint
		8 fluid ounces
		16 tablespoons
1 pint	=	2 cups
		16 fluid ounces
1 quart	=	2 pints
		4 cups
		32 fluid ounces
1 gallon	=	4 quarts
		8 pints

WEIGHT

1 ounce	=	28.35 grams
100 grams	=	3.5 ounces
4 ounces	=	¼ pound
8 ounces	=	½ pound
12 ounces	=	¾ pound
1 pound	=	16 ounces
		454 grams

A

Food and Description	Amount	Fat Grams	Total Calories	% Fat Calories
ABALONE				
fried	3 oz	5.8	161	32%
raw	3 oz	1.0	90	10%
ACEROLA /raw	1 medium	–	2	–
	1 cup	–	31	–
ACEROLA JUICE	8 fl oz	0.7	51	12%
ACORN				
dried	1 oz	8.9	145	55%
raw	1 oz	6.8	105	58%
ACORN FLOUR (See FLOUR)				
ADZUKI BEAN				
(Arrowhead Mills) raw	¼ cup	0.5	160	3%
(Eden)	½ cup	–	110	–
generic				
boiled	½ cup	<1.0	147	3%
raw	½ cup	<1.0	325	1%
sweetened/canned	½ cup	<1.0	351	1%
Yokan	¼" slice	–	35	–
AGAR (See SEAWEED)				
ALBACORE (See TUNA)				
ALE (See BEER, ALE, & MALT LIQUOR)				
ALEWIFE/HERRING /raw	4 oz	5.6	144	35%
ALFALFA SPROUTS /raw	1 cup	–	10	–
ALLIGATOR /raw	3 oz	3.0	200	14%
ALLSPICE	1 tsp	–	6	–
ALMOND				
(Azar)				
sliced	1 oz	15.0	170	79%
slivered	1 oz	15.0	170	79%
(Beer Nuts)	1 oz	14.0	180	70%
(Blue Diamond)				
blanched/whole	1 oz	15.0	190	71%
chopped/natural	1 oz	15.0	180	75%
dried/whole	1 oz	15.0	180	75%
roasted/salted	1 oz	17.0	190	81%
slivered	1 oz	15.0	190	71%
Smokehouse	1 oz	17.0	180	85%
(Diamond of California)				
sliced	¼ cup	15.0	190	71%
slivered	¼ cup	15.0	190	71%

Food and Description	Amount	Fat Grams	Total Calories	% Fat Calories
whole	¼ cup	15.0	190	71%
(Dole)				
chopped natural	¼ cup	15.0	170	79%
sliced natural	⅓ cup	15.0	170	79%
slivered blanched	⅓ cup	15.0	180	75%
whole				
blanched	¼ cup	15.0	170	79%
natural	¼ cup	15.0	170	79%
(Fisher) Snack'N Serve Nut Bowl				
chocolate covered	1.42 oz	16.0	220	65%
generic				
dried				
blanched				
pieces	1 cup	76.0	850	80%
whole	1 oz	15.0	166	81%
unblanched				
pieces	1 cup	49.0	555	79%
slivered/packed	1 cup	70.5	795	80%
whole	1 oz	15.0	167	81%
dry-roasted	1 oz	15.0	167	81%
blanched	1 oz	15.0	167	81%
hickory smoked	1 oz	15.0	166	81%
unblanched	1 oz	15.0	167	81%
oil-roasted				
blanched	1 oz	16.0	174	83%
toasted	1 oz	14.0	167	75%
unblanched	1 oz	16.0	176	82%
(Planters)	1 oz	15.0	170	79%
Gold Measure/slivered	2 oz	31.0	340	82%
honey-roasted	1 oz	14.0	160	79%
ALMOND BUTTER				
(Arrowhead Mills)	2 Tbs	20.0	210	86%
(Erewhon)	1 Tbs	8.0	90	80%
generic				
honey & cinnamon	1 Tbs	8.0	96	75%
	½ cup	65.0	755	77%
plain	1 Tbs	9.5	100	86%
	1 cup	74.0	790	84%
(Hain)				
natural/raw	2 Tbs	18.0	190	85%
toasted-blanched	2 Tbs	19.0	220	78%
(Kettle) Roaster Fresh				
salted	1 oz	16.0	184	78%
unsalted	1 oz	16.0	184	78%
(Spanky's)	1 oz	17.0	190	80%
(Westbrae Natural)				
crunchy	2 Tbs	17.0	190	80%
smooth	2 Tbs	17.0	190	80%
ALMOND FILLING				
(Odom) marizipan	2 Tbs	4.0	500	7%
(Solo)	2 Tbs	2.5	120	19%

Food and Description	Amount	Fat Grams	Total Calories	% Fat Calories
ALMOND MEAL /partially defatted	1 oz	5.0	116	39%
ALMOND PASTE	1 Tbs	7.7	127	55%
	1 cup	62.0	1010	55%
ALMOND POWDER				
full-fat	1 oz	15.0	168	80%
	1 cup	34.0	385	80%
partially defatted	1 oz	5.0	112	40%
	1 cup	10.0	255	35%
ALOE VERA JUICE	2 oz	–	5	–
AMARANTH				
(Arrowhead Mills) Seeds	¼ cup	2.0	170	11%
generic				
cooked	½ cup	–	14	–
raw	1 cup	–	7	–
AMARANTH FLOUR (*See* FLOUR)				
ANASAZI BEAN				
(Arrowhead Mills) dry	¼ cup	0.5	150	3%
(Bean Cuisine) dry	½ cup	1.0	115	8%
ANCHOVY, EUROPEAN				
canned/in oil	5 fish	1.9	42	41%
fresh/raw	3 oz	4.0	62	58%
ANCHOVY PASTE	1 tsp	0.8	14	51%
ANISE	1 tsp	–	7	–
APPLE (*See also* APPLE, CARAMEL)				
canned				
generic/sliced/sweetened	½ cup	0.5	68	7%
(Luck's) fried				
plain	½ cup	–	130	–
w/cinnamon	½ cup	–	120	–
(Musselman's)				
chips	4 oz	–	50	–
diced	4 oz	–	50	–
rings/green or red	4 oz	–	100	–
sliced				
dessert	4 oz	–	70	–
sweetened				
in syrup	4 oz	–	50	–
in water	4 oz	–	50	–
unpeeled	4 oz	–	90	–
whole				
baked	1 apple	–	110	–
sweetened/peeled-cored	1 apple	–	90	–
(S&W)				
rings	2 pieces	–	25	–
spiced crab	1 piece	–	35	–
(TreeTop) sliced	5 oz	–	40	–
dried				
(Del Monte) sliced	⅓ cup	–	80	–
generic				
cooked				
w/sugar	1 cup	–	232	–

Food and Description	Amount	Fat Grams	Total Calories	% Fat Calories
w/o sugar	1 cup	–	144	–
uncooked	10 rings	–	155	–
	1 cup	–	209	–
(Mariani)	¼ cup	–	150	–
(Nature's Favorite) apple chips				
cinnamon	1 oz	5.0	120	38%
golden delicious	1 oz	5.0	120	38%
original	1 oz	5.0	120	38%
(Seneca) apple chips				
caramel	1 oz	7.0	140	45%
cinnamon	1 oz	7.0	140	45%
golden delicious	1 oz	7.0	140	45%
Granny Smith	1 oz	8.0	150	48%
honey apple	1 oz	7.0	140	45%
original	1 oz	7.0	140	45%
red hot cinnamon	1 oz	7.0	140	45%
(Sun Maid) chunks	¼ cup	–	110	–
fresh				
cooked/w/o skin	1 cup	0.6	91	6%
microwaved/sliced				
peeled	½ cup	0.5	65	7%
unpeeled	½ cup	0.5	50	9%
raw				
(Dole)	1 medium	1.0	80	11%
w/skin				
sliced	1 cup	–	64	6%
whole	1 medium	0.5	81	6%
w/o skin				
sliced	1 cup	–	62	–
whole	1 medium	–	72	–

APPLE, CARAMEL

Food and Description	Amount	Fat Grams	Total Calories	% Fat Calories
(Classic Kettle)				
almond chocolate	¼ apple	16.0	320	45%
peanut chocolate	¼ apple	12.0	260	42%
pecan chocolate	¼ apple	17.0	320	48%
toffee walnut chocolate	¼ apple	14.0	310	41%
triple chocolate chunk	¼ apple	12.0	300	36%

APPLE BUTTER

Food and Description	Amount	Fat Grams	Total Calories	% Fat Calories
(Dutch Girl)	1 Tbs	–	35	–
(Eden)	1 Tbs	–	25	–
generic	1 Tbs	<1.0	33	3%
	1 cup	2.0	525	3%
(Kozlowski Farms)	1 Tbs	–	30	–
(Mary Ellen)	1 Tbs	–	35	–
(Smuckers)				
cider	1 Tbs	–	45	–
Simply Fruit	1 Tbs	–	45	–
spiced	1 Tbs	–	45	–

APPLE CIDER (*See* CIDER)
APPLE DUMPLING (*See* PASTRY)

Food and Description	Amount	Fat Grams	Total Calories	% Fat Calories
APPLE JUICE/NECTAR				
bottled, boxed, or canned				
(Campbell's) Juice Bowl/apple	6 fl oz	–	110	–
(Dole)	10 fl oz	–	160	–
(Indian Summer)	6 fl oz	–	90	–
(Knudsen)				
apple	8 fl oz	–	110	–
Thirst Quencher				
natural apple	8 fl oz	–	120	–
nectar	8 fl oz	–	120	–
(Kraft) pure 100%	6 fl oz	–	80	–
(Libby's)				
Juicy Juice	4.23 fl oz	–	60	–
Juicy Pouch	4.23 fl oz	–	60	–
(Martinelli's) sparkling	6 fl oz	–	100	–
(Minute Maid)	8 fl oz	–	110	
	8.45 fl oz	–	120	–
	10 fl oz	–	140	–
	11.5 fl oz	–	160	–
(Mott's)				
natural	8 fl oz	–	120	–
	9.5 fl oz	–	140	–
	10 fl oz	–	150	–
(Musselman's)				
enriched, w/100% vitamin C	6 fl oz	–	90	–
original	6 fl oz	–	90	–
(Red Cheek)				
natural style	8 fl oz	–	120	–
100% pure	8 fl oz	–	120	–
(Season's) best	6 fl oz	–	80	–
	8 fl oz	–	120	–
	10 fl oz	–	140	–
	11.5 fl oz	–	160	–
(Seneca)	8 fl oz	–	110	–
country apple	8 fl oz	–	110	–
Granny Smith	8 fl oz	–	110	–
(Sippin' Pak) from concentrate	8.45 fl oz	–	110	–
(Snapple Farms)	12 fl oz	–	180	–
(TreeTop)				
country style	8.45 fl oz	–	120	–
	10 fl oz	–	140	–
	11.5 fl oz	–	170	–
fiber rich	4 fl oz	–	70	–
	8 fl oz	–	150	–
(TreeSweet)	8 fl oz	–	120	–
(Tropicana) Season's Best	6 fl oz	–	80	–
	8 fl oz	–	110	–
	10 fl oz	–	140	–
	11.5 fl oz	–	160	–

Food and Description	Amount	Fat Grams	Total Calories	% Fat Calories
(Welch's)				
juice	5.5 fl oz	–	80	–
	8 fl oz	–	120	–
	10 fl oz	–	140	–
	11.5 fl oz	–	160	–
Juicemakers	8 fl oz	–	120	–
frozen				
(Birds Eye)	6 fl oz	–	80	–
(Minute Maid)	8 fl oz	–	110	–
(Seneca)	8 fl oz	–	120	–
country style	8 fl oz	–	120	–
Granny Smith	8 fl oz	–	110	–
(Sunkist)	8 fl oz	–	80	–
(TreeTop)				
country style	8 fl oz	–	120	–
original	8 fl oz	–	120	–
(Welch's) juice cocktail	8 fl oz	–	160	–

APPLE JUICE BLEND/DRINK

(NOTE: Unless stated otherwise, data are for prepared serving amounts.)

Food and Description	Amount	Fat Grams	Total Calories	% Fat Calories
bottled, boxed, or canned				
(Betty Crocker) Squeezit 100	7 fl oz	–	90	–
(Dole)				
Apple Berry Burst	8 fl oz	–	120	–
apple-cranberry	10 fl oz	–	160	–
(Fruitopia) Apple Raspberry Embrace	8 fl oz	–	75	–
(Hi-C) Jammin' Apple	8.45 fl oz	–	120	–
(Knudsen)				
apple-boysenberry juice	8 fl oz	–	120	–
Thirst Quencher/apple-cranberry	8 fl oz	–	130	–
(Libby's) Juicy Juice				
apple-grape	8 fl oz	–	100	–
	8.45 fl oz	–	130	–
(Minute Maid) apple-grape	8 fl oz	–	125	–
(Mott's)				
apple juice drink	9.5 fl oz	–	150	–
	10 fl oz	–	160	–
apple-cranberry juice	8 fl oz	–	120	–
	9.5 fl oz	–	150	–
	10 fl oz	–	180	–
apple-grape juice	8 fl oz	–	120	–
apple-raspberry juice	6 fl oz	–	85	–
	8.45 fl oz	–	125	–
	9.5 fl oz	–	135	–
	10 fl oz	–	140	–
(Seneca)				
apple juice cocktail	8 fl oz	–	110	–
apple-cranberry juice	8 fl oz	–	120	–
(TreeTop)				
apple-apricot juice	4 fl oz	–	90	–
	8 fl oz	–	160	–

Food and Description	Amount	Fat Grams	Total Calories	% Fat Calories
apple-cranberry juice	10 fl oz	–	190	–
	11.5 fl oz	–	230	–
apple-grape juice	5.5 fl oz	–	90	–
	8.45 fl oz	–	140	–
	11.5 fl oz	–	190	–
apple-orange-banana juice	4 fl oz	–	80	–
	8 fl oz	–	170	–
apple-pear juice	5.5 fl oz	–	80	–
	8 fl oz	–	120	–
	8.45 fl oz	–	120	–
	10 fl oz	–	140	–
	11.5 fl oz	–	170	–
apple-raspberry juice	5.5 fl oz	–	80	–
	8.45 fl oz	–	120	–
	10 fl oz	–	140	–
	11.5 fl oz	–	160	–
(Tropicana) Twister/apple-raspberry-	8 fl oz	–	130	–
blackberry	11.5 fl oz	–	180	–
(Welch's)				
apple-cranberry drink	11.5 fl oz	–	210	–
apple-orange-pineapple drink	11.5 fl oz	–	210	–
Cocktail-In-A-Box				
apple-grape-cherry	8.45 fl oz	–	150	–
apple-grape-raspberry	8.45 fl oz	–	150	–
Juice Cocktail				
apple	8 fl oz	–	140	–
apple-cranberry	8 fl oz	–	150	–
apple-grape-cherry	8 fl oz	–	150	–
apple-orange-pineapple	8 fl oz	–	150	–
frozen				
(Dole) Apple Berry Burst	8 fl oz	–	120	–
(Mott's) Fruit Basket Juice Cocktail				
apple	8 fl oz	–	120	–
apple-raspberry	8 fl oz	–	130	–
(TreeTop)				
apple-cranberry juice	8 fl oz	–	130	–
apple-grape juice	8 fl oz	–	130	–
apple-pear juice	8 fl oz	–	120	–
apple-raspberry juice	8 fl oz	–	110	–
(Welch's) Orchard Juice Blend				
apple-grape-cherry	8 fl oz	–	140	–
apple-grape-raspberry	8 fl oz	–	140	–
APPLESAUCE				
(Del Monte)				
lite	½ cup	–	50	–
sweetened	½ cup	–	90	–
generic/canned				
sweetened	1 cup	–	194	–
unsweetened	1 cup	–	106	–

Food and Description	Amount	Fat Grams	Total Calories	% Fat Calories
(Mott's)				
chunky	5 oz	–	110	–
cinnamon	5 oz	–	120	–
fruit snacks				
cinnamon	4 oz	–	90	–
Dutch apple spice	4 oz	–	70	–
strawberry	4 oz	–	80	–
sweetened	4 oz	–	90	–
(Musselman's)				
applesauce				
chunky	½ cup	–	110	–
deluxe cinnamon	½ cup	–	120	–
natural	½ cup	–	50	–
sweetened	½ cup	–	110	–
unsweetened	½ cup	–	50	–
(Seneca)				
cinnamon	4.5 oz	–	100	–
Golden Delicious	4.5 oz	–	100	–
McIntosh	4.5 oz	–	60	–
100% natural	4.5 oz	–	100	–
regular	4.5 oz	–	100	–
(TreeTop)				
cinnamon	4 oz	–	90	–
	½ cup	–	100	–
original	4 oz	–	90	–
	½ cup		100	
unsweetened	4 oz	–	70	–
	½ cup	–	70	–
(Wilderness)				
raspberry	½ cup	–	82	–
strawberry	½ cup	–	90	–
APRICOT				
candied	1 oz		96	–
canned				
(Del Monte) halves/unpeeled				
almond-flavored	½ cup	–	90	–
in heavy syrup	½ cup	–	100	–
lite	½ cup	–	60	–
generic				
peeled				
in juice	1 cup	–	119	–
in water	1 cup	–	51	–
unpeeled				
in heavy syrup	1 cup	–	214	–
in light syrup	1 cup	–	160	–
in water	1 cup	–	65	–
(Libby's) unpeeled/lite	½ cup	–	60	–
(S&W) whole/peeled/in heavy syrup	½ cup	–	110	–
dried				
(Ann's House of Nuts) Turkish	5 pieces		90	–

Food and Description	Amount	Fat Grams	Total Calories	% Fat Calories
(Del Monte) sun-dried	⅓ cup	–	80	–
(Dole) Sun Giant Turkish	6 pieces	–	90	–
generic				
cooked	½ cup	<1.0	106	2%
uncooked	½ cup	0.6	155	3%
(Mariani)				
California	¼ cup	–	140	–
Mediterranean	¼ cup	–	140	–
(Sonoma)	10 pieces	–	120	–
(Sun Maid)	¼ cup	–	140	–
fresh	3 medium	0.5	51	9%
	1 cup	0.6	74	7%
frozen/sweetened	½ cup	–	119	–
APRICOT FILLING (Solo)	2 Tbs	–	80	–
APRICOT JUICE/NECTAR /bottled, boxed, or canned				
(Del Monte)	6 fl oz	–	100	–
generic				
juice/unsweetened	8 fl oz	–	123	–
nectar	8 fl oz	–	140	–
(Kern's)	6 fl oz	–	110	–
(Knudsen)	8 fl oz	–	105	–
(Libby's)	6 fl oz	–	110	–
	11.5 fl oz	–	220	–
(S&W)	5.5 fl oz	–	100	–
	8 fl oz	–	140	–
	12 fl oz	–	210	–
APRICOT JUICE/NECTAR BLEND /bottled or canned				
(Kern's)				
apricot-mango	11.5 fl oz	–	220	–
apricot-pineapple	11.5 fl oz	–	220	–
(Seneca) apricot nectar cocktail	8 fl oz	–	140	–
ARMADILLO /raw	3 oz	4.0	150	24%
ARROWHEAD /plant				
cooked	medium corm	0.5	9	50%
raw	medium corm	0.5	12	38%
ARTICHOKE (See also JERUSALEM ARTICHOKE)				
canned or jarred				
(Cara Mia) marinated				
crowns	1 oz	–	12	–
hearts	1 oz	2.0	27	67%
(Progresso) hearts				
in brine	3 oz	–	30	–
marinated	1.1 oz	5.0	60	75%
regular	2 pieces	–	35	–
(Reese)				
bottoms	2 pieces	–	35	–
hearts	3 pieces	–	30	–

Food and Description	Amount	Fat Grams	Total Calories	% Fat Calories
(S&W)				
bottoms/in water	3 pieces	–	25	–
hearts				
in water	3 pieces	–	30	–
marinated	2 pieces	2.0	20	90%
fresh				
(Dole)	1 large	–	23	–
generic				
cooked	1 medium	–	53	–
hearts/cooked	½ cup	–	37	–
raw	1 medium	–	65	–
frozen				
(Birds Eye) hearts/deluxe	½ cup	–	30	–
(C&W) hearts	3 oz	–	25	–
ARTICHOKE HEART (See ARTICHOKE)				
ARUGULA				
fresh/chopped	½ cup	<1.0	2	13%
	1 lb	1.5	105	13%
ASIAN FOOD (See also FROZEN ENTRÉE/DINNER; PASTA ENTRÉE/DINNER; RICE DISH; VEGETARIAN FOODS; individual listings)				
■ **BEEF DISHES** (See also Chow Mein; Fried Rice; Sweet & Sour in this section)				
(Chun King)				
beef pepper Oriental/divider pak entrée/prepared	1 cup	2.5	100	23%
generic/canned				
beef pepper Oriental	¾ cup	2.0	80	23%
(LaChoy) prepared				
beef pepper/bi-pack	¾ cup	2.0	80	23%
beef pepper Oriental entrée/prepared	¾ cup	4.0	100	36%
■ **CHICKEN DISHES** (See also Chow Mein; Fried Rice; Sweet & Sour in this section)				
(Chun King) frozen entrée				
imperial chicken	13 oz	10.0	460	20%
walnut chicken	13 oz	19.0	460	37%
(La Choy) canned/prepared				
chicken teriyaki/bi-pack	¾ cup	2.0	85	21%
sweet & sour				
bi-pack	¾ cup	2.0	120	15%
entrée	¾ cup	2.0	240	8%
■ **CHOP SUEY**				
homemade/USDA Standard Home Recipe				
w/beef & pork	1 cup	17.0	300	51%
w/beef w/o noodles	1 cup	17.0	300	51%
■ **CHOW MEIN** (See also Vegetables in this section)				
beef				
(Chun King) canned/prepared				
divider pak entrée	1 cup	1.5	110	12%
stir-fry entrée	6 oz	19.0	290	59%
generic/canned	¾ cup	1.0	70	13%
homemade				
USDA Standard Home Recipe	1 cup	17.0	300	51%

Food and Description	Amount	Fat Grams	Total Calories	% Fat Calories
chicken				
(Chun King) canned/prepared				
divider pak entrée	1 cup	4.5	110	37%
stir-fry entrée	1 cup	11.0	220	45%
homemade/USDA Standard Home Recipe	¾ cup	10.0	255	35%
(La Choy)				
bi-pack/canned/prepared	¾ cup	3.0	80	34%
dinner	¾ pkg	17.0	300	51%
entrée	¾ cup	4.0	70	51%
pork				
(Chun King) canned/prepared	1 cup	4.5	110	37%
homemade/USDA Standard Home Recipe				
w/noodles	1 cup	24.7	432	51%
w/o noodles	¾ cup	14.0	223	57%
(La Choy)				
bi-pack/canned/prepared	¾ cup	4.0	80	45%
shrimp				
(Chun King) canned/prepared	1 cup	2.5	110	37%
homemade/USDA Standard Home Recipe				
w/noodles	¾ cup	3.9	141	25%
(La Choy) canned/prepared	¾ cup	1.0	70	13%
■ CRAB RANGOON				
(Pagoda Cafe)/frozen	5.2 oz	22.0	440	45%
■ EGG FOO YOUNG				
(Chun King) canned/prepared	5 oz	8.0	140	51%
homemade/USDA Standard Home Recipe	~5 oz	10.0	150	60%
■ EGG ROLL				
(Chun King) frozen				
chicken				
mini	6 pieces	9.0	210	39%
restaurant style	1 piece	9.0	190	43%
pork & shrimp/mini	6 pieces	9.0	210	39%
shrimp				
mini	6 pieces	6.0	190	28%
restaurant style	1 piece	7.0	180	35%
Homemade/USDA Standard Home Recipe/w/o meat	2.25 oz	5.9	102	52%
(La Choy) frozen				
bite-size				
pork & shrimp	12 pieces	10.0	210	43%
mini				
chicken	6 pieces	9.0	210	39%
pork & shrimp	6 pieces	9.0	210	39%
shrimp	6 pieces	6.0	190	28%
vegetable w/lobster	6 pieces	7.0	190	33%
restaurant style/6 oz				
chicken	1 piece	9.0	210	39%
pork	1 piece	11.0	220	45%

Food and Description	Amount	Fat Grams	Total Calories	% Fat Calories
shrimp	1 piece	7.0	180	35%
sweet & sour	1 piece	9.0	220	37%
(Minh) frozen				
chicken white meat	3 oz	5.0	150	30%
pork	3 oz	8.0	170	37%
seafood	3 oz	4.5	140	29%
(Pagoda Cafe) frozen				
chicken	1 piece	6.0	160	34%
Hunan style pork	1 piece	9.0	190	43%
pork	1 piece	8.0	170	42%
pork & shrimp	1 piece	8.0	180	40%
vegetable	1 piece	4.0	140	26%
(Schwan's) frozen				
chicken	2 pieces	7.0	220	29%
pork	2 pieces	11.0	240	41%
shrimp	2 pieces	4.5	180	23%
(Yu Sing) frozen				
chicken	6 rolls	7.0	180	35%
pork & shrimp	6 rolls	9.0	200	41%
shrimp	6 rolls	7.0	180	35%
sweet & sour chicken	6 rolls	7.0	190	33%
sweet & sour pork	6 rolls	9.0	210	39%
■ EGG ROLL WRAPPER				
(Azumaya Pasta)	2 wrappers	–	130	–
(Nasoya)	2 wrappers	–	120	–
■ FORTUNE COOKIE				
(La Choy)	4 cookies	–	112	–
■ FRIED RICE (*See also* RICE DISH and YU SING in this section)				
(Chun King) frozen				
w/chicken	8 oz	6.0	270	20%
w/pork	8 oz	5.0	290	19%
(Kan Tong) dry				
chicken	2 oz	3.5	190	17%
pork	2 oz	1.0	190	5%
shrimp	2 oz	1.0	190	5%
spicy chicken	2 oz	1.0	190	5%
traditional	2 oz	3.0	190	14%
vegetable	2 oz	0.5	190	2%
(La Choy)	1 cup	1.0	235	4%
(Ling Ling) frozen				
vegetable	1 cup	4.0	140	26%
■ NOODLE (*See also* PASTA; PASTA ENTRÉE/DINNER)				
(Chun King) chow mein/dry	1 oz	7.0	140	45%
generic				
Chinese cellophane/long rice/dry	2 oz	–	200	–
chow mein/cooked	1 cup	14.0	240	53%
rice/canned	½ cup	5.0	130	35%
soba/buckwheat				
cooked	4 oz	–	115	–
dry	2 oz	0.5	195	2%

Food and Description	Amount	Fat Grams	Total Calories	% Fat Calories
somen/wheat				
cooked	4 oz	–	149	–
dry	2 oz	0.5	205	2%
udon/wheat				
cooked	4 oz	0.5	115	4%
dry	2 oz	0.7	160	4%
(La Choy)				
chow mein	½ cup	6.0	135	40%
crispy wide	½ cup	8.0	150	35%
rice	½ cup	3.0	120	23%
■ POTSTICKERS				
(Ling Ling) frozen				
chicken & vegetable dumplings				
dumplings only	5 pieces	7.0	280	23%
w/1 Tbs sauce	1 serving	7.0	300	21%
(Pagoda Cafe) frozen				
pork & vegetable	5.2 oz piece	24.0	420	51%
■ SAUCES & SEASONINGS (See also SAUCE; SEASONINGS)				
(Chun King)				
hot teriyaki sauce	1 Tbs	–	17	–
soy sauce	1 Tbs	–	10	–
(Contadina) Sweet 'N Sour Sauce	2 Tbs	1.0	40	23%
w/pineapple				
generic/soy sauce				
shoyu	1 Tbs	–	9	–
	¼ cup	–	30	–
tamari	1 Tbs	–	11	–
	¼ cup	–	35	–
(House Of Tsang)				
oil				
hot chili sesame	1 tsp	5.0	45	100%
Mongolian Fire Oil	1 tsp	5.0	45	100%
pure sesame	1 tsp	5.0	45	100%
Singapore curry	1 tsp	5.0	45	100%
wok	1 Tbs	14.0	130	100%
sauce				
Bangkok padang	1 Tbs	2.5	45	50%
classic stir-fry	1 Tbs	1.0	25	36%
hoisin sauce	1 tsp	–	15	–
Hong Kong BBQ	1 tsp	–	10	–
Korean teriyaki	1 Tbs	0.5	30	15%
Mandarin marinade	1 Tbs	–	25	–
Saigon sizzle	1 Tbs	1.0	40	23%
soy sauce				
dark	1 Tbs	–	17	–
ginger-flavored				
low-sodium	1 Tbs	–	10	–
regular	1 Tbs	–	20	–
light	1 Tbs	–	5	–
low-sodium	1 Tbs	–	5	–

Food and Description	Amount	Fat Grams	Total Calories	% Fat Calories
spicy brown bean	1 tsp	–	15	–
sweet & sour concentrate	1 tsp	–	10	–
sweet & sour stir-fry	1 Tbs	–	35	–
Szechuan spicy stir-fry	1 Tbs	0.5	20	23%
vegetables & sauce				
Hong Kong sweet & sour	½ cup	1.0	160	6%
Szechaun hot & spicy	½ cup	1.0	70	13%
Tokyo teriyaki	½ cup	–	100	–
(Kikkoman)				
chow mein seasoning				
lite	1 Tbs	–	10	–
regular	1 pkg	–	100	–
soy sauce				
lite	1 Tbs	–	10	–
regular	1 Tbs	–	10	–
teriyaki/baste & glaze	1 Tbs	–	25	–
(La Choy)				
bead molasses	1 Tbs	–	50	–
brown gravy sauce	¼ cup	–	275	–
plum	1 Tbs	–	25	–
soy sauce/lite	1 Tbs	–	15	–
stir-fry				
Mandarin soy sauce	½ cup	–	70	–
sweet & sour	½ cup	–	140	–
Szechwan	½ cup	–	80	–
teriyaki	½ cup	–	95	–
sweet & sour				
duck sauce	2 Tbs	–	60	–
original	2 Tbs	–	60	–
teriyaki				
lite	1 Tbs	–	18	–
original	1 Tbs	–	16	–
(S&B Sunbird)				
Oriental seasonings/dry				
beef & broccoli	¾ Tbs	–	20	–
Chinese barbecue	½ Tbs	–	10	–
Chinese chicken salad	½ Tbs	–	15	–
chop suey	1 Tbs	–	20	–
chow mein	2 tsp	–	15	–
fried rice	½ Tbs	–	12	–
honey teriyaki	2 tsp	–	15	–
hot & spicy	½ Tbs	–	14	–
kung pao chicken	¾ Tbs	–	20	–
lemon chicken stir-fry	½ Tbs	–	10	–
orange beef	½ Tbs	–	13	–
stir-fry	1 Tbs	–	15	–
sukiyaki	½ tsp	–	15	–
sweet & sour	½ Tbs	–	15	–
tomato beef	¾ Tbs	–	25	–
teriyaki marinade	½ Tbs	–	10	–

Food and Description	Amount	Fat Grams	Total Calories	% Fat Calories
■ SEA VEGETABLES				
(Eden)				
hiziki sea vegetable	¼ cup	–	30	–
sushi nori sea vegetable	1 sheet	–	10	–
■ SEAFOOD DISHES (*See also* Chow Mein; Fried Rice in this section)				
homemade/USDA Standard Home recipe				
teriyaki shrimp	¾ cup	1.0	174	5%
■ SEASONINGS (*See* SAUCES & SEASONINGS in this section)				
■ STIR-FRY (*See also* VEGETABLES, MIXED)				
(Birds Eye) Easy Recipe Creations/frozen/as packaged				
Oriental lo mein	2¼ cups	3.5	230	14%
spicy Szechuan w/cashews	2¼ cups	4.5	180	23%
sweet & sour w/pineapple tidbits	2¼ cups	0.5	200	2%
teriyaki/sesame ginger	2¼ cups	1.5	140	10%
(C&W) frozen/vegetable stir-fry dinner				
w/basmati rice	1 cup	–	220	–
w/Oriental noodles	1 cup	2.5	200	11%
(Green Giant) frozen/Create A Meal!/as packaged				
beef & broccoli	2⅓ cups	3.5	120	26%
garlic & ginger	1⅔ cups	1.5	130	10%
lo mein	2⅓ cups	1.5	170	8%
sweet & sour	1½ cups	–	180	–
Szechuan	1¾ cups	5.0	150	30%
teriyaki	1¾ cups	0.5	100	5%
(Pictsweet) frozen/International Combinations				
Chinese	¾ cup	–	30	–
Oriental	¾ cup	–	30	–
Singapore	¾ cup	–	30	–
■ SUSHI				
homemade/USDA Standard Home Recipe/w/vegetables	4.5 oz	–	181	–
■ SWEET & SOUR				
generic/canned/prepared	¾ cup	2.0	120	15%
(La Choy) canned/prepared				
chicken entrée	¾ cup	2.0	240	8%
pork entrée	¾ cup	4.0	250	14%
homemade/USDA Standard Home Recipe	¾ cup	7.7	187	37%
■ VEGETABLES/VEGETABLE DISHES (*See also* Chow Mein; Fried Rice; Sea Vegetables; Stir-Fry in this section)				
(Birds Eye) Frozen stir-fry vegetables/as packaged				
asparagus	2 cups frozen	0.5	90	5%
broccoli	1 cup frozen	–	30	–
pepper	3 oz frozen	–	25	–
sugar snap	¾ cup frozen	–	35	–
whole bean	5.4 oz frozen	0.5	100	5%
(Chun King)				
Chinese pea pods	3 oz	1.5	35	38%
chow mein vegetables/divider pak entrée/prepared	⅔ cup	–	15	–

Food and Description	Amount	Fat Grams	Total Calories	% Fat Calories
water chestnuts				
sliced	16 slices	–	10	–
	8 oz	0.5	179	3%
whole	8.5 oz	0.5	190	2%
(Empress)				
bamboo shoots/sliced	2 oz	–	13	–
water chestnuts				
sliced	2 oz	–	14	–
whole	2 oz	–	14	–
generic				
bamboo shoots	1 cup	<1.0	25	18%
water chestnuts/sliced	½ cup	–	35	–
(La Choy)				
bamboo shoots	2 Tbs	–	3	–
	¼ cup	–	6	–
bean sprouts	1 cup	–	10	–
water chestnuts				
sliced	2 Tbs	–	10	–
	¼ cup	–	18	–
whole	2 medium	–	10	–
■ **WON TON**				
generic/fried	½ cup	8.0	110	65%
■ **WON TON SOUP** (*See* SOUP)				
■ **WON TON WRAPPER**				
(Azumaya)	1 wrapper	–	23	–
(Nasoya)	1 wrapper	–	23	–
■ **(YU SING)** (*See also* **EGG ROLL** *in this section*)				
Frozen Entrées				
beef				
ginger beef w/rice	1 meal	9.0	290	28%
Cantonese w/rice	1 meal	7.0	270	23%
Oriental beef & peppers	1 meal	7.0	290	22%
teriyaki w/rice	1 meal	2.0	240	8%
chicken				
& almonds w/rice	1 meal	6.0	300	18%
chow mein w/rice	1 meal	6.0	270	20%
fried rice	1 meal	7.0	360	18%
garlic w/rice	1 meal	3.0	240	11%
ginger w/rice	1 meal	5.0	250	18%
lo mein	1 meal	2.5	220	10%
Mandarin w/rice	1 meal	4.0	300	12%
sweet & sour w/rice	1 meal	3.5	340	9%
pork				
& shrimp fried rice	1 meal	11.0	410	24%
chop suey w/rice	1 meal	8.0	320	23%
fried rice	1 meal	13.0	450	26%
shrimp				
fried rice	1 meal	6.0	350	15%
lo mein	1 meal	1.5	210	6%

Food and Description	Amount	Fat Grams	Total Calories	% Fat Calories
ASPARAGUS				
canned				
(Del Monte) tender green				
cut spears	½ cup	–	20	–
extra-long spears	½ cup	–	20	–
salad tips	½ cup	–	20	–
spears	½ cup	–	20	–
tips	½ cup	–	20	–
(Green Giant)				
cut spears				
50% less sodium	½ cup	–	20	–
regular	½ cup	–	20	–
extra-long spears	4.5 oz	–	20	–
Harvest Fresh				
cuts	⅔ cup	–	25	–
spears	4.5 oz	–	20	–
(LeSueur) extra-large spears	4.5 oz	–	20	–
(Reese) white spears	⅓ can	–	20	–
(S&W)				
blended	6 pieces	–	15	–
colossal	3 pieces	–	10	–
(Seneca)	½ cup	–	20	–
(Stokely)				
green	½ cup	–	20	–
no salt or sugar added	½ cup	–	20	–
(Thank You) whole spears	½ cup	–	25	–
fresh				
cooked				
cuts w/tips	½ cup	–	22	–
(Dole) spears	5 spears	–	18	–
spears	4 spears	–	15	–
raw				
cuts w/tips	½ cup	–	15	–
spears	4 spears	–	13	–
frozen				
(Birds Eye)				
cuts	3.3 oz	–	25	–
spears	3.3 oz	–	25	–
(C&W) spears	2.6 oz	–	20	–
ASPARAGUS SOUP, CREAM OF (*See* SOUP)				
AVOCADO				
fresh/raw				
California				
mashed	1 cup	36.0	407	80%
whole	1 medium	30.8	324	86%
Florida	1 medium	27.0	340	72%

B

Food and Description	Amount	Fat Grams	Total Calories	% Fat Calories
BABY FOOD (*See also* BABY/INFANT FORMULA)				

(NOTE: The nutritional needs of young children differ from those of older children and adults. A low-fat nutrition program is not recommended for any child under two years of age, as it may interfere with his or her development)

■ **(Beech-Nut)**
Stage 1
Cereal-Instant

Food and Description	Amount	Fat Grams	Total Calories	% Fat Calories
barley/dry	¼ cup	–	60	–
oatmeal/dry	¼ cup	2.0	60	30%
rice/dry	¼ cup	–	60	–
fruit				
applesauce/Golden Delicious	2.5 oz	–	90	–
bananas				
Chiquita	2.5 oz	–	70	–
	4 oz	–	100	–
w/pears & apples	4 oz	–	90	–
peaches/yellow cling	2.5 oz	–	50	–
	4 oz	–	60	–
pears/Bartlett	4 oz	–	70	–
juice				
apple	4 fl oz	–	60	–
pear	4 fl oz	–	60	–
white grape	4 fl oz	–	100	–
meat				
beef & broth	2.5 oz	6.0	95	57%
chicken & broth	2.5 oz	3.0	70	39%
lamb & broth	2.5 oz	3.0	60	45%
turkey & broth	2.8 oz	6.0	90	60%
veal & broth	2.5 oz	2.0	70	30%
vegetables				
carrots/sweet	4 oz	–	35	–
green beans	4 oz	–	45	–
peas/tender sweet	4 oz	–	60	–
squash/butternut	4 oz	–	40	–
sweet potatoes	4 oz	–	60	–
Stage 2				
Cereal-dry				
mixed/dry-instant	¼ cup	1.0	60	15%
oatmeal & bananas	4 oz	–	70	–
rice cereal & apples	4 oz	–	70	–

Food and Description	Amount	Fat Grams	Total Calories	% Fat Calories
rice cereal & bananas	4 oz	–	70	–
Cereal-Jarred				
Mixed & apples	4 oz	1	60	15%
Oatmeal & apples	4 oz	2	60	30%
Peach, Oat, & bananas	4 oz	1	85	10%
Rice & apples	4 oz	2	60	30%
desserts				
apple, peach, & strawberry	4 oz	–	100	–
apple, strawberry	4 oz	–	90	–
banana pudding	2.5 oz	–	90	–
banana yogurt	4 oz	2.0	120	15%
banana-pineapple	4 oz	–	100	–
Dutch apple	4 oz	–	100	–
fruit	4 oz	–	80	–
guava	2.5 oz	–	90	–
island fruit	2.5 oz	–	80	–
mango	2.5 oz	–	90	–
mixed fruit w/yogurt	4 oz	–	100	–
papaya	2.5 oz	–	90	–
vanilla custard pudding	4 oz	3.0	120	23%
dinners				
apples & beef	4 oz	6.0	110	49%
apples & chicken	4 oz	6.0	100	54%
beef & egg noodle	4 oz	6.0	100	54%
beef supreme	4 oz	9.0	130	62%
broccoli & turkey	4 oz	3.0	70	39%
chicken & rice	4 oz	3.0	80	34%
chicken noodle	4 oz	4.0	70	51%
chicken soup	4 oz	4.0	90	40%
macaroni & beef w/vegetables	4 oz	6.0	110	49%
sweet potatoes & chicken	4 oz	2.0	120	15%
turkey rice	4 oz	3.0	70	39%
vegetable beef	4 oz	5.0	100	45%
vegetable chicken	4 oz	3.0	80	34%
vegetable ham	4 oz	3.0	80	34%
vegetable turkey	4 oz	3.0	80	34%
fruit				
apples & bananas	4 oz	–	60	–
apples & blueberries	4 oz	–	70	–
apples & cherries	4 oz	–	80	–
apples & pears	4 oz	–	80	–
apples & plums	4 oz	–	70	–
apples, pears, & bananas	4 oz	–	90	–
apricots w/pears & apples	4 oz	–	90	–
peaches & bananas	4 oz	–	70	–
pears & raspberries	4 oz	–	80	–
juice				
apple-banana	4 fl oz	–	70	–
apple-cherry	4 fl oz	–	70	–
apple-cranberry	4 fl oz	–	60	–

Food and Description	Amount	Fat Grams	Total Calories	% Fat Calories
apple-grape	4 fl oz	–	60	–
apple-pear	4 fl oz	–	60	–
apple-white grape	4 fl oz	–	70	–
mixed	4 fl oz	–	70	–
vegetables				
corn & sweet potatoes	4 oz	1.0	80	11%
garden vegetables	4 oz	–	50	–
Stage 3				
Cereal/jarred				
cinnamon raisin granola	6 oz	2.0	120	15%
oatmeal & pears w/cinnamon	6 oz	–	90	–
rice & pears	6 oz	–	90	–
desserts				
apple cobbler	6 oz	–	110	–
apple, peach, & strawberry	6 oz	–	120	–
fruit	6 oz	–	120	–
mixed fruit w/yogurt	6 oz	–	170	–
vanilla custard pudding	6 oz	6.0	190	28%
dinners				
beef & noodle	6 oz	6.0	130	42%
chicken & stars	6 oz	3.0	100	27%
chicken lasagna	6 oz	4.0	110	33%
chicken noodle	6 oz	4.0	110	33%
macaroni & beef	6 oz	6.0	130	42%
pasta & cheese	6 oz	5.0	120	38%
spaghetti & beef	6 oz	6.0	130	42%
turkey rice	6 oz	3.0	100	27%
vegetable chicken	6 oz	4.0	110	33%
vegetable turkey	6 oz	4.0	110	33%
fruit				
apples & bananas	6 oz	–	90	–
apples & cherries	6 oz	–	110	–
applesauce	6 oz	–	100	–
apricots w/pears & apples	6 oz	–	130	–
bananas/Chiquita	6 oz	–	160	–
peaches	6 oz	–	100	–
pears/Bartlett	6 oz	–	110	–
pears & raspberry	6 oz	–	90	–
juice/orange	4 fl oz	–	60	–
vegetables				
carrots	6 oz	–	70	–
sweet potatoes	6 oz	–	110	–
Table Time/microwave				
chicken & stars	6 oz	7.0	150	42%
chicken stew w/alphabets	6 oz	7.0	150	42%
lasagna w/meat sauce	6 oz	7.0	150	42%
macaroni & cheese	6 oz	12.0	200	54%
seashells primavera	6 oz	3.0	120	23%
spaghetti rings in meat sauce	6 oz	6.0	160	34%
turkey stew w/rice	6 oz	7.0	150	42%

Food and Description	Amount	Fat Grams	Total Calories	% Fat Calories
vegetable stew w/beef	6 oz	3.0	110	25%
■ **(Earth's Best)**				
baby foods				
cereal				
brown rice	0.5 oz	–	60	–
mixed grain	0.5 oz	–	60	–
dinner/meat				
sweet potato & chicken	4 oz	4.0	80	45%
vegetable beef	4 oz	4.0	80	45%
vegetable turkey	4 oz	2.0	60	30%
dinner/vegetarian				
macaroni & cheese	4 oz	5.0	100	45%
pasta dinner	4 oz	3.0	70	39%
potato & green bean	4 oz	3.0	80	34%
rice & lentil	4 oz	1.0	60	15%
spaghetti w/cheese	6 oz	4.0	120	30%
spring vegetables & pasta	6 oz	2.0	90	20%
summer vegetables	4 oz	2.0	70	26%
fruit				
apples	4 oz	–	50	–
apples & apricots	4 oz	–	60	–
apples & bananas	4 oz	–	50	–
apples & blueberries	4 oz	–	50	–
apples & plums	4 oz	–	50	–
bananas	4 oz	–	70	
pears	4 oz	–	50	–
pears & raspberries	4 oz	–	50	–
fruit & grains				
peaches, oatmeal, & bananas	4 oz	1.0	60	15%
plums, bananas, & rice	4 oz	–	70	–
prunes & oatmeal	4 oz	–	90	–
juice				
apple	4 fl oz	–	70	–
apple-banana	4 fl oz	–	70	–
apple-grape	4 fl oz	–	70	–
pear	4 fl oz	–	70	–
vegetables				
carrots	4 oz	–	25	–
corn & butternut squash	4 oz	1.0	60	15%
potatoes & vegetables/country	6 oz	2.0	90	20%
green beans & rice	4 oz	–	45	–
peas & brown rice	4 oz	1.0	70	13%
spinach & potatoes	4 oz	–	50	–
squash/winter	4 oz	–	35	–
sweet potatoes	4 oz	–	50	–
yogurt breakfasts				
apple yogurt	4 oz	2.0	90	20%
blueberry yogurt	4 oz	2.0	90	20%
junior foods				
apple cinnamon oatmeal	6 oz	1.0	100	9%

Food and Description	Amount	Fat Grams	Total Calories	% Fat Calories
chunky orchard fruit	6 oz	–	80	–
country potatoes & vegetables	6 oz	2.0	90	20%
garden harvest vegetables	6 oz	1.0	80	11%
peach apricot meusli	6 oz	1.0	100	9%
spaghetti w/cheese	6 oz	4.0	120	30%
spring vegetables & pasta	6 oz	2.0	90	20%
sweet potato pudding	6 oz	2.0	130	14%
tender chicken & stars	6 oz	2.0	100	18%
vegetable beef pilaf	6 oz	2.0	100	18%
vegetable soufflé	6 oz	3.0	105	26%
■ (Gerber)				
baked goods Graduates				
Bakery products				
Biter Biscuits	1 serving	0.5	45	10%
Zwieback Toast	1 serving	1.0	30	30%
1st Foods				
cereal				
fruit cereal w/fruit crisps				
oatmeal w/mixed fruit	4 Tbs	1.5	60	23%
rice w/apple bits	4 Tbs	1.0	60	15%
mixed and fruit				
mixed	4 Tbs	1.0	60	15%
oatmeal w/bananas	4 Tbs	1.0	60	15%
rice w/apples	4 Tbs	.5	60	8%
rice w/bananas	4 Tbs	.5	60	8%
rice w/mixed fruit	4 Tbs	.5	60	8%
single grain cereal				
barley	4 Tbs	0.5	60	8%
oatmeal	4 Tbs	1.0	60	15%
rice	4 Tbs	0.5	60	8%
fruits				
applesauce	2.5 oz	–	40	–
bananas	2.5 oz	–	70	–
peaches	2.5 oz	–	30	–
pears	2.5 oz	–	40	–
prunes	2.5 oz	–	70	–
juices				
fruit & vegetable				
apple carrot	4 fl oz	–	60	–
apple sweet potato	4 fl oz	–	70	–
mixed fruits				
apple banana	4 fl oz	–	60	–
apple cherry	4 fl oz	–	60	–
apple cranberry	4 fl oz	–	60	–
apple grape	4 fl oz	–	60	–
apple prune	4 fl oz	–	70	–
banana strawberry juice medley	4 fl oz	–	70	–
mixed fruit	4 fl oz	–	60	–
tropical blend	4 fl oz	–	70	–
single fruit				
apple	4 fl oz	–	60	–

Food and Description	Amount	Fat Grams	Total Calories	% Fat Calories
orange	4 fl oz	–	60	–
pear	4 fl oz	–	60	–
white grape	4 fl oz	–	80	–
special w/yogurt				
banana juice medley	4 fl oz	2.0	110	16%
mixed fruit	4 fl oz	2.0	110	18%
vegetables				
carrots	2.5 oz	–	25	–
green beans	2.5 oz	–	25	–
peas	2.5 oz	–	35	–
potatoes	2.5 oz	–	35	–
squash	2.5 oz	–	25	–
sweet potatoes	2.5 oz	–	45	–
2nd Foods				
cereal/jarred				
mixed w/applesauce & bananas	4 oz	1.0	100	18%
oatmeal w/applesauce & bananas	4 oz	1.0	90	10%
rice w/applesauce	4 oz	–	100	–
desserts				
banana-apple	4 oz	–	80	–
banana-yogurt	4 oz	1.0	90	10%
cherry-vanilla pudding	4 oz	–	80	–
Dutch apple	4 oz	–	90	–
Fruit medley	4 oz	–	90	–
Hawaiian delight	4 oz	–	100	–
mixed fruit yogurt	4 oz	0.5	90	5%
peach cobbler	4 oz	–	90	–
vanilla custard pudding	4 oz	2	110	16%
dinners				
regular				
chicken noodle	4 oz	2.5	80	28%
macaroni & cheese	4 oz	2.5	80	28%
macaroni tomato beef	4 oz	1.0	70	13%
turkey rice	4 oz	1.5	60	23%
vegetable bacon	4 oz	3.5	80	39%
vegetable beef	4 oz	2.5	70	32%
vegetable chicken	4 oz	2.0	70	26%
vegetable ham	4 oz	2.5	70	32%
vegetable turkey	4 oz	1.0	60	15%
simple recipe				
apples & chicken	4 oz	1.5	70	19%
apples & ham	4 oz	2.0	80	23%
broccoli & chicken	4 oz	2.0	45	40%
carrots & beef	4 oz	3.0	70	39%
pears & chicken	4 oz	2.5	80	28%
sweet potatoes & turkey	4 oz	2.0	80	23%
fruits				
applesauce	4 oz	–	60	–
applesauce-apricot	4 oz	–	60	–
apple-blueberry	4 oz	–	60	–

Food and Description	Amount	Fat Grams	Total Calories	% Fat Calories
apricots w/mixed fruit	4 oz	–	70	–
bananas	4 oz	–	100	–
bananas w/apples & pears	4 oz	–	90	–
peaches	4 oz	–	70	–
pear-pineapple	4 oz	–	60	–
pears	4 oz	–	80	–
plums	4 oz	–	80	–
prunes	4 oz	–	90	–
juices				
apple-banana	4 fl oz	–	60	–
apple-cherry	4 fl oz	–	60	–
apple-cranberry	4 fl oz	–	60	–
apple-grape	4 fl oz	–	60	–
apple-peach	4 fl oz	–	60	–
apple-plum	4 fl oz	–	60	–
apple-prune	4 fl oz	–	70	–
mixed fruit	4 fl oz	–	60	–
orange	4 fl oz	–	60	–
juice w/low fat yogurt				
apple	4 oz	1.0	90	10%
banana	4 oz	1.5	110	12%
mixed fruit	4 oz	1.5	90	15%
meat w/gravy				
beef	2.5 oz	3.5	70	45%
chicken	2.5 oz	4.5	80	51%
ham	2.5 oz	3.0	70	39%
lamb	2.5 oz	3.0	70	39%
turkey	2.5 oz	4.0	70	51%
veal	2.5 oz	6.0	90	60%
vegetables				
carrots	4 oz	–	35	–
corn/creamed	4 oz	0.5	70	19%
creamed spinach	4 oz	1.0	50	18%
garden vegetables	4 oz	–	35	–
green beans	4 oz	–	35	–
mixed vegetables	4 oz	–	45	–
peas	4 oz	0.5	60	8%
spinach/creamed	4 oz	1.0	50	18%
squash	4 oz	–	35	–
sweet potatoes	4 oz	–	70	–
3rd Foods				
cereal/jarred				
mixed w/apples & bananas	6 oz	1.0	130	7%
oatmeal w/apples & cinnamon	6 oz	1.0	110	8%
desserts				
apple banana	6 oz	–	130	–
blueberry buckle	6 oz	–	120	–
Dutch apple	6 oz	–	130	–
Fruit medley	6 oz	–	130	–
Hawaiian delight	6 oz	–	150	–

Food and Description	Amount	Fat Grams	Total Calories	% Fat Calories
peach cobbler	6 oz	–	130	–
vanilla custard pudding	6 oz	1.5	150	9%
dinners				
beef egg noodle	6 oz	4.0	130	28%
chicken noodle	6 oz	3.5	110	29%
lasagna w/meat sauce	6 oz	3.5	130	24%
spaghetti in tomato sauce w/beef/Italian	6 oz	4.5	140	29%
turkey rice & garden vegetable	6 oz	3.5	100	32%
vegetable beef	6 oz	3.5	110	29%
vegetable chicken	6 oz	3.0	100	27%
vegetable ham	6 oz	4.0	120	30%
vegetable pasta	6 oz	2.0	120	15%
vegetable stew	6 oz	3.5	130	24%
vegetable turkey	6 oz	3.5	110	29%
fruits				
applesauce	6 oz	–	90	–
apricots w/mixed fruit	6 oz	–	100	–
bananas	6 oz	–	160	–
w/pineapple	6 oz	–	130	–
w/strawberries	6 oz	–	160	–
fruit salad	6 oz	–	110	–
peaches	6 oz	–	110	–
pears	6 oz	–	120	–
plums	6 oz	–	120	–
juices				
apple-carrot	4 fl oz	–	50	–
apple-sweet potato	4 fl oz	–	60	–
orange-carrot	4 fl oz	–	50	–
pineapple-carrot	4 fl oz	–	60	–
meat				
beef	2.5 oz	3.0	70	39%
chicken	2.5 oz	6.0	100	54%
turkey	2.5 oz	5.0	90	50%
vegetables				
broccoli-carrots-cheese	6 oz	2.0	80	23%
carrots	6 oz	–	50	–
green beans w/rice	6 oz	–	70	–
peas w/rice	6 oz	1.0	90	10%
squash	6 oz	–	60	–
sweet potatoes	6 oz	–	100	–
Graduates				
baked finger snacks				
animal crackers	1 serving	1.0	35	26%
apple cinnamon cookies	1 serving	1.0	40	23%
Arrowroot Cookies	1 serving	1.0	25	36%
Banana cookies	1 serving	1.0	35	26%
cinnamon graham	1 serving	1.0	40	23%
pretzels	1 serving	–	25	–
strawberry fruit bars	1 serving	1.0	35	26%

Food and Description	Amount	Fat Grams	Total Calories	% Fat Calories
veggie crackers	1 serving	1.5	35	39%
beverages				
apple	6 fl oz	–	80	–
apple banana	6 fl oz	–	100	–
apple grape	6 fl oz	–	90	–
berry punch	6 fl oz	–	100	–
fruit punch	6 fl oz	–	100	–
spring water	6 fl oz	–	–	–
cereal/instant hot				
apple multigrain	1 serving+			
	2% milk	1.0	80	11%
Finger foods				
Dinner Dices				
carrots & white turkey	2.1 oz	1.0	35	26%
corn & chicken	2.5 oz	2.0	70	26%
green beans & white turkey	2.3 oz	1.0	40	23%
peas & chicken	2.3 oz	2.0	60	30%
Finger Sticks				
chicken	2.5 oz	5.0	100	45%
meat	2.5 oz	7.0	100	63%
turkey	2.5 oz	7.0	100	63%
Fruit Dices				
apples	4.5 oz	–	60	–
mixed	4.5 oz	–	60	–
peaches	4.5 oz	–	60	–
pears	4.5 oz	–	70	–
Vegetable Dices				
carrots	2.5 oz	–	20	–
green beans	2.5 oz	–	20	–
mixed	2.5 oz	–	35	–
juice, fruit/snack	1 fl oz	–	100	–
microwavable meals				
chicken & broccoli in cheese sauce	6 oz	4.0	100	36%
chicken ravioli w/tomato sauce	6 oz	3.0	160	17%
chicken stew w/noodles	6 oz	3.0	120	23%
macaroni & beef	6 oz	3.0	140	19%
pasta shells & cheese	6 oz	4.5	140	29%
potatoes & ham au gratin	6 oz	3.0	130	21%
spaghetti w/mini meatballs & sauce	6 oz	4.0	150	24%
tomato sauce w/cheese ravioli	6 oz	3.5	170	19%
turkey stew w/rice	6 oz	2.0	100	18%
vegetable stew w/beef	6 oz	2.5	120	19%
white turkey stew w/rice	6 oz	3.0	110	25%
Tender Harvest				
Dinners				
chicken & wild rice	4 oz	1.5	70	19%
minestrone dinner	4 oz	2.5	70	32%
pasta primavera	4 oz	2.5	70	32%
vegetable pilaf	4 oz	2.0	80	23%
vegetables turkey & barley	4 oz	1.5	60	23%

Food and Description	Amount	Fat Grams	Total Calories	% Fat Calories
Fruits				
apple mango kiwi	4 oz	–	70	–
apple strawberry	4 oz	–	70	–
banana oatmeal & peach	4 oz	–	90	–
pear & wild blueberry	4 oz	–	70	–
tropical fruit blend	4 oz	–	80	–
Fruits & Vegetables				
apple sweet potato	4 oz	–	70	–
pears & winter squash	4 oz	–	60	–
100% Juices				
orchard fruit blend	4 fl oz	–	60	–
white grape kiwi	4 fl oz	–	80	–
vegetables				
butternut squash & corn	4 oz	0.5	70	6%
garden carrots & brown rice	4 oz	1.5	50	27%
green beans & potatoes	4 oz	2.0	70	26%
spring garden vegetables	4 oz	–	40	–
Tropical Fruit Desserts				
Fruit medley	4 oz	–	70	
guava	4 oz	–	80	–
mango	4 oz	–	80	–
papaya	4 oz	–	70	–
■ (Heinz)				
Building Block #1				
applesauce	2.5 oz	–	45	–
bananas	2.5 oz	–	70	–
carrots	2.5 oz	–	20	–
green beans	2.5 oz	–	25	–
peaches	2.5 oz	–	50	–
pears	2.5 oz	–	50	–
peas	2.5 oz	–	35	–
sweet potatoes	2.5 oz	–	30	–
squash	2.5 oz	–	40	–
Building Block #2				
Dessert Varieties				
banana apple dessert	3.5 oz	–	75	–
banana pudding	3.5 oz	0.5	80	6%
dutch apple dessert	3.5 oz	1.0	85	11%
fruit dessert	3.5 oz	–	70	–
hawaiian delight	3.5 oz	–	70	–
mixed fruit yogurt dessert	3.5 oz	0.5	80	6%
peach cobbler	3.5 oz	–	80	–
tutti-fruitti dessert	3.5 oz	–	75	–
vanilla custard pudding	3.5 oz	2.0	90	30%
Dinner Varieties				
beef egg noodle dinner	1 jar	2.0	50	36%
chicken noodle dinner	1 jar	2.0	65	38%
macaroni & cheese	1 jar	2.0	80	23%
macaroni/tomato beef dinner	1 jar	3.0	60	45%
turkey rice dinner	1 jar	1.0	50	18%
vegetable bacon dinner	1 jar	2.5	55	41%

Food and Description	Amount	Fat Grams	Total Calories	% Fat Calories
vegetable beef dinner	1 jar	2.0	55	33%
vegetable beef dumpling	1 jar	1.5	60	23%
vegetable chicken dinner	1 jar	2.0	55	33%
vegetable ham dinner	1 jar	0.5	40	11%
vegetable turkey dinner	1 jar	2.0	50	36%
Jarred Cereal				
Mixed cereal w/apples & bananas	1 jar	–	80	–
oatmeal cereal w/apples & bananas	1 jar	0.5	90	5%
rice cereal w/applesauce	1 jar	–	80	–
Meat Varieties				
beef w/beef broth	1 jar	5.0	90	50%
chicken w/chicken broth	1 jar	6.0	90	60%
turkey w/turkey broth	1 jar	4.0	70	51%
Simple & Delicious				
apples & chicken	1 jar	1.0	70	13%
apples & ham	1 jar	1.0	80	11%
broccoli & chicken	1 jar	1.0	45	20%
carrots & beef	1 jar	3.0	70	39%
green beans & turkey	1 jar	1.0	45	20%
Simple Goodness				
fruits				
apples & apricots	1 jar	–	60	–
apples & blueberries	1 jar	–	60	–
apples & cranberries	1 jar	–	60	–
apples & pears	1 jar	–	50	–
applesauce	1 jar	–	80	–
apricots w/pears & apples	1 jar	–	80	–
bananas	1 jar	–	100	–
bananas w/apples & pears	1 jar	–	100	–
peaches	1 jar	–	65	–
pears	1 jar	–	60	–
pears & pineapples	1 jar	–	70	–
plums w/apples	1 jar	–	90	–
prunes w/pears	1 jar	–	110	–
vegetables				
carrots	1 jar	–	25	–
corn & sweet potatoes	1 jar	–	90	–
green beans	1 jar	–	30	–
mixed vegetables	1 jar	–	35	–
peas	1 jar	–	60	–
squash	1 jar	–	50	–
sweet potatoes	1 jar	–	70	–
Building Blocks #3				
cereals/jarred				
oatmeal w/apples & cinnamon	1 jar	1.5	130	10%
rice cereal w/apples & bananas	1 jar	0.5	120	4%
desserts				
banana apple desert	1 jar	1.0	110	8%
dutch apple dessert	1 jar	1.5	120	11%
fruit dessert	1 jar	–	100	–

Food and Description	Amount	Fat Grams	Total Calories	% Fat Calories
peach cobbler	1 jar	0.5	125	4%
tutti-frutti	1 jar	–	110	–
vanilla custard pudding	1 jar	2.5	125	18%
dinner varieties				
broccoli, carrots, & cheese	1 jar	2.0	85	21%
chicken noodle dinner	1 jar	1.0	95	9%
turkey rice dinner	1 jar	1.0	75	12%
vegetable bacon dinner	1 jar	3.0	90	30%
vegetable beef dinner	1 jar	3.0	100	27%
vegetable chicken dinner	1 jar	1.0	90	10%
vegetable ham dinner	1 jar	2.0	85	21%
vegetable turkey dinner	1 jar	3.0	80	34%
fruits				
applesauce	1 jar	–	80	–
apple-blueberry	1 jar	–	60	–
apricots w/tapioca	1 jar	–	125	–
bananas w/tapioca	1 jar	–	120	–
bananas & pineapple w/tapioca	1 jar	–	100	–
bananas & strawberries w/tapioca	1 jar	–	130	–
peaches	1 jar	–	120	–
pears	1 jar	0.5	85	5%
plums w/tapioca	1 jar	1.0	135	7%
strawberries w/tapioca	1 jar	–	100	–
tropical fruit	1 jar	1.0	140	6%
homestyle desserts				
apple pie a la mode	1 jar	1.5	150	9%
banana cream pie	1 jar	2.0	160	11%
blueberry cobbler	1 jar	1.0	125	7%
cherry cobbler	1 jar	1.0	145	6%
strawberry shortcake	1 jar	2.0	150	12%
homestyle recipes				
beef & vegetable stew	1 jar	3.0	110	25%
chicken & vegetable stew	1 jar	4.0	95	38%
chicken w/rice & garden vegetable	1 jar	2.5	100	23%
macaroni & cheese	1 jar	4.0	130	28%
macaroni & beef	1 jar	2.0	100	18%
pasta & vegetables in cheese sauce	1 jar	3.0	120	23%
spaghetti w/meat sauce	1 jar	3.5	130	24%
turkey w/rice & garden vegetables	1 jar	1.0	90	10%
vegetables				
peas	1 jar	1.0	95	9%
squash	1 jar	1.0	60	15%
sweet potatoes	1 jar	–	95	–

BABY/INFANT FORMULA

(NOTE: A low-fat nutrition program is not recommended for any child under two years of age, as the nutritional needs of young children differ from those of older children and adults.)

Food and Description	Amount	Fat Grams	Total Calories	% Fat Calories
(Alimentum) hypoallergenic/ liquid ready to feed	5 fl oz	5.5	100	50%
(Bonamil)				
liquid	5 fl oz	5.4	100	49%

Food and Description	Amount	Fat Grams	Total Calories	% Fat Calories
liquid ready to feed	5 fl oz	5.4	100	49%
powder/prepared	5 fl oz	5.4	100	49%
(Carnation)				
Alsoy				
liquid	5 fl oz	5.5	100	50%
powder/prepared	5 fl oz	5.5	100	50%
Good Start				
liquid	5 fl oz	5.1	100	46%
liquid ready to feed	5 fl oz	5.1	100	46%
powder/prepared	5 fl oz	5.1	100	46%
Follow-Up				
liquid	5 fl oz	4.1	100	37%
liquid ready to feed	5 fl oz	4.1	100	37%
powder/prepared	5 fl oz	4.1	100	37%
soy/prepared	5 fl oz	5.5	100	50%
(Enfamil)				
liquid ready to feed				
w/iron	5 fl oz	5.3	100	48%
w/low iron	5 fl oz	5.3	100	48%
Next Step/toddler				
regular	5 fl oz	5.0	100	45%
soy	5 fl oz	4.4	100	40%
powder/prepared				
w/iron	5 fl oz	5.3	100	48%
w/low iron	5 fl oz	5.3	100	48%
(Gerber) powder/prepared				
regular	5 fl oz	5.3	100	48%
soy	5 fl oz	5.3	100	48%
(Isomil)				
liquid	5 fl oz	5.5	100	50%
liquid ready to feed	5 fl oz	5.5	100	50%
powder/prepared	5 fl oz	5.5	100	50%
(Lactofree)				
liquid	5 fl oz	5.5	100	50%
powder/prepared	5 fl oz	5.5	100	50%
(Nursoy) liquid concentrate	5 fl oz	5.3	100	48%
(ProSobee)				
liquid	5 fl oz	5.3	100	48%
liquid ready to feed	5 fl oz	5.3	100	48%
powder/prepared	5 fl oz	5.3	100	48%
(Similac)				
liquid ready to feed				
w/iron	5 fl oz	5.4	100	49%
w/low iron	5 fl oz	5.4	100	49%
powder/prepared				
w/iron	5 fl oz	5.4	100	49%
w/low iron	5 fl oz	5.4	100	49%
Toddler's Best Beverage				
berry	8 fl oz	8.0	160	45%
chocolate	8 fl oz	8.0	160	45%
vanilla	8 fl oz	8.0	160	45%

Food and Description	Amount	Fat Grams	Total Calories	% Fat Calories
BACON (*See also* BACON, CANADIAN STYLE; BACON BITS, CHIPS, & PIECES; BACON SUBSTITUTE; LUNCHEON MEAT)				
(Butterball) turkey bacon	2 slices	2.5	70	32%
(Country Creek)				
cracklins	½ oz	7.0	80	79%
peppered	2 slices	7.0	90	70%
regular	2 slices	7.0	90	70%
generic				
pork breakfast strips/medium-sliced				
cooked	3 slices	12.0	160	68%
raw	3 slices	24.0	265	82%
regular				
all types/cooked/yield from 1 lb raw	4.5 oz	59.5	735	73%
medium-sliced				
cooked	3 slices	9.0	110	74%
raw	3 slices	37.0	380	88%
thick-sliced/raw	1 slice	20.5	210	88%
(Hillshire Farm) country smoked	1 slice	12.0	120	90%
(Hormel) cooked				
Black Label				
center cut	3 slices	5.5	70	71%
low-salt	2 slices	7.0	80	79%
regular	2 slices	7.0	80	79%
Canadian style	2 oz	3.0	70	39%
microwave	4 slices	5.0	70	64%
Old Smokehouse	2 slices	7.0	80	79%
original	2.5 slices	5.0	70	64%
Range	2 slices	9.0	110	74%
Red Label	2 slices	7.0	80	79%
(Kahn's) American Beauty/cooked	2 slices	9.0	100	81%
(Louis Rich) turkey bacon	1 slice	2.5	35	64%
(Mr. Turkey) turkey bacon	1 slice	2.0	25	72%
(Oscar Mayer) cooked				
⅛" thick cut	1 slice	5.0	60	75%
center cut	2 slices	4.5	60	68%
lower sodium	2 slices	5.0	70	64%
original	2 slices	6.0	70	77%
(Schwan's) thick-sliced	1 slice	6.0	70	77%
BACON, CANADIAN STYLE				
generic/1-oz slices				
cold	2 slices	4.0	89	40%
heated	2 slices	3.9	86	41%
(Hormel) 1-oz slices/cooked	2 slices	3.0	70	39%
(Jones) Canadian style/uncooked	3 slices	3.0	70	39%
(Oscar Mayer) cooked	2 slices	1.5	50	27%
BACON BITS, CHIPS, & PIECES				
imitation				
(Betty Crocker) BacOs				
bits	1½ Tbs	1.5	35	39%

Food and Description	Amount	Fat Grams	Total Calories	% Fat Calories
chips	1½ Tbs	1.5	35	39%
(Durkee)				
bits	1 Tbs	1.0	25	36%
chips	1 Tbs	1.0	25	36%
(McCormick/Schilling)				
Bac'n Bits	1 Tbs	<1.0	25	18%
Bac'n Chips	1 Tbs	<1.0	25	18%
(Molly McButter) sprinkles	½ tsp	−	4	−
(Tone's) bits	1 Tbs	1.0	30	30%
real				
(Hormel)				
Bits	1 Tbs	1.5	30	30%
Pieces	1 Tbs	1.5	25	54%
(Oscar Mayer)				
Bits	1 Tbs	1.5	25	54%
Pieces	1 Tbs	1.5	25	54%
BACON SUBSTITUTE (*See also* BACON BITS, CHIPS, & PIECES; VEGETARIAN FOODS)				
(Sizzlean) cooked	2 strips	5.0	70	64%
(Swift Premium) Sizzling breakfast, lunch, & dinner strips				
beef & turkey	1 slice	6.0	70	77%
pork & turkey	1 slice	6.0	70	77%
BAGEL				
(Dunkin' Donuts)				
blueberry	1 bagel	1.0	340	3%
cinnamon-raisin	1 bagel	1.0	340	3%
egg	1 bagel	1.5	350	4%
everything	1 bagel	2.0	360	5%
garlic	1 bagel	1.0	360	3%
onion	1 bagel	1.0	340	3%
plain	1 bagel	1.0	330	3%
poppyseed	1 bagel	2.5	360	6%
pumpernickel	1 bagel	1.5	350	4%
salt	1 bagel	1.0	340	3%
sesame	1 bagel	4.5	380	11%
wheat	1 bagel	1.5	330	4%
(Intenational-Bailys)				
garlic	1.5 oz	<1.0	110	4%
onion	1.5 oz	<1.0	110	4%
plain	1.5 oz	<1.0	110	4%
(Lender's)				
frozen				
cinnamon-raisin				
Big 'N Crusty	1 bagel	2.0	230	8%
original	1 bagel	1.0	150	6%
egg				
Big 'N Crusty	1 bagel	2.0	230	8%
New York Style	1 bagel	2.0	220	8%
original	1 bagel	1.0	150	6%
garlic	1 bagel	1.0	150	6%
oat bran	1 bagel	1.0	150	6%

Food and Description	Amount	Fat Grams	Total Calories	% Fat Calories
onion				
Big 'N Crusty	1 bagel	2.0	230	8%
New York Style	1 bagel	2.0	220	8%
original	1 bagel	1.0	150	6%
plain				
Big 'N Crusty	1 bagel	2.0	230	8%
New York Style	1 bagel	2.0	220	8%
poppy	1 bagel	1.0	150	6%
pumpernickel	1 bagel	1.0	150	6%
raisins/New York Style	1 bagel	2.0	220	8%
raisin & honey	1 bagel	1.0	150	6%
rye	1 bagel	1.0	150	6%
sesame	1 bagel	1.0	150	6%
soft				
egg	1 bagel	3.0	200	14%
plain	1 bagel	3.0	200	14%
raisin	1 bagel	3.0	200	14%
(Otis Spunkmeyer) Thaw & Serve frozen				
3 oz bagels				
blueberry	1 bagel	1.0	210	4%
cinnamon raisin	1 bagel	1.0	210	4%
onion	1 bagel	1.0	210	4%
plain	1 bagel	1.0	210	4%
4 oz bagels				
blueberry	1 bagel	1.0	290	3%
cinnamon raisin	1 bagel	1.0	280	3%
onion	1 bagel	1.0	280	3%
(Pepperidge Farm) food service/Bountiful Bagels				
cinnamon-raisin	1 bagel	1.5	300	5%
onion	1 bagel	1.5	290	5%
plain	1 bagel	1.5	300	5%
poppy	1 bagel	1.5	300	5%
sesame	1 bagel	1.0	300	3%
The Works	1 bagel	1.5	300	5%
(Roman Meal) original	1 bagel	1.0	220	4%
(Rubschlager) sandwich	1 bagel	2.0	90	20%
(Sara Lee) Frozen				
blueberry	1 bagel	1.0	210	4%
cinnamon-raisin	1 bagel	2.0	220	4%
egg	1 bagel	0.5	210	2%
oatbran	1 bagel	1.0	210	4%
onion	1 bagel	–	210	–
plain	1 bagel	0.5	210	2%
poppyseed	1 bagel	1.0	210	4%
sesame seed	1 bagel	1.5	210	4%
(Thomas')				
Gourmet pre-sliced				
apple cinnamon brown sugar	1 bagel	1.5	280	5%
cranberry orange	1 bagel	1.5	280	5%
wildberry blueberry	1 bagel	1.5	180	5%

Food and Description	Amount	Fat Grams	Total Calories	% Fat Calories
New York Style				
cinnamon raisin				
2.16 oz	1 bagel	1.0	140	6%
3.66 oz	1 bagel	2.0	280	6%
egg/2.16 oz	1 bagel	1.0	160	6%
plain				
2.16 oz	1 bagel	1.0	150	6%
3.66 oz	1 bagel	2.0	280	6%
(Western) Big Bagels				
blueberry	4.3 oz	1.0	330	3%
cinnamon-raisin	4.3 oz	1.0	315	3%
plain	4.3 oz	1.0	330	3%
(Wonder)				
Beefsteak Rye	1 bagel	1.0	220	4%
blueberry	1 bagel	1.0	220	4%
cinnamon raisin	1 bagel	1.0	210	4%
onion	1 bagel	1.0	210	4%
plain	1 bagel	1.0	210	4%
wheat	1 bagel	1.0	210	4%
BAGEL CHIPS				
(Burns & Ricker)				
Bagel Chip Mix	1 oz	3.5	120	26%
Bagel Crisps				
cinnamon-raisin	5 chips	3.5	130	24%
fat-free original	5 chips	–	100	–
garlic				
fat-free	5 chips	–	100	–
regular	5 chips	4.0	130	28%
onion	5 chips	4.0	130	28%
plain	5 chips	4.0	130	28%
sea salt	5 chips	4.0	130	28%
sesame	5 chips	6.0	130	36%
(New York Style)				
Chip Mix				
Baked				
fat-free	1 oz	–	100	–
original	1 oz	3.5	120	26%
Chips				
cinnamon-raisin	3 chips	4.0	130	28%
garlic				
baked	3 chips	3.0	130	21%
bite-size	1 oz	0.5	120	4%
regular	3 chips	4.0	130	28%
original	3 chips	6.0	140	39%
sea salt	3 chips	4.0	140	29%
(Rondel´e)				
cinnamon raisin w/honey	13 chips	4.0	130	28%
roasted garlic				
original	13 chips	5.0	140	32%
reduced-fat	13 chips	3.0	130	21%
toasted onion & parsley	13 chips	5.0	140	32%

Food and Description	Amount	Fat Grams	Total Calories	% Fat Calories
very plain	13 chips	5.0	140	32%
(Sara Lee)				
cinnamon-raisin	6 chips	5.0	130	35%
garlic	6 chips	5.0	130	35%
plain	6 chips	5.0	130	35%
sour cream & onion	6 chips	5.0	130	35%
BAKE & FRY MIX (See also SEASONINGS; TEMPURA BATTER)				
(Arrowhead) All purpose baking mix/dry				
regular	¼ cup	0.5	140	3%
wheat-free	¼ cup	0.5	120	4%
(Bisquick) Dry mix only				
original	⅓ cup	6.0	170	32%
reduced fat	⅓ cup	2.5	150	15%
sweet	¼ cup	4.0	170	21%
(Calhoun Bend Mill) mix only				
chicken & shrimp fry	4 Tbs	–	35	–
fish fry				
mild	4 Tbs	–	35	–
spicy	4 Tbs	–	30	–
(Fearn) Dry mix only				
brown rice	½ cup	2.0	215	8%
rice	½ cup	1.0	260	4%
whole wheat	½ cup	2.0	210	9%
(Golden Dipped) Dry mix only				
Breadings & Batters				
all-purpose batter mix	¼ cup	1.0	140	6%
blossoming onion	¼ cup	1.0	140	6%
breakable breader	¼ cup	6.5	155	38%
Cantonese batter/breader	¼ cup	1.0	130	7%
hush puppy w/onion	¼ cup	0.5	135	3%
light n' crunchy bread crumbs	¼ cup	–	45	–
pressure fry all purpose	¼ cup	1.0	130	7%
tempura batter	¼ cup	1.0	145	6%
Gourmet Coating/Natural texture fish & seafood coatings				
fish batter	¼ cup	1.0	140	6%
fish n' chips-English style	¼ cup	1.0	130	7%
old south fish fry meal	¼ cup	1.0	140	6%
seafood breader	¼ cup	1.0	140	6%
Poultry Coatings				
chicken fry	¼ cup	1.0	130	7%
dustless breader	¼ cup	1.0	140	6%
spicy chicken coater	¼ cup	1.0	140	6%
Pre-Dip Egg & Milk Replacement	¼ cup	1.0	140	6%
(Hain) Whole Wheat/dry	⅓ cup	1.0	140	6%
(Jiffy) Dry mix only	1 oz	3.0	115	24%
(Krusteaz) bake & fry mix	¼ cup	1.0	100	9%
(Martha White) Recip-Ease	½ cup	8.0	240	30%
BAKING BITS, CHIPS, CHUNKS, & PIECES				
(Baker's) baking chocolate				
bars				
bittersweet	½ square	6.0	70	77%

Food and Description	Amount	Fat Grams	Total Calories	% Fat Calories
German sweet	2 squares	3.5	60	52%
semisweet	½ square	4.5	70	58%
unsweetened	½ square	7.0	70	90%
white	½ square	4.5	80	51%
chips				
Chocolate-flavored/semi-sweet	½ oz	3.5	70	45%
Real				
milk chocolate, 55 chips per ounce	½ oz	4.0	70	51%
semisweet, 55 chips per ounce	½ oz	3.5	60	52%
(Ghirardelli) baking chocolate				
bars				
bittersweet	3 sections	15.0	210	64%
classic white	3 sections	15.0	240	56%
dark w/mint	5 squares	11.0	190	52%
milk	3 sections	9.0	150	54%
blocks				
milk	1 section	8.0	140	51%
semisweet	3 sections	14.0	210	60%
sweet dark	3 sections	14.0	210	60%
unsweetened	3 sections	23.0	210	99%
chips				
classic white	2 Tbs	4.0	70	51%
milk chocolate	2 Tbs	3.5	70	45%
semisweet	2 Tbs	4.0	70	51%
(Hershey)				
bits for baking				
candy-coated holiday	1 Tbs	3.0	70	39%
chocolate & Reese's peanut butter	1 Tbs	3.0	70	39%
Skor English toffee	1 Tbs	4.5	70	58%
chips				
butterscotch	1 Tbs	4.0	80	45%
chocolate				
milk	1 Tbs	4.5	80	51%
mint	1 Tbs	4.0	80	45%
semisweet				
mini	1 Tbs	4.0	80	45%
regular	1 Tbs	4.0	80	45%
sweet	1 Tbs	4.5	80	51%
Premier white milk	1 Tbs	4.0	80	45%
raspberry	1 Tbs	4.0	80	45%
Reese's peanut butter	1 Tbs	4.0	80	45%
Kisses, mini for baking	11 pieces	4.5	80	51%
(M&M * Mars) M&M Baking Bits				
milk chocolate	0.5 oz	3.0	70	39%
semisweet chocolate	0.5 oz	3.5	70	45%
(Nestlé)				
baking bars/chocolate				
Choco Bake	½ oz	8.0	80	56%
Premier white	½ oz	5.0	80	56%
semisweet	½ oz	4.0	70	51%

Food and Description	Amount	Fat Grams	Total Calories	% Fat Calories
unsweetened	½ oz	7.0	80	79%
baking morsels				
butterscotch	1 Tbs	4.0	70	51%
chocolate				
milk	1 Tbs	4.0	70	51%
mint	1 Tbs	4.0	70	51%
Premier white	1 Tbs	4.0	80	45%
Semisweet				
mega	1 Tbs	4.0	70	51%
mini	1 Tbs	4.0	70	51%
regular	1 Tbs	4.0	70	51%
pieces/Nestlé Crunch baking	1½ Tbs	3.5	80	39%
raisins/chocolate-covered semi-sweet	1⅓ Tbs	3.0	70	39%
BAKING CHOCOLATE (*See* BAKING BITS, CHIPS, CHUNKS, & PIECES)				
BAKING POWDER				
(Calumet)	1 tsp	–	4	–
(Davis)	1 Tbs	–	15	–
generic	1 tsp	–	5	–
BAKING SODA	1 tsp	–	5	–
BALSAM PEAR/raw	1 cup	–	15	–
leaf tips				
cooked	½ cup	–	10	–
raw	½ cup	–	7	–
pods				
cooked	½ cup	–	12	–
raw	½ cup	–	8	–
BAMBOO SHOOT (*See also* ASIAN FOOD)				
canned	1 cup	<1.0	25	18%
fresh				
cooked	1 cup	–	15	–
raw	½ cup	–	21	–
BANANA				
dried	¼ cup	0.5	90	5%
freeze-dried/chips	½ cup	8.0	250	29%
fresh				
red				
whole	1 medium	<1.0	120	2%
sliced	½ cup	<1.0	70	3%
yellow				
mashed	1 cup	1.0	210	4%
whole	1 medium	0.5	105	4%
(Chiquita)	1 medium	–	110	–
(Dole)	1 medium	1.0	120	8%
powdered	1 Tbs	–	20	–
BANANA, COOKING OR BAKING (*See* PLANTAIN)				
BANANA NECTAR/NECTAR BLEND				
(Kern's)				
banana	11.5 fl oz	–	190	–
banana-pineapple	11.5 fl oz	–	220	–
BARBECUE LOAF (*See* LUNCHEON MEAT)				

Food and Description	Amount	Fat Grams	Total Calories	% Fat Calories
BARBECUE SAUCE (*See also* SAUCE; SEASONINGS)				
(Bill Johnson's)				
hickory	2 Tbs	–	40	–
hot & spicy	2 Tbs	–	40	–
mesquite	2 Tbs	–	40	–
original	2 Tbs	–	40	–
(Bull's Eye)				
original	2 Tbs	–	60	–
steakhouse style	2 Tbs	–	50	–
(Chris' & Pitt's)	1 Tbs	–	15	–
(Estee)	1 Tbs	–	18	–
(Featherweight)	1 Tbs	–	14	–
(French's) Cattleman's				
mild	1 Tbs	–	25	–
smoky	1 Tbs	–	25	–
(Healthy Choice)				
hickory	2 Tbs	–	25	–
hot & spicy	2 Tbs	–	25	–
original	2 Tbs	–	25	–
(Heinz)				
Barbecue Select				
hickory	2 Tbs	–	35	–
original	2 Tbs	–	40	–
Thick & Rich				
Cajun	2 Tbs	–	35	–
chunky	2 Tbs	–	30	–
Hawaiian	2 Tbs	–	40	–
hickory smoke	2 Tbs	–	35	–
mesquite	2 Tbs	–	30	–
mushroom	2 Tbs	–	30	–
old-fashioned	2 Tbs	–	35	–
onion	2 Tbs	–	30	–
original	2 Tbs	–	35	–
Texas Hot	2 Tbs	–	30	–
(Hunt's)				
Dijon/mild	2 Tbs	–	40	–
hickory				
bold	2 Tbs	–	45	–
regular	2 Tbs	–	40	–
hickory & brown sugar	2 Tbs	–	75	–
honey				
hickory	2 Tbs	–	40	–
mustard	2 Tbs	–	50	–
hot & spicy	2 Tbs	–	50	–
light	2 Tbs	–	25	–
mesquite	2 Tbs	–	40	–
mild	2 Tbs	–	40	–
original				
bold	2 Tbs	–	45	–

Food and Description	Amount	Fat Grams	Total Calories	% Fat Calories
regular	2 Tbs	–	40	–
teriyaki	2 Tbs	–	50	–
(K.C. Masterpiece)				
bold	2 Tbs	–	60	–
hickory	2 Tbs	–	60	–
honey Dijon	2 Tbs	1.0	50	18%
honey teriyaki	2 Tbs	1.0	60	15%
mesquite	2 Tbs	–	60	–
original				
no salt	2 Tbs	–	60	–
regular	2 Tbs	–	60	–
spicy	2 Tbs	–	60	–
(Kingsford) Masterpiece				
mesquite	1 Tbs	–	30	–
original	1 Tbs	–	30	–
(Kraft)				
regular				
Char-Grill	2 Tbs	–	60	15%
extra rich original	2 Tbs	–	50	–
hickory smoke				
regular	2 Tbs	–	40	–
w/onion bits	2 Tbs	–	45	–
honey				
hickory	2 Tbs	–	60	–
mustard	2 Tbs	–	60	–
regular	2 Tbs	–	50	–
hot				
hickory smoke	2 Tbs	–	50	–
regular	2 Tbs	–	40	–
Kansas City style	2 Tbs	–	45	–
mesquite smoke	2 Tbs	–	40	–
molasses	2 Tbs	–	70	–
onion bits	2 Tbs	–	45	–
original	2 Tbs	–	40	–
roasted garlic	2 Tbs	–	50	–
spicy honey	2 Tbs	–	60	–
teriyaki	2 Tbs	–	60	–
Thick 'N Spicy				
brown sugar	2 Tbs	–	60	–
hickory				
bacon	2 Tbs	–	60	–
smoke	2 Tbs	–	50	–
honey	2 Tbs	–	60	–
Kansas City style	2 Tbs	–	60	–
mesquite smoke	2 Tbs	–	50	–
original	2 Tbs	–	50	–
(Lawry's) California Grill/orange	¼ cup	1.0	35	26%
(Lea & Perrins)				
bold & spicy	2 Tbs	–	50	–
original	2 Tbs	–	50	–

Food and Description	Amount	Fat Grams	Total Calories	% Fat Calories
tomato, garlic, & herbs (Maull's)	2 Tbs	–	40	–
beer-flavor (nonalcoholic)	1 Tbs	<1.0	20	23%
	3.5 oz	3.5	140	23%
genuine	1 Tbs	<1.0	20	23%
Kansas City style	1 Tbs	<1.0	30	15%
lite	1 Tbs	<1.0	12	38%
onion	1 Tbs	<1.0	20	23%
smoky	1 Tbs	<1.0	20	23%
	3.5 oz	3.5	140	23%
sweet/mild	1 Tbs	<1.0	30	15%
	3.5 oz	3.5	210	15%
sweet/smoky	1 Tbs	<1.0	30	15%
	3.5 oz	3.5	210	15%
w/onion bits	1 Tbs	<1.0	20	23%
	3.5 oz	3.5	140	23%
(Newman's Own) Bandito Diavalo/spicy	2 Tbs	2.0	70	26%
(Open Pit)				
hickory smoke	1 Tbs	–	25	–
hickory thick 'n tangy	1 Tbs	–	25	–
hot 'n tangy	1 Tbs	–	25	–
mesquite 'n tangy	1 Tbs	–	25	–
original				
regular	1 Tbs	–	25	–
w/onions	1 Tbs	–	25	–
sweet 'n tangy	1 Tbs	–	25	–
(Texas Best)				
Cajun	2 Tbs	–	50	–
mesquite	2 Tbs	–	50	–
original recipe	2 Tbs	2.5	40	56%
BARLEY (See also BABY FOOD; CEREAL)				
(Arrowhead Mills)				
flakes/rolled	¼ cup	1.0	110	8%
flour	¼ cup	0.5	93	5%
hulless	¼ cup	1.0	140	6%
pearled	¼ cup	0.5	170	3%
generic				
pearled				
cooked	4 oz	0.5	139	2%
	1 cup	0.7	193	3%
dry	1 oz	<1.0	100	4%
	1 cup	2.0	704	3%
raw	1 oz	0.7	100	6%
	1 cup	4.0	651	6%
(Manischewitz) egg/plain	¼ cup	3.0	220	12%
(Quaker/Scotch)				
pearled/quick	⅓ cup	1.0	170	5%
regular/medium	¼ cup	1.0	170	5%
BARLEY MALT				
(Eden)	1 Tbs	–	60	–

Food and Description	Amount	Fat Grams	Total Calories	% Fat Calories
BARRACUDA				
baked or broiled	3 oz	5.0	135	33%
breaded & fried	3 oz	7.5	169	40%
BASIL				
dried				
generic				
crumbled	1 tsp	–	3	–
	1 Tbs	–	10	–
ground	1 tsp	–	5	–
(McCormick/Schilling)	¼ tsp	–	1	–
fresh	2 Tbs	–	1	–
BASS				
black				
cooked-dry heat	3 oz	14.5	215	61%
raw	3 oz	1.0	80	11%
freshwater/raw	3 oz	3.0	97	28%
mixed species/raw	3 oz	3.0	97	28%
striped/cooked-dry heat	3 oz	2.0	82	22%
BAY LEAF/crumbled	1 tsp	–	5	–
BEAN (See individual bean listings)				
BEAN DISH (See also BEANS, BAKED & VARIETY; FROZEN ENTRÉE/DINNER; MEXICAN FOOD; individual bean listings)				
can, jar, or microwave container				
generic				
four-bean salad	½ cup	–	100	–
three-bean salad	½ cup	7.0	153	41%
(Green Giant) three bean salad	½ cup	–	90	–
(Hanover) four-bean salad	½ cup	–	80	–
(Hormel) beef & wieners	7.5 oz	12.0	290	37%
(Kid's Kitchen) beans & wieners microwave cup	1 cup	13.0	310	38%
(Libby's) Diner beans w/franks	1 container	16.0	330	44%
(Luck's)				
beans w/sliced hot dogs	1 cup	16.0	390	37%
mixed bean salad seasoned w/pork	7.25 oz	5.0	200	23%
(Read) four-bean salad	½ cup	–	110	–
(S&W) bean salad				
deli style	½ cup	–	80	–
dill garden	½ cup	–	50	–
marinated	½ cup	–	70	–
marinated garden	½ cup	–	50	–
(Seneca) three-bean salad	½ cup	–	60	–
homemade/USDA Standard Home Recipe				
three-bean salad	1 cup	15.0	300	45%
BEAN SOUP (See SOUP)				
BEAN SPROUTS (See also individual bean listings)				
canned				
(LaChoy) drained	⅔ cup		8	

Food and Description	Amount	Fat Grams	Total Calories	% Fat Calories
fresh				
kidney				
boiled	4 oz	<1.0	37	12%
raw	1 cup	<1.0	53	8%
mung				
boiled	½ cup	–	13	–
canned				
(Arrowhead Mills)	½ cup	–	25	–
raw	4 oz	–	40	–
stir-fried	½ cup	–	31	–
navy				
boiled	1 cup	<1.0	88	5%
raw	4 oz	<1.0	70	6%
pinto				
boiled	4 oz	–	25	–
raw	4 oz	1.0	70	13%
soy				
boiled	½ cup	2.0	38	47%
raw	10 sprouts	0.6	12	45%
stir-fried	4 oz	8.0	143	50%
BEANS, BAKED & VARIETY (See also BEAN DISH; MEXICAN FOOD)				
(B&M) baked beans				
barbecue	½ cup	1.0	210	4%
bacon & onion	½ cup	2.0	190	9%
original	½ cup	2.0	170	5%
red kidney	½ cup	1.0	170	5%
vegetarin	½ cup	1.0	150	6%
w/honey	½ cup	1.5	170	8%
yellow eye	½ cup	3.0	180	15%
(Bush's Best)				
baked beans				
homestyle	½ cup	2.0	160	11%
w/onions	½ cup	2.0	150	12%
pork & beans/deluxe	½ cup	2.0	160	11%
vegetarian	½ cup	1.0	140	6%
(Campbell's)				
baked beans				
brown sugar & bacon	½ cup	3.0	170	16%
New England	½ cup	3.0	180	15%
Old Fashioned/in molasses & brown sugar sauce	½ cup	3.0	180	15%
pork & beans	½ cup	3.0	130	21%
(Friend's) baked				
maple	8 oz	2.0	240	8%
original	½ cup	1.0	170	5%
generic/baked				
w/beef	½ cup	4.6	160	26%
w/brown sugar	½ cup	2.5	145	16%
w/crumbled bacon	½ cup	4.0	160	23%
w/franks	½ cup	8.0	180	40%

Food and Description	Amount	Fat Grams	Total Calories	% Fat Calories
w/molasses & brown sugar	½ cup	1.5	135	10%
w/pork	½ cup	2.0	135	13%
w/pork & sweet sauce	½ cup	2.0	140	13%
(Green Giant)				
baked				
in sauce	½ cup	1.5	160	8%
w/onions	½ cup	1.5	150	9%
barbecue	½ cup	0.5	140	3%
honey bacon flavored	½ cup	0.5	160	3%
pork & beans w/tomato sauce	½ cup	1.0	120	8%
(Hanover)				
baked beans				
barbecue	½ cup	2.0	140	13%
brown sugar & bacon	½ cup	1.0	120	8%
honey mustard	½ cup	1.0	170	5%
vegetarian	½ cup	–	130	–
pork & beans	½ cup	1.5	120	11%
(Health Valley)				
Boston Baked				
no salt	7.5 oz	–	190	–
regular	7.5 oz	–	190	–
vegetarian w/miso	7.5 oz	1.0	180	5%
(Heinz) vegetarian in tomato sauce	½ cup	0.5	130	3%
homemade/USDA Standard Home Recipe				
baked/made w/white beans, molasses, brown sugar, salt pork & spices	½ cup	6.5	190	31%
barbecue	½ cup	<1.0	120	4%
(Hunt's)				
Big John's Beans & Fixins	½ cup	4.0	130	28%
pork & beans	½ cup	1.0	130	7%
(Joan of Arc)				
baked				
in sauce	½ cup	1.5	160	8%
w/onions	½ cup	1.5	150	9%
barbecue	½ cup	0.5	140	3%
honey bacon flavored	½ cup	0.5	160	3%
pork & beans w/tomato sauce	½ cup	1.0	120	8%
(Libby's)				
pork & molasses	½ cup	2.0	140	13%
pork & tomato sauce	½ cup	2.0	140	13%
vegetarian	½ cup	1.0	130	7%
(Luck's) pork & beans in tomato sauce	½ cup	1.0	150	6%
(S&W)				
baked				
barbecue/Texas Style	½ cup	1.5	140	10%
brick oven	½ cup	0.5	160	3%
honey mustard	½ cup	–	130	–
maple sugar	½ cup	0.5	150	33%
sweet bacon	½ cup	1.5	140	10%
Pinquitos	½ cup	0.5	80	6%

Food and Description	Amount	Fat Grams	Total Calories	% Fat Calories
(Van Camp's)				
baked				
fat-free	½ cup	–	130	–
Premium	½ cup	1.0	140	6%
Beanee Weenee/BBQ	z cup	14.0	340	37%
brown sugar	½ cup	3.0	170	16%
pork & beans	½ cup	2.0	110	9%
vegetarian style	½ cup	1.0	110	8%
BEAR				
simmered	4 oz	15.0	295	46%
simmered/diced	1 cup	19.0	365	47%
BEAVER				
roasted	4 oz	6.0	190	28%
roasted/diced	1 cup	7.5	230	29%
BEECHNUT/dried	1 oz	14.0	164	77%
BEEF				

(NOTE: All serving sizes are for cooked portions, unless otherwise stated. "Lean" means beef trimmed of separable fat before cooking. "Lean & fat" means untrimmed and cooked or eaten as purchased. In most cases, 4 ounces of raw beef yields approximately 3 ounces cooked. Prime cuts have the most fat; choice cuts less; and select cuts the least.)

■ BEEF CUTS/FRESH	Amount	Fat Grams	Total Calories	% Fat Calories
brisket/all grades/braised				
flat half				
lean				
0" fat	3 oz	5.0	160	28%
¼" fat	3 oz	8.0	190	38%
lean & fat				
¼" fat	3 oz	24.0	310	70%
½" fat	3 oz	25.0	315	71%
whole				
lean				
0" fat	3 oz	9.0	185	44%
¼" fat	3 oz	11.0	210	47%
lean & fat				
¼" fat	3 oz	27.0	330	74%
½" fat	3 oz	28.0	330	76%
chuck				
arm pot roast/braised				
lean				
0" fat				
choice	3 oz	7.5	187	36%
select	3 oz	5.0	170	26%
¼" fat				
choice	3 oz	8.0	190	38%
select	3 oz	6.0	175	31%
lean & fat				
¼" fat				
choice	3 oz	16.0	250	58%
select	3 oz	12.0	220	49%

Food and Description	Amount	Fat Grams	Total Calories	% Fat Calories
½" fat				
choice	3 oz	23.0	305	68%
select	3 oz	20.0	280	64%
blade roast/braised				
lean				
0" fat				
choice	3 oz	12.0	225	48%
select	3 oz	10.0	205	44%
¼" fat				
choice	3 oz	12.0	225	48%
select	3 oz	10.0	205	44%
lean & fat				
¼" fat				
choice	3 oz	24.0	310	70%
select	3 oz	20.0	280	64%
½" fat				
choice	3 oz	26.0	330	71%
select	3 oz	24.0	310	70%
roast or steak/braised				
lean				
choice	3 oz	15.6	218	64%
select	3 oz	8.7	187	42%
lean & fat				
choice	3 oz	31.0	364	77%
select	3 oz	25.8	321	72%
stew meat				
boneless/braised or stewed				
lean	3 oz	8.0	183	39%
lean & fat	3 oz	20.0	279	65%
corned beef				
boneless/roasted	3 oz	25.8	316	74%
flank/braised				
lean/0" fat/choice	3 oz	8.5	175	44%
lean & fat/0" fat/choice	3 oz	10.5	195	48%
ground				
extra-lean				
baked				
medium	3 oz	14.0	215	59%
well-done	3 oz	13.5	235	52%
broiled				
medium	3 oz	14.0	215	59%
well-done	3 oz	13.0	225	52%
pan-fried				
medium	3 oz	14.0	220	57%
well-done	3 oz	14.0	225	56%
lean				
baked				
medium	3 oz	15.5	230	61%
well-done	3 oz	15.5	250	56%
broiled				
medium	3 oz	15.5	230	61%

Food and Description	Amount	Fat Grams	Total Calories	% Fat Calories
well-done	3 oz	15.0	240	56%
pan-fried				
medium	3 oz	16.0	235	61%
well-done	3 oz	15.0	235	57%
regular				
baked				
medium	3 oz	18.0	245	66%
well-done	3 oz	18.0	270	60%
broiled				
medium	3 oz	17.5	245	64%
well-done	3 oz	16.5	250	59%
pan-fried				
medium	3 oz	19.0	260	66%
well-done	3 oz	16.0	245	59%
loin/top/broiled				
lean				
¼" fat				
choice	3 oz	8.5	185	41%
select	3 oz	6.5	165	35%
½" fat				
choice	3 oz	8.0	175	41%
select	3 oz	6.5	165	35%
lean & fat				
¼" fat				
choice	3 oz	18.0	255	64%
select	3 oz	14.5	225	58%
½" fat				
choice	3 oz	16.5	245	61%
select	3 oz	14.0	220	57%
London broil/100% lean				
choice/braised	3 oz	6.0	167	32%
porterhouse/braised				
lean/¼" fat/choice	3 oz	9.0	185	44%
lean & fat/¼" fat/choice	3 oz	19.0	260	66%
rib				
large end/roasted				
lean/0" fat				
choice	3 oz	13.0	215	54%
select	3 oz	10.0	190	47%
lean & fat				
¼" fat				
choice	3 oz	27.0	326	76%
select	3 oz	23.0	290	71%
½" fat				
choice	3 oz	26.0	315	74%
select	3 oz	25.0	305	74%
small end/broiled				
lean				
0" fat				
choice	3 oz	10.0	190	47%

Food and Description	Amount	Fat Grams	Total Calories	% Fat Calories
select	3 oz	7.5	170	40%
¼" fat				
choice	3 oz	11.0	200	50%
select	3 oz	8.0	180	40%
lean & fat				
¼" fat				
choice	3 oz	24.0	300	72%
select	3 oz	20.5	275	67%
whole/roasted				
lean				
¼" fat				
choice	3 oz	12.0	210	54%
select	3 oz	9.0	180	45%
½" fat				
choice	3 oz	12.0	200	54%
select	3 oz	10.0	190	47%
lean & fat				
¼" fat				
choice	3 oz	26.0	320	73%
select	3 oz	22.5	290	70%
½" fat				
choice	3 oz	27.5	330	75%
select	3 oz	25.0	310	73%
rib eye/broiled				
lean/0" fat/choice	3 oz	10.0	190	47%
lean & fat/0" fat/choice	3 oz	19.0	260	66%
ribs/short/braised				
lean/choice	3 oz	15.0	250	54%
lean & fat/choice	3 oz	36.0	400	81%
round				
bottom/roasted				
lean				
0" fat				
choice	3 oz	6.5	167	35%
select	3 oz	4.5	145	28%
¼" fat				
choice	3 oz	7.0	170	37%
select	3 oz	5.0	155	29%
lean & fat				
0" fat				
choice	3 oz	8.0	175	41%
select	3 oz	5.0	150	30%
¼" fat				
choice	3 oz	14.0	220	57%
select	3 oz	11.0	200	50%
eye of/roasted				
lean				
¼" fat				
choice	3 oz	5.0	150	30%
select	3 oz	3.5	140	23%

Food and Description	Amount	Fat Grams	Total Calories	% Fat Calories
½" fat				
choice	3 oz	6.0	160	34%
select	3 oz	5.0	150	30%
lean & fat				
¼" fat				
choice	3 oz	12.0	205	53%
select	3 oz	9.5	185	46%
½" fat				
choice	3 oz	12.0	210	51%
select	3 oz	11.5	200	52%
full cut/broiled				
lean				
¼" fat				
choice	3 oz	6.5	165	35%
select	3 oz	4.5	145	28%
lean & fat/¼" fat/choice	3 oz	11.5	205	50%
tip/roasted				
lean				
0" fat				
choice	3 oz	5.5	155	32%
select	3 oz	4.5	145	28%
¼" fat				
choice	3 oz	6.0	160	34%
select	3 oz	5.5	155	32%
lean & fat				
¼" fat				
choice	3 oz	12.5	210	54%
select	3 oz	10.5	195	48%
½" fat				
choice	3 oz	13.0	220	53%
select	3 oz	12.0	205	53%
top/broiled				
lean				
¼" fat				
choice	3 oz	5.0	160	28%
select	3 oz	3.5	145	22%
½" fat				
choice	3 oz	5.5	165	30%
select	3 oz	4.5	155	26%
lean & fat				
¼" fat				
choice	3 oz	9.0	190	47%
select	3 oz	7.0	175	36%
½" fat				
choice	3 oz	8.0	180	40%
select	3 oz	7.0	180	35%
rump roast/roasted				
lean				
choice	3 oz	7.9	177	40%
select	3 oz	6.0	162	33%

Food and Description	Amount	Fat Grams	Total Calories	% Fat Calories
lean & fat				
choice	3 oz	23.0	295	70%
select	3 oz	19.9	269	67%
shank crosscuts/simmered				
lean/choice	3 oz	5.5	175	28%
lean & fat/¼" fat/choice	3 oz	12.5	225	50%
sirloin				
top/broiled				
lean				
¼" fat				
choice	3 oz	7.0	175	36%
select	3 oz	5.5	160	31%
½" fat choice	3 oz	8.0	180	40%
select	3 oz	6.5	170	34%
lean & fat				
¼" fat				
choice	3 oz	14.0	230	55%
select	3 oz	12.0	219	51%
½" fat				
choice	3 oz	16.0	240	60%
select	3 oz	15.0	235	57%
wedge-bone/broiled				
lean				
choice	3 oz	6.0	178	30%
prime	3 oz	10.0	201	45%
select	3 oz	7.0	170	37%
lean & fat				
choice	3 oz	16.0	240	56%
prime	3 oz	19.0	271	63%
select	3 oz	15.0	232	58%
steak/broiled				
club/choice				
lean & fat	3 oz	34.5	386	30%
porterhouse/choice				
lean	3 oz	9.0	185	44%
lean & fat	3 oz	18.0	254	64%
T-bone/choice				
lean	3 oz	9.0	185	44%
lean & fat/¼" fat	3 oz	18.0	255	64%
tenderloin/roasted				
lean				
¼" fat				
choice	3 oz	14.5	265	49%
select	3 oz	9.0	180	43%
½" fat				
choice	3 oz	10.0	190	47%
select	3 oz	8.5	180	43%
lean & fat				
¼" fat				
choice	3 oz	22.5	290	70%

Food and Description	Amount	Fat Grams	Total Calories	% Fat Calories
select	3 oz	21.0	275	69%
½" fat				
choice	3 oz	19.5	265	66%
select	3 oz	17.5	245	64%
■ BEEF CUTS, LEAN/BRAND NAME				
(Dakota Lean) raw				
chuck roast	3 oz	2.0	80	23%
eye of round	3 oz	2.0	80	23%
flank	3 oz	1.0	80	11%
ground	3 oz	2.0	90	20%
rib eye	3 oz	2.0	90	20%
round/outside	3 oz	1.0	80	11%
round/top	3 oz	1.0	80	11%
sirloin tip	3 oz	3.0	90	30%
strip loin	3 oz	2.0	90	20%
tenderloin	3 oz	1.0	70	13%
(Lean & Free) raw				
burger	4 oz	9.5	175	49%
cube steak	4 oz	1.0	110	8%
rib eye	4 oz	2.5	120	19%
round steak	4 oz	1.0	110	8%
sirloin steak	4 oz	1.5	110	12%
sirloin tip	4 oz	1.0	110	8%
strip steak/loin	4 oz	2.0	115	16%
T-bone	4 oz	2.5	125	18%
tenderloin steak/fillet	4 oz	2.5	120	19%
top round	4 oz	4.5	135	30%
■ BEEF CUTS, ORGAN/OTHER				
brain				
fried	3 oz	13.5	167	73%
simmered	3 oz	10.6	136	70%
heart/braised	3 oz	4.8	148	29%
kidney/simmered	3 oz	2.9	122	21%
liver				
braised	3 oz	4.0	137	26%
fried	3 oz	6.8	184	33%
lung/braised	3 oz	3.0	102	27%
pancreas/braised	3 oz	14.7	232	57%
spleen/braised	3 oz	4.0	123	29%
sweetbread/braised	3 oz	19.7	272	65%
thymus/braised	3 oz	21.0	273	69%
tongue				
braised/medium fat	3 oz	22.0	208	95%
simmered	3 oz	17.6	241	66%
tripe				
(Armour Star) canned	3 oz	2.0	90	20%
raw	4 oz	4.0	111	32%
BEEF, DRIED/SMOKED (See also JERKY STRIPS & STICKS; LUNCHEON MEAT)				
dried or chipped	2.5 oz	4.0	145	25%
smoked/chopped	1 oz	1.0	38	24%

Food and Description	Amount	Fat Grams	Total Calories	% Fat Calories
BEEF BROTH (*See* SOUP)				
BEEF DISH/ENTRÉE (*See also* ASIAN FOOD; FROZEN ENTRÉE/DINNER; HAMBURGER; MEXICAN FOOD; PASTA ENTRÉE/DINNER; RICE DISH; individual listings)				
Canned				
(Armour Star)				
beef stew	1 cup	12.0	220	49%
corned beef hash	1 cup	30.0	440	61%
roast beef hash	1 cup	25.0	400	56%
roast beef in gravy	½ cup	4.0	150	24%
(Chef Boyardee)				
ABC'S & 123'S w/mini meatballs	7.5 oz	9.0	230	35%
beef stew	1 can	13.0	220	53%
Beefaroni w/beef	1 cup	9.0	260	31%
mini ravioli	1 cup	5.0	230	20%
(Dinty Moore)				
American Classics				
beef ravioli	1 bowl	9.0	300	27%
beef stew	1 bowl	11.0	250	40%
pot roast	1 bowl	3.0	200	14%
roast beef w/mashed potatoes	1 bowl	5.0	240	19%
Salisbury steak	1 bowl	13.0	300	39%
Spaghetti w/meatballs	2 bowl	7.0	290	22%
other				
beef stew				
canned	1 cup	8.0	180	40%
individual serving	1 cup	10.0	190	47%
meatball stew	1 cup	15.0	250	54%
sliced potatoes & beef	7.5 oz	9.0	230	35%
(Heinz)				
beef stew	7.5 oz	9.0	210	34%
goulash	7.5 oz	11.0	240	41%
(Hormel)				
beef goulash	7.5 oz	11.0	230	43%
corned beef	2 oz	7.0	120	53%
roast beef w/gravy	½ cup	4.0	150	24%
(Mary Kitchen)				
corned beef hash				
50% less fat	1 cup	12.0	280	39%
original	7.5 oz	22.0	350	57%
	1 cup	24.0	390	55%
Fiesta hash	1 cup	23.0	410	50%
roast beef hash	7.5 oz	21.0	348	54%
	1 cup	24.0	390	55%
Frozen				
(Armanino) cocktail meatballs	7 pieces	17.0	220	70%
(Schwan's)				
Convenience Meats				
beef crumble	2 oz	8.0	130	55%

Food and Description	Amount	Fat Grams	Total Calories	% Fat Calories
beef patties				
4-oz patty	1 patty	22.0	280	71%
90/10 patty	1 patty	11.0	180	55%
beef tips & gravy	1 cup	7.0	240	26%
chopped BBQ beef	½ cup	8.0	220	33%
burgers				
beef steak hoagie	4 oz	20.0	280	64%
"E-Z Fix"	3 oz	16.0	220	65%
chopped BBQ beef	½ cup	6.0	180	30%
creamed chipped beef	1 cup	17.0	310	49%
Italian meat balls	6 pieces	17.0	230	67%
roast/burgundy peppercorn	4 oz	5.0	120	38%
steaks/beef				
Big Sam	6 oz	7.0	200	32%
chopped	5.3 oz	31.0	390	72%
cubed/foured	4 oz	26.0	390	60%
filet mignon	5 oz	3.0	140	19%
New York strip	8 oz	37.0	520	64%
sirloin ball tip	6 oz	13.0	260	45%
sirloin fillet of beef steak	4 oz	4.0	130	28%
sirloin steak tips	4 oz	4.0	130	28%
top sirloin	10 oz	44.0	640	62%
Homemade/USDA Standard Home Recipe				
beef bourguignon	¾ cup	8.0	194	37%
beef pot pie/9" dia.	⅓ pie	30.0	515	52%
beef stew	1 cup	11.0	220	45%
beef stroganoff w/noodles	1 cup	20.0	342	53%
beef Wellington	4 oz	18.0	325	50%
corned beef hash	1 cup	21.5	344	56%
creamed dried beef	¾ cup	18.0	275	59%
stuffed green pepper				
w/beef & bread crumbs	1 medium	10.5	325	29%
w/beef, bread crumbs, & rice	½ pepper	13.0	219	53%
Microwave container				
(Chef Boyardee) microwave bowl				
beef ravioli/main meal	1 bowl	5.0	270	17%
beef stew	1 bowl	11.0	220	45%
Beefaroni				
w/beef	1 bowl	3.0	190	14%
w/meat sauce	1 bowl	3.0	180	15%
chili w/beans	1 bowl	14.0	300	42%
meat tortellini				
main meal	1 bowl	4.0	300	12%
regular	1 bowl	2.5	220	10%
rice w/beef & vegetables	1 bowl	7.0	250	25%
Sir Chomps-A-Lot	1 bowl	2.0	180	10%
(Dinty Moore) microwave cup				
beef stew	1 cup	7.0	160	39%
burger stew/hearty	1 cup	13.0	240	49%

Food and Description	Amount	Fat Grams	Total Calories	% Fat Calories
(Hormel) micro cup meal				
beef stew	1 cup	6.0	150	36%
Mix				
(Betty Crocker) Hamburger Helper				
BBQ				
mix only	½ cup	1.0	170	5%
prepared	1 cup	10.0	320	28%
beef pasta				
mix only	⅔ cup	1.5	120	11%
prepared	1 cup	10.0	270	33%
beef Romanoff				
mix only	⅔ cup	1.5	150	9%
prepared	1 cup	11.0	300	33%
beef stew/homestyle				
mix only	½ cup	0.5	110	4%
prepared	1 cup	10.0	260	35%
beef taco				
mix only	½ cup	1.5	150	9%
prepared	1 cup	10.0	280	32%
beef teriyaki				
mix only	⅓ cup	0.5	150	3%
prepared	1 cup	10.0	290	31%
cheddar 'n bacon				
mix only	⅔ cup	5.0	170	26%
prepared	1 cup	15.0	330	41%
cheddar and broccoli				
mix only	½ cup	5.0	190	24%
prepared	1 cup	13.0	300	39%
cheeseburger macaroni				
mix only	⅓ cup	4.5	180	23%
prepared	1 cup	16.0	360	40%
cheesy hashbrowns				
mix only	½ cup	1.5	170	8%
prepared	1 cup	19.0	400	43%
cheesy Italian				
mix only	½ cup	3.0	150	18%
prepared	1 cup	14.0	320	39%
cheesy shells				
mix only	½ cup	5.0	170	26%
prepared	1 cup	15.0	330	41%
chili macaroni				
mix only	⅓ cup	1.0	140	6%
prepared	1 cup	10.0	290	31%
fettuccine Alfredo				
mix only	½ cup	3.5	140	23%
prepared	1 cup	13.0	310	38%
four cheese lasagne				
mix only	⅔ cup	4.0	160	23%
prepared	1 cup	14.0	330	38%
Italian Parmesan w/rigatoni				
mix only	⅓ cup	1.5	160	8%

Food and Description	Amount	Fat Grams	Total Calories	% Fat Calories
prepared	1 cup	11.0	300	33%
lasagna				
mix only	⅔ cup	1.0	130	7%
prepared	1 cup	10.0	270	33%
meat loaf				
mix only	1.5 Tbs	0.5	50	9%
prepared	⅛ loaf	14.0	270	47%
meaty spaghetti & cheese				
mix only	½ cup	1.5	150	9%
prepared	1 cup	10.0	290	31%
mushroom & wild rice				
mix only	¼ cup	2.5	150	15%
prepared	1 cup	12.0	310	35%
nacho cheese				
mix only	½ cup	2.5	160	14%
prepared	1 cup	13.0	320	37%
pizza pasta w/cheese topping				
mix only	½ cup	1.5	140	10%
prepared	1 cup	10.0	280	32%
Pizzabake				
mix only	⅓ cup	1.5	140	10%
prepared	½ pizza	10.0	270	33%
ravioli				
mix only	½ cup	1.0	140	6%
prepared	1 cup	10.0	280	32%
ravioli w/white cheese topping				
mix only	½ cup	1.0	160	6%
prepared	1 cup	10.0	310	82%
rice Oriental				
mix only	¼ cup	0.5	160	3%
prepared	1 cup	10.0	310	29%
Salisbury/homestyle				
mix only	⅔ cup	1.0	130	7%
prepared	1 cup	10.0	270	33%
spaghetti				
mix only	½ cup	1.0	130	7%
prepared	1 cup	10.0	270	33%
stroganoff				
mix only	⅔ cup	3.0	160	17%
prepared	1 cup	13.0	320	37%
Swedish meatballs/homestyle				
mix only	⅔ cup	4.5	150	27%
prepared	1 cup	14.0	290	43%
three cheese				
mix only	½ cup	4.5	180	23%
prepared	1 cup	15.0	340	42%
zesty Italian				
mix only	⅓ cup	1.0	150	6%
prepared	1 cup	15.0	340	40%

Food and Description	Amount	Fat Grams	Total Calories	% Fat Calories
zesty Mexican				
mix only	⅔ cup	1.5	140	10%
prepared	1 cup	10.0	280	32%
BEEF JERKY, STICKS, & STRIPS (*See* JERKY STICKS & STRIPS)				
BEEF SAUSAGE (*See* LUNCHEON MEAT; SAUSAGE)				
BEEF SOUP (*See* SOUP)				
BEEF TALLOW (*See also* SUET, BEEF)	1 Tbs	12.8	115	100%
	1 cup	205.0	1849	100%
BEER, ALE, & MALT LIQUOR				
(Amber Key) light				
repeal	12 fl oz	–	106	–
3.2	12 fl oz	–	106	–
(Amstel) Light	12 fl oz	–	95	–
(Anheuser-Busch)				
ice	12 fl oz	–	172	–
light	12 fl oz	–	75	–
natural light	12 fl oz	–	110	–
non-alcoholic	12 fl oz	–	60	–
regular	12 fl oz	–	133	–
(Augsburger)				
bock	12 fl oz	–	169	–
dark	12 fl oz	–	169	–
golden	12 fl oz	–	169	–
red	12 fl oz	–	159	–
(Beck's)				
dark	12 fl oz	–	156	–
light	12 fl oz	–	132	–
regular	12 fl oz	–	143	–
(Black Horse)	12 fl oz	–	158	–
(Blatz LA) Old Style	12 fl oz	–	73	–
(Blue Moon)	12 fl oz	–	171	–
(Budweiser)				
dry	12 fl oz	–	130	–
ice	12 fl oz	–	148	–
ice light	12 fl oz	–	110	–
light	12 fl oz	–	110	–
regular	12 fl oz	–	148	–
(Busch)				
light	12 fl oz	–	110	–
nonalcoholic	12 fl oz	–	60	–
regular	12 fl oz	–	143	–
(Carling's) Black Label	12 fl oz	–	136	–
(Carlsburg)				
light	12 fl oz	–	110	–
regular	12 fl oz	–	149	–
(Champale) extra dry	12 fl oz	–	169	–
(Cheers) nonalcoholic	12 fl oz	–	55	–
(Classic)	12 fl oz	–	144	–
(Colt 45)	12 fl oz	–	156	–

Food and Description	Amount	Fat Grams	Total Calories	% Fat Calories
(Coors)				
Extra Gold	12 fl oz	–	147	–
light	12 fl oz	–	105	–
non-alcoholic	12 fl oz	–	73	–
original	12 fl oz	–	148	–
(Coqui) malt liquor	12 fl oz	–	208	–
(Corona) light	12 fl oz	–	105	–
(Cutter) non-alcoholic	12 fl oz	–	76	–
(Elephant) malt liquor	12 fl oz	–	208	–
(Elk Mountain)				
amber ale	12 fl oz	–	201	–
red	12 fl oz	–	159	–
(Foster's) lager	12 fl oz	–	120	–
(Gablinger's)	12 fl oz	–	96	–
generic				
ale	12 fl oz	–	155	–
light	12 fl oz	–	100	–
near beer	12 fl oz	–	32	–
regular	12 fl oz	–	146	–
stout	12 fl oz	–	120	–
(Genesee)				
bock	12 fl oz	–	156	–
Genny Ice	12 fl oz	–	156	–
Genny				
Cream Ale	12 fl oz	–	162	–
Ice	12 fl oz	–	156	–
Light	12 fl oz	–	96	–
N/A/nonalcoholic	12 fl oz	–	70	–
Red	12 fl oz	–	148	–
original	12 fl oz	–	148	–
12 Horse Ale	12 fl oz	–	152	–
(Goebel)	12 fl oz	–	131	–
(George Killian's) Irish Red	12 fl oz	–	163	–
(Guinness) extra stout	12 fl oz	–	192	–
(Hamm's)				
light	12 fl oz	–	96	–
regular	12 fl oz	–	136	–
(Heidelberg) light	12 fl oz	–	115	–
(Heileman's)				
Black Label	12 fl oz	–	156	–
Old Style				
light	12 fl oz	–	110	–
regular	12 fl oz	–	147	–
Special Export				
dark	12 fl oz	–	155	–
light	12 fl oz	–	115	–
regular	12 fl oz	–	152	–
special dark	12 fl oz	–	192	–
(Heineken)				
regular	12 fl oz		152	

Food and Description	Amount	Fat Grams	Total Calories	% Fat Calories
special dark	12 fl oz	–	192	–
(Herman Joseph's)	12 fl oz	–	157	–
(Hofbrau) dark reserve	12 fl oz	–	204	–
(JW Dundee's)				
Dundee's classic lager	12 fl oz	–	150	–
honey brown lager	12 fl oz	–	150	–
(Keystone)				
dry	12 fl oz	–	125	–
ice	12 fl oz	–	129	–
light	12 fl oz	–	100	–
original	12 fl oz	–	122	–
(KGA)				
ice	12 fl oz	–	154	–
regular	12 fl oz	–	138	–
(KGAL)	12 fl oz	–	110	–
(King Cobra)	12 fl oz	–	182	–
(Kingsbury) nonalcoholic malt	12 fl oz	–	60	–
(Knickerbocker)	12 fl oz	–	140	–
(Koch's) Golden anniversary				
ice	12 fl oz	–	154	–
original	12 fl oz	–	138	–
(Kronenbourg)	12 fl oz	–	170	–
(LA)	12 fl oz	–	112	–
(Lite)				
genuine draft	12 fl oz	–	98	–
ultra	12 fl oz	–	77	–
(Löwenbrau)				
dark special	12 fl oz	–	158	–
regular	12 fl oz	–	157	–
special	12 fl oz	–	158	–
(Michael Shea's)				
Irish amber	12 fl oz	–	145	–
Black & tan	12 fl oz	–	150	–
(Michelob)				
amber block	12 fl oz	–	166	–
black & tan	12 fl oz	–	171	–
classic dark	12 fl oz	–	163	–
dry	12 fl oz	–	133	–
golden draft	12 fl oz	–	151	–
golden draft light	12 fl oz	–	110	–
hefeweizen	12 fl oz	–	180	–
honey lager	12 fl oz	–	175	–
light	12 fl oz	–	134	–
regular	12 fl oz	–	155	–
(Miller)				
genuine draft	12 fl oz	–	147	–
High Life	12 fl oz	–	147	–
Lite	12 fl oz	–	96	–
Magnum	12 fl oz	–	162	–
Sharp's/nonalcoholic	12 fl oz	–	58	–

Food and Description	Amount	Fat Grams	Total Calories	% Fat Calories
(Milwaukee's Best) light	12 fl oz	–	98	–
(Minnesota's Best)	12 fl oz	–	138	–
(Molson) light	12 fl oz	–	109	–
(Moussy) nonalcoholic	11.1 fl oz	–	50	–
(MSB&T)	12 fl oz	–	150	–
(Msia)	12 fl oz	–	145	–
(MS Blonde) lager	12 fl oz	–	150	–
(Nordik Wolf) light	12 fl oz	–	110	–
(O'Doul's)	12 fl oz	–	70	–
amber	12 fl oz	–	90	–
original	12 fl oz	–	70	–
(Old Milwaukee)				
ice	12 fl oz	–	154	–
light	12 fl oz	–	110	–
nonalcoholic	12 fl oz	–	72	–
red	12 fl oz	–	136	–
lager	12 fl oz	–	145	–
(Old Style) Lager	12 fl oz	–	133	–
(Olympia) gold light	12 fl oz	–	70	–
(Pabst)				
Blue Ribbon	12 fl oz	–	135	–
Lager	12 fl oz	–	133	–
low-calorie	12 fl oz	–	110	–
nonalcoholic	12 fl oz	–	55	–
Old English malt liquor	12 fl oz	–	151	–
(Piels)				
light	12 fl oz	–	127	–
regular	12 fl oz	–	133	–
(Pilsner) natural	12 fl oz	–	145	–
(Primo)	12 fl oz	–	138	–
(Prior) double dark	12 fl oz	–	171	–
(Rainier)	12 fl oz	–	142	–
(Red Bull) malt liquor	12 fl oz	–	192	–
(Red Light)	12 fl oz	–	106	–
(Red River Valley) lager	12 fl oz	–	163	–
(Red While & Blue) light	12 fl oz	–	115	–
(Red Wolf)	12 fl oz	–	157	–
(Rheingold)				
light	12 fl oz	–	96	–
regular	12 fl oz	–	148	–
(St. Pauli Girl)				
dark	12 fl oz	–	156	–
light	12 fl oz	–	144	–
(Schaefer)				
light	12 fl oz	–	112	–
regular	12 fl oz	–	138	–
(Schlitz)				
ice	12 fl oz	–	145	–
ice light	12 fl oz	–	121	–
light	12 fl oz	–	120	–

Food and Description	Amount	Fat Grams	Total Calories	% Fat Calories
malt liquor	12 fl oz	–	176	–
regular	12 fl oz	–	145	–
(Schmidt)				
light	12 fl oz	–	96	–
regular	12 fl oz	–	142	–
select nonalcoholic malt	12 fl oz	–	80	–
(Silver Thunder)	12 fl oz	–	165	–
(Steinlager)	12 fl oz	–	138	–
(Stroh's)				
American lager	12 fl oz	–	145	–
light	12 fl oz	–	115	–
Signature	12 fl oz	–	158	–
(Tiger Head) ale	12 fl oz	–	166	–
(XXXX)	12 fl oz	–	133	–
(Ziegen) bock	12 fl oz	–	152	–
(Zima)				
gold	12 fl oz	–	185	–
Citrix	12 fl oz	–	185	–
BEERWURST (*See* SAUSAGE)				
BEET				
canned or jarred				
(Del Monte)				
pickled/sliced/crinkle style	½ cup	–	80	–
regular				
sliced	½ cup	–	35	–
whole	½ cup	–	35	–
(Freshlike)				
pickled/small	½ cup	–	40	–
regular				
sliced	½ cup	–	40	–
small	½ cup	–	40	–
whole	½ cup	–	40	–
generic				
Harvard/sliced	½ cup	–	89	–
pickled	½ cup	–	75	–
(Green Giant)				
Harvard	⅓ cup	–	60	–
sliced				
no salt added	½ cup	–	35	–
regular	½ cup	–	35	–
whole	½ cup	–	35	–
(LeSueur) baby/whole	½ cup	–	35	–
(Libby's)				
pickled				
sliced	½ cup	–	80	–
whole	½ cup	–	35	–
regular/sliced	½ cup	–	35	–
(S&W)				
pickled				
party sliced	1 oz	–	15	–

Food and Description	Amount	Fat Grams	Total Calories	% Fat Calories
sliced	½ cup	–	30	–
whole	1 oz	–	15	–
regular				
julienne	½ cup	–	30	–
whole/small	½ cup	–	30	–
(Seneca)				
Harvard	½ cup	–	90	–
pickled	2 Tbs	–	20	–
pickled w/onions	2 Tbs	–	20	–
(Stokely)				
pickled				
canned	½ cup	–	100	–
jar	½ cup	–	90	–
regular				
cut	½ cup	–	40	–
diced	½ cup	–	40	–
sliced	½ cup	–	40	–
whole	½ cup	–	40	–
fresh				
cooked				
sliced	½ cup	–	26	–
whole	2 medium	–	30	–
raw				
sliced	½ cup	–	38	–
whole	2 medium	–	70	–
BEET GREENS/fresh				
cooked	½ cup	–	20	–
raw	½ cup	–	4	–
BEET JUICE	6 oz	–	75	–
BERLINER SAUSAGE (*See* SAUSAGE)				
BERRY DRINK/BLEND (*See also* BERRY JUICE/JUICE BLEND; FRUIT PUNCH; SOFT DRINK; SOFT DRINK MIX; individual drink listings)				
bottled, boxed, or canned				
(Betty Crocker)				
Squeezit Berry B. Wild	7 fl oz	–	110	–
Squeezit 100	7 fl oz	–	190	–
(Hawaiian Punch)				
Very Berry	6 fl oz	–	90	–
(Hi-C)				
Boppin' Berry				
can	7.7 fl oz	–	110	–
drink box	8.45 fl oz	–	130	–
pet	8 fl oz	–	120	–
wild berry				
pet	8 fl oz	–	120	–
BERRY JUICE/JUICE BLEND (*See also* BERRY DRINK/BLEND; individual juice listings)				
bottled, boxed, or canned				
(Capri Sun)				
red berry	6.75 fl oz	–	100	–
Yo Yogi Berry	6.75 fl oz	–	100	–

Food and Description	Amount	Fat Grams	Total Calories	% Fat Calories
(Heinke's) nectar	8 fl oz	–	120	–
(Knudsen) Oregon berry	8 fl oz	–	100	–
(Libby's) Juicy Juice	8 fl oz	–	130	–
frozen				
(Hi-C) Five Alive/berry citrus	8 fl oz	–	120	–
BIRCH BEER (*See* SOFT DRINK)				
BISCOTII (*See* COOKIE)				
BISCUIT (*See also* BAKE & FRY MIX: BREAKFAST SANDWICH)				
homemade (USDA Standard Home Recipe)				
buttermilk/1½" high/2½" dia	1 biscuit	9.0	212	38%
plain/1½" high/2½" dia	1 biscuit	9.0	212	38%
mix				
(Arrowhead Mills) biscuit mix				
mix only	¼ cup	1.0	120	8%
(Betty Crocker) Gold Medal				
mix only	⅓ cup	6.0	170	32%
prepared	2 biscuits	6.0	180	30%
generic				
buttermilk	1 biscuit	7.0	190	38%
plain	1 biscuit	7.0	190	38%
(Bisquick)				
original	⅓ cup	6.0	170	32%
reduced fat	⅓ cup	2.5	150	15%
sweet	¼ cup	4.0	170	21%
(General Mills) Value Mixes				
prepared	1 biscuit	5.0	160	28%
(Jiffy) buttermilk				
mix only	⅓ cup	5.0	130	35%
prepared	1 biscuit	7.0	150	42%
(Krusteaz)				
baking mix				
mix only	⅓ cup	6.0	180	30%
prepared	2 biscuits	6.0	180	30%
(Martha White) Bix Mix	⅓ cup	5.0	160	28%
packaged ready to serve				
(Arnold) old-fashioned	1 biscuit	3.0	60	45%
(Awrey's)				
country	1 biscuit	5.0	160	28%
round	1 biscuit	3.0	80	34%
sliced	1 biscuit	5.0	160	28%
square	1 biscuit	3.0	80	34%
unsliced	1 biscuit	5.0	160	28%
(Oroweat)				
Australian toaster	1 biscuit	4.5	180	23%
cinnamon-raisin	1 biscuit	5.0	200	23%
refrigerated				
(Pillsbury)				
1869/buttermilk	1 biscuit	5.0	100	45%
Big Country				
butter tastin'	1 biscuit	4.0	100	36%

Food and Description	Amount	Fat Grams	Total Calories	% Fat Calories
buttermilk	1 biscuit	4.0	100	36%
Southern style	1 biscuit	4.0	100	36%
Grands!				
blueberry	1 biscuit	9.0	210	39%
butter	1 biscuit	9.0	190	43%
buttermilk				
original	1 biscuit	9.0	190	43%
reduced-fat	1 biscuit	6.5	170	34%
extra rich	1 biscuit	11.0	220	45%
flaky	1 biscuit	9.0	200	9%
golden corn	1 biscuit	7.0	190	33%
homestyle	1 biscuit	8.0	180	40%
Southern style	1 biscuit	9.0	190	43%
Wheat/reduced-fat	1 biscuit	7.0	190	33%
Hungry Jack				
butter tastin' flaky	1 biscuit	4.5	100	41%
buttermilk	1 biscuit	4.5	100	41%
cinnamon & sugar	1 biscuit	4.0	110	33%
flaky	1 biscuit	4.5	100	41%
honey butter	1 biscuit	4.0	110	33%
Southern style flaky	1 biscuit	4.5	100	41%
Pillsbury				
buttermilk	3 biscuits	2.0	150	12%
country	3 biscuits	2.0	150	12%
tender layer buttermilk	3 biscuits	4.5	160	25%
BLACK BEAN				
(Eden)				
black soy	½ cup	1.5	90	15%
original	½ cup	–	100	–
generic				
boiled	½ cup	<1.0	113	4%
raw	½ cup	1.5	330	4%
(Goya) frijoles negros	½ cup	0.5	90	5%
(Green Giant)	½ cup	–	100	–
(Joan of Arc)	½ cup	–	100	–
(Progresso)	½ cup	1.0	110	8%
(S&W)				
50% less salt	½ cup	–	70	–
regular	½ cup	–	70	–
BLACK BEAN SOUP (See SOUP)				
BLACK CHERRY DRINK /bottled	8 fl oz	–	130	–
BLACK CHERRY JUICE /bottled, boxed, or canned				
(Knudsen) Thirst Quencher	8 fl oz	–	180	–
(Smucker's)	8 fl oz	–	130	–
BLACK TURTLE BEAN				
(Bean Cuisine) Mix	½ cup	1.0	115	8%
(Hain)	4 oz	–	170	–
BLACK TURTLE BEAN SOUP (See SOUP)				
BLACKBERRY				
canned				
in heavy syrup	½ cup	<1.0	94	5%

Food and Description	Amount	Fat Grams	Total Calories	% Fat Calories
in juice	½ cup	<1.0	41	11%
in water	1 cup	1.5	60	23%
fresh	½ cup	<1.0	40	7%
	1 lb	2.0	240	7%
frozen				
(Big Valley) no sugar	⅔ cup	–	70	–
BLACKBERRY JUICE				
generic/canned	8 fl oz	2.0	92	20%
(Smucker's)	8 fl oz	1.5	91	15%
BLACK-EYED PEA				
canned				
(Bush's Best)				
regular	½ cup	–	70	–
seasoned w/bacon	½ cup	1.0	190	5%
(Glory) Southern style	½ cup	0.5	60	8%
(Green Giant)	½ cup	1.0	90	10%
(Luck's) seasoned w/pork	½ cup	3.0	130	21%
(Trappey's)				
w/bacon	½ cup	2.0	120	15%
w/bacon & jalapeño	½ cup	2.0	110	16%
dried				
mature				
boiled	½ cup	0.6	100	5%
raw	½ cup	1.0	131	7%
young pods w/seeds				
boiled	1 cup	–	32	–
raw	1 cup	–	42	–
frozen				
(Freshlike)	3.3 oz	1.0	130	7%
generic/cooked	½ cup	1.0	114	8%
	10 oz	2.0	400	5%
(Pictsweet)	½ cup	1.0	110	8%
(Veg-All)	3.3 oz	1.0	130	7%
BLINTZ (See FROZEN ENTRÉE/DINNER)				
BLOOD SAUSAGE (See SAUSAGE)				
BLUEBERRY				
canned				
generic				
in heavy syrup	1 cup	<1.0	225	2%
in water	2 cup	<1.0	94	5%
(S&W) wild Maine/in heavy syrup	⅓ cup	–	70	–
fresh	2 cups	<1.0	82	6%
frozen				
(C&W)	¾ cup	–	70	–
generic				
no sugar added	1 cup	<1.0	88	5%
	3.5 oz	<1.0	50	9%
sweetened	1 cup	<1.0	190	2%
BLUEBERRY JUICE				
(Knudsen) Thirst Quencher/Maine coast	8 fl oz	–	90	

Food and Description	Amount	Fat Grams	Total Calories	% Fat Calories
BLUEFISH/raw	3 oz	3.6	105	31%
BOLOGNA (*See* LUNCHEON MEAT)				
BORAGE/fresh				
cooked	½ cup	1.0	25	36%
raw	½ cup	<1.0	9	50%
BORSCHT (*See* SOUP)				
BOYSENBERRY				
canned				
in heavy syrup	1 cup	–	226	–
in water	1 cup	–	90	–
fresh	½ lb	–	125	–
frozen				
no sugar added	1 cup	–	66	–
sweetened	1 cup	–	144	–
BOYSENBERRY JUICE/NECTAR				
(Knudsen) nectar	8 fl oz	–	110	–
(Smucker's) juice	8 fl oz	–	120	–
BRAN (*See also* CEREAL)				
corn/dry	½ cup	0.5	85	5%
oat				
generic				
cooked	¼ cup	1.0	45	20%
dry	½ cup	3.0	115	23%
(Golden Harvest)	1 oz	2.0	90	20%
(Hodgson Mill)	¼ cup	3.0	120	23%
(Mother's) prepared	½ cup	3.0	150	18%
(Quaker) prepared	½ cup	3.0	150	18%
rice				
generic/dry	½ cup	8.5	130	59%
(Golden Harvest)	½ cup	8.0	120	60%
(Uncle Ben's)	½ cup	9.0	100	81%
wheat				
(Arrowhead Mills)	⅓ cup	1.0	30	30%
generic/dry	½ cup	1.5	65	21%
(Hodgson Mill)	¼ cup	1.0	30	30%
(Kretchmer) toasted	¼ cup	1.0	30	30%
BRANDY (*See* LIQUEUR)				
BRATWURST (*See* SAUSAGE)				
BRAZIL NUT				
dried	1 oz	19.0	186	91%
shelled	1 oz	19.0	190	90%
	1 cup	93.0	920	91%
(Diamond)	1 oz	19.0	190	90%
BREAD (*See also* BAGEL; BISCUIT; BREADSTICK; CROISSANT; MUFFIN; ROLL)				
■ **BROWN & SERVE**				
(Arnold) Francisco sourdough	1 oz	0.5	70	6%
(Colombo)				
sourdough				
French/round	½" slice	0.5	120	4%

Food and Description	Amount	Fat Grams	Total Calories	% Fat Calories
French sourdough	1½" slice	–	130	–
garlic/plain	3" slice	9.0	190	43%
Luigi's loaves	1" slice	1.0	130	7%
(Earth Grains) pizza rounds	1 round	4.0	210	17%
(Pepperidge Farm) European Bake Shoppe				
Italian	⅑ loaf	2.0	130	14%
(Wonder) du jour				
Austrian	1 slice	1.0	70	13%
French/twin loaves	3" slice	1.0	140	6%
■ CANNED				
(B&M)				
plain	½" slice	0.5	130	3%
raisin	½" slice	0.5	130	3%
(Friends)				
plain	½" slice	0.5	130	3%
raisin	½" slice	0.5	130	3%
generic				
Boston/3¼" x ½" slice	1 slice	1.0	95	10%
(S&W) New England recipe	½" slice	1.0	90	10%
■ FROZEN				
(Bridgeford) dough/baked				
French	2 slices	1.0	150	6%
honey wheat	1 slice	1.0	75	12%
white	1 slice	1.0	75	12%
(Cole's) mini loaf/garlic butter-flavored	1 slice	3.0	90	39%
(Mama Bella) homestyle garlic				
original/1" slice	2 slices	8.0	150	48%
Romano cheese/1" slice	2 slices	9.0	160	51%
(Marie Callender's)				
cornbread	1 piece	3.0	150	18%
honey butter added	1 Tbs	5.0	50	90%
(New York)				
garlic bread	2-1" slices	7.0	190	33%
garlic loaf				
reduced-fat	2-1" slices	3.0	160	17%
original	2-1" slices	7.0	190	33%
Texas garlic toast				
Parmesan	1" slice	11.0	190	55%
plain	1" slice	10.0	170	53%
w/cheese	1" slice	11.0	180	55%
(Pepperidge Farm)				
garlic	⅙ loaf	10.0	160	56%
garlic & olive oil loaves/reduced fat	2½" slice	7.0	170	37%
garlic Parmesan	⅙ loaf	7.0	160	39%
Monterey Jack/jalapeño cheese	⅙ loaf	10.0	200	45%
mozzarella garlic	⅙ loaf	10.0	200	45%
sourdough garlic	⅙ loaf	9.0	180	45%
two cheddar cheese	⅙ loaf	11.0	210	47%
(Rhodes) dough/baked				
honey wheat	1 slice	2.0	130	14%

Food and Description	Amount	Fat Grams	Total Calories	% Fat Calories
Italian	1 slice	2.0	130	14%
raisin	1 slice	2.0	140	13%
sweet	1 slice	3.0	150	18%
white	1 slice	2.0	140	13%
(Rich's) dough/baked				
white	1 slice	2.0	150	12%
(Schwan's)				
dough/baked				
wheat/honey	2 oz	1.5	130	10%
white	2 oz	1.5	140	10%
ready to heat French Baguette	¼ loaf	–	130	–

■ HOMEMADE
USDA Standard Home Recipe (Note: If milk was an ingredient, whole milk was used in preparation)

banana	1 slice	6.0	195	28%
corn pone/9" dia	⅛ pone	3.0	122	22%
cornbread/3" square	1 piece	5.0	170	26%
date nut	1 slice	3.0	100	27%
Irish soda	1 slice	3.0	175	15%
pumpkin	1 slice	7.0	200	32%
raisin	1 slice	2.0	135	13%
spoonbread w/whole ground cornmeal	2 oz	7.0	117	54%
white	1 slice	2.0	110	16%
whole wheat	1 slice	2.0	125	14%

■ MIX
(Arrowhead Mills) mix only

cornbread	¼ cup	1.0	120	8%
multigrain	⅓ cup	1.0	160	6%
rye	⅓ cup	0.5	160	3%
spelt	⅓ cup	1.0	150	6%
white	⅓ cup	0.5	150	3%
whole wheat	⅓ cup	1.0	150	3%
(Aunt Patsy) mix only				
cornbread	¼ cup	–	130	–
sourdough beer	¼ cup	–	130	–
(Ballard)				
cornbread				
mix only	⅟₁₈ pkg	1.5	110	12%
prepared	1 piece	2.5	130	17%
(Betty Crocker) Quickbread Mixes/pouch/prepared				
banana	1 slice	7.0	170	37%
cinnamon streusel	1 slice	7.0	180	35%
cranberry orange	1 slice	6.0	180	30%
lemon poppyseed	1 slice	7.0	170	37%
(Calhoun Bend Mill)				
cornbread/country style/prepared	1 piece	<1.0	146	3%
hushpuppy/mix only	2 Tbs	–	150	–
Mexican/mix only	¼ cup	0.5	120	4%
(Daily Bread Co.) Quick Loaf/fat-free/mix only				
cinnamon-raisin	3 Tbs	–	120	–

Food and Description	Amount	Fat Grams	Total Calories	% Fat Calories
garlic & herb	3 Tbs	–	120	–
honey oatmeal	3 Tbs	–	120	–
onion dill	3 Tbs	–	120	–
nine-grain	3 Tbs	–	120	–
wheat/cracked/hearty	3 Tbs	–	120	–
(Dromedary) mix only				
cheddar cheese	1/9 pkg	2.5	140	16%
cornbread	1/10 pkg	2.5	140	16%
date nut	1/12 pkg	7.0	180	35%
gingerbread	1/6 pkg	4.0	260	14%
Italian herb	1/9 pkg	2.5	140	16%
sourdough	1/9 pkg	2.0	140	13%
wheat/stone-ground	1/9 pkg	2.0	140	13%
white/country	1/9 pkg	1.0	140	6%
(Krusteaz)				
Bread Machine Mixes/prepared				
Classic Hearth				
Bavarian pumpernickel rye	1 slice	2.0	170	11%
Hawaiian royal sweet	1 slice	2.5	170	13%
Mediterranean black olive	1 slice	2.5	150	15%
New England cracked pepper	1 slice	2.5	140	16%
Parisian toasted onion	1 slice	2.0	140	13%
Provencal sun dried tomato & basil	1 slice	2.0	150	12%
Southwestern jalapeño cheese	1 slice	2.5	160	15%
Other				
cinnamon raisin bread	1 slice	2.5	180	13%
honey wheat berry	1 slice	2.0	150	12%
Italian herb	1 slice	2.0	150	12%
oat bran	1 slice	2.5	150	15%
savory rye	1 slice	2.0	150	12%
sourdough	1 slice	2.0	150	12%
12-Grain	1 slice	2.5	170	13%
wheat/cracked	1 slice	2.0	150	12%
white/country	1 slice	2.0	150	12%
Cornbread/original				
mix only	1/4 cup	2.5	110	20%
prepared/2" x 2" piece	1 piece	3.0	120	23%
Cornbread & muffin/fat-free honey				
mix only	1/4 cup	–	120	–
prepared/2" x 2" piece	1 piece	–	120	–
(Marie Callender's) cornbread/mix only	1/4 cup	4.0	150	24%
(Martha White) cornbread				
buttermilk/prepared	1/5 pan	3.0	140	19%
Cotton Pickin				
mix only	1/4 pkg	3.0	140	19%
prepared	1/5 loaf	3.0	140	19%
Mexican/prepared	1/6 pan	3.0	120	23%
(Pillsbury)				
bread machine mix/prepared				
wheat/cracked	1/12 loaf	2.0	130	14%

Food and Description	Amount	Fat Grams	Total Calories	% Fat Calories
white/crusty	½12 loaf	2.0	130	14%
gingerbread mix/prepared	⅛ pkg	5.0	220	20%
quickbread mix				
apple-cinnamon				
mix only	½12 pkg	1.5	140	10%
prepared	1 slice	6.0	180	30%
banana				
mix only	½12 pkg	1.5	130	10%
prepared	1 slice	7.0	180	35%
carrot				
mix only	½12 pkg	1.0	110	8%
prepared	1 slice	5.0	140	32%
chocolate chip				
mix only	½16 pkg	4.0	140	26%
prepared	1 slice	7.0	170	37%
cinnamon swirl				
mix only	½12 pkg	5.0	180	25%
prepared	1 slice	9.0	220	37%
cranberry				
mix only	½12 pkg	1.5	140	10%
prepared	1 slice	4.0	160	23%
date				
mix only	½12 pkg	1.5	150	9%
prepared	1 slice	4.0	180	20%
lemon poppyseed				
mix only	½12 pkg	3.0	150	18%
prepared	1 slice	6.0	180	30%
nut				
mix only	½12 pkg	3.5	150	21%
prepared	1 slice	6.0	170	32%
pecan swirl				
mix only	½12 pkg	6.0	180	30%
prepared	1 slice	11.0	230	43%
pumpkin				
mix only	½12 pkg	1.5	130	10%
prepared	1 slice	6.0	170	32%
(Zia Foods) cornbread/blue cornmeal	1 piece	6.0	110	49%
■ PACKAGED/READY TO SERVE				
(Arnold)				
Arnold Brand				
bakery light				
country bran	2 slices	1.0	80	11%
golden wheat	2 slices	0.5	80	6%
Italian	2 slices	1.0	80	11%
oatmeal	2 slices	1.0	80	11%
soft rye	2 slices	1.0	80	11%
sourdough	2 slices	0.5	80	6%
white/premium	2 slices	0.5	80	6%
bakery soft				
rye				
seeded	1 slice	1.0	80	11%

Food and Description	Amount	Fat Grams	Total Calories	% Fat Calories
unseeded	1 slice	1.0	80	11%
Bran'nola				
country oat	1 slice	2.5	90	25%
honey wheat berry	1 slice	1.5	90	15%
nutty grains	1 slice	2.5	90	25%
original	1 slice	2.0	90	20%
7-grain white	1 slice	2.0	90	20%
12-grain	1 slice	2.0	90	20%
wheat				
dark	1 slice	2.0	90	20%
hearty	1 slice	3.0	90	30%
Brick Oven				
wheat				
8-oz loaf	2 slices	2.5	110	20%
1-lb loaf	2 slices	3.0	110	25%
2-lb loaf	1 slice	2.0	80	23%
white				
8-oz loaf	2 slices	2.5	120	19%
1-lb loaf	2 slices	2.5	130	17%
2-lb loaf	1 slice	1.5	80	17%
Country				
buttermilk	1 slice	2.0	100	18%
potato	1 slice	2.0	100	18%
soft rye	1 slice	1.0	70	13%
soft white	1 slice	1.5	80	17%
wheat	1 slice	1.5	90	15%
white	1 slice	1.5	100	14%
Francisco				
French bread	1 oz	1.0	70	13%
French stick	1 oz	1.0	70	13%
Italian sliced bread	2 slices	1.0	110	8%
Italian sliced stick	1 slice	0.5	70	6%
Italian stick	1 oz	1.0	70	13%
sourdough/24-oz loaf	1 slice	1.0	90	10%
Levy's				
melba thin sliced rye	1 slice	1.0	90	10%
pumpernickel	1 slice	0.5	80	6%
Real Jewish Rye				
w/seeds	1 slice	1.0	70	13%
w/o seeds	1 slice	0.5	70	6%
Other				
cranberry	1 slice	1.0	70	13%
honey wheat berry	1 slice	1.0	70	13%
100% stone-ground whole wheat				
1-lb-4-oz loaf	1 slice	1.0	60	15%
2-lb loaf	1 slice	1.5	100	14%
pumpernickel	1 slice	1.0	80	11%
raisin & cinnamon	1 slice	1.0	70	13%
rye				
deli	1 slice	0.5	80	6%
dill	1 slice	1.0	80	11%

Food and Description	Amount	Fat Grams	Total Calories	% Fat Calories
Real Jewish/rye				
Dijon	1 slice	1.0	80	11%
melba thin	2 slices	1.0	90	10%
regular				
w/seeds	1 slice	1.0	70	13%
w/o seeds/1-lb loaf	1 slice	1.0	70	13%
w/o seeds/2-lb loaf	1 slice	0.5	70	6%
(August Brothers)				
onion rye				
plain	1 slice	1.0	80	11%
w/seeds	1 slice	1.0	90	10%
pumpernickel				
16-oz loaf	1 slice	1.0	80	11%
24-oz loaf	1 slice	1.0	90	10%
rye				
thin w/o seeds	2 slices	1.0	90	10%
w/seeds				
16-oz loaf	1 slice	1.0	80	11%
24-oz loaf	1 slice	1.0	90	10%
w/o seeds				
16-oz loaf	1 slice	1.0	80	11%
24-oz loaf	1 slice	1.0	90	10%
rye n' pump	1 slice	1.0	90	10%
sliced stick	2 slices	1.0	110	8%
sourdough	1 slice	1.0	110	8%
Texas toast	1 slice	3.0	150	18%
(Aunt Hattie's)				
buttermilk	1 slice	–	70	–
potato/homestyle	1 slice	1.5	80	17%
wheat				
homestyle	1 slice	2.0	80	23%
soft	1 slice	1.0	70	13%
stone-ground whole	1 slice	1.0	100	9%
white/homestyle	1 slice	2.0	80	23%
Bran'nola (See (Arnold); (Brownberry) in this section)				
(Brownberry)				
bakery light				
country bran	2 slices	1.0	80	11%
golden wheat	2 slices	0.5	80	6%
Italian	2 slices	1.0	80	11%
oatmeal	2 slices	1.0	80	11%
soft rye	2 slices	1.0	80	6%
white/premium	2 slices	0.5	80	6%
Bran'nola				
country oat	1 slice	2.5	90	25%
nutty grains	1 slice	2.5	90	25%
original				
24-oz loaf	1 slice	2.0	90	20%
3-lb loaf	1 slice	2.0	90	20%
7-grain white	1 slice	2.0	90	20%

Food and Description	Amount	Fat Grams	Total Calories	% Fat Calories
wheat				
dark	1 slice	2.0	90	20%
hearty	1 slice	3.0	90	20%
Francisco International				
French/twin	1 slice	1.0	80	11%
Italian/thick-sliced	2 slices	1.0	110	8%
sliced stick	1 slice	–	100	–
sourdough	1 slice	1.0	90	10%
Hearth				
grain	1 slice	1.5	90	15%
rye	1 slice	1.5	90	15%
wheat	1 slice	1.0	90	10%
Natural				
cinnamon	1 slice	2.0	80	23%
dill	1 slice	1.0	70	13%
health nut	1 slice	1.5	70	19%
oatmeal	1 slice	1.0	70	13%
pumpernickel rye	1 slice	0.5	70	6%
rye				
caraway	1 slice	1.0	70	13%
unseeded				
regular	1 slice	1.0	70	13%
thin-sliced	2 slices	1.0	100	9%
12-grain	2 slices	2 3	110	20%
wheat				
24-oz loaf	1 slice	1.0	80	11%
3-lb loaf	1 slice	1.0	80	11%
white	2 slices	1.5	120	11%
whole bran	1 slice	1.0	60	15%
Other				
orange-raisin	1 slice	1.0	70	13%
raisin-cinnamon	1 slice	1.0	70	13%
raisin-walnut	1 slice	2.5	80	28%
soft oatmeal	1 slice	1.5	70	19%
wheat				
apple honey	1 slice	1.0	60	15%
country	1 slice	1.5	90	15%
soft				
16-oz loaf	2 slices	2.0	110	16%
24-oz loaf	1 slice	–	80	–
3-lb loaf	1 slice	2.0	80	23%
white				
country	1 slice	1.5	90	15%
soft				
16-oz loaf	2 slices	2.0	110	16%
24-oz loaf	1 slice	1.5	80	17%
(Cedar Lane) Pita/low-fat				
whole wheat	1 pita	1.0	150	6%
unbleached wheat	1 pita	1.0	150	6%
(Country Hearth)				
European butter sesame	1 slice	1.0	70	13%

Food and Description	Amount	Fat Grams	Total Calories	% Fat Calories
granola	1 slice	1.0	75	12%
honey nugget	1 slice	1.0	70	13%
Indian	1 slice	1.0	100	9%
old-fashioned buttermilk	1 slice	1.0	70	13%
old-fashioned sandwich	1 slice	1.0	75	12%
old-fashioned wheat	1 slice	1.0	70	13%
7 whole grain	1 slice	1.0	80	11%
stone-ground whole wheat	1 slice	1.0	70	13%
wheat berry	1 slice	1.0	70	13%
(Earth Grains)				
barley bran	1 slice	1.0	70	13%
Canadian oat	1 slice	1.0	70	13%
French	1 slice	1.0	70	13%
gold'n bran	1 slice	1.0	70	13%
honey 'n bran	1 slice	1.0	70	13%
honey multigrain	1 slice	1.0	70	13%
honey oat & nut	1 slice	2.0	80	23%
honey oatberry	1 slice	1.0	70	13%
oat & nut	1 slice	2.0	80	23%
oat bran	1 slice	2.0	80	23%
raisin-cinnamon swirl	1 slice	2.0	80	23%
rye				
dark	1 slice	1.0	70	13%
deli	1 slice	1.0	70	13%
extra sour	1 slice	1.0	80	11%
Jewish	1 slice	1.5	80	17%
Russian style	1 slice	1.0	80	11%
sourdough	1 slice	1.0	70	13%
wheat berry	1 slice	1.5	100	14%
yogurt bran	1 slice	1.0	70	13%
(Father Sam's) pocket bread				
cinnamon-raisin	1 pita	–	150	–
Magic Pockets	1 pita	–	170	–
wheat				
medium	½ pita	–	110	–
mini	1 pita	–	100	–
white				
large	¼ pita	–	140	–
medium	½ pita	–	110	–
mini	1 pita	–	110	–
Francisco (See (Arnold); (Brownberry) in this section)				
generic				
black	1 slice	–	64	–
bran	1 slice	2.9	110	24%
buttermilk/homestyle	1 slice	1.0	75	12%
cheese	1 slice	1.0	72	13%
cinnamon-raisin	1 slice	1.0	80	11%
cracked wheat	1 slice	1.0	75	12%
egg	1 slice	2.0	115	16%
French/5" x 2½" x 1"	1 slice	1.0	80	11%

Food and Description	Amount	Fat Grams	Total Calories	% Fat Calories
garlic	2 slices	3.8	100	34%
gluten	1 slice	1.0	70	13%
high-calcium				
dark	1 slice	<1.0	60	8%
light	1 slice	<1.0	65	7%
hushpuppies	1 piece	7.0	145	43%
Indian (Navajo) fry				
5" dia	1 piece	8.0	295	24%
10.5" dia	1 piece	14.0	525	24%
Italian/4½" x 3¼" x ¾"	1 slice	1.0	85	11%
low-sodium	1 slice	0.8	70	10%
mixed-grain	1 slice	1.0	70	13%
oat bran				
reduced calorie	1 slice	<1.0	55	8%
regular	1 slice	1.0	70	13%
oatmeal				
reduced calorie	1 slice	<1.0	60	8%
regular	1 slice	1.0	70	13%
pita				
sesame/ 6½" dia	1 pita	1.0	140	6%
white				
6½" dia	1 pita	0.5	165	3%
8½" dia	1 pita	1.0	232	4%
whole wheat				
6½" dia	1 pita	1.0	170	6%
8½" dia	1 pita	2.0	200	9%
potato	1 slice	0.8	70	10%
pumpernickel	1 slice	1.0	80	11%
raisin	1 slice	1.0	80	11%
rice bran	1 slice	1.0	70	13%
rye				
reduced calorie	1 slice	<1.0	55	8%
regular	1 slice	1.0	80	11%
seven-grain	1 slice	1.0	65	14%
sourdough	1 slice	0.8	72	10%
triticale	1 slice	0.5	60	8%
Vienna/4¾" x 4" x ½"	1 slice	1.0	70	13%
wheat berry	1 slice	1.0	75	12%
wheat bran	1 slice	1.0	90	10%
wheat germ	1 slice	1.0	75	13%
white				
reduced calorie	1 slice	<1.0	60	8%
regular	1 slice	1.0	65	14%
whole wheat	1 slice	1.0	70	13%
(Grant's Farm)				
buttermilk	1 slice	1.0	80	11%
honey cracked	1 slice	1.0	70	13%
oat bran	1 slice	1.0	70	13%
oatmeal & toasted almonds	1 slice	2.0	80	11%
pumpernickel rye	1 slice	1.0	70	13%

Food and Description	Amount	Fat Grams	Total Calories	% Fat Calories
stone-ground wheat & 7 grain	1 slice	1.0	70	13%
wheat berry	1 slice	1.0	70	13%
(Hearth Farms)				
buttermilk wheat	1 slice	0.5	60	8%
buttermilk white	1 slice	0.5	70	6%
deli rye	1 slice	1.0	100	9%
honey 'n nut oat bran	1 slice	1.0	100	9%
honey wheat berry	1 slice	1.0	90	10%
multigrain	1 slice	1.5	100	14%
whole wheat	1 slice	1.0	90	10%
(Kangaroo) pocket bread				
breakfast				
cinnamon-raisin	1 loaf	–	65	–
wheat-oat bran	1 loaf	–	60	–
sandwich	1 loaf	–	75	–
(King's Hawaiian) center slice	½" slice	4.0	180	20%
Levy's (See (Arnold) in this section)				
Master's Best (See (Orowheat) in this section)				
Middle East pita pocket bread				
garlic	1 pita	2.0	160	11%
onion	1 pita	2.0	150	12%
white				
4" dia	1 pita	–	70	–
4 per pkg	1 pita	1.0	210	4%
6 per pkg	1 pita	0.5	140	3%
wheat/4" dia	1 pita	–	70	–
whole wheat				
4 per pkg	1 pita	1.5	200	7%
6 per pkg	1 pita	1.0	140	6%
(Monk's Bread)				
cinnamon	1 slice	2.0	70	26%
golden rice bran	1 slice	1.0	70	13%
Hi-Fibre	1 slice	1.0	50	18%
raisin	1 slice	2.0	70	26%
sunflower & bran	1 slice	1.0	70	13%
(Mrs. Wright's)				
French/enriched	1 slice	1.0	70	13%
grain/unsalted	1 slice	1.0	70	13%
honey bran	1 slice	1.0	90	10%
honey wheat berry	1 slice	1.0	70	13%
Jewish rye w/seeds	1 slice	1.0	60	15%
lite	1 slice	–	40	–
multimeal/sandwich	1 slice	1.0	70	13%
old fashioned Italian	1 slice	1.0	100	9%
Old World style black	1 slice	1.0	60	15%
raisin	1 slice	1.0	70	13%
sandwich				
supersoft	1 slice	1.0	60	15%
wheat	1 slice	1.0	80	11%

Food and Description	Amount	Fat Grams	Total Calories	% Fat Calories
wheat				
crushed				
regular	1 slice	1.0	80	11%
sandwich	1 slice	1.0	70	13%
homestyle butter top	1 slice	1.0	70	13%
roundtop	1 slice	1.0	80	11%
white				
homestyle butter top	1 slice	1.0	80	11%
supersoft	1 slice	1.0	80	11%
unsalted	1 slice	1.0	80	11%
(Natural Hearth)				
buttermilk	1 slice	1.0	70	13%
7-grain	1 slice	1.5	100	14%
stone-ground whole wheat	1 slice	1.0	60	15%
wheat berry	1 slice	1.0	70	13%
(Oroweat)				
Master's Best				
deli rye	2 slices	1.5	130	10%
northern oat	1 slice	3.0	100	27%
3-seed	1 slice	3.5	90	35%
winter wheat	1 slice	3.0	90	30%
Oroweat				
country oat/light	1 slice	–	40	–
oatnut	1 slice	2.0	100	18%
100% whole wheat/light	1 slice	–	40	–
rye				
dark	1 slice	1.0	70	13%
extra sour	1 slice	1.0	70	13%
hearty/light	1 slice	–	40	–
Jewish	1 slice	1.0	70	13%
Russian	1 slice	1.0	70	13%
9-grain/light	1 slice	–	40	–
sourdough/light	1 slice	–	40	–
(Pepperidge Farm)				
Bakery Breads				
cinnamon	1 slice	3.0	90	30%
cracked wheat/thin sliced	1 slice	1.0	70	13%
crunchy oat	2 slices	4.0	190	19%
date walnut	2 slices	3.0	90	30%
French				
fully baked	2 oz	2.0	150	12%
twin	1 oz	1.0	80	11%
honey bran	1 slice	1.0	90	10%
honey wheat berry/hearty	1 slice	1.5	100	14%
Italian				
brown & serve	1 oz	1.0	80	11%
regular/sliced	1 slice	1.0	70	13%
oatmeal				
light	1 slice	–	45	–
1½ lb loaf	1 slice	1.0	90	10%
regular	1 slice	1.0	70	13%

Food and Description	Amount	Fat Grams	Total Calories	% Fat Calories
very thin sliced	1 slice	1.0	40	23%
pumpernickel				
classic dark	1 slice	1.0	80	11%
party slices	4 slices	1.0	60	15%
raisin w/cinnamon	1 slice	2.0	90	20%
rye				
Dijon				
regular	1 slice	1.0	50	18%
thick-sliced	1 slice	1.0	70	13%
family	1 slice	1.0	80	11%
Jewish				
seeded	1 slice	1.0	80	11%
seedless family	1 slice	1.0	80	11%
onion	1 slice	1.0	80	11%
party rye slices	4 slices	1.0	80	11%
soft	1 slice	1.0	70	13%
7-grain				
hearty slice	2 slices	2.0	180	10%
light	1 slice	–	40	–
Vienna				
light	1 slice	–	45	–
thick-sliced	1 slice	1.0	70	13%
wheat				
light	1 slice	–	45	–
natural	1 slice	1.5	90	15%
regular				
family 2-lb loaf	1 slice	1.0	70	13%
1.5-lb loaf	1 slice	2.0	90	20%
sesame/hearty	1 slice	1.5	95	14%
sprouted	1 slice	2.0	70	26%
very thin	1 slice	–	35	–
white				
country/hearty	1 slice	1.0	95	9%
large family thin	1 slice	1.0	70	13%
sandwich	2 slices	2.0	130	14%
thin	1 slice	2.0	80	23%
toasting	1 slice	1.0	90	10%
very thin	1 slice	–	40	–
whole wheat thin	1 slice	1.0	60	15%
(Rainbo)				
family recipe split top				
grain	1 slice	1.0	70	13%
oat	1 slice	1.0	70	13%
wheat				
honey buttered	1 slice	1.0	70	13%
regular	1 slice	1.0	70	13%
stone-ground	1 slice	1.0	70	13%
white	1 slice	1.0	80	11%
regular				
milk/old-fashioned	1 slice	1.0	70	13%

Food and Description	Amount	Fat Grams	Total Calories	% Fat Calories
sourdough/light	1 slice	0.5	40	11%
thin	1 slice	1.0	70	13%
wheat/light	1 slice	<1.0	40	11%
white				
Iron kids	1 slice	1.0	60	15%
light	1 slice	<1.0	40	11%
(Roman Meal)				
light				
oat bran	2 slices	1.0	80	11%
100% whole wheat	2 slices	1.0	80	11%
7-grain	2 slices	1.0	80	11%
wheat				
hearty	2 slices	1.0	80	11%
regular	2 slices	1.0	80	11%
wheat berry	2 slices	1.0	80	11%
white	2 slices	1.0	80	11%
original				
round top	1 slice	1.0	70	13%
sandwich	2 slices	1.0	110	8%
w/oat bran	1 slice	1.0	70	13%
premium variety				
country potato	1 slice	1.0	90	10%
hearty oat	2 slice	2.0	100	18%
honey nut oat bran	1 slice	2.5	100	23%
honey oat bran	1 slice	3.0	100	27%
honey wheatberry	1 slice	1.0	100	9%
multi-grain w/calcium	1 slice	2.0	100	18%
100% whole wheat	1 slice	1.0	90	10%
100% whole-grain	1 slice	1.5	90	15%
potato wheat	1 slice	1.0	70	13%
7-grain	1 slice	1.0	100	9%
sun grain	1 slice	2.0	100	18%
super seed	1 slice	3.0	100	27%
twelve grain	1 slice	1.5	100	14%
(Rubschlager)				
cocktail breads				
honey whole grain	3 slices	1.0	80	11%
pumpernickel	3 slices	1.0	80	11%
rye	3 slices	1.5	80	17%
regular				
Komissbrot/German-style	1 slice	1.0	70	13%
pumpernickel				
Danish	1 slice	1.0	70	13%
Westphalian	1 slice	0.5	70	6%
rye				
Jewish deli	1 slice	1.0	70	13%
marble	2 slices	1.5	110	12%
sandwich	1 slice	2.0	90	20%
Swedish limpa	1 slice	1.0	60	15%

Food and Description	Amount	Fat Grams	Total Calories	% Fat Calories
sandwich				
malt	1 slice	2.0	90	20%
rye	1 slice	2.0	90	20%
wheat	1 slice	2.0	90	20%
whole-grain/European-style	1 slice	2.0	80	23%
(Sahara) (*See* (Thomas') in this section)				
(Sara Lee) pita bread				
plain	1 pita	1.0	160	6%
whole wheat	1 pita	1.0	160	6%
(Sunbeam)				
family	2 slices	2.0	120	15%
king				
round top	2 slices	2.0	120	15%
sandwich	2 slices	2.0	120	15%
w/buttermilk	2 slices	2.0	120	15%
one-pound	1 slice	1.0	70	13%
(The Great Dakotas Baking Co.)				
blueberry walnut	1 slice	3.5	100	32%
pesto	1 slice	1.0	80	11%
raisin walnut-wheat	1 slice	3.5	100	32%
(Thomas')				
date nut loaf	1 slice	2.0	80	23%
Sahara pita bread				
oat bran	1 pita	1.0	130	7%
onion	1 pita	0.5	140	3%
original				
large, 4 per pkg	1 pita	1.0	220	4%
mini, 8 per pkg	1 pita	–	70	–
regular, 6 or 12 per pkg	1 pita	1.0	150	6%
sourdough	1 pita	0.5	150	3%
whole wheat				
mini, 8 per pkg	1 pita	0.5	60	9%
regular, 6 per pkg	1 pita	1.0	130	7%
(Wolferman's) toasting breads				
cinnamon & raisin	1 slice	1.0	120	8%
heartland harvest	1 slice	1.0	110	8%
honey nut	1 slice	1.5	120	11%
oatmeal cinnamon	1 slice	2.0	120	15%
original	1 slice	–	110	–
sourdough	1 slice	–	110	–
(Wonder)				
cinnamon raisin	1 slice	1.0	70	13%
Good Hearth				
honey wheat	1 slice	1.0	70	13%
multigrain	1 slice	1.5	70	19%
Home Pride				
wheat	1 slice	1.0	80	11%
white	1 slice	1.0	80	11%
potato	1 slice	1.0	70	13%

Food and Description	Amount	Fat Grams	Total Calories	% Fat Calories
Italian				
Light	2 slices	1.0	80	11%
regular	1 slice	1.5	120	11%
Kid's	1 slice	1.0	70	13%
Multigrain/fat-free	1 slice	–	70	–
Oat bran 'n fiber	1 slice	1.0	100	9%
Oatmeal Goodness				
oat & bran	1 slice	1.0	80	11%
oat & sunflower	1 slice	1.5	90	15%
potato				
fat-free	1 slice	–	70	–
regular	1 slice	1.0	70	13%
pumpernickel	1 slice	1.5	80	17%
rye				
Beefsteak				
hearty	1 slice	1.0	70	13%
light/soft	1 slice	1.0	80	11%
soft	1 slice	1.5	80	17%
Jewish	1 slice	1.5	80	17%
sourdough				
light	2 slices	1.0	80	11%
regular	1 slice	0.5	60	8%
Texas toast	1 slice	1.5	120	11%
wheat				
family	1 slice	1.0	70	13%
honey	1 slice	1.0	70	13%
light	2 slices	0.5	80	6%
100% stone ground	1 slice	1.0	70	13%
split-top	1 slice	1.0	70	13%
white				
butter bread	1 slice	1.5	80	17%
buttermilk	1 slice	1.0	70	13%
enriched				
light	2 slices	1.5	120	11%
regular	1 slice	1.0	70	13%
honey white/fat-free	1 slice	–	70	–
light	2 slices	0.5	80	6%
old fashioned	1 slice	1.5	120	11%
■ REFRIGERATED				
(Bread Du Jour)				
Twin French Loaves	3" slice	1.0	140	6%
(Pillsbury)				
cornbread twists	1 twist	6.0	140	39%
French loaf	⅕ loaf	2.0	150	12%
homestyle loaf				
wheat	⅙ loaf	2.5	150	15%
white	⅙ loaf	2.5	150	15%
BREAD COATING (See BAKE & FRY MIX; SEASONINGS)				
BREAD CRUMBS (See also BAKE & FRY MIX; SEASONINGS)				
(Contadina)	¼ cup	1.5	100	14%

Food and Description	Amount	Fat Grams	Total Calories	% Fat Calories
(Devonsheer)				
Italian	¼ cup	2.0	100	18%
plain	¼ cup	1.5	100	14%
(Friday's) seasoned	1 oz	–	56	–
generic				
plain	1 oz	1.0	110	8%
	1 cup	5.0	425	12%
seasoned	1 oz	1.0	105	9%
	1 cup	3.0	440	6%
(Golden Dipt)				
Modern Maid				
American style/fine	¼ cup	1.0	140	6%
oriental	¼ cup	–	45	–
Panko				
plain	¼ cup	–	45	–
seasoned	¼ cup	–	45	–
(Kellogg's) corn flake crumbs	2 Tbs	–	40	–
(Old London)				
plain	¼ cup	1.5	100	14%
seasoned	¼ cup	2.0	100	18%
(Progresso)				
garlic-herb	¼ cup	1.5	100	14%
Italian	¼ cup	1.5	110	12%
parmesan	¼ cup	1.5	110	12%
plain	¼ cup	1.5	110	12%
BREAD CUBES (See CROUTONS; STUFFING/DRESSING)				
BREAD PUDDING (See PUDDING & MOUSSE)				
BREAD STUFFING (See STUFFING/DRESSING)				
BREADFRUIT /raw	¼ small	–	99	–
	1 cup	0.5	227	2%
BREADSTICK				
(Angonoa)				
mini				
cheese	1 oz	2.0	110	16%
pizza	1 oz	2.0	120	15%
sesame	1 oz	4.0	120	30%
whole wheat	1 oz	4.0	120	30%
regular				
cheese	1 oz	2.0	110	16%
garlic	1 oz	2.0	120	15%
Italian	1 oz	2.0	120	15%
onion	1 oz	3.0	120	23%
sesame royal	1 oz	4.0	120	30%
(Bread du Jour) brown & serve				
original	1 piece	1.0	130	7%
sourdough	1 piece	1.0	130	7%
(Fattorie & Pandea)				
traditional	3 pieces	1.0	60	15%
whole wheat	3 pieces	1.0	60	15%

Food and Description	Amount	Fat Grams	Total Calories	% Fat Calories
generic/brown & serve				
garlic	1 piece	<1.0	70	6%
Italian soft	1 piece	1.0	80	11%
(Lance)				
cheese	4 pieces	1.0	50	18%
garlic	4 pieces	1.0	50	18%
plain	4 pieces	1.0	50	18%
sesame	4 pieces	2.0	60	30%
(New York) frozen				
garlic parmesan	1 piece	5.0	180	25%
(Oroweat)				
cheese	1 oz	2.0	110	16%
garlic	1 oz	2.0	113	16%
plain	1 oz	2.0	110	16%
sesame	1 oz	2.0	120	15%
(Pepperidge Farm)				
brown & serve	1 piece	1.5	150	9%
cheddar cheese/thin	7 pieces	2.5	70	32%
onion/thin	7 pieces	2.0	70	26%
sesame/thin	7 pieces	1.5	60	23%
(Pillsbury) soft/refrigerated				
garlic and herb	2 pieces	7.0	180	35%
parmesan	2 pieces	7.0	180	35%
plain	2 pieces	2.5	140	16%
(Stella D'Oro)				
garlic				
deli/fat-free	5 pieces	–	60	–
Grissini/fat-free	3 pieces	–	60	–
regular	1 piece	1.0	35	26%
traditional/fat-free	2 pieces	–	70	–
onion	1 piece	1.0	40	23%
original				
deli/fat-free	5 pieces	–	60	–
Grissini/fat-free	3 pieces	–	60	–
traditional/fat-free	2 pieces	–	70	–
pizza	1 piece	1.0	43	21%
sesame				
low-fat	2 pieces	1.0	70	13%
sodium-free	1 piece	3.0	50	54%
wheat	1 piece	1.0	40	21%
(Toufayan)				
Grissini Style				
cheese	3 sticks	1.0	50	18%
garlic	3 sticks	0.5	50	9%
plain	3 sticks	0.5	50	9%
Soft				
cinnamon-raisin	1 piece	2.0	110	16%
pizza	1 piece	2.0	110	16%
plain	1 piece	2.0	110	16%

BREAKFAST BAR (*See* GRANOLA/GRANOLA-TYPE BAR)

Food and Description	Amount	Fat Grams	Total Calories	% Fat Calories

BREAKFAST DRINK (*See also* NUTRITIONAL SUPPLEMENT)
(NOTE: Unless otherwise noted, mixes are prepared according to package directions)

Food and Description	Amount	Fat Grams	Total Calories	% Fat Calories
(Alba) Dairy Shake				
chocolate	8 fl oz	–	70	–
double fudge	8 fl oz	–	70	–
vanilla	8 fl oz	–	70	–
(Carnation) Instant Breakfast				
liquid ready to drink				
milk chocolate/creamy	10 fl oz	2.5	220	10%
French vanilla	10 fl oz	3.0	200	14%
strawberry creme	10 fl oz	3.0	220	12%
powdered mix				
cafe mocha				
mix only	1 envelope	0.5	130	3%
prepared w/8 oz skim milk	9 fl oz	1.0	216	4%
chocolate malt/classic				
no sugar added				
mix only	1 envelope	1.5	80	17%
prepared w/8 oz skim milk	9 fl oz	2.0	166	11%
regular				
mix only	1 envelope	1.5	130	10%
prepared w/8 oz skim milk	9 fl oz	2.0	216	8%
French vanilla				
no sugar added				
mix only	1 envelope	–	70	–
prepared w/8 oz skim milk	9 fl oz	0.5	156	3%
regular				
mix only	1 envelope	–	130	–
prepared w/8 oz skim milk	9 fl oz	0.5	216	2%
milk chocolate/creamy				
no sugar added				
mix only	1 envelope	1.0	70	13%
prepared w/8 oz skim milk	9 fl oz	1.4	156	8%
regular				
mix only	1 envelope	1.0	130	7%
prepared w/8 oz skim milk	9 fl oz	1.4	216	6%
strawberry creme				
no sugar added				
mix only	1 envelope	–	70	–
prepared w/8 oz skim milk	9 fl oz	0.4	156	2%
regular				
mix only	1 envelope	–	130	–
prepared w/8 oz skim milk	9 fl oz	0.5	216	2%
(Lucerne) Instant Breakfast				
chocolate	1 serving	1.0	130	7%
coffee	1 serving	–	130	–
vanilla	1 serving	–	130	–

BREAKFAST SANDWICH (*See also* FROZEN ENTRÉE/DINNER; individual FAST FOOD listings; VEGETARIAN FOOD)

Food and Description	Amount	Fat Grams	Total Calories	% Fat Calories
(Bob Evans)				
sandwich				
sausage & biscuits	2 biscuits	14.0	200	63%
sausage, egg, & cheese biscuits	2 biscuits	15.0	230	59%
Snackwich				
ham & cheese bagel	2 bagels	6.0	240	23%
sausage biscuits	2 biscuits	23.0	370	56%
sausage & cheese	2 biscuits	21.0	320	59%
sausage burritos	2 burritos	19.0	340	50%
(Don Miguel) frozen				
bacon & egg	1 sandwich	27.0	520	47%
sausage	1 sandwich	27.0	510	48%
smoked ham	1 sandwich	17.0	420	36%
(Owens)				
burrito				
sausage	2 burritos	11.0	330	30%
sandwiches				
ham 'n cheese biscuits	2 sandwiches	16.0	320	45%
hot sausage & biscuits	2 biscuits	23.0	370	56%
sausage & biscuit/large	1 sandwich	18.0	280	58%
sausage & biscuits	2 sandwiches	23.0	370	56%
sausage, egg, & cheese biscuits				
large	1 sandwich	23.0	370	56%
regular	2 sandwiches	26.0	410	57%
sausage burrito	2 burritos	11.0	330	30%
smoked sausage	1 sandwich	12.0	200	54%
(Schwan's) frozen				
sausage breakfast bagel	1 bagel	11.0	300	33%
sausage & biscuit	1 twin pack	22.0	340	58%
BREATH MINT (*See* CANDY)				
BREWER'S YEAST (*See* YEAST)				
BROAD BEAN				
canned	½ cup	<1.0	91	5%
fresh				
boiled	½ cup	<1.0	93	5%
raw				
immature	8 oz	1.0	238	4%
mature	8 oz	3.8	766	5%
BROCCOLI (*See also* BROCCOLI DISH; VEGETABLES, MIXED)				
fresh				
chopped				
generic				
cooked	½ cup	–	23	–
raw	½ cup	–	12	–
(Dole)				
florets	3 oz	0.5	25	18%
spears	1 medium	1.0	40	23%
frozen				
(Birds Eye)				
chopped	½ cup		25	

Food and Description	Amount	Fat Grams	Total Calories	% Fat Calories
cuts	½ cup	–	25	–
florets	3 oz	–	25	–
spears				
baby deluxe	3 oz	–	30	–
regular	3 oz	–	25	–
(C&W)				
florets	4 florets	–	30	–
microwave Brocclettes	1 cup	–	30	–
(Cascadian Farm)	½ cup	–	25	–
generic				
chopped	10 oz	<1.0	75	10%
spears	10 oz	1.0	85	11%
(Green Giant)				
chopped/select poly bag	¾ cup	–	25	–
cuts				
plain poly bag	1 cup	–	25	–
regular	⅔ cup	–	25	–
florets	1⅓ cups	–	25	–
spears				
regular	3.5 oz	–	25	–
select poly bag	3 oz	–	25	–
	4 oz	1.5	50	27%
(Pictsweet) spears	3.3 oz	–	25	–
(Seneca)	1 cup	–	25	–
(Stokely) cuts	3 oz	–	25	–

BROCCOLI DISH (*See also* FROZEN ENTRÉE/DINNER: VEGETABLES, MIXED; VEGETARIAN FOODS)

frozen				
(Birds Eye)				
broccoli stir-fry	1 cup	–	30	–
(Cascadian Farm) Broccoli in cheese sauce	½ cup	2.5	60	38%
generic/spears w/butter sauce	½ cup	–	58	–
(Green Giant)				
broccoli in cheese-flavored sauce	⅔ cup	2.5	70	32%
spears in butter sauce	4 oz	1.5	50	27%
(Pepperidge Farm) vegetables in pastry				
broccoli w/cheese	1 pastry	14.0	240	53%
(Stokely) Singles				
broccoli in cheese sauce	4 oz	4.0	80	45%

BROCCOLI SOUP (*See* SOUP)
BROTWURST (*See* SAUSAGE)
BROWNIE/BLONDIE (*See also* CAKE; CAKE, SNACK; COOKIE)

frozen				
(Weight Watchers)				
à la mode	1 brownie	4.0	190	19%
homemade/USDA Standard Home Recipe				
butterscotch/1¾" x 1¾" x ⅞"	1 brownie	5.0	115	39%
plain	~1 oz	7.0	115	55%
w/nuts	~1 oz	8.0	105	69%

Food and Description	Amount	Fat Grams	Total Calories	% Fat Calories
mix				
(Arrowhead Mills) prepared				
fat-free	1 brownie	–	120	–
regular	1 brownie	–	110	110%
wheat-free	1 brownie	2.0	120	15%
(Betty Crocker)				
Pouch				
dark chocolate fudge				
mix only	⅑ pkg	1.5	130	10%
prepared	1 brownie	8.0	190	38%
fudge				
mix only	⅑ pkg	1.5	130	10%
prepared	1 brownie	8.0	190	38%
Supreme				
chocolate chunk				
mix only	½₀ pkg	3.0	130	21%
prepared	1 brownie	9.0	180	45%
dark chocolate fudge				
mix only	½₀ pkg	1.5	110	12%
prepared	1 brownie	7.0	170	37%
dark chocolate w/Hershey's Syrup				
mix only	½₀ pkg	1.5	120	11%
prepared	1 brownie	7.0	170	37%
fall frosted				
mix only	½₀ pkg	3.0	150	18%
prepared	1 brownie	9.0	210	39%
frosted				
mix only	½₀ pkg	3.0	150	18%
prepared	1 brownie	9.0	210	39%
fudge/prepared				
family size	1 brownie	7.0	170	37%
mega-pack/four pouches	1 brownie	7.0	170	37%
regular size				
original	1 brownie	7.0	190	33%
reduced-fat recipe	1 brownie	4.0	140	26%
German chocolate				
mix only	½₀ pkg	3.0	150	18%
prepared	1 brownie	8.0	200	36%
hot fudge				
mix only	½₀ pkg	2.0	110	16%
prepared	1 brownie	8.0	170	42%
peanut butter chunk w/Reese's Pieces				
mix only	½₀ pkg	3.0	130	21%
prepared	1 brownie	9.0	180	45%
turtle				
mix only	½₀ pkg	2.5	120	19%
prepared	1 brownie	8.0	170	42%
walnut				
mix only	½₀ pkg	3.5	120	26%
prepared	1 brownie	9.0	180	45%

Food and Description	Amount	Fat Grams	Total Calories	% Fat Calories
Sweet Rewards				
fudge/low-fat				
mix only	1/18 pkg	2.5	130	17%
supreme/reduced-fat				
mix only	1/20 pkg	1.0	120	8%
prepared	1 brownie	3.5	140	23%
(Duncan Hines)				
chewy recipe fudge				
original				
mix only	1/12 pkg	2.0	120	15%
prepared	1 brownie	7.0	170	37%
Premium family-size				
mix only	1/20 pkg	2.0	120	15%
Prepared	1 brownie	8.0	170	42%
Dark'N Chunky Chocolate Lover's Premium				
mix only	1/20 pkg	4.0	140	26%
prepared	1 brownie	7.0	160	39%
Dark'N Fudgy Chocolate Lover's Premium				
regular				
mix only	1/18 pkg	3.0	120	23%
prepared	1 brownie	8.0	170	42%
double fudge				
mix only	1/20 pkg	3.0	140	20%
prepared	1 brownie	6.0	170	32%
milk chocolate chunk				
mix only	1/20 pkg	4.0	140	26%
prepared	1 brownie	7.0	170	37%
Mississippi mud chocolate lover's premium				
mix only	1/20 pkg	2.5	130	17%
prepared	1 brownie	6.0	160	34%
raspberry fudge				
mix only	1/20 pkt	3.0	120	23%
prepared	1 brownie	7.0	150	42%
walnut				
mix only	1/20 pkg	4.5	130	31%
prepared	1 brownie	10.0	190	47%
(Estee) prepared	2 brownies	4.0	100	36%
(Gold Medal) Chocolate				
Original	2x3" brownie	5.0	190	24%
Sweet Rewards	2x3" brownie	2.0	170	11%
(Krusteaz) Prepared				
fudge brownie				
fat free	2x2" brownie	–	120	–
original	2x2" brownie	7.0	190	33%
swirl brownie/fat-free	2.5x2" brownie	–	150	–
(Pamela's)				
ultra chocolate				
mix only	2 Tbs	1.0	100	9%
prepared				
oil-free	1 brownie	1.5	110	12%

Food and Description	Amount	Fat Grams	Total Calories	% Fat Calories
traditional	1 brownie	5.0	130	35%
(Pillsbury) prepared				
fudge				
15 oz. box	1 brownie	5.0	140	32%
19.5 oz. box	1 brownie	9.0	190	43%
Thick'n Fudgy				
cheesecake swirl	1 brownie	7.0	150	42%
chocolate chunk	1 brownie	7.0	160	39%
double chocolate	1 brownie	6.0	150	36%
caramel swirl	1 brownie	7.0	160	39%
hot fudge swirl	1 brownie	8.0	170	42%
walnut	1 brownie	10.0	190	47%
Ready-to-serve				
(Dolly Madison)				
low-fat	1.48 oz	3.0	150	18%
regular				
individual	2.96 oz	11.0	340	29%
multi-pack	1.6 oz	6.0	180	30%
(Drake's) fudge nut/reduced fat	1 brownie	2.5	170	13%
(Eagle) fudge w/chocolate chips	1 brownie	11.0	260	38%
(Entenmann's) fudge/fat-free	⅒ strip	–	110	–
(Famous Amos) chocolate/fat-free	1 brownie	–	130	–
(Frookie) fudge/fat-free	1 brownie	–	110	–
generic				
chocolate w/frosting	~¾ oz	4.0	100	36%
plain	1 oz	5.0	115	39%
	2 oz	9.0	230	35%
w/nuts	1 oz	10.0	250	36%
(Health Valley) w/fudge filling/fat-free	1 brownie	–	110	–
(Hostess)				
Brownie Bites				
plain	3 brownies	9.0	170	48%
regular				
light	1 brownie	2.5	140	16%
original fudge	1 brownie	11.0	330	30%
(Lance) Fudge Nut	2¾ oz	11.0	310	32%
(Little Debbie)				
fudge	1.2 oz	13.0	270	43%
	2.5 oz	15.0	310	44%
	3.59 oz	21.0	450	42%
light, low-fat	1.9 oz	3.0	190	14%
(Otis Spunkmeyer)				
half sheet brownies	2 oz brownie	11.5	260	40%
(Tastykake) fudge walnut	1 brownie	17.0	370	41%
refrigerated				
(Pillsbury) fudge	1 brownie	8.0	180	40%
BRUSSELS SPROUTS				
fresh				
cooked	½ cup	–	30	–
raw	½ cup	–	20	–

Food and Description	Amount	Fat Grams	Total Calories	% Fat Calories
(Dole)	½ cup	–	19	–
frozen				
(Birds Eye)				
baby	3 oz	–	35	–
regular	3 oz	–	35	–
(C&W) petite	10 sprouts	–	30	–
(Green Giant)	½ cup	–	25	–
(Freshlike)	3.3 oz	–	35	–
(Pictsweet)				
regular	3.3 oz	–	35	–
express microwave	2.5 oz	–	30	–
(Stokely)	3 oz	–	35	–
BRUSSELS SPROUTS DISH				
(Green Giant) baby, in butter sauce	⅔ cup	1.5	50	27%
(Stokely) singles, in butter sauce	4 oz	1.0	50	18%
BUCKWHEAT GROATS/KASHA				
(Arrowhead Mills) brown	¼ cup	1.0	140	6%
(Wolff's) roasted kernels/cooked	½ cup	1.0	170	5%
BUFFALO/BISON				
cooked				
(Denver Buffalo Co.)				
buffalo burgers	4 oz	5.2	130	36%
ground	4 oz	17.0	250	61%
dried	4 oz	2.0	149	12%
raw	4 oz	1.6	112	13%
roasted	3 oz	2.0	148	12%
BULGUR/HARD RED WINTER WHEAT				
cooked				
(Arrowhead Mills)	¼ cup	0.5	150	3%
generic	1 cup	< 1.0	152	3%
dry/canned				
seasoned	1 cup	4.5	246	17%
unseasoned	1 serving	0.9	227	4%
uncooked	1 cup	3.0	600	5%
BUN (See PASTRY; ROLL)				
BURBOT /raw	3 oz	0.7	76	8%
BURDOCK ROOT				
cooked	1 cup	<1.0	110	4%
raw	1 cup	<1.0	85	5%
BURGER (See BEEF; BUFFALO; HAMBURGER; TURKEY; VEGETARIAN FOODS)				
BURGER MIX (See BEEF DISH/ENTRÉE; VEGETARIAN FOODS)				
BURRITO (See BREAKFAST SANDWICH; MEXICAN FOOD; VEGETARIAN FOODS)				
BUTTER (See BUTTER BLEND, BUTTER-FLAVORED SEASONING; MARGARINE, MARGARINE SPREAD, & SPRAY)				
(Breakstone)				
stick/salted or unsalted	1 Tbs	11.0	100	100%
whipped/salted or unsalted	1 Tbs	7.0	70	100%
(Darigold)				
stick/salted or unsalted	1 tsp	4.0	35	100%
whipped/salted or unsalted	1 tsp	3.0	25	100%

Food and Description	Amount	Fat Grams	Total Calories	% Fat Calories
generic				
stick/salted or unsalted	1 pat	4.0	36	100%
	1 Tbs	11.0	100	100%
	½ cup	92.0	810	100%
whipped/salted or unsalted	1 pat	3.0	27	100%
	1 Tbs	9.0	81	100%
	½ cup	61.0	542	100%
(Hotel Bar)	1 tsp	4.0	35	100%
(Keller's)	1 tsp	4.0	35	100%
(Land O'Lakes)				
honey butter	1 Tbs	8.0	90	90%
light				
stick/salted or unsalted	1 Tbs	6.0	50	100%
whipped	1 Tbs	3.5	35	100%
regular				
stick/salted or unsalted	1 Tbs	11.0	100	100%
whipped/salted or unsalted	1 Tbs	7.0	60	100%
roasted garlic butter	1 Tbs	11.0	100	100%
BUTTER BEAN (*See also* LIMA BEAN)				
canned				
(Aunt Nellie's) Reber	½ cup	1.0	140	6%
(Bush Bros)				
baby	½ cup	–	120	–
green	½ cup	–	110	–
large	½ cup	–	100	–
speckled	½ cup	–	110	–
(Green Giant)	½ cup	–	90	–
(Joan of Arc)	½ cup	–	90	–
(Luck's) speckled/seasoned w/pork	½ cup	3.0	140	19%
(S&W) tender cooked/dry	½ cup	–	70	–
(Trappey's) large white	½ cup	1.0	80	11%
(Van Camp's)	1 cup	1.0	160	6%
BUTTER BLEND/SPREAD (*See also* MARGARINE, MARGARINE SPREAD & SPRAY)				
(Blue Bonnet)				
stick w/tub	1 Tbs	11.0	90	100%
	4 oz	44.0	360	100%
(Buttery Blend) liquid	1 Tbs	14.0	120	100%
(Downey's) honey butter				
cinnamon	1 Tbs	1.0	50	18%
original	1 Tbs	1.0	50	18%
(Kraft) Touch of Butter				
bowl	1 Tbs	6.0	50	100%
squeeze bottle	1 Tbs	9.0	80	100%
stick/50% fat	1 Tbs	10.0	90	100%
(Land O'Lakes)				
Country Morning Blend				
stick				
light	1 Tbs	6.0	50	100%
regular/salted or unsalted	1 Tbs	11.0	100	100%

Food and Description	Amount	Fat Grams	Total Calories	% Fat Calories
tub				
light	1 Tbs	6.0	50	100%
regular	1 Tbs	11.0	100	100%
BUTTERBUR				
cooked	½ cup	<1.0	8	56%
raw	1 cup	<1.0	13	35%
BUTTERFISH /raw	3 oz	6.8	124	49%
BUTTER-FLAVORED SEASONING (*See also* SEASONINGS)				
(Best O' Butter)				
cheddar cheese flavor	½ tsp	<1.0	6	60%
garlic buttery	½ tsp	<1.0	4	90%
original	½ tsp	<1.0	4	90%
sour cream flavor	½ tsp	<1.0	4	90%
(Butter Buds)				
butter-flavored mix	1 Tbs	–	6	–
butter-flavored salt	any amount	–	–	–
(Molly McButter) sprinkles				
butter	1 tsp	–	5	–
cheese	1 tsp	–	5	–
garlic & herb	1 tsp	–	5	–
BUTTERNUT /dried	1 oz	16.0	174	83%

C

Food and Description	Amount	Fat Grams	Total Calories	% Fat Calories
CABBAGE (*See also* SWAMP CABBAGE)				
canned or jarred				
(Aunt Nellie's)				
pickled	1 cup	<1.0	260	2%
red/sweet & sour	2 Tbs	–	20	–
(S&W) red/sweet & sour	2 Tbs	–	15	–
fresh				
Chinese/bok choy/napa				
cooked	½ cup	–	10	–
raw/shredded	½ cup	–	5	–
(Dole)	½ cup	–	5-6	–
Danish				
shredded	½ cup	–	20	–
whole/2-lb head	1 head	2.0	225	8%

Food and Description	Amount	Fat Grams	Total Calories	% Fat Calories
red/raw/shredded	½ cup	–	10	–
(Dole)	3 oz	–	25	–
Savoy/raw	1 cup	–	12	–
spoon/raw	1 cup	–	37	–
white				
cooked	½ cup	–	16	–
raw/shredded	½ cup	–	12	–

CABBAGE DISH (*See also* ASIAN FOOD; FROZEN ENTRÉE/DINNER)
homemade/USDA Standard Home Recipe

coleslaw/made w/regular mayonnaise	⅔ cup	10.0	150	60%
stuffed cabbage	~5 oz	18.0	310	52%

CACTUS

(Embassa)	⅔ cup	–	5	–
(La Costena)				
Napolitos tender cactus	1 cup	–	20	–

CAKE (*See also* BROWNIE; CAKE, SNACK; DONUT; MUFFIN; PASTRY; POPCORN BARS & CAKES; RICE CAKES)

■ **FROZEN OR REFRIGERATED**
(Chef Pierre) food service products
cheesecake/10" dia

French cream	¹⁄₁₀ cake	28.0	410	61%
dessert cups				
Boston cream pie	1 cup	11.0	310	32%
strawberry shortcake	1 cup	9.0	210	39%
layer cake/9" dia				
apple spice	¹⁄₂₁ cake	17.0	310	49%
carrot	¹⁄₁₈ cake	20.0	340	53%
chocolate cream	¹⁄₁₈ cake	11.0	260	38%
chocolate gold	¹⁄₁₈ cake	12.0	300	36%
coconut	¹⁄₁₈ cake	14.0	310	41%
double chocolate	¹⁄₂₀ cake	14.0	320	39%
German chocolate	¹⁄₂₀ cake	15.0	310	44%
lemon cream	¹⁄₁₆ cake	12.0	290	37%
walnut cream	¹⁄₁₆ cake	12.0	290	37%
(Pepperidge Farm)				
layer cake				
chocolate decadence	1 piece	18.0	300	54%
chocolate fudge	1 piece	11.0	250	40%
chocolate fudge stripe	1 piece	9.0	170	48%
chocolate supreme	1 piece	16.0	300	48%
coconut classic	1 piece	11.0	250	40%
devil's food	1 piece	10.0	180	20%
German chocolate	1 piece	12.0	250	43%
golden	1 piece	9.0	180	45%
strawberry stripe	1 piece	8.0	160	45%
vanilla	1 piece	8.0	190	38%
Pound cake/all butter	1 piece	7.0	130	48%
Special Recipe Cake				
Boston creme pie	1 piece	14.0	290	43%
carrot w/cream cheese icing	1 piece	9.0	150	54%

Food and Description	Amount	Fat Grams	Total Calories	% Fat Calories
chocolate mousse	1 piece	9.0	190	43%
lemon				
coconut supreme	1 piece	13.0	280	42%
cream supreme	1 piece	9.0	170	48%
pineapple cream	1 piece	7.0	190	33%
strawberry cream	1 piece	7.0	190	33%
Supreme Dessert Lights				
lemon	1 piece	5.0	170	26%
peach parfait	1 piece	5.0	150	30%
raspberry vanilla swirl	1 piece	5.0	160	28%
strawberry shortcake	1 piece	5.0	170	26%
(Sara Lee)				
cheesecake				
cherry cream	¼ cake	12.0	350	31%
chocolate chip	¼ cake	21.0	410	46%
chocolate mousse	⅕ cake	25.0	400	56%
French	⅙ cake	21.0	350	54%
original	¼ cake	18.0	350	46%
reduced-fat/25%	¼ cake	13.0	310	38%
strawberry cream	¼ cake	12.0	330	33%
strawberry French	⅙ cake	14.0	320	39%
cheesecake bites				
chocolate dipped original	1 piece	7.0	100	63%
	5 pieces	34.0	500	61%
chocolate praline pecan	1 piece	6.0	100	54%
	5 pieces	31.0	480	58%
toasted almond crunch	1 piece	6.0	100	54%
	5 pieces	30.0	470	57%
layer cake				
double chocolate	⅛ cake	13.0	260	45%
flaky coconut	⅛ cake	14.0	260	48%
fudge golden	⅛ cake	13.0	260	45%
German chocolate	⅛ cake	14.0	280	45%
harvest pumpkin spice	⅛ cake	15.0	280	48%
red, white, & blueberry	⅒ cake	8.0	210	65%
strawberry shortcake	⅛ cake	7.0	180	35%
vanilla	⅛ cake	14.0	260	48%
pound cake				
all butter				
family size	⅙ cake	9.0	310	26%
regular	¼ cake	16.0	320	45%
chocolate swirl	¼ cake	16.0	330	44%
free & light	¼ cake	4.0	200	18%
reduced-fat	¼ cake	11.0	280	35%
strawberry	¼ cake	11.0	290	34%
strawberry swirl	¼ cake	11.0	290	34%
■ **HOMEMADE**				
USDA Standard Home Recipe				
angel food	1/12 cake	–	140	–
Boston creme pie	⅙ cake	12.0	290	37%

Food and Description	Amount	Fat Grams	Total Calories	% Fat Calories
caramel/8" dia				
w/caramel icing	1/12 cake	12.0	315	34%
w/o icing	1/12 cake	10.0	218	42%
carrot w/cream cheese frosting/ 10" dia	1/10 cake	21.0	385	49%
cheesecake/9" dia	1/12 cake	18.0	280	58%
chocolate/9" dia				
w/chocolate icing	1/12 cake	16.0	385	40%
w/o icing	1/12 cake	13.0	272	43%
chocolate torte/8½" dia	1/16 cake	22.0	317	63%
coffeecake				
cheese w/crumb topping	1/6 cake	12.0	260	42%
cinnamon w/crumb topping	1/9 cake	15.0	260	52%
fruit	1/8 cake	5.0	160	28%
cottage pudding				
w/chocolate sauce	3 oz	8.7	315	25%
w/o sauce	3 oz	8.0	251	29%
devil's food w/chocolate icing/9" dia	1/16 cake	8.0	235	31%
fruitcake/dark/7½" dia	1/32 cake	7.0	165	38%
gingerbread/8" square	1/9 cake	4.0	175	21%
pineapple upside down	1/9 cake	14.0	365	35%
pound cake/8½" x 3½" x 3¼"	1/17 cake	5.0	120	38%
prune whip/baked				
cold	1 cup	–	203	–
hot	1 cup	–	140	–
sheet cake/9" square				
w/no-cook white frosting	1/9 cake	14.0	445	28%
w/o frosting	1/9 cake	12.0	314	33%
spice w/brown sugar frosting/9" dia	1/10 cake	16.0	411	35%
sponge/tube/9¾" dia	1/12 cake	3.8	196.0	17%
white/9" dia				
w/coconut frosting	1/16 cake	10.0	289	31%
w/white frosting	1/16 cake	9.0	260	28%
yellow/9" dia				
w/caramel frosting	1/16 cake	9.5	293	29%
w/chocolate frosting	1/16 cake	11.0	245	40%
■ MIX				
(Betty Crocker)				
Classic Dessert				
gingerbread				
mix only	1/12 pkg	6.0	150	36%
prepared	1/12 cake	6.0	230	23%
pineapple upside down cake				
mix only	1/6 pkg	10.0	350	26%
prepared	1/6 cake	15.0	400	34%
pound cake				
mix only	1/6 pkg	7.0	240	26%
prepared	1/6 cake	15.0	400	34%
Stir'n Bake				
carrot cake w/cream cheese	1/6 cake	7.0	250	25%

Food and Description	Amount	Fat Grams	Total Calories	% Fat Calories
cinnamon streusel coffee cake	⅛ cake	6.0	200	27%
devil's food cake w/chocolate frosting	⅙ cake	7.0	240	26%
yellow cake w/chocolate frosting	⅙ cake	7.0	240	26%
SuperMoist				
angel food/prepared				
chocolate swirl	½12 cake	–	150	–
confetti	½12 cake	–	150	–
easy angel (pouch)	½12 cake	–	170	–
one-step white	½12 cake	–	140	–
traditional	½12 cake	–	130	–
butter chocolate				
mix only	½12 pkg	2.5	170	13%
prepared	½12 cake	11.0	225	44%
butter pecan				
mix only	½12 pkg	3.0	170	16%
prepared	½12 cake	10.0	240	38%
butter yellow				
mix only	½12 pkg	2.0	170	11%
prepared	½12 cake	11.0	260	38%
carrot cake				
mix only	½10 pkg	3.0	200	14%
prepared	½10 cake	15.0	320	42%
cherry chip				
mix only	½10 pkg	4.5	210	19%
prepared	½10 cake	13.0	300	39%
chocolate chip				
mix only	½12 pkg	4.0	180	20%
prepared	½12 cake	11.0	250	40%
chocolate fudge				
mix only	½12 pkg	2.5	170	13%
prepared	½12 cake	12.0	270	40%
chocolate w/creamy swirls of fudge				
mix only	⅛ pkg	2.5	160	14%
prepared	⅛ cake	8.0	210	34%
devil's food				
mix only	½12 pkg	2.5	170	13%
prepared	½12 cake	13.0	270	43%
double chocolate swirl				
mix only	½12 pkg	2.5	170	13%
prepared	½12 cake	13.0	270	43%
French vanilla				
mix only	½12 pkg	3.0	170	16%
prepared	½12 cake	10.0	240	38%
fudge marble				
mix only	½10 pkg	3.5	210	15%
prepared	½10 cake	12.0	290	37%
German chocolate				
mix only	½12 pkg	2.5	170	13%
prepared	½12 cake	13.0	270	43%

Food and Description	Amount	Fat Grams	Total Calories	% Fat Calories
golden vanilla				
mix only	½₂ pkg	3.0	170	16%
prepared	½₂ cake	10.0	240	38%
lemon				
mix only	½₂ pkg	3.0	170	16%
prepared	½₂ cake	10.0	240	38%
milk chocolate				
mix only	½₂ pkg	3.0	170	16%
prepared	½₂ cake	9.0	230	35%
party swirl				
mix only	½₂ pkg	3.5	180	18%
prepared	½₂ cake	11.0	250	40%
pineapple				
mix only	½₂ pkg	3.0	170	16%
prepared	½₂ cake	10.0	250	36%
rainbow chip				
mix only	⅟₁₀ pkg	4.5	210	19%
prepared	⅟₁₀ cake	13.0	300	39%
sour cream white				
mix only	⅟₁₀ pkg	5.0	210	21%
prepared	⅟₁₀ cake	13.0	300	39%
spice				
mix only	½₂ pkg	3.0	170	16%
prepared	½₂ cake	10.0	240	38%
strawberry				
mix only	½₂ pkg	3.0	170	16%
prepared	½₂ cake	10.0	250	36%
strawberry swirl				
mix only	⅟₁₀ pkg	4.5	210	19%
prepared	⅟₁₀ cake	11.0	280	35%
white				
mix only	½₂ pkg	4.0	180	20%
prepared	½₂ cake	10.0	230	39%
white chocolate swirl				
mix only	½₂ pkg	3.5	180	18%
prepared	½₂ cake	11.0	250	40%
yellow				
mix only	½₂ pkg	3.0	170	16%
prepared	½₂ cake	10.0	250	36%
yellow w/creamy swirls of fudge				
mix only	⅑ pkg	2.5	160	14%
prepared	⅑ cake	8.0	210	34%
Supreme Dessert Bar				
chocolate peanut butter				
mix only	½₂ pkg	6.0	160	34%
prepared	1 bar	9.0	200	41%
easy layer				
mix only	⅟₁₆ pkg	4.0	120	30%
prepared	1 bar	6.0	140	39%
Hershey Cookie Bars				
mix only	⅟₁₆ pkg	2.5	110	20%

Food and Description	Amount	Fat Grams	Total Calories	% Fat Calories
prepared	1 bar	6.0	150	36%
Sunkist lemon				
mix only	⅟₁₆ pkg	3.5	130	24%
prepared	1 bar	4.5	140	29%
Sweet Rewards /prepared				
Cakes/prepared/Reduced-Fat				
devil's food	⅟₁₂ cake	5.0	200	23%
white	⅟₁₂ cake	4.0	190	19%
yellow	⅟₁₂ cake	4.5	200	20%
Snack Bars/Fat-Free				
blueberry w/drizzle	1 bar	–	120	–
double fudge supreme	1 bar	–	110	–
homestyle brownie	1 bar	–	100	–
raspberry	1 bar	–	120	–
strawberry w/drizzle	1 bar	–	120	–
Snack Cakes/Fat-Free				
apple cinnamon	⅛ cake	–	170	–
banana	⅛ cake	–	170	–
chocolate	⅛ cake	–	170	–
lemon	⅛ cake	–	170	–
(Dromedary) pound cake				
carrot	⅟₁₂ cake	15.0	232	58%
date nut	⅟₁₂ cake	8.0	183	39%
gingerbread	1 piece	2.0	100	18%
pound cake	½" slice	6.0	150	36%
(Duncan Hines)				
angel food				
mix only	⅟₁₂ pkg	–	140	–
prepared	⅟₁₂ cake	–	140	–
banana supreme				
mix only	⅟₁₂ pkg	4.0	180	20%
prepared	⅟₁₂ cake	11.0	250	40%
butter recipe fudge				
mix only	⅟₁₀ pkg	6.0	220	25%
prepared	⅟₁₀ cake	17.0	320	48%
butter recipe golden				
mix only	⅟₁₀ pkg	5.0	230	20%
prepared	⅟₁₀ cake	16.0	320	45%
butterscotch				
mix only	⅟₁₂ pkg	4.0	180	20%
prepared	⅟₁₂ cake	11.0	250	40%
caramel deluxe				
mix only	⅟₁₂ pkg	4.0	180	20%
prepared	⅟₁₂ cake	11.0	250	40%
dark chocolate fudge				
mix only	⅟₁₂ pkg	4.0	180	20%
prepared	⅟₁₂ cake	15.0	290	47%
devil's food				
mix only	⅟₁₂ pkg	4.0	180	20%
prepared	⅟₁₂ cake	15.0	290	47%

Food and Description	Amount	Fat Grams	Total Calories	% Fat Calories
French vanilla				
mix only	1/12 pkg	4.0	180	20%
prepared	1/12 cake	11.0	250	40%
fudge marble				
mix only	1/12 pkg	4.0	180	20%
prepared	1/12 cake	11.0	250	40%
lemon supreme				
mix only	1/12 pkg	4.0	180	20%
prepared	1/12 cake	11.0	250	40%
orange supreme				
mix only	1/12 pkg	4.0	180	20%
prepared	1/12 cake	11.0	250	40%
pineapple supreme				
mix only	1/12 pkg	4.0	180	20%
prepared	1/12 cake	11.0	250	40%
spice				
mix only	1/12 pkg	4.0	180	20%
prepared	1/12 cake	11.0	250	40%
strawberry supreme				
mix only	1/12 pkg	4.0	180	20%
prepared	1/12 cake	11.0	250	40%
Swiss chocolate				
mix only	1/12 pkg	4.0	180	20%
prepared	1/12 cake	15.0	290	47%
white				
mix only	1/12 pkg	3.5	170	19%
prepared	1/12 cake	10.0	240	38%
wild cherry vanilla				
mix only	1/12 pkg	4.0	180	20%
prepared	1/12 cake	11.0	250	40%
yellow				
mix only	1/12 pkg	4.0	180	20%
prepared	1/12 cake	10.0	240	38%
(Estee) prepared				
chocolate	1/5 cake	4.0	190	19%
lemon	1/5 cake	4.0	200	18%
pound cake	1/5 cake	4.0	200	18%
white	1/5 cake	4.0	200	18%
(Jell-0) No-Bake/prepared				
cheesecake snack cups	13 oz	6.0	160	34%
double-layer desserts				
cookies & crean	1/6 dessert	19.0	390	44%
chocolate	1/8 dessert	12.0	260	42%
lemon	1 serving	12.0	260	42%
no-bake cheesecake				
cherry	1/8 pie	12.0	340	32%
homestyle	1/6 cake	15.0	360	38%
peanut butter cup	1/8 dessert	23.0	380	54%
real	1/6 cake	16.0	360	40%
strawberry	1/8 cake	12.0	340	32%

Food and Description	Amount	Fat Grams	Total Calories	% Fat Calories
strawberry swirl/reduced-fat (Pillsbury) Moist Supreme	⅛ cake	6.0	250	21%
angel food/prepared	¹⁄₁₂ cake	–	140	–
banana				
mix only	¹⁄₁₂ pkg	4.0	180	20%
prepared	¹⁄₁₂ cake	11.0	250	40%
butter recipe				
mix only	¹⁄₁₂ pkg	3.0	170	16%
prepared	¹⁄₁₂ cake	12.0	260	42%
butter recipe chocolate				
mix only	¹⁄₁₂ pkg	4.0	180	20%
prepared	¹⁄₁₂ cake	13.0	270	43%
chocolate				
mix only	¹⁄₁₂ pkg	5.0	180	25%
prepared	¹⁄₁₂ cake	12.0	250	43%
chocolate chip				
mix only	¹⁄₁₂ pkg	5.0	190	24%
prepared	¹⁄₁₂ cake	10.0	240	38%
dark chocolate				
mix only	¹⁄₁₂ pkg	4.0	180	20%
prepared	¹⁄₁₂ cake	11.0	250	40%
devil's food				
mix only	¹⁄₁₂ pkg	4.0	180	20%
prepared	¹⁄₁₂ cake	14.0	270	47%
Easter funfetti				
mix only	¹⁄₁₂ pkg	4.5	190	21%
prepared	¹⁄₁₂ cake	10.0	240	38%
French vanilla				
mix only	¹⁄₁₂ pkg	4.0	180	20%
prepared	¹⁄₁₂ cake	11.0	250	40%
Funfetti				
mix only	¹⁄₁₂ pkg	4.0	190	19%
prepared	¹⁄₁₂ cake	10.0	250	36%1
German chocolate				
mix only	¹⁄₁₂ pkg	4.0	180	20%
prepared	¹⁄₁₂ cake	11.0	250	40%
Halloween Funfetti				
mix only	¹⁄₁₂ pkg	4.5	190	21%
prepared	¹⁄₁₂ cake	10.0	240	38%
Holiday Funfetti				
mix only	¹⁄₁₂ pkg	4.5	190	21%
prepared	¹⁄₁₂ cake	10.0	240	38%
lemon				
mix only	¹⁄₁₂ cake	3.0	170	16%
prepared	¹⁄₁₀ cake	11.0	250	40%
strawberry				
mix only	¹⁄₁₂ pkg	4.0	180	20%
prepared	¹⁄₁₂ cake	11.0	250	40%
Valentine's Funfetti				
mix	¹⁄₁₂ cake	4.5	190	21%

Food and Description	Amount	Fat Grams	Total Calories	% Fat Calories
prepared	1/12 cake	10.0	240	38%
white				
mix only	1/12 pkg	4.0	180	20%
prepared	1/12 cake	9.0	230	35%
yellow				
mix only	1/12 pkg	4.0	180	20%
prepared	1/12 cake	10.0	240	38%
Streusel Coffee Cake				
chocolate chip				
mix only	1/16 cake	6.0	210	26%
prepared	1/16 cake	12.0	270	40%
cinnamon				
mix only	1/16 cake	5.0	190	24%
prepared	1/16 cake	11.0	260	38%
(Robin Hood) pouch				
devil's food				
mix only	1/5 pkg	5.0	190	50%
prepared	1/5 cake	17.0	310	49%
yellow				
mix only	1/5 pkg	4.0	190	19%
prepared	1/5 cake	13.0	280	42%
(Royal) No-Bake cheesecake				
lite/whipped	1/8 cake	3.0	130	21%
Real/original	1/8 cake	3.0	160	17%
(Vermont Country Maple) prepared				
chocolate	1 slice	2.0	290	6%
gingerbread	1 slice	1.0	270	3%
■ **READY TO SERVE**				
(Awrey's)				
Best Wishes/6" dia	1/4 cake	9.0	150	54%
Black Forest torte	1/14 cake	21.0	350	54%
carrot cake				
supreme/iced	1 slice	12.0	210	51%
3-layer/cream cheese icing	1/12 cake	23.0	390	53%
chocolate/2-layer w/white icing	1/12 cake	15.0	270	50%
coconut & yellow cake/3-layer	1/12 cake	21.0	350	54%
coconut butter cream cake	1 slice	9.0	160	51%
double chocolate cake				
iced	1 slice	6.0	130	42%
3-layer	1/12 cake	14.0	310	41%
2-layer	1/12 cake	11.0	250	40%
double chocolate torte	1/14 cake	15.0	340	40%
German chocolate cake				
iced	2" square	9.0	260	31%
3-layer	1/12 cake	18.0	350	46%
golden pound cake	1/14 loaf	5.0	130	35%
lemon & yellow cake/2-layer	1/12 cake	17.0	290	53%
lemon cake/3-layer	1/12 cake	19.0	320	53%
milk chocolate & yellow cake/2-layer	1/12 cake	17.0	290	53%
Neapolitan torte	1/14 cake	22.0	380	52%

Food and Description	Amount	Fat Grams	Total Calories	% Fat Calories
orange cake				
frosty w/icing	1 slice	8.0	150	
3-layer	1/12 cake	17.0	320	48%
pistachio torte	1/12 cake	22.0	370	54%
sponge cake	2" square	3.0	80	34%
strawberry supreme torte	1/14 cake	12.0	270	40%
walnut torte	1/14 cake	19.0	320	53%
(Entenmann's)				
fat-free				
apple topped	1/6 cake	–	180	–
banana crunch	1/8 cake	–	150	–
blackberry topped	1/6 cake	–	180	–
carrot cake	1/8 cake	–	170	–
chocolate chip	1/8 cake	–	130	–
French crumb	1/8 cake	–	140	–
fudge iced chocolate cake	1/6 cake	–	210	–
fudge iced gold cake	1/6 cake	–	220	
golden loaf	1/8 loaf	–	130	–
Louisiana crunch	1/8 cake	–	130	–
marble loaf	1/8 loaf	–	130	–
marshmallow iced devil's food	1/6 cake	–	200	–
pineapple				
cheese cake	1/5 cake	–	200	–
crunch	1/8 cake	–	140	–
topped	1/5 cake	–	170	–
raspberry-filled cheesecake	1/5 cake	–	200	–
original				
all butter French crumb	1 serving	8.0	180	40%
all butter pound loaf	1 serving	5.0	110	41%
almond topped coffee cake	1 serving	9.0	180	45%
banana crunch	1 serving	9.0	220	37%
carrot cake	1 serving	16.0	290	50%
cheese coffeecake	1 serving	8.0	190	39%
cheese filled crumb coffeecake	1 serving	10.0	210	43%
chocolate fudge	1 serving	7.0	150	42%
crumb coffeecake	1 serving	7.0	160	40%
fudge-iced devil's food	1 serving	5.0	130	35%
Louisiana crunch	1 serving	8.0	180	40%
marble loaf	1 serving	10.0	200	45%
sour cream loaf	1 serving	7.0	120	53%
thick fudge golden cake	1 serving	6.0	130	42%
reduced-fat				
butter loaf	1/8 loaf	4.0	140	26%
chocolate crumb cake	1/8 cake	2.5	140	16%
fudge gold	1/8 cake	6.0	270	20%
golden lemon delight	1/8 cake	7.0	210	30%
sour cream chip loaf	1/8 loaf	6.0	180	30%
(Formagg) Le Creme				
amaretto almond	2 oz	6.0	115	47%
pineapple	2 oz	6.0	115	47%

Food and Description	Amount	Fat Grams	Total Calories	% Fat Calories
plain	2 oz	6.0	115	47%
strawberry	2 oz	6.0	115	47%

CAKE, SNACK
■ HOMEMADE
USDA Standard Home Recipe (Note: Homemade cakes were made with vegetable shortening. Homemade frostings were made with margarine.)

Food and Description	Amount	Fat Grams	Total Calories	% Fat Calories
cupcake				
chocolate				
w/chocolate frosting	1 cupcake	8.0	175	41%
w/o frosting	1 cupcake	5.0	103	44%
white				
w/chocolate frosting	1 cupcake	8.0	186	39%
w/white frosting	1 cupcake	6.0	165	33%
w/o frosting	1 cupcake	5.0	114	35%
yellow				
w/chocolate frosting	1 cupcake	8.0	195	37%
w/o frosting	1 cupcake	5.0	125	36%

■ READY TO SERVE
(Dolly Madison)

Food and Description	Amount	Fat Grams	Total Calories	% Fat Calories
angel food ring	2 oz	1.5	160	8%
apple crumb cake				
2 per pkg	2 piece	10.0	330	27%
6 per pkg	1 piece	5.0	170	26%
barcakes				
angel food				
mini	1 piece	1.5	180	8%
regular	2 oz	1.5	160	8%
devil's food	2.8 oz	14.0	330	38%
spice	2.8 oz	17.0	350	44%
white	2.8 oz	14.0	320	39%
buttercrumb cake				
2 per pkg	2 pieces	11.0	340	29%
3 per pkg	1 piece	6.0	180	30%
6 per pkg	1 piece	6.0	170	32%
cake delights				
2 per pkg	2 pieces	12.0	280	39%
6 per pkg	1 piece	6.0	140	39%
carrot cake/individual	1 piece	8.0	360	20%
cinnamon swirl coffee	1 piece	6.0	170	32%
coconut layer cake	3 oz	9.0	300	27%
coffeecake	2 pieces	11.0	270	37%
creme boat				
2 per pkg	2 pieces	9.0	300	27%
3 per pkg	1 piece	13.0	430	27%
4 per pkg	2 pieces	10.0	320	28%
creme cakes				
3 per pkg	3 pieces	12.0	340	32%
4 per pkg	4 pieces	15.0	420	32%
7 per pkg	3 pieces	12.0	320	34%
10 per pkg	3 pieces	12.0	330	33%

Food and Description	Amount	Fat Grams	Total Calories	% Fat Calories
crumb cake/low-fat				
2 per pkg	2 pieces	3.0	280	9%
6 per pkg	1 piece	1.5	140	10%
cupcakes				
chocolate				
2 per pkg	2 pieces	10.0	.390	23%
3 per pkg	1 piece	5.0	190	24%
6 per pkg	1 piece	5.0	190	24%
8 per pkg	1 piece	5.0	190	24%
spice				
2 per pkg	2 pieces	20.0	470	38%
3 per pkg	1 piece	10.0	230	39%
6 per pkg	1 piece	10.0	230	39%
dessert roll				
lemon	1 piece	2.5	260	8%
plain	1 piece	2.0	230	8%
Flips				
banana flip	1 piece	15.0	410	33%
devil's food flip	1 piece	14.0	380	33%
sweet potato flip	1 piece	15.0	310	44%
German chocolate cake				
6 per pkg	1 piece	9.0	220	37%
2 per pkg	2 pieces	19.0	450	38%
Goggles	2 pieces	10.0	420	21%
Koo Koo's	2 pieces	17.0	400	38%
pound cake				
mini	1 piece	13.0	370	32%
½ ring	3 oz	13.0	360	33%
whole ring	2.5 oz	11.0	310	32%
shortcake	1 piece	2.0	110	16%
squares				
raspberry				
2 per pkg	2 pieces	15.0	370	36%
3 per pkg	3 pieces	22.0	560	35%
6 per pkg	1 piece	7.0	190	33%
snack				
2 per pkg	2 pieces	19.0	400	43%
3 per pkg	3 pieces	29.0	610	43%
6 per pkg	1 piece	10.0	210	43%
Zingers				
chocolate				
4 per pkg	4 pieces	14.0	470	27%
7 per pkg	2 pieces	8.0	280	26%
12 per pkg	2 pieces	8.0	260	26%
raspberry				
3 per pkg	3 pieces	17.0	440	35%
4 per pkg	2 pieces	11.0	300	33%
7 per pkg	2 pieces	11.0	290	34%
12 per pkg	2 pieces	11.0	300	33%

Food and Description	Amount	Fat Grams	Total Calories	% Fat Calories
yellow				
3 per pkg	3 pieces	12.0	400	27%
4 per pkg	4 pieces	15.0	530	25%
(Drake)				
Boston creme	1 piece	8.0	170	42%
coffee cakes				
low-fat	1 piece	1.5	100	14%
original	1 piece	6.0	130	42%
Devil Dogs				
original	1 piece	7.0	170	37%
reduced-fat	1 piece	4.0	160	23%
Funny Bones	2 pieces	12.0	300	36%
Ring Dings	2 pieces	14.0	320	39%
Sunny Doodles	2 pieces	8.0	220	33%
Yankee Doodles	2 pieces	9.0	220	37%
Yodels	2 pieces	16.0	280	51%
generic				
devil's food cupcake w/creme filling	1 cake	4.0	105	34%
(Hostess)				
angel food cake	⅛ cake	1.5	160	8%
apple spice lights	1 cake	1.0	130	7%
Brownie Bites				
plain	5 pieces	14.0	260	48%
walnut	5 pieces	15.0	270	50%
Brownie/light	1 brownie	2.5	140	16%
Chocodiles	1 cake	11.0	240	41%
Chocolicious	1 cake	7.0	190	33%
crumb coffeecake				
light	1 cake	0.5	90	5%
regular	1 cake	5.0	130	35%
cupcakes				
chocolate				
light	1 cupcake	1.5	140	10%
regular	1 cupcake	6.0	180	30%
golden	1 cupcake	7.0	200	32%
orange	1 cupcake	5.0	160	28%
Ding Dongs	2 cakes	19.0	360	48%
Ho Ho's	2 cakes	12.0	250	43%
King Dons	2 cakes	19.0	360	48%
Leopards	1 cake	8.0	210	34%
Shortcake Dessert Cups	1 cake	2.0	100	18%
Snoballs	1 cake	5.0	180	25%
Suzy Q's	1 cake	9.0	230	35%
Twinkies				
lights	1 cake	1.5	130	10%
original	1 cakes	5.0	150	30%
(Lance) fig				
fat-free	½ piece	–	100	–
original	½ piece	2.0	110	16%

Food and Description	Amount	Fat Grams	Total Calories	% Fat Calories
(Little Debbie)				
angel cake/low-fat				
lemon	1 pkg	0.5	130	3%
low-fat	1 pkg	1.0	120	8%
raspberry	1 pkg	0.5	130	3%
apple coffee streusel cake	1 pkg	7.0	230	27%
banana twins	1 pkg	10.0	250	36%
Be My Valentine cake				
chocolate				
boxed	1 pkg	13.0	180	65%
individual pkg	1 pkg	18.0	360	45%
vanilla/boxed	1 pkg	14.0	290	43%
cherry cordial	1 pkg	8.0	170	42%
chocolate chip cake	1 pkg	15.0	310	44%
chocolate chip cupcake	1 pkg	9.0	180	45%
Christmas tree cake	1 pkg	10.0	190	47%
coconut rounds	1 pkg	7.0	150	42%
devil creme cake				
boxed	1 pkg	8.0	190	38%
individual pkg	1 pkg	16.0	370	39%
devil squares	1 pkg	13.0	270	43%
Easter basket cakes				
chocolate	1 pkg	14.0	290	43%
vanilla	1 pkg	15.0	310	44%
fancy cakes	1 pkg	15.0	300	45%
Fig Bars/low-fat	1 pkg	3.5	150	21%
frosted fudge cake				
boxed	1 pkg	10.0	200	45%
individual pkg	1 pkg	12.0	260	42%
fudge rounds	1 pkg	6.0	140	39%
golden creme cake				
boxed	1 pkg	5.0	150	30%
individual pkg	1 pkg	12.0	280	39%
holiday cake roll				
cherry creme	1 pkg	12.0	270	40%
chocolate	1 pkg	14.0	300	42%
vanilla	1 pkg	15.0	320	42%
Jelly Creme	1 pkg	7.0	150	42%
marshmallow supreme	1 pkg	5.0	130	35%
Nutty Bar	1 pkg	18.0	310	52%
oatmeal creme pie	1 pkg	7.0	170	48%
oatmeal lights/low-fat	1 pkg	2.5	130	17%
PB&J oatmeal	1 pkg	5.0	130	35%
peanut butter bar	1 pkg	15.0	270	50%
peanut cluster	1 pkg	11.0	190	52%
raisin creme pie	1 pkg	5.0	140	32%
snack cake/chocolate	1 pkg	15.0	310	44%
Star Crunch	1 pkg	6.0	140	39%
strawberry shortcake roll				
boxed	1 pkg	8.0	230	31%

Food and Description	Amount	Fat Grams	Total Calories	% Fat Calories
individual pkg	1 pkg	13.0	340	34%
Swiss cake roll				
boxed	1 pkg	12.0	270	40%
2.7-oz pkg	1 pkg	15.0	330	41%
Zebra Cake				
boxed	1 pkg	19.0	370	46%
individual pkg	1 pkg	16.0	330	44%
(TastyKake)				
Creamies				
banana	1 cake	7.0	170	37%
bunny trail treats	1 cake	6.0	150	36%
chocolate	1 cake	8.0	180	40%
cupid	1 cake	6.0	150	34%
Kringle Kake	1 cake	6.0	150	34%
Sparkle Kake	1 cake	6.0	150	34%
vanilla	1 cake	9.0	190	43%
witchy treats	1 cake	6.0	150	36%
cupcakes				
butter cream iced/creme filled	2 cakes	8.0	240	30%
chocolate				
iced/creme-filled	2 cakes	8.0	230	31%
low-fat creme-filled	2 cakes	3.0	200	14%
plain	2 cakes	6.0	200	27%
	3 cakes	9.0	330	26%
Koffee Kake				
apple-filled	2 cakes	2.0	170	11%
creme filled				
plain	2 cakes	10.0	240	38%
raspberry/low-fat	2 cakes	2.0	170	11%
lemon-filled	2 cakes	3.0	180	15%
Kreepy Kakes	2 cakes	8.0	240	30%
Santa snacks	2 cakes	8.0	240	30%
Tasty Tweets	2 cakes	8.0	240	30%
Tropical Delights				
coconut	2 cakes	9.0	190	43%
guava	2 cakes	7.0	190	33%
papaya	2 cakes	7.0	200	32%
pineapple	2 cakes	7.0	200	32%
Juniors				
chocolate	1 cake	12.0	330	33%
coconut	1 cake	8.0	310	23%
Koffee Kake	1 cake	9.0	270	30%
Pound Kake	1 cake	13.0	320	37%
Kandy Kakes				
chocolate	3 cakes	13.0	250	47%
coconut	2 cakes	18.0	330	49%
peanut butter	2 cakes	9.0	180	45%
	3 cakes	14.0	280	45%
Krimpets				
butterscotch iced	2 cakes	5.0	210	21%

Food and Description	Amount	Fat Grams	Total Calories	% Fat Calories
	3 cakes	8.0	310	23%
jelly filled	2 cakes	3.0	190	14%
	3 cakes	4.0	280	13%
Kreme Krimpies	2 cakes	9.0	230	35%
	3 cakes	13.0	340	34%
strawberry iced	2 cakes	5.0	210	21%
	3 cakes	8.0	310	23%
Tasty Too				
jelly-filled	2 cakes	1.5	180	8%
lemon-filled	2 cakes	2.0	180	10%
	4 cakes	15.0	350	39%

CAKE FROSTING/ICING (*See also* CAKE/COOKIE DECORATION)
(Betty Crocker)
Mix
  creamy frosting
    coconut pecan

Food and Description	Amount	Fat Grams	Total Calories	% Fat Calories
mix only	3 Tbs	4.0	120	30%
prepared	2 Tbs	8.0	160	45%

    fluffy frosting/white

Food and Description	Amount	Fat Grams	Total Calories	% Fat Calories
mix only	3 Tbs	–	100	–
prepared	6 Tbs	–	100	–

Ready-to-spread
  creamy deluxe

Food and Description	Amount	Fat Grams	Total Calories	% Fat Calories
butter cream	2 Tbs	5.0	140	32%
cherry	2 Tbs	5.0	140	32%
chocolate	2 Tbs	5.0	130	35%
coconut pecan	2 Tbs	8.0	140	51%
cream cheese	2 Tbs	5.0	140	32%
dark chocolate	2 Tbs	5.0	130	35%
French vanilla	2 Tbs	5.0	140	32%
lemon	2 Tbs	5.0	140	32%
milk chocolate	2 Tbs	5.0	130	35%
rainbow chip	2 Tbs	5.0	140	32%
sour cream chocolate	2 Tbs	5.0	130	35%
sour cream white	2 Tbs	5.0	140	32%
strawberry cream cheese	2 Tbs	5.0	140	32%
vanilla	2 Tbs	5.0	140	32%
white chocolate	2 Tbs	5.0	140	32%

Ready-to-spread Party Frostings

Food and Description	Amount	Fat Grams	Total Calories	% Fat Calories
chocolate w/stars	2 Tbs	5.0	140	32%
vanilla w/stars	2 Tbs	5.0	140	32%
vanilla w/Hershey's Toppers	2 Tbs	5.0	140	32%

Ready-to-Spread Sweet Rewards

Food and Description	Amount	Fat Grams	Total Calories	% Fat Calories
chocolate	2 Tbs	2.0	120	15%
milk chocolate	2 Tbs	2.0	120	15%
vanilla	2 Tbs	2.0	130	14%

Ready-to-spread Whipped Deluxe

Food and Description	Amount	Fat Grams	Total Calories	% Fat Calories
chocolate	2 Tbs	5.0	100	45%
cream cheese	2 Tbs	4.5	100	41%
fluffy white	2 Tbs	4.5	100	41%
lemon	2 Tbs	5.0	100	45%

Food and Description	Amount	Fat Grams	Total Calories	% Fat Calories
milk chocolate	2 Tbs	4.5	100	41%
strawberry	2 Tbs	5.0	100	45%
vanilla	2 Tbs	4.5	100	41%
(Duncan Hines) Creamy Homestyle/ready to spread				
butter cream	2 Tbs	5.0	140	32%
caramel	2 Tbs	5.0	140	32%
cream cheese	2 Tbs	5.0	140	32%
chocolate	2 Tbs	5.0	130	35%
chocolate mocha	2 Tbs	5.0	130	35%
dark chocolate	2 Tbs	5.0	130	35%
milk chocolate	2 Tbs	5.0	130	35%
strawberries & cream	2 Tbs	5.0	140	32%
vanilla	2 Tbs	5.0	140	32%
wild cherry vanilla	2 Tbs	5.0	140	32%
(Estee) mix/all flavors/mix only	⅕ pkg	–	80	–
homemade/USDA Standard Home Recipe				
boiled	¼ cup	–	74	–
caramel	¼ cup	6.0	306	18%
chocolate	¼ cup	9.5	259	33%
coconut	¼ cup	5.0	300	15%
white	¼ cup	5.0	300	15%
(Jiffy) mix/prepared				
fudge	¼ cup	4.0	150	24%
white	¼ cup	4.0	150	24%
(Pillsbury) ready to spread				
Creamy Supreme				
Banana creme	2 Tbs	6.0	150	48%
chocolate	2 Tbs	6.0	140	39%
chocolate fudge	2 Tbs	6.0	140	39%
chocolate mocha	2 Tbs	6.0	140	39%
coconut pecan	2 Tbs	10.0	160	56%
cookies & creme	2 Tbs	6.0	150	36%
cream cheese	2 Tbs	6.0	150	36%
French vanilla	2 Tbs	6.0	160	34%
Funfetti				
Easter	2 Tbs	6.0	150	36%
Halloween	2 Tbs	6.0	150	36%
Holiday	2 Tbs	6.0	150	36%
pink vanilla	2 Tbs	6.0	150	36%
Valentines	2 Tbs	6.0	150	36%
vanilla	2 Tbs	6.0	150	34%
hot fudge	2 Tbs	6.0	140	39%
lemon creme	2 Tbs	6.0	150	36%
milk chocolate	2 Tbs	6.0	140	39%
milk chocolate swirl w/fudge glaze	2 Tbs	6.0	140	39%
strawberry creme	2 Tbs	6.0	150	36%
vanilla swirl	2 Tbs	6.0	150	36%
(Robin Hood) mix				
chocolate				
mix only	2 Tbs	1.5	110	12%
prepared	2 Tbs	5.0	140	32%

Food and Description	Amount	Fat Grams	Total Calories	% Fat Calories
(Vermont Country Maple) mix/prepared				
delectable cocoa	1 Tbs	–	50	–
maple butter cream	1 Tbs	–	40	–
CAKE/COOKIE DECORATION (*See also* CAKE FROSTING/ICING)				
(Dec-A-Cake)				
all sugar crystals	1 tsp	–	15	–
bats/pumpkins	1 tsp	–	20	–
candy cards	4 gm	–	15	–
choco mint trims	1 tsp	0.5	15	30%
choco trims	1 tsp	0.5	15	30%
confetti	1 tsp	–	15	–
dec-a-cone	1 tsp	0.5	15	30%
decorating icing				
chocolate	1 tsp	0.5	20	23%
all other colors	1 tsp	0.5	25	18%
fruit cocktail	9 pieces	–	15	–
fun sprinkles	1 tsp	0.5	15	30%
harvest mix	1 tsp	0.5	15	30%
holiday sprinkles	1 tsp	0.5	15	30%
nonpareils	1 tsp	–	15	–
party imperials	9 pieces	–	15	–
pastel trims	1 tsp	0.5	15	30%
rainbow mix	1 tsp	0.5	15	30%
red/green trim	1 tsp	0.5	15	30%
red/white trim	1 tsp	0.5	15	30%
red/white/pink hearts	1 tsp	–	20	–
variety pack	1 tsp	0.5	15	30%
(McCormick/Schilling)				
decorating gel/all colors	1 tsp	–	25	–
decorating icing/all colors	1 tsp	1.0	35	26%
decors				
chocolate-flavored	1 tsp	1.0	20	45%
cinnamon	1 tsp	–	25	–
fruit flavored	1 tsp	–	25	–
nonpareil	1 tsp	–	15	–
snowflake	1 tsp	–	15	–
sugar crystals/all colors	1 tsp	–	–	–
CALAMARI (*See* SQUID)				
CALIFORNIA RED BEAN /boiled	½ cup	–	109	–
CALZONE (*See* PIZZA)				
CANADIAN BACON (*See* BACON, CANADIAN STYLE)				
CANDY				
■ **ABRA CA BUBBLE** (*See* (Brach's) in this section)				
■ **(Allen Wertz)**				
Coffee Time				
assorted	1 piece	1.0	30	30%
decaffeinated	1 piece	1.0	20	45%
■ **ALMOND JOY** (*See* (Hershey) in this section)				
■ **ALMOND ROCA** (*See* (Brown & Haley) in this section)				

Food and Description	Amount	Fat Grams	Total Calories	% Fat Calories
■ **ALPINE WHITE** (*See* (Nestlé) in this section)				
■ **(Andes)**				
cherry jubilee thins	8 pieces	13.0	210	56%
creme de menthe wafers	8 pieces	13.0	210	56%
nut & honey thins	8 pieces	13.0	210	56%
orange mint thins	8 pieces	13.0	200	59%
parfait mints	8 pieces	13.0	210	56%
toasted coconut	8 pieces	13.0	210	56%
toffee crunch thins	8 pieces	12.0	210	51%
■ **(Andre Prost)**				
Honees Bars				
Eu-Mint	1 piece	–	20	–
Milk-N-Honees	1 piece	–	20	–
original	1 piece	–	20	–
Swedish peppermint creams	14 pieces	3.0	70	16%
Zotz				
Lotz-A-Zotz	1 piece	–	40	–
Mega Zotz	1 piece	–	15	–
pops	1 pop	–	40	–
strings	1 piece	–	15	–
■ **Ann's House of Nuts)**				
chocolate covered raisins	3 Tbs	8.0	200	36%
double dip chocolate covered peanuts	5 pieces	15.0	230	59%
jelly beans	32 pieces	–	150	–
sour gummies	16 pieces	–	140	–
yougurt-covered				
peanuts	3 Tbs	16.0	220	65%
pretzels	⅔ cup	10.0	170	53%
raisins	3 Tbs	5.0	150	30%
■ **A-OK** (*See* (Nature's Warehouse) in this section)				
■ **BABY RUTH** (*See* (Nestlé) in this section)				
■ **(Beich)**				
Laffy Taffy chews				
apple	1 oz	1.0	110	8%
banana	1 oz	1.0	110	8%
grape	1 oz	1.0	110	8%
passion punch	1 oz	1.0	110	8%
strawberry	1 oz	1.0	110	8%
sweet & sour cherry	1 oz	1.0	110	8%
watermelon	1 oz	1.0	110	8%
■ **BIT-O-HONEY** (*See* (Concorde) in this section)				
■ **BLACK COW** (*See* (Clark) in this section)				
■ **BOUNTY** (*See* (M&M * Mars) in this section)				
■ **(Brach's)**				
A&W root beer barrells	3 pieces	–	70	–
Abra Ca Bubble	1 piece	–	45	–
bells/solid chocolate/foiled	1 oz	8.0	150	48%
bridge mix	14 pieces	8.0	180	40%
butterscotch disks	3 pieces	–	70	–
California chocolate-covered raisins	34 pieces	7.0	170	37%

Food and Description	Amount	Fat Grams	Total Calories	% Fat Calories
candy corn				
chickens	6 pieces	–	160	–
corn	26 pieces	–	140	–
rabbits	6 pieces	–	160	–
Sue Bee honey	26 pieces	–	140	–
Chelsea Chips/chocolate-covered	1 oz	6.0	140	39%
cherries				
chocolate creme	1 oz	2.0	110	16%
chocolate-covered	1 oz	2.0	110	16%
dark chocolate covered	2 pieces	3.0	140	19%
milk chocolate covered	2 pieces	3.0	140	19%
cherry disks	3 pieces	–	70	–
Christmas ornaments	1 oz	8.0	150	48%
cinnamon candy				
disks	3 pieces	–	70	–
imperials	52 pieces	–	60	–
coffee candy	3 pieces	1.5	80	8%
cookie bits/chocolate covered	38 pieces	10.0	200	45%
Cookie Delites	40 pieces	10.0	210	43%
Crazy Pumpkin Heads	1 oz	1.0	100	9%
cream drops/dark chocolate	3 pieces	3.0	160	17%
Dem Bones	19 pieces	–	60	–
Double Dippers	15 pieces	14.0	220	57%
Easter eggs				
buttercream/chocolate-covered	1 oz	3.0	120	23%
cherry cream/chocolate-covered	1 oz	2.0	110	16%
coconut cream/chocolate-covered	1 oz	3.0	110	25%
fruit & nut cream/chocolate-covered	1 oz	2.0	110	16%
malted milk				
chocolate	5 pieces	5.0	180	25%
fiesta	5 pieces	5.0	180	25%
maple cream/chocolate-covered	1 oz	2.0	110	16%
marshmallow	1 oz	3.0	120	23%
pastel fiesta	1 oz	3.0	120	23%
PBM	1 oz	10.0	160	56%
solid chocolate	1 oz	8.0	150	48%
solid milk chocolate	8 pieces	11.0	200	50%
Fruit Bunch	3 pieces	–	150	–
Fruit Chews	5 pieces	3.0	160	17%
Fruit slices	3 pieces	–	150	–
fruity hard candies	3 pieces	–	70	–
Gumdinger gum balls	1 oz	2.0	110	16%
Gummi Bears				
regular	18 pieces	–	130	–
wild 'n fruity	15 pieces	–	130	–
Gummi Squirms				
regular	5 pieces	–	120	–
sugar-free	16 pieces	–	100	–
wild'n fruity	5 pieces	–	120	–
heart box candies	1 oz	2.0	110	16%

Food and Description	Amount	Fat Grams	Total Calories	% Fat Calories
hearts				
PBM	1 oz	9.0	150	54%
Valentine	1 oz	2.0	110	16%
Hi-C Gummy Fruits	13 pieces	–	120	–
Hulachews/dark chocolate covered	1 oz	8.0	140	51%
jelly beans	24 pieces	–	150	–
jelly bird eggs	14 pieces	–	150	–
Jots				
chocolate	1 oz	5.0	130	35%
Christmas	1 oz	5.0	130	35%
Milk chocolate	38 pieces	7.0	190	33%
mint	1 oz	2.0	120	15%
peanut	17 pieces	9.0	190	43%
Jube Jets	1 oz	–	100	–
Kisses				
peanut butter	4 pieces	6.0	170	32%
peppermint	4 pieces	2.0	150	12%
Valentine nougat	1 oz	2.0	110	16%
lemon drops	3 pieces	–	60	–
licorice				
red laces	1 oz	–	100	–
red twists	5 pieces	–	150	–
twists	1 oz	1.0	100	9%
Lip Smackers	6 pieces	–	140	–
Lollydrops	3 pieces	–	70	–
malt balls				
malted milk	15 pieces	9.0	190	43%
milk chocolate covered	15 pieces	9.0	190	43%
maple nut goodies	7 pieces	9.0	190	43%
Milk Maid caramels				
chocolate covered	4 pieces	4.0	150	24%
original	4 pieces	4.0	160	23%
Royals	5 pieces	3.5	130	24%
vanilla	5 pieces	6.0	190	28%
mint-filled straws	1 oz	1.0	110	8%
mints				
chocolate mint cremes	3 pieces	3.0	190	14%
creme de menthe	1 oz	9.0	150	54%
cremes/chocolate-covered	1 oz	2.0	110	16%
dessert	37 pieces	–	160	–
holiday	1 oz	1.0	110	8%
Kentucky	17 pieces	0.5	150	3%
patties/chocolate-covered	3 pieces	2.0	130	14%
pearls				
Christmas	1 oz	1.0	110	8%
regular	1 oz	2.0	120	15%
starlight				
regular	3 pieces	–	60	–
spearmint	3 pieces	–	60	–
thin/chocolate-covered	1 oz	2.0	110	16%

Food and Description	Amount	Fat Grams	Total Calories	% Fat Calories
Mr. Pretzel/yogurt-covered	9 pieces	8.0	190	38%
Neapolitan coconuts	3 pieces	5.0	160	28%
nonpareils/dark chocolate				
Christmas	1 oz	6.0	140	39%
regular	1 oz	6.0	140	39%
sprinkles	17 pieces	9.0	200	41%
nougat				
Christmas	1 oz	2.0	110	16%
jelly	4 pieces	2.0	170	11%
nut goodies/chocolate	8 pieces	10.0	190	47%
orange slices	3 pieces	–	150	–
orange sticks/chocolate-covered	1 oz	2.0	110	16%
Orangettes	2 pieces	–	130	–
parfait				
mint	1 oz	9.0	150	54%
peanut	1 oz	10.0	160	56%
party mix/Chocolate Selections	29 pieces	9.0	190	43%
PBM squares	1 oz	9.0	150	54%
peanut clusters				
milk chocolate covered	3 pieces	14.0	220	57%
peanut-caramel	3 pieces	13.0	220	53%
regular	3 pieces	15.0	230	59%
peanuts				
chocolate-covered	1 oz	10.0	160	56%
circus	11 pieces	–	260	–
Double Dippers	15 pieces	14.0	220	57%
filled	1 oz	1.0	110	8%
French burnt	28 pieces	9.0	190	43%
milk chocolate covered	1 oz	9.0	150	54%
panned	1 oz	7.0	140	45%
petite	1 oz	9.0	150	54%
Putters/milk chocolate covered	1 oz	9.0	150	54%
rabbits				
chocolate-covered	4 pieces	7.0	200	32%
marshmallow	1 oz	3.0	120	23%
Rainbow Bears	4 pieces	–	150	–
Raisins/California yogurt covered	28 pieces	7.0	180	35%
Rich & Dreamy chocolate cremes	3 pieces	3.5	190	17%
robin's eggs/solid milk chocolate	6 pieces	8.0	200	36%
Rocks	7 pieces	–	150	–
Royals	5 pieces	4.0	150	24%
salt water taffy	4 pieces	2.0	140	13%
Santas				
assortment	1 oz	2.0	110	16%
foiled/tray of 8	1 oz	7.0	140	45%
marshmallow	1 oz	3.0	120	23%
PBM	1 oz	10.0	160	56%
Snappy Tarts	6 pieces	–	150	–
Sour Balls	3 pieces	–	70	–
Sour Crackers	10 pieces	–	130	–

Food and Description	Amount	Fat Grams	Total Calories	% Fat Calories
Sour Sea Creatures	16 pieces	–	140	–
spearmint leaves	5 pieces	–	140	–
Special Treasures International				
amaretto	3 pieces	2.0	80	23%
French vanilla	3 pieces	2.0	80	23%
golden butter toffee	3 pieces	2.0	80	23%
Suisse mocha	3 pieces	2.0	80	23%
spice drops	12 pieces	–	130	–
Spicettes	12 pieces	–	130	–
Star Brites				
fruit candies	3 pieces	–	45	–
peppermint	3 pieces	–	60	–
stars				
Christmas	10 pieces	11.0	200	50%
chocolate	10 pieces	11.0	200	50%
milk chocolate	1 oz	8.0	150	48%
Sundaes Neapolitan/coconut	3 pieces	5.0	160	28%
Super Premium International	3 pieces	2.0	80	23%
Targets	4 pieces	4.0	160	23%
Ting-A-Ling	1 oz	8.0	150	48%
Trail Mix				
Big River	¼ cup	6.0	120	45%
Nut Berry	¼ cup	8.0	130	55%
Twisters/cherry	1 oz pkg	1.0	100	9%
vanilla cream/chocolate-covered	1 oz	2.0	110	16%
wild 'n fruity	5 pieces	–	120	–
■ (Breath Savers)				
breath mints/sugar-free				
cinnamon	1 piece	–	10	–
iced mint	1 piece	–	10	–
peppermint	1 piece	–	10	–
spearmint	1 piece	–	10	–
vanilla mint	1 piece	–	10	–
wintergreen	1 piece	–	10	–
■ (Brown & Haley)				
Almond Roca	3 pieces	15.0	210	64%
■ BUNCHA CRUNCH (See (Nestlé in this section)				
■ BUTTERFINGER (See (Nestlé) in this section)				
■ (Cadbury)				
Caramello/5-oz bar	5 blocks	9.0	190	43%
chocolate creme egg	1 egg	6.0	180	30%
dairy milk chocolate bar/5 oz	9 blocks	12.0	220	49%
fruit & nut bar/5 oz	9 blocks	11.0	210	47%
roasted almond bar/5 oz	9 blocks	13.0	220	53%
■ (Cambridge)				
Charleston Chew/all flavors	1.875 oz	7.0	230	27%
Junior Mints	1.6 oz	4.0	190	19%
Pom Poms	1.58 oz	6.0	200	27%
Sugar Babies	1.7 oz	2.0	190	9%
Sugar Daddy	1.7 oz	3.0	200	14%

Food and Description	Amount	Fat Grams	Total Calories	% Fat Calories
■ **CARAMELLO** (*See* (Cadbury) in this section)				
■ **(Cellas)**				
chocolate-covered cherries				
dark chocolate	2 pieces	4.0	110	33%
milk chocolate	2 pieces	4.0	110	33%
■ **(Certs)**				
breath mints/sugar-free				
assorted	1 piece	–	5	–
extra flavor peppermint	1 piece	–	5	–
peppermint	1 piece	–	5	–
spearmint	1 piece	–	5	–
wintergreen	1 piece	–	5	–
■ **CHARLESTON CHEW** (*See* (Cambridge) in this section)				
■ **(Charms)**				
blow pop	1 pop	–	80	–
flat pop	1 pop	–	70	–
■ **CHUCKLES** (*See* (Hershey) in this section)				
■ **CHUNKY** (*See* (Nestlé) in this section)				
■ **(Chupa Chups)**				
ice-cream-flavored lollipops				
choco vanilla	1 piece	–	50	–
strawberry vanilla	1 piece	–	50	–
vanilla	1 piece	–	50	–
■ **(Clark)**				
Black Cow/sucker	1 oz	3.0	127	21%
Clark bar	1.76 oz	10.0	240	38%
Slo Poke	1 sucker	2.0	124	15%
■ **COFFEE TIME** (*See* (Allen Wertz) in this section)				
■ **(Concorde)**				
Bit-O-Honey				
bar	1 bar	4.0	200	18%
pieces				
jar	1 piece	0.6	32	17%
	5 pieces	3.0	160	17%
twist-wrap	1 piece	0.5	28	16%
	6 pieces	3.0	170	16%
Laffy Taffy	1 piece	0.5	38	12%
	4 pieces	2.0	150	12%
Shock Tarts	1 piece	–	8	–
	8 pieces	0.5	60	8%
Taffy Tarts	1 piece	–	2	–
	27 pieces	0.5	60	8%
■ **CRUNCH BAR** (*See* (Nestlé) in this section)				
■ **(Demet's)**				
turtles	1 piece	4.5	80	51%
■ **DOVE** (*See* (M&M * Mars) in this section)				
■ **(Estee)**				
candy-coated peanuts	¼ cup	9.0	200	41%
caramel/chocolate & vanilla	5 pieces	5.0	115	39%

Food and Description	Amount	Fat Grams	Total Calories	% Fat Calories
chocolate bar				
dark chocolate	7 squares	14.0	200	63%
milk chocolate				
crisp rice	1 bar	26.0	370	63%
plain	7 squares	17.0	230	67%
w/almonds	7 squares	17.0	230	67%
w/fruit & nuts	7 squares	16.0	220	65%
mint	7 squares	14.0	200	63%
chocolate-covered raisins	¼ cup	6.0	180	60%
fruit & nut mix	¼ cup	12.0	210	51%
peanut brittle	⅓ box	9.0	160	51%
peanut butter cups	5 candies	12.0	200	54%
sugar-free				
gourmet jelly beans	26 pieces	–	70	–
gumdrops				
fruit	23 pieces	–	80	–
licorice	11 pieces	–	90	–
gummy				
apple rings	5 pieces	–	70	–
assorted fruit	17 pieces	–	100	–
bears/assorted	17 pieces	–	100	–
hard candy				
butterscotch	2 pieces	–	25	–
fruit/assorted	5 pieces	–	30	–
tropical/assorted	5 pieces	–	30	–
peppermint swirl	3 pieces	–	30	–
toffee candies	5 pieces	–	30	–
sour citrus slices	9 pieces	–	60	–
■ (Farley)				
bridge mix/chocolate	18 pieces	8.0	180	40%
butter toffee	3 pieces	1.0	70	13%
butterscotch discs	3 pieces	–	70	–
candy corn	24 pieces	–	150	–
candy roll	1 roll	–	25	–
chocolate-covered raisins	37 pieces	8.0	180	40%
cinnamon discs	3 pieces	–	70	–
Clearly Fruit hard candies	3 pieces	–	70	–
fruit slices	3 pieces	–	150	–
fruit snacks				
cherry	15 pieces	–	90	–
strawberry	13 pieces	–	90	–
giant jellies	3 pieces	–	120	–
gummy bears	17 pieces	–	130	–
gummy dinos	7 pieces	–	120	–
jelly beans				
itsy bitsy	32 pieces	–	140	–
regular	17 pieces	–	150	–
Kid Pops	1 pop	–	45	–
Kiddie Mix	0.67 oz	–	70	–
orange slices	3 pieces	–	150	–

Food and Description	Amount	Fat Grams	Total Calories	% Fat Calories
party mix	3 pieces	–	60	–
peanut clusters/chocolate	3 pieces	16.0	230	63%
peanuts				
chocolate-dipped	17 pieces	13.0	220	53%
circus	5 pieces	–	160	–
French burnt	25 pieces	5.0	180	25%
spice drops	10 pieces	–	140	–
starlight mints	3 pieces	–	60	–
■ (Featherweight)				
Sweet Pretenders				
chewy caramels	5 pieces	5.0	115	39%
hard candy				
berry patch	5 pieces	–	30	–
butterscotch	2 pieces	–	30	–
orchard blend	5 pieces	–	30	–
peppermint swirls	3 pieces	–	30	–
milk chocolate				
w/almonds	7 squares	17.0	230	67%
w/crisp rice	1 bar	26.0	370	63%
■ 5TH AVENUE (See (Hershey) in this section)				
■ GENERIC				
almonds/chocolate-covered	1 oz	12.0	161	67%
butternut	2 oz	13.0	270	43%
butterscotch	1 oz	1.0	113	8%
candy corn	¼ cup	1.0	180	5%
cherries/chocolate-covered	1 piece	3.0	90	30%
chocolate bar				
dark sweet chocolate	1 oz	10.0	150	60%
milk chocolate				
plain	1 oz	9.0	145	50%
w/almonds	1 oz	10.0	150	60%
w/peanuts	1 oz	11.0	155	64%
chocolate discs/sugar-coated	1 oz	5.6	132	38%
chocolate mint patty	1 piece	1.0	50	18%
fudge				
caramel & peanuts	1 oz	5.0	123	37%
chocolate	1 oz	4.5	122	33%
chocolate w/nuts	1 oz	5.9	128	42%
vanilla	1 oz	3.0	113	24%
vanilla w/nuts	1 oz	5.0	120	38%
gumdrops/all flavors	1 oz	–	100	–
hard candy	1 oz	–	110	–
jaw breaker	1 piece	–	20	–
jelly beans/all flavors	1 oz	–	100	–
	1 cup	1.0	807	1%
licorice/black	1 oz	<1.0	100	5%
malt balls/milk chocolate covered	2 pieces	4.0	50	72%
nonpareils/mint	1 oz	9.0	150	54%
peanuts/yogurt-covered	1 oz	9.0	125	65%
penuche	1 oz	4.0	120	30%

Food and Description	Amount	Fat Grams	Total Calories	% Fat Calories
pralines	1 oz	3.0	90	30%
stars/milk chocolate	1 oz	8.0	160	45%
taffy	1 oz	1.0	100	9%
vanilla cream	1 oz	4.8	123	35%
■ **(Ghirardelli)** chocolate bars				
Baby Premier/1.25 oz				
cookies & cream	1 bar	11.0	190	52%
dark chocolate				
plain	1 bar	12.0	180	60%
w/almonds	1 bar	12.0	180	60%
w/raspberries	1 bar	12.0	180	60%
double chocolate mocha	1 bar	10.0	180	50%
milk chocolate				
plain	1 bar	11.0	190	52%
w/almonds	1 bar	12.0	190	57%
w/crisp	1 bar	10.0	180	50%
w/macadamia	1 bar	13.0	190	62%
mint	1 bar	12.0	180	60%
Premier/2.5 oz				
cookies & cream	1 bar	21.0	380	50%
milk				
w/macadamias	1 bar	26.0	380	62%
Premier/3 oz				
double chocolate mocha	1 bar	19.0	350	49%
	4 sections	12.0	210	51%
cookies & cream	1 bar	21.0	370	51%
dark chocolate				
plain	6 sections	14.0	210	60%
w/almonds	6 sections	16.0	220	65%
w/raspberries	6 sections	14.0	210	60%
milk chocolate				
plain	6 sections	14.0	220	57%
raspberries & cream	6 sections	14.0	230	55%
w/almonds	6 sections	15.0	230	59%
w/crisp	1 bar	21.0	360	53%
w/macadamias	1 bar	26.0	380	62%
mint chocolate	6 sections	14.0	220	57%
raspberries & cream	6 sections	14.0	230	55%
Legend Boxes				
milk chocolate wafers	11 pieces	12.0	210	51%
mint chocolate wafers	11 pieces	14.0	220	57%
nonpareils	10 pieces	9.0	190	43%
■ **(Godiva)**				
almond butter dome	3 pieces	17.0	240	64%
bouchee au chocolat	1 piece	11.0	210	47%
bouchee ivory raspberry	1 piece	9.0	160	51%
gold ballotin	3 pieces	10.0	210	43%
truffles				
amaretto di Saronno	2 pieces	12.0	210	51%
deluxe liqueur	2 pieces	13.0	210	43%

Food and Description	Amount	Fat Grams	Total Calories	% Fat Calories
■ **GOOBERS** (*See* (Nestlé) in this section)				
■ **GOOD 'N PLENTY** (*See* (Hershey) in this section)				
■ **GUMMI BEARS** (*See* (Brach's) in this section)				
■ **(GuyLian)**				
chocolate bars/no sugar added				
dark chocolate	8 squares	9.0	112	72%
milk chocolate				
plain	8 squares	9.0	125	65%
w/hazelnuts	8 squares	10.0	132	68%
■ **(Hershey)**				
Almond Joy	0.69 oz bar	5.0	90	50%
	0.48 oz bar	4.0	70	51%
Carmello	0.66 oz bar	4.0	90	40%
Classic Caramels				
chocolate creme filled	3 pieces	3.0	80	34%
soft & chewy	3 pieces	2.25	80	25%
Chuckles				
jellied candies	2 pieces	–	70	–
Jujubees	7 pieces	–	80	–
Cookies 'n' Creme bar/0.6 oz	2 bars	10.0	180	50%
Cookies 'n' Mint				
bar/0.6 oz	1 bar	4.5	90	45%
nuggets/0.35 oz	1 piece	2.5	45	50%
Crispy Rice Snacks/peanut butter	1 bar	2.5	70	32%
5th Avenue	0.58 oz bar	3.5	80	39%
Golden Collection solitaires/almonds	1 piece	1.0	15	60%
Good 'N Fruity/snack size	1 box	–	60	–
Good 'N Plenty	1 box	–	60	–
Gummy Bears/amazin' fruit	1 pouch	–	60	–
Heath Bar				
regular	1.4 oz bar	13.0	210	56%
snack bar	5 pieces	15.0	240	56%
	1 piece	3.0	50	54%
Heide Jujubes	45 pieces	–	100	–
Hershey's				
Bites				
almond joy	7 pieces	6.0	90	60%
milk chocolate w/almond	7 pieces	6.0	90	60%
Reese's peanut butter	7 pieces	6.0	90	60%
Cookies 'n' Creme	8 pieces	5.0	90	50%
York Peppermint Patty	9 pieces	1.5	90	15%
Candy-coated milk chocolate eggs	4 pieces	4.0	90	40%
Miniatures/chocolate bars:				
special dark	1 piece	2.5	45	50%
milk chocolate	1 piece	2.5	45	50%
Krackel	1 piece	2.5	45	50%
Mr. Goodbar	1 piece	3.0	45	60%
Nuggets				
Cookies 'n' Mint	1 piece	2.5	50	45%
Cookies 'n' Creme	1 piece	3.0	50	54%

Food and Description	Amount	Fat Grams	Total Calories	% Fat Calories
dark chocolate w/almonds	1 piece	3.0	50	54%
milk chocolate				
plain	1 piece	3.0	50	54%
w/almonds	1 piece	3.0	50	54%
w/almonds & toffee	1 piece	3.5	50	63%
w/raisins & almonds	1 piece	2.5	50	45%
Sweet Escapes/bars				
caramel & peanut butter crispy	0.7 oz	2.5	70	32%
chocolate toffee crisp	0.66 oz	3.5	80	39%
crispy caramel fudge	0.7 oz	2.0	80	23%
crunchy peanut butter	0.7 oz	2.5	80	28%
triple chocolate wafer	0.56 oz	2.5	80	28%
Tastetations/hard candy				
butterscotch	3 pieces	1.5	60	23%
caramel	3 pieces	1.5	60	23%
chocolate	3 pieces	1.5	60	23%
chocolate mint	3 pieces	1.5	60	23%
peppermint	3 pieces	–	60	–
Hugs/chocolate				
plain	1 piece	1.5	25	54%
w/almonds	1 piece	1.5	25	54%
Jolly Ranchers				
hard assorted candies	1 piece	–	40	–
lollipops	1 piece	–	60	–
Juicyfruits	2 boxes	–	80	–
Kisses				
plain	1 piece	1.5	25	54%
w/almonds	1 piece	1.5	25	54%
Kit-Kat	0.56 oz	4.0	80	45%
Krackel	0.3 oz bar	2.5	45	50%
	0.6 oz bar	4.5	90	45%
Mexican Hats	9 pieces	–	100	–
milk chocolate bar				
plain	0.3 oz	2.5	45	50%
	0.6 oz	5.0	90	50%
w/almond nuggets	0.35 oz	3.5	60	53%
w/almonds	0.6 oz	6.0	90	60%
Milk Duds	7 pieces	3.5	90	35%
	1.85 oz	8.0	230	31%
Mr. Goodbar	0.3 oz bar	3.0	50	54%
	0.6 oz bar	6.0	100	54%
Mounds	0.69 oz bar	5.0	90	50%
Nibs				
cherry	1 pouch/ 8 pieces	–	45	–
licorice	1 pouch/ 8 pieces	–	40	–
Pay Day	1.83 oz	12.0	240	45%
	Snack bar	5.0	100	45%
Rainblo bubble gum balls	1 piece		10	–

Food and Description	Amount	Fat Grams	Total Calories	% Fat Calories
Red Hot Dollars	7 pieces	–	100	–
Reese's				
Nutrageous	0.6 oz	5.0	90	50%
	1.6 oz	14.0	240	53%
peanut butter				
cup/miniatures	0.275 oz	2.5	40	56%
eggs	1 piece	5.0	90	50%
Pieces	0.7 oz	4.5	90	45%
Robin Eggs				
large	2 pieces	2.0	70	26%
medium	4 pieces	3.0	90	30%
mini	10 pieces	2.5	70	32%
Rolo chocolate caramels in milk chocolate	3 pieces	2.5	80	28%
Sixlets	24 pieces	3.5	90	35%
Soft Drops	9 pieces	–	100	–
Super Bubble bubble gum	1 piece	–	15	–
Symphony				
milk chocolate				
plain	0.6 oz	6.0	100	54%
w/almonds & toffee chips	0.6 oz	5.0	80	56%
Twizzlers				
cherry	1 piece	–	30	–
Pull'n'Peel	1 piece	1.0	90	10%
regular				
chocolate	1 piece	–	25	–
licorice	1 piece	–	30	–
strawberry	1 piece	–	30	–
Whatchamacallit	0.58 oz bar	4.5	80	51%
Whoppers	10 pieces	4.0	100	36%
Wunderbeans/gourmet jelly beans	33 pieces	–	100	–
York Peppermint Patty	0.58 oz piece	1.0	50	18%
Zagnut	1.8 oz bar	9.0	230	35%
	Snack bar	3.0	70	39%
Zero	0.6 oz bar	2.5	70	32%
■ HOMEMADE				
USDA Standard Home Recipe				
divinity/plain	1 oz	–	98	–
truffles	0.5 oz	4.0	59	61%
■ (Jelly Belly) Jelly Beans				
A&W				
cream soda	35 pieces	–	140	–
rootbeer	35 pieces	–	140	–
buttered popcorn	35 pieces	–	140	–
canteloupe	35 pieces	–	140	–
champagne punch	35 pieces	–	140	–
chocolate pudding	35 pieces	–	140	–
cotton candy	35 pieces	–	140	–
grape jelly	35 pieces	–	140	–
green apple	35 pieces	–	140	–
jalapeño	35 pieces	–	140	–

Food and Description	Amount	Fat Grams	Total Calories	% Fat Calories
margarita	35 pieces	–	140	–
peanut butter	35 pieces	–	140	–
strawberry cheesecake	35 pieces	–	140	–
toasted marshmallow	35 pieces	–	140	–

■ **JOLLY RANCHERS** (*See* (Hershey) in this section)
■ **JUNIOR MINTS** (*See* (Cambridge) in this section)
■ **KIT-KAT** (*See* (Hershey) in this section)
■ **KRACKEL** (*See* (Hershey) in this section)
■ **KUDOS** (*See* (M&M * Mars) in this section)
■ **LAFFY TAFFY** (*See* (Beich); (Concorde) in this section)
■ **(Lance)**

Food and Description	Amount	Fat Grams	Total Calories	% Fat Calories
chews/11 pieces per pkg				
cinnamon	1 pkg	0.5	120	4%
fruit	1 pkg	0.5	120	4%
mint	1 pkg	0.5	120	4%
strawberry	1 pkg	0.5	120	4%
chocolaty peanut bar	1 bar	15.0	270	50%
gum ball pops	1 piece	–	45	–
K-Nuts	4 pieces	15.0	240	56%
mints/soft	2 pieces	–	40	–
peanut bar	1 bar	15.0	270	50%
Pop-A-Lance	1 piece	–	45	–
popcorn 'n' caramel bar	1 bar	–	90	–
starlight mints	3 pieces	–	60	–
suckers/assorted	3 pieces	–	50	–
whistle pop	1 piece	–	70	–

■ **LIFE SAVERS** (*See* (Planters) in this section)
■ **(Lindt)**

Food and Description	Amount	Fat Grams	Total Calories	% Fat Calories
chocoletti milk bar	7 pieces	12.0	210	51%
chocoletti mint bar	7 pieces	10.0	190	47%
Lindor Swiss chocolate	3 balls	16.0	220	65%
mocca bar	14 blocks	13.0	210	56%
Swiss milk chocolate				
w/cherry	6 blocks	9.0	180	45%
w/orange	6 blocks	10.0	190	47%
w/raspberry	6 blocks	9.0	180	45%
Swiss milk filled	7 pieces	18.0	240	68%

■ **(M&M * Mars)**

Food and Description	Amount	Fat Grams	Total Calories	% Fat Calories
Dove				
dark chocolate				
miniatures	7 pieces	14.0	220	55%
single	1.3 oz	12.0	200	54%
6-oz bar	¼ bar	14.0	230	55%
milk chocolate				
miniatures	7 pieces	13.0	230	51%
single	1.3 oz	12.0	200	54%
6-oz bar	¼ bar	13.0	230	51%
Kudos				
chocolate chip	1 bar	4.5	120	34%
chocolate fudge	1 bar	4.5	120	34%

Food and Description	Amount	Fat Grams	Total Calories	% Fat Calories
M&M's milk chocolate mini's	1 bar	2.5	90	25%
peanut butter	1 bar	5.0	130	35%
Snickers Bar	1 bar	3.5	100	32%
M&M's				
almond	Singles bag	11.0	200	50%
baking & decorating pack	0.5 oz	3.0	70	38%
crispy	Singles bag	9.0	200	41%
peanut	Singles bag	13.0	250	47%
peanut butter	Singles bag	13.0	240	49%
plain	Singles bag	10.0	240	38%
Mars Bar/Singles	1 bar	13.0	240	49%
Milky Way/Singles				
Midnight	1 bar	8.0	220	33%
lite bar	1 bar	5.0	170	26%
milk chocolate	1 bar	10.0	270	33%
reduced fat	1 bar	7.0	140	45%
Skittles				
original				
fun size	2 bags	2.0	180	10%
single	2.8 oz	3.0	250	8%
tropical				
fun size	2 bags	2.0	160	11%
single	2.2 oz	3.0	250	8%
wild berry				
fun size	2 bags	2.0	160	11%
single	2.2 oz	3.0	250	8%
Snickers/Singles				
munch bar	1 bar	15.0	230	59%
original	1 bar	14.0	280	45%
Starburst				
California fruits	8 pieces	3.0	160	17%
original fruits	8 pieces	3.0	160	17%
strawberry fruits	8 pieces	3.0	160	17%
tropical fruits	8 pieces	3.0	160	17%
3 Musketeers	1 bar	8.0	260	28%
■ MILK DUDS (See (Hershey) in this section)				
■ MILKY WAY (See (M&M * Mars) in this section)				
■ MR. GOODBAR (See (Hershey) in this section)				
■ MOUNDS (See (Hershey) in this section)				
■ (Nabisco)				
Peppermint Patty	1 oz	1.0	110	8%
Thin Mint	1 piece	1.0	42	21%
■ (Natural Touch)				
Caroby Bars				
almond	4 sections	10.0	150	60%
milk	4 sections	9.0	150	54%
milk-free	4 sections	11.0	160	62%
mint	4 sections	9.0	150	54%
■ (Nature's Warehouse)				
A-OK	1 oz	6.0	130	42%

Food and Description	Amount	Fat Grams	Total Calories	% Fat Calories
My O My	1 oz	1.5	105	13%
No-How	1 oz	10.0	140	64%
Nut Wit	1 oz	6.0	135	40%
■ (Nestlé)				
Baby Ruth				
fun size	1 bar	6.0	130	42%
regular	2.1 oz	13.0	270	43%
Buncha Crunch	1.4 oz	10.0	200	45%
Butterfinger				
BB's	1.7 oz	9.0	230	31%
Bittyfinger	2 bars	7.0	170	37%
fun size	1 bar	3.5	100	32%
regular	2.1 oz	11.0	270	37%
Chunky Bar	1.4 oz	11.0	210	47%
Crunch				
bar				
fun size	4 bars	11.0	210	47%
regular	1.55 oz	12.0	230	47%
Flipz/2 oz. pkg				
milk chocolate	1 oz	6.0	130	42%
peanut butter	1 oz	6.0	140	39%
white fudge	1 oz	6.0	130	42%
Goobers	1.38 oz bag	13.0	210	56%
milk chocolate bar	1.45 oz	13.0	220	53%
mocha crunch bar	1.3 oz	12.0	200	54%
Nips				
Butter rum	2 pieces	1.5	60	23%
chocolate	2 pieces	1.5	60	23%
chocolate parfait	2 pieces	2.0	60	30%
coffee	2 pieces	1.5	50	27%
peanut butter parfait	2 pieces	2.0	60	30%
vanilla almond cafe	2 pieces	1.0	50	18%
Oh Henry!	1.8 oz bar	5.0	120	38%
Raisinets	1.58 oz bag	8.0	190	38%
Sno Caps	2.3 oz box	13.0	320	37%
Thousand Grand Bar	1.5 oz	8.0	200	36%
Treasures				
butterfinger	3 pieces	9.0	180	45%
caramel	3 pieces	9.0	180	45%
peanut butter	4 pieces	17.0	250	61%
Turtles	2 pieces	9.0	160	51%
White Crunch Bar	1.5 oz	13.0	220	53%
■ (Newman's Own)				
Organics bars				
crisp rice				
espresso sweet dark chocolate	½ bar	15.0	240	56%
milk chocolate	½ bar	17.0	250	61%
milk chocolate	½ bar	16.0	240	60%
■ NUTRAGEOUS (See (Hershey) in this section)				

Food and Description	Amount	Fat Grams	Total Calories	% Fat Calories
■ **OH HENRY!** (*See* (Nestlé) in this section)				
■ **(Panda)**				
licorice	3.5 oz	<1.0	340	1%
raspberry-flavored chew	3.5 oz	<1.0	340	1%
■ **PAY DAY** (*See* (Hershey) in this section)				
■ **(PB Max)**				
fun size	2 pieces	12.0	180	60%
regular	2 pieces	15.0	240	56%
■ **(Pearson's)**				
butter rum	2 pieces	1.5	60	23%
caramel nip	2 pieces	1.5	60	23%
chocolate mint	2 pieces	1.5	60	23%
chocolate parfait	2 pieces	1.5	60	23%
coffee nip	2 pieces	1.5	60	23%
licorice nip	2 pieces	1.5	60	23%
mint patties	5 pieces	2.5	150	15%
peanut buffer parfait	2 pieces	1.5	60	23%
■ **(Pez)**	1 roll	–	30	–
■ **(Planters)**				
Life Savers				
candy cane, big tablet	4 pieces	–	60	–
cards 'n candy	4 pieces	–	40	–
Gummy Savers				
five flavor	11 pieces	–	130	–
mixed berry	11 pieces	–	130	–
tangy fruit	11 pieces	–	130	–
variety bag	2 bags	–	120	–
wacky frootz	11 pieces	–	130	–
Holes				
five flavor	20 pieces	–	20	–
island fruits	20 pieces	–	20	–
sour 'n sweet	16 pieces	–	20	–
sunshine fruits	20 pieces	–	20	–
super tart	20 pieces	–	20	–
wild fruits super	20 pieces	–	20	–
Life Savers/regular roll				
butter rum	2 pieces	–	20	–
candy cane	4 pieces	–	40	–
cryst-o-mint	2 pieces	–	20	–
egg-sortment	1 roll	–	40	–
five flavor	2 pieces	–	20	–
fruits on fire	2 pieces	–	20	–
pep-o-mint	3 pieces	–	20	–
spear-o-mint	3 pieces	–	20	–
sunshine fruits	2 pieces	–	20	–
tangy fruit swirls	4 pieces	–	40	–
tangy fruits	2 pieces	–	20	–
tropical fruits	2 pieces	–	20	–
watermelon	2 pieces	–	20	–
wint-o-green	3 pieces	–	20	–

Food and Description	Amount	Fat Grams	Total Calories	% Fat Calories
lollipops/assorted	1 pop	–	40	–
Sack'it				
butter rum	4 pieces	–	60	–
Christmas tin	4 pieces	–	60	–
five flavor	4 pieces	–	60	–
holiday tin	4 pieces	–	60	–
pep-o-mint	4 pieces	–	60	–
tangy fruits	4 pieces	–	60	–
wild cherry	4 pieces	–	60	–
wint-o-green	4 pieces	–	60	–
peanutbar	1.6 oz	14.0	230	54%
peanut brittle	½ cup	7.0	180	35%
peanut butter chocolates	4 pieces	15.0	230	59%
sweet 'n crunchy	1 oz	7.0	140	45%
■ POM POMS (*See* (Cambridge) in this section)				
■ RAISINETS (*See* (Nestlé) in this section)				
■ REESE's (*See* (Hershey) in this section)				
■ RIESEN (*See* (Storck) in this section)				
■ ROLO (*See* (Hershey) in this section)				
■ (Russell Stover)				
almond delights	2 pieces	12.0	210	51%
Ambassadors miniature chocolates	6 pieces	9.0	190	43%
candy jar chocolates	4 pieces	9.0	190	43%
caramels	3 pieces	7.0	170	37%
assorted	3 pieces	8.0	190	38%
English	6 pieces	6.0	180	30%
Santas	1 Santa	11.0	230	43%
squares/soft & creamy	3 pieces	10.0	190	47%
cherry cordials	3 pieces	7.0	170	37%
chocolate assortments				
dark chocolate	3 pieces	8.0	190	38%
gift box				
gold bow	2 pieces	10.0	200	45%
regular	3 pieces	8.0	180	40%
milk chocolate	3 pieces	8.0	190	38%
chocolate-covered nuts	3 pieces	16.0	230	63%
coconut clusters	3 pieces	14.0	230	55%
fudge/German chocolate	1 piece	10.0	190	47%
mints				
French chocolate				
boxed	4 pieces	14.0	220	57%
individual	1 bar	15.0	240	56%
Mint Dream	1 bar	8.0	160	45%
patties/dark chocolate covered	6 pieces	6.0	180	30%
pecan delights				
boxed	2 pieces	14.0	220	57%
individual	1 bar	20.0	310	58%
pecan roll	1.5 oz	20.0	300	60%
truffles	3 pieces	11.0	200	50%
whips/assorted	2 pieces	7.0	210	30%

Food and Description	Amount	Fat Grams	Total Calories	% Fat Calories
■ (Sherwood)				
Cows				
butter 'n cream	3 pieces	1.5	71	19%
butter 'n toffees				
chocolate-filled	6 pieces	11.0	240	41%
plain	6 pieces	7.0	180	35%
■ SHOCK TARTS (*See* (Concorde) in this section)				
■ SKITTLES (*See* (Hershey) in this section)				
■ SLO POKE (*See* (Clark) in this section)				
■ SNO CAPS (*See* (Nestlé) in this section)				
■ (Spangler)				
candy cane	1 piece	–	60	–
chocolate-coated creme center	1 piece	2.0	80	23%
caramel w/nuts	1 piece	6.0	100	54%
cherry w/nuts	1 piece	5.0	110	41%
fudge w/nuts	1 piece	6.0	140	39%
fudge w/pecans	1 piece	7.0	140	45%
maple w/nuts	1 piece	5.0	110	41%
vanilla w/nuts	1 piece	5.0	110	41%
circus peanuts	4 pieces	–	110	–
lollipops				
Dum Dums/all flavors	1 lollipop	–	25	–
Saf-T-Pops	1 lollipop	–	45	–
w/bubble gum center/all flavors	1 lollipop	–	60	–
mint/dark chocolate covered	1 piece	2.0	80	23%
■ STARBURST (*See* (Hershey) in this section)				
■ (Storck)				
Chocolate Riesen	5 pieces	7.0	180	35%
Riesen chocolate chew	1 bar	7.0	180	35%
Werther's original	3 pieces	1.0	60	15%
■ SUGAR BABIES (*See* (Cambridge) in this section)				
■ SUGAR DADDY (*See* (Cambridge) in this section)				
■ (Sweet 'N Low)				
hard candies				
butterscotch	4 pieces	–	30	–
cinnamon	4 pieces	–	30	–
coffee	4 pieces	–	30	–
fancy fruit	4 pieces	–	30	–
fruit	4 pieces	–	30	–
peppermint	4 pieces	–	30	–
watermelon	4 pieces	–	30	–
■ SWEET PRETENDERS (*See* (Featherweight) in this section)				
■ SYMPHONY (*See* (Hershey) in this section)				
■ TAFFY TARTS (*See* (Concorde) in this section)				
■ 3 MUSKETEERS (*See* (M&M * Mars) in this section)				
■ (Tootsie Roll)				
Tootsie Pop				
caramel apple	1 pop	0.5	70	6%
regular	1 pop	–	60	–

Food and Description	Amount	Fat Grams	Total Calories	% Fat Calories
Tootsie Roll				
midgees	6 pieces	3.0	160	17%
regular	1 oz	2.0	110	16%
■ **WERTHER's** (*See* (Storck) in this section)				
■ **(Whitman's)**				
assorted	3 pieces	8.0	190	38%
dark chocolate	3 pieces	10.0	200	45%
Little Ambassadors	7 pieces	9.0	190	43%
Pecan Delight Bar	1 bar	20.0	310	58%
Pecan Roll	1 bar	20.0	300	60%
■ **(WHATCHAMACALLIT** (*See* (Hershey) in this section)				
■ **WHOPPERS** (*See* (Hershey) in this section)				
■ **(Woody's)**				
fudge				
chocolate w/nuts	1 piece	4.0	120	30%
maple walnut	1 piece	4.0	120	30%
mint w/walnuts	1 piece	4.0	120	30%
vanilla w/walnuts	1 piece	4.0	120	30%
■ **(YORK)** (*See* (Hershey) in this section)				
■ **(Zachary)**				
creme drops/old-fashioned milk chocolate	3 pieces	3.0	170	16%
■ **ZOTZ** (*See* (Andre Prost) in this section)				
CANDY APPLE (*See* APPLE, CARAMEL)				
CANNELLINI BEAN (*See* KIDNEY BEAN)				
CANTALOUPE/MUSKMELON				
fresh				
cubed	1 cup	<1.0	57	8%
whole/~ 9.5 oz	½ melon	0.7	94	7%
CAPERS				
(Progresso) drained	1 tsp	–	5	–
CAPON				
giblets/simmered	5 oz	7.8	238	30%
meat & skin/roasted	3.5 oz	11.7	229	46%
	~1.5 lb	74.0	1457	46%
meat only/roasted	3.5 oz	8.8	178	44%
CARAMBOLA (*See* STAR FRUIT)				
CARAWAY SEEDS	1 tsp	–	8	–
CARDAMOM SEEDS				
ground	1 Tbs	0.5	20	23%
whole	1 tsp	–	6	–
CARDOON				
cooked	3 oz	–	19	–
raw/shredded	1 cup	–	35	–
CARIBOU /boneless				
raw	3 oz	5.0	160	28%
roasted	4 oz	5.0	190	24%
roasted/diced	1 cup	6.0	235	23%
CARISSA/NATAL PLUM				
raw	1 medium	–	12	–

Food and Description	Amount	Fat Grams	Total Calories	% Fat Calories
CAROB CHIPS				
regular	1 oz	7.0	140	45%
mini	1 oz	7.0	140	45%
CAROB POWDER				
(Chatfield's)	¼ cup	–	96	–
(El Molino)	¼ cup	–	110	–
CARP (See CARP ROE)				
breaded & fried	3 oz	12.0	226	48%
cooked-dry heat	3 oz	6.0	138	39%
raw	3 oz	4.8	108	40%
smoked	1 oz	1.8	50	32%
CARP ROE /raw	3 oz	1.7	111	14%
CARROT (See also VEGETABLES, MIXED)				
canned				
(Del Monte) sliced	½ cup	–	35	–
(Freshlike) sliced/crinkle cut	½ cup	–	30	–
generic/sliced/cooked	½ cup	–	35	–
(Green Giant) sliced	½ cup	–	25	–
(LeSueur) whole baby	½ cup	–	35	–
(Libby's)				
diced	½ cup	–	20	–
sliced	½ cup	–	20	–
(S&W)				
julienne	½ cup	0.5	25	18%
sliced	½ cup	0.5	25	18%
whole tiny	½ cup	0.5	25	18%
(Seneca) all styles	½ cup	–	30	–
(Stokely)				
diced/no salt or sugar added	½ cup	–	30	–
sliced	½ cup	–	30	–
(Thank You) fingerling	½ cup	–	30	–
(Veg-All) crinkle cut	½ cup	–	30	–
fresh				
cooked	1 small	–	21	–
raw				
shredded	½ cup	–	24	–
(Dole)	3 oz	1.0	50	18%
whole	1 medium	–	31	–
(Dole)	1 medium	1.0	40	23%
frozen				
(Birds Eye)				
sliced	½ cup	–	35	–
whole baby	½ cup	–	40	–
(C&W)				
Parisienne	⅔ cup	–	40	–
whole baby	⅔ cup	–	35	–
generic	½ cup	–	26	–
(Green Giant) baby cut				
Harvest Fresh	⅔ cup	–	20	–
regular	¾ cup	–	30	–
(Seneca)	¾ cup	–	30	–

Food and Description	Amount	Fat Grams	Total Calories	% Fat Calories
(Stokely)				
diced	½ cup	–	35	–
sliced	½ cup	–	35	–
whole baby	⅔ cup	–	35	–
CARROT JUICE /canned				
generic	6 fl oz	–	75	–
(Hain)	6 fl oz	–	80	–
(Hollywood)	12 fl oz	–	120	–
CASABA MELON /fresh				
cubed	1 cup	–	45	–
whole/8" melon	2" slice	–	45	–
CASHEW				
(Beer Nuts)	1 oz	13.0	170	69%
(Eagle)				
honey-roasted	1 oz	14.0	180	70%
lightly salted	1 oz	14.0	190	66%
(Fisher)				
honey-roasted	1 oz	13.0	150	78%
oil-roasted	1 oz	15.0	170	79%
Snack'N Serve Nut Bowl	1 oz	15.0	170	79%
whole	1 oz	13.0	160	73%
(Frito Lay)	1 oz	15.0	180	75%
generic				
dry-roasted/salted or unsalted	1 oz	13.0	163	72%
	1 cup	64.0	790	73%
oil-roasted/salted or unsalted	1 oz	14.0	163	77%
	1 cup	63.0	750	76%
(Guys) Whole Salted	1 oz	14.0	170	74%
(Lance)	1½ oz	22.0	270	73%
	1 oz-¼ cup	14.0	180	70%
(Planters)				
honey-roasted				
Munch 'N Go	2 oz	24.0	310	70%
regular	1 oz	12.0	150	72%
	2 oz	24.0	310	70%
oil-roasted				
fancy	1 oz	14.0	170	74%
	2 oz	29.0	340	77%
halves	1 oz	14.0	170	74%
lightly salted	1 oz	13.0	160	73%
Munch 'N Go	2 oz	28.0	330	76%
nut bag	1 oz	14.0	160	79%
regular	1.5 oz	21.0	250	76%
CASHEW BUTTER				
generic/plain	1 Tbs	8.0	94	77%
	1 oz	14.0	167	75%
(Hain)				
raw	2 Tbs	15.0	190	71%
toasted	2 Tbs	17.0	210	73%
unsalted	2 Tbs	19.0	210	81%
(Kettle) Roaster Fresh/unsalted	1 oz	14.0	165	76%

Food and Description	Amount	Fat Grams	Total Calories	% Fat Calories
(Westbrae) natural				
raw	2 Tbs	17.0	190	81%
roasted	2 Tbs	17.0	190	81%
CASSAVA				
raw/trimmed	3.5 oz	<1.0	120	3%
	1 lb	2.0	525	3%
CATFISH (*See also* SEAFOOD ENTRÉE/DINNER)				
channel/fresh/meat only				
baked or broiled	3 oz	7.0	149	42%
breaded & fried	3 oz	11.0	194	51%
raw	3 oz	3.6	99	33%
CATSUP/KETCHUP				
(Del Monte) tomato	1 Tbs	–	15	–
generic	1 Tbs	–	15	–
	1 cup	1.0	290	3%
(Hain) natural				
no salt added	1 Tbs	–	16	–
regular	1 Tbs	–	16	–
(Healthy Choice)	1 Tbs	–	10	–
(Heinz)				
hot	1 Tbs	–	15	–
lite	1 Tbs	–	10	–
regular	1 Tbs	–	15	–
w/onions	1 Tbs	–	20	–
(Hunt's)				
no salt added	1 Tbs	–	15	–
regular	1 Tbs	–	15	–
(Smucker's)	1 Tbs	–	25	–
(Stokely)	1 Tbs	–	20	–
(Weight Watchers)	1 Tbs	–	15	–
(Westbrae) fruit-sweetened				
no salt	1 Tbs	–	10	–
regular	1 Tbs	–	10	–
CAULIFLOWER				
fresh				
cooked	½ cup	–	17	–
raw				
chopped	½ cup	–	12	–
(Dole)	3 oz	0.5	20	23%
whole/medium head	⅙ head	–	18	–
frozen				
(Birds Eye)	½ cup	–	25	–
(Green Giant) florets	1 cup	–	2o	–
(Seneca)	1 cup	–	20	–
jarred				
(Mrs. Klein's) hot	1 oz	–	–	–
(Vlasic)				
hot & spicy	1 oz	–	4	–
sweet	1 oz	–	35	–
CAULIFLOWER DISH (*See also* FROZEN ENTRÉE/DINNER; VEGETABLES, MIXED)				
(Birds Eye) frozen w/cheese sauce	½ pkg	5.0	90	50%

Food and Description	Amount	Fat Grams	Total Calories	% Fat Calories
(Green Giant) frozen in cheese-flavored sauce	½ cup	2.5	60	38%
CAULIFLOWER SOUP (See SOUP)				
CAVIAR				
general/black or red				
granular	1 Tbs	3.0	40	68%
	1 oz	5.0	71	63%
pressed	1 Tbs	2.8	54	47%
	1 oz	4.7	90	47%
(Romanoff)				
black lumpfish	1 Tbs	1.0	15	60%
black whitefish	1 Tbs	1.5	25	54%
red lumpfish	1 Tbs	1.0	15	60%
CELERIAC/CELERY ROOT/WILD CELERY				
raw	½ cup	–	31	–
	4-5 medium	–	40	–
CELERY				
fresh/medium stalks				
cooked	½ cup	–	11	–
raw	1 stalk	–	6	–
	½ cup	–	9	–
(Dole)	2 stalks	–	20	–
frozen				
(Freshlike)	3.5 oz	–	14	–
(Seneca)	¾ cup	–	10	–
CELERY ROOT (See CELERIAC)				
CELERY SEED /whole	1 tsp	0.5	8	56%
	1 Tbs	1.5	25	54%

CELERY SOUP (See SOUP)
CEREAL (See also BABY FOOD; BARLEY; BULGUR; CORN GRITS)

QUICK REFERENCE: MILK	Amount	Fat Grams	Total Calories	% Fat Calories
Skim/fat-free	¼ cup	–	23	–
	½ cup	–	45	–
1% fat/light	¼ cup	0.5	26	17%
	½ cup	1.0	55	16%
2% fat/reduced fat	¼ cup	1.0	31	29%
	½ cup	2.5	61	37%
Whole	¼ cup	2.0	38	47%
	½ cup	4.0	75	48%

■ COLD/READY TO EAT

	Amount	Fat Grams	Total Calories	% Fat Calories
(Alpen) Swiss style				
low-fat	⅔ cup	3.0	200	14%
original	⅓ cup	2.0	110	16%
	⅔ cup	4.0	220	16%
Alpha-Bits (See (Post) in this section)				
(Arrowhead Mills)				
amaranth flakes	1 cup	1.0	128	7%

Food and Description	Amount	Fat Grams	Total Calories	% Fat Calories
bran flakes	1 cup	1.0	90	10%
corn flakes	1 cup	–	130	–
kamut flakes	1 cup	1.0	110	8%
maple buckwheat flakes	1 cup	1.0	160	6%
multigrain flakes	1 cup	1.5	140	10%
Nature O's	1 cup	2.0	130	14%
oat bran flakes	1 cup	2.5	140	16%
puffed corn	1 cup	0.5	60	8%
puffed kamut	1 cup	–	50	–
puffed millet	1 cup	0.5	60	8%
puffed rice	1 cup	0.5	60	8%
puffed wheat	1 cup	0.5	60	8%
raisin bran	1 cup	1.5	190	7%
rice flakes	1 cup	1.0	80	11%
shredded wheat				
sweetened	1 cup	1.0	200	5%
unsweetened	1 cup	0.5	180	3%
spelt flakes	1 cup	0.5	100	5%
wheat bran	¼ cup	0.5	30	15%
wheat germ/raw	3 Tbs	1.5	50	27%
(Back To Nature) granola				
apple blueberry	½ cup	3.0	170	16%
apple strawberry	½ cup	3.0	190	14%
natural	½ cup	3.0	170	16%
raisin	½ cup	2.5	170	13%
(Barbara's)				
Apple Cinnamon Toasted O's	¾ cup	1.0	110	8%
Cocoa crunch Stars	1 cup	0.5	110	4%
Frosted Corn flakes	1 cup	–	110	–
fruit sweetened				
Breakfast O's	1 cup	2.0	120	15%
Brown Rice Crisps	1 cup	1.0	120	8%
corn flakes	1 cup	–	110	–
Honey Crunch Stars	1 cup	–	110	–
Honey Nut Toasted O's	¾ cup	2.0	120	15%
Organic Fruity Punch	1 cup	0.5	110	4%
Puffins				
cinnamon	¾ cup	1.0	100	9%
plain	¾ cup	1.0	90	105
shredded				
oats/bite size	1¼ cups	2.5	220	10%
Spoonfuls/multigrain	¾ cup	1.5	120	11%
wheat biscuits	2 biscuits	1.0	140	6%
Startoons frosted cocoa crunch	1 cup	0.5	110	4%
Basic 4 (See (General Mills) in this section)				
(Breadshop)				
Cinnamon Grins	¾ cup	0.5	110	4%
granola				
blueberries 'n cream	½ cup	7.5	220	31%
crunchy oat bran	½ cup	8.5	210	36%
raspberries 'n cream	½ cup	7.5	220	31%

Food and Description	Amount	Fat Grams	Total Calories	% Fat Calories
strawberries 'n cream	½ cup	7.5	220	31%
super natural w/almonds	½ cup	9.0	220	37%
Kamut 'n Honey	1 cup	0.5	110	4%
Puffs 'n Honey	¾ cup	3.0	120	23%
Cap'n Crunch (*See* (Quaker) in this section)				
Cheerios (*See* (General Mills) in this section)				
Crispix (*See* (Kellogg's) in this section)				
(El Molino)				
puffed corn	¾ cup	–	50	–
puffed millet	¾ cup	–	50	–
puffed rice	¾ cup	–	50	–
puffed wheat	¾ cup	–	50	–
(Erewhon)				
amaranth/Aztec Corn	1 cup	–	110	–
Apple Stroodles	¾ cup	0.5	110	4%
Banana O's	¾ cup	–	110	–
corn flakes	1¼ cup	2.5	210	11%
crisp brown doe				
low-sodium	1 oz	1.0	110	8%
regular	1 oz	1.0	110	8%
Fruit 'n Wheat	¾ cup	1.0	100	9%
Galaxy Grahams	¾ cup	0.5	100	5%
kamut flakes	1 oz	–	90	–
Poppels	1 cup	1.0	120	8%
raisin bran	1 cup	1.0	170	5%
Right Start				
original	1 cup	–	90	–
w/raisins	1 cup	–	90	–
Super O's	1 oz	–	110	–
wheat flakes	1 oz	1.0	110	8%
(Familia) Swiss style muesli				
chocolate	½ cup	10.0	250	36%
no sugar	½ cup	3.0	200	9%
original	½ cup	3.0	210	13%
(Featherweight) corn flakes	1 cup	–	110	–
Froot Loops (*See* (Kellogg's) in this section)				
Fruit & Fibre (*See* (Post) in this section)				
(General Mills)				
Basic 4	¾ cup	1.5	120	11%
Booberry	1 cup	1.0	120	8%
Cheerios				
apple cinnamon	¾ cup	2.5	120	19%
frosted	1 cup	1.0	120	8%
honey nut	1 cup	1.5	120	11%
multigrain plus	1 cup	1.0	110	8%
original	1 cup	2.0	110	16%
Team	1 cup	1.0	120	8%
Cinnamon Grahams	¾ cup	1.0	120	8%
Cinnamon Toast Crunch	¾ cup	3.5	130	24%
Clusters	1 cup	4.0	220	16%

Food and Description	Amount	Fat Grams	Total Calories	% Fat Calories
w/almonds/walnuts/pecans	½ cup	2.0	110	16%
Cocoa Puffs	1 cup	1.0	120	8%
Cookie Crisp	1 cup	1.0	120	8%
Corn Chex	1 cup	–	110	–
Count Chocula	1 cup	1.0	120	8%
Country Corn Flakes	1 cup	–	110	–
Fiber One	½ cup	1.0	60	15%
Frankenberry	1 cup	1.0	120	8%
French Toast Crunch	¾ cup	1.0	120	8%
Golden Grahams	¾ cup	1.0	120	8%
Honey Nut Clusters	1 cup	2.0	210	9%
Kaboom	1¼ cups	1.0	120	8%
Kix				
berry berry	¾ cup	1.5	120	11%
original	1⅓ cups	0.5	120	4%
Lucky Charms	1 cup	1.0	120	8%
Millenios	1 cup	1.0	120	8%
Multi-bran Chex	1 cup	1.5	200	7%
Nature Valley low-fat fruit granola	⅔ cup	2.5	210	11%
Nesquick chocolate	¾ cup	2.0	120	15%
Oatmeal Crisp				
almond	1 cup	4.5	220	19%
apple cinnamon	1 cup	2.0	210	9%
raisin	1 cup	2.0	210	9%
Raisin Nut Bran	¾ cup	4.0	200	20%
Reese's Peanut Butter Puffs	¾ cup	3.0	130	21%
Rice Chex	1¼ cups	–	120	–
Total				
brown sugar & oat	¾ cup	1.0	110	8%
corn flakes	1⅓ cup	–	110	–
raisin bran	1 cup	1.0	180	5%
whole wheat	¾ cup	1.0	110	8%
Trix	1 cup	1.0	120	8%
Wheat Chex	1 cup	1.0	180	5%
Wheaties				
honey frosted	¾ cup	–	110	–
original	1 cup	1.0	110	8%
raisin bran	1 cup	1.0	180	5%
(Golden Temple)				
almond raisin/low-fat	1 oz	1.5	110	12%
apple cinnamon/low-fat	1 cup	1.5	110	12%
granola				
cashew almond	1 oz	3.5	130	24%
cinnamon apple raisin	1 oz	3.5	125	25%
coconut almond	1 oz	7.0	145	43%
fruit 'n nut	1 oz	4.5	130	31%
golden	1 oz	6.0	140	39%
Hawaiian	1 oz	4.0	125	29%
high protein	1 oz	3.5	125	25%
honey almond	1 oz	3.5	130	24%

Food and Description	Amount	Fat Grams	Total Calories	% Fat Calories
honey blueberry apple	1 oz	3.5	130	24%
lite 'n crunchy	1 oz	4.5	130	31%
low-fat/sweet home farm	1 oz	2.0	110	16%
maple almond	1 oz	3.5	130	24%
natural blueberry				
coconut-free	1 oz	4.5	130	31%
regular	1 oz	5.0	130	35%
natural delite	1 oz	3.5	130	24%
oat bran				
berries	1 oz	3.5	120	25%
raisins & almonds	1 oz	3.5	120	25%
orange almond	1 oz	4.0	135	27%
raisin apricot date	1 oz	3.5	130	24%
hazelnut boysenberry				
muesli				
lite	1 oz	1.0	100	9%
oat bran				
dates & almonds	1 oz	1.5	110	12%
raisins & hazelnuts	1 oz	1.5	105	14%
sweet home farm crunchy/low-fat	1 oz	2.0	105	17%
Swiss style	1 oz	1.5	105	13%
35% fruit	1 oz	1.0	100	9%
natural foods/low-fat				
apple cinnamon	1 oz	1.0	110	8%
raisin almond	1 oz	1.0	110	8%
strawberry/raspberry	1 oz	1.0	110	8%
oat bran flakes				
almond	1 cup	3.5	120	26%
apple	1 oz	3.5	110	29%
muesli				
dates & almonds	1 cup	1.5	110	12%
raisins & hazelnuts	1 cup	1.5	100	14%
100% natural				
almond	1 oz	4.0	125	29%
apple cinnamon	1 oz	4.0	120	30%
oat bran	1 oz	2.5	70	32%
raisin & almond	1 oz	4.0	120	30%
organic oats	1 oz	5.5	135	37%
6 Grain Crisp/fruit & flaxseed	1 oz	3.5	120	26%
Sweet Home Farm				
almond	1 oz	4.0	125	29%
raisin	1 oz	1.5	105	13%
Grape-Nuts (*See* (Post) in this section)				
(Grist Mill) Natural				
Apple Cinnamon	½ cup	10.0	160	56%
Bran Oat & Honey	½ cup	8.0	250	29%
Oat Honey & Raisin	½ cup	12.0	270	40%
(Health Valley)				
Amaranth				
cereal w/bananas	½ cup	2.0	110	16%

Food and Description	Amount	Fat Grams	Total Calories	% Fat Calories
crunch w/raisins	¼ cup	3.0	110	25%
flakes/100% organic	½ cup	–	90	–
Blue-corn Flakes/100% organic	½ cup	–	90	–
Bran Cereal/100% organic				
w/dates	¼ cup	1.0	100	9%
w/raisins	¼ cup	1.0	100	9%
Fiber 7 Flakes/100% organic				
regular	½ cup	–	90	–
w/raisins	½ cup	–	90	–
Fruit & Fitness	1 cup	4.0	220	16%
Fruit Lites				
corn	½ cup	–	45	–
rice	½ cup	1.0	45	20%
wheat	½ cup	1.0	45	20%
Healthy Crunch				
almond date	¼ cup	3.0	110	25%
apple Cinnamon	¼ cup	3.0	110	25%
Healthy O's/100% organic	¾ cup	1.0	90	10%
Lites				
puffed corn	½ cup	–	50	–
puffed rice	½ cup	–	50	–
puffed wheat	½ cup	–	50	–
Oat Bran Flakes/100% organic				
regular	½ cup	–	100	–
w/almonds & dates	1½ cup	–	100	–
w/raisins	½ cup	–	100	–
Oat Bran Natural				
apples & cinnamon	¼ cup	–	100	–
raisins & spice	¼ cup	–	100	–
Oat Bran O's				
100% organic	½ cup	–	110	–
fruit & nuts	½ cup	3.0	100	25%
Orangeola				
almonds & dates	¼ cup	3.0	110	25%
bananas & Hawaiian fruit	¼ cup	4.0	120	30%
Raisin Bran Flakes/100% organic	½ cup	–	100	–
Real Oat Bran				
almond crunch	¼ cup	3.0	110	25%
Hawaiian fruit	¼ cup	3.0	130	21%
raisin nut	¼ cup	3.0	130	21%
Rice Bran O's				
regular	½ cup	1.0	100	8%
w/almonds & dates	½ cup	3.0	110	25%
Sprouts 7				
bananas & Hawaiian fruit	¼ cup	1.0	90	9%
raisin	¼ cup	1.0	90	9%
Swiss Breakfast				
raisin nut	¼ cup	3.0	100	27%
tropical fruit	¼ cup	3.0	100	27%

Food and Description	Amount	Fat Grams	Total Calories	% Fat Calories
Healthy Choice (*See* (Kellogg's) in this section)				
Heartland (*See* (Pillsbury) in this section)				
homemade/USDA Standard Home Recipe				
granola	¼ cup	7.7	138	50%
(Kashi) puffed cereal				
chocolate pillows	¾ cup	1.0	200	5%
medley	½ cup	1.0	100	9%
regular	1 cup	1.5	70	6%
(Kellogg's)				
All Bran				
Bran Buds	⅓ cup	0.5	80	6%
original	½ cup	1.0	80	11%
w/extra fiber	½ cup	1.0	50	18%
Apple Jacks	1 cup	–	120	–
Cocoa Frosted Flakes	¾ cup	–	120	–
Cocoa Krispies	¾ cup	1.0	120	8%
Complete				
Oat Bran Flakes	¾ cup	1.0	110	8%
Wheat Bran Flakes	¾ cup	0.5	90	5%
corn flakes	1 cup	–	100	–
Corn Pops	1 cup	–	120	–
Country Inn Specialties				
Green Gables Inn	½ cup	6.0	210	26%
Greyfield Inn	¾ cup	6.0	210	26%
Inn at Ormsby Hill	1 cup	2.0	220	8%
Cracklin Oat Bran	¾ cup	7.0	190	33%
Crispix	1 cup	–	110	–
Froot Loops				
Marshmallow blasted	1 cup	0.5	120	4%
original	1 cup	1.0	120	80%
Frosted Flakes	¾ cup	–	120	–
Healthy Choice from Kellogg's				
Almond crunch w/raisins	1 cup	2.5	210	11%
Low-fat Granola				
w/raisins	½ cup	3.0	220	12%
w/o raisins	½ cup	3.0	190	14%
Mueslix/raisin & almond crunch w/dates	⅔ cup	3.0	200	14%
Toasted Brown Sugar Squares	1 cup	1.0	190	5%
Honey Crunch corn Flakes	¾ cup	1.0	120	8%
Just Right w/fruit & nuts	1 cup	2.0	220	8%
Mini-Wheats				
apple cinnamon	¾ up	1.0	180	5%
blueberry	¾ cup	1.0	180	5%
frosted bite-size	~24 biscuits	1.0	200	5%
frosted original	~5 biscuits	1.0	180	5%
frosted raisin	¾ cup	1.0	180	5%
strawberry	¾ cup	1.0	170	5%
Product 19	1 cup	–	100	–

Food and Description	Amount	Fat Grams	Total Calories	% Fat Calories
Raisin Bran	1 cup	1.5	190	7%
Raisin Bran Crunch	1 cup	1.0	190	5%
Rice Krispies				
original	1¼ cup	–	120	–
Razzle Dazzle	¾ cup	–	110	–
Treats	¾ cup	1.5	120	11%
Smacks	¾ cup	0.5	100	5%
Smart Start	1 cup	0.5	180	3%
Special K				
original	1 cup	–	110	–
Plus	1 cup	2.0	210	9%
(Kretschmer)				
toasted wheat bran	¼ cup	1.0	30	30%
wheat germ				
honey crunch	5 tsp	1.0	50	18%
plain	2 Tbs	1.0	50	18%
(Krusteaz)				
corn flakes	1 cup	–	130	–
Crisp Rice	1 cup	–	130	–
Frosted Flakes	¾ cup	–	110	–
Fruit Whirls	¾ cup	1.0	120	8%
raisin bran	¾ cup	1.5	210	6%
Toasted Oats				
apple cinnamon	¾ cup	2.0	130	14%
honey nut	¾ cup	2.0	120	15%
original	1 cup	2.0	120	15%
Life (See (Quaker) in this section)				
(Lifestream)				
Berry granola	¾ cup	3.0	210	13%
8-Grain flakes	¾ cup	1.0	130	7%
Flax Plus	¾ cup	2.0	120	15%
Multigrain honey puffs	¾ cup	3.0	120	23%
SmartBran	½ cup	1.5	120	11%
Wild Berry Muesli	½ cup	3.0	210	13%
(Lundberg Family)				
8-Grain Flakes	¾ cup	1.0	130	7%
Berry Granola	¾ cup	3.0	210	13%
Flax Plus	¾ cup	2.0	120	15%
Multigrain Honey Puffs	¾ cup	3.0	120	23%
Smartbran	½ cup	1.5	120	9%
Wild Berry Muesli	1 cup	1.0	130	7%
Morning Traditions (See (Post) in this section)				
(Mother's)				
Cinnamon Oat crunch	2 oz	3.0	230	12%
Groovy Grahams	1 oz	0.5	100	5%
Harvest Oat Flakes				
original	1 oz	1.0	110	8%
w/apples & almonds	1 oz	1.5	120	9%
Honey Roundups	1 oz	0.5	110	4%
Toasted Oat Bran	1 oz	1.5	120	11%

Food and Description	Amount	Fat Grams	Total Calories	% Fat Calories
Peanut Butter Bumpers	1 oz	2.5	130	17%
(Nabisco)				
100 % Bran Cereal	⅓ cup	0.5	80	6%
Shredded Wheat				
bite size				
frosted	1 cup	1.0	190	5%
Honey-Nut	1 cup	2.0	200	9%
original				
regular	2 biscuits	0.5	160	3%
spoon size	1 cup	0.5	170	3%
wheat 'n Bran	1¼ cups	1.0	200	5%
Nature Valley (*See* (General Mills) in this section)				
(Nature's Path)				
Fruit Juice Corn Flakes	¾ cup	1.0	115	8%
Heritage Flakes	¾ cup	–	120	–
Heritage O's	¾ cup	–	115	–
Honey'd				
corn flakes	¾ cup	–	115	–
raisin bran	¾ cup	–	110	–
Millet Rice	¾ cup	2.0	120	15%
Muesli				
blueberry	½ cup	6.0	220	25%
Sunrise	½ cup	2.0	120	15%
tropical	½ cup	5.0	215	21%
Multigrain Flakes	⅔ cup	–	110	–
Multigrain & Raisin	⅔ cup	2.0	120	15%
(Nectar Sweet)				
granola				
blueberry 'n cream	⅓ cup	4.0	110	33%
raspberry 'n cream	⅓ cup	4.0	110	33%
strawberry 'n cream	⅓ cup	4.0	110	33%
Crunch Oat Bran	⅓ cup	5.0	110	41%
(Pacific Grain)				
Nutty Corn	¾ cup	10.0	220	41%
Nutty Wheat	¾ cup	5.0	220	20%
(Pillsbury) Heartland				
coconut	1 oz	5.0	130	35%
plain	1 oz	4.0	130	28%
w/raisins	1 oz	4.0	130	28%
(Post)				
Alpha-Bits				
original	1 cup	1.5	130	10%
w/marshmallows	1 cup	1.0	120	7%
Bran flakes	¾ cup	0.5	100	5%
Cocoa Pebbles	¾ cup	1.0	120	8%
Crispy Critters	1⅓ cup	–	120	–
Fruit & Fibre				
dates/raisins/walnuts	1 cup	3.0	210	13%
peaches/raisins/almonds	1 cup	3.0	210	13%
Fruity Pebbles	¾ cup	1.0	110	8%

Food and Description	Amount	Fat Grams	Total Calories	% Fat Calories
Golden Crisp	¾ cup	–	110	–
Grape-Nuts				
flakes	¾ cup	1.0	100	9%
original	½ cup	1.0	200	5%
Honey Bunches of Oats				
honey roasted	¾ cup	1.5	120	11%
w/almonds	¾ cup	3.0	130	21%
Honeycomb	1⅓ cup	0.5	110	4%
Morning Traditions				
Banana Nut Crunch	1 cup	6.0	250	22%
Blueberry Morning	1¼ cups	3.0	220	12%
Cranberry Almond Crunch	1 cup	3.0	220	12%
Great Grains				
crunchy pecan	⅔ cup	6.0	220	25%
raisins, dates, & pecans	⅔ cup	5.0	210	21%
Post Toasties	1 cup	–	100	–
Raisin bran	1 cup	1.0	190	5%
Waffle Crisp	1 cup	3.0	130	21%
Product 19 (See (Kellogg's) in this section)				
(Quaker)				
Apple Zaps	1 cup	1.0	120	8%
Bran/Unprocessed	⅓ cup	0.5	35	13%
Cinnamon Crunch	1 cup	2.0	120	15%
Cap'n Crunch				
Crunchberries	¾ cup	1.5	100	14%
Oops! All Berries	1 cup	1.5	130	10%
peanut butter	¾ cup	2.5	110	20%
regular	¾ cup	1.5	110	12%
Cocoa Blasts	1 cup	1.0	130	7%
Crispy Corn Puffs	1 cup	1.0	110	8%
Crunchy Corn bran	¾ cup	1.0	90	10%
Frosted				
Flakes	¾ cup	–	120	–
Oats	1 cup	1.5	110	12%
Fruitangy Oh's	1 cup	1.0	120	8%
Honey Crisp Corn Flakes	¾ cup	–	110	–
Honey Dipps	1¼ cup	1.5	130	10%
Honey Graham Oh's	¾ cup	1.5	110	12%
Honey Nut Oats	¾ cup	1.0	110	8%
King Vitaman	1½ cups	1.0	120	8%
Life				
cinnamon	¾ cup	1.0	120	8%
plain	¾ cup	1.5	120	11%
Marshmallow Safari	¾ cup	2.0	140	13%
Oat Bran High Fiber	1¼ cups	3.0	210	13%
Oat Squares				
cinnamon	1 cup	2.5	230	10%
original	1 cup	3.0	220	12%
100% Natural Granola				
low-fat w/raisins	1⅔ cup	3.0	210	13%

Food and Description	Amount	Fat Grams	Total Calories	% Fat Calories
regular				
oats & honey	½ cup	9.0	220	37%
w/raisins	½ cup	9.0	230	35%
Popeye Puffed				
rice	1¼ cups	–	50	–
wheat	1¼ cups	–	50	–
Quisp	1 cup	1.5	110	12%
Rice Crisps	1 cup	–	110	–
Shredded Wheat				
frosted	1 cup	1.0	190	5%
original	3 biscuits	1.5	220	6%
Sugar Frosted Flakes	¾ cup	–	110	–
Sweet Crunch	1 cup	1.5	110	12%
Sweet Puffs	1 cup	1.0	130	7%
Toasted Oatmeal				
Honey Nut	1 cup	2.5	190	12%
original	1 cup	2.5	190	12%
Toasted Oatmeal Squares				
cinnamon	1 cup	2.5	210	11%
original	1 cup	2.5	230	10%
Toasted Oats	1 cup	1.5	110	12%
U.S. Soccer Golden Goals	1 cup	1.0	110	8%
(Quinoa) quinoa flakes	⅓ cup	1.0	105	9%
(Ralston)				
Almond Delight	1 cup	3.0	210	13%
Bran Flakes	¾ cup	1.0	110	8%
Chex Multi-Bran	1¼ cups	2.0	220	8%
Cocoa Crispy Rice	1 cup	1.0	200	5%
Cocoa Crunchies	¾ cup	1.0	120	8%
Cookie Crisp/chocolate chip	1 cup	1.5	120	11%
Corn Bran	1 cup	2.0	120	15%
Corn Flakes	1¼ cups	–	120	–
Crisp Crunch	¾ cup	1.0	120	8%
Crisp Rice	1¼ cups	–	130	–
Frosted Flakes	¾ cup	–	120	–
Fruit Rings	¾ cup	1.0	100	9%
fruit muesli				
blueberry pecan	1 cup	3.0	200	14%
cranberry walnut	¾ cup	3.0	200	14%
peach pecan	¾ cup	3.0	200	14%
raspberry almond	¾ cup	3.0	200	14%
strawberry pecan	1 cup	3.0	200	14%
Nutty Nuggets	½ cup	2.0	180	10%
Raisin Bran	¾ cup	1.0	190	5%
Spiderman	1 cup	–	120	–
Sun Flakes	¾ cup	1.0	110	8%
Tasteeos				
apple cinnamon	1 cup	2.0	130	14%
honey nut	1 cup	2.0	130	14%
original	1¼ cups	3.0	130	21%

Food and Description	Amount	Fat Grams	Total Calories	% Fat Calories
Wheat Chex/100% whole wheat	¾ cup	1.0	190	5%
Rice Krispies (*See* (Kellogg's) in this section)				
Special K (*See* (Kellogg's) in this section)				
(Sunbelt)				
five whole grains muesli	½ cup	2.0	210	9%
granola				
banana nut	½ cup	9.0	250	32%
berry basic	½ cup	6.0	220	25%
fruit & nut	½ cup	7.0	240	26%
low-fat cinnamon raisin	½ cup	3.0	200	14%
(S.W. Graham)				
cinnamon	½ cup	–	100	–
plain	½ cup	–	100	–
Total (*See* (General Mills) in this section)				
(U.S. Mills) Uncle Sam	1 cup	1.0	110	8%
(Weetabix) whole wheat	2 biscuits	<1.0	100	5%
Wheaties (*See* (General Mills) in this section)				

■ HOT/COOKED

(NOTE: All cereals are either dry or prepared with water per directions on packaging. If milk is used, calorie and fat content increase accordingly. Data on milk are shown in the Quick Reference on page 155. For additional information on milk, see MILK.)

Food and Description	Amount	Fat Grams	Total Calories	% Fat Calories
(Arrowhead Mills) Dry				
Bear Mush	¼ cup	1.0	160	6%
Bits of Barley	⅓ cup	1.0	140	6%
bulgur	¼ cup	0.5	150	3%
corn grits				
white	¼ cup	–	140	–
yellow	¼ cup	–	130	–
couscous	¼ cup	–	170	–
cracked wheat	¼ cup	0.5	140	3%
4 grain plus flax	¼ cup	2.0	150	12%
oat bran	⅓ cup	2.5	150	16%
oats/oatmeal				
instant				
cinnamon raisin almond	1 pkg	2.0	130	14%
maple apple	1 pkg	2.0	130	14%
regular	1 pkg	2.0	110	16%
regular/steel-cut	¼ cup	3.0	170	16%
Rice & Shine	¼ cup	1.0	150	6%
rolled wheat flakes	¼ cup	0.5	110	4%
seven-grain cereal				
regular	⅓ cup	1.5	140	10%
wheat-free	¼ cup	1.5	120	11%
wheat bran	¼ cup	1.0	35	26%
wheat germ/raw	3 Tbs	1.5	50	27%
(Erewhon)				
Barley Plus	1 serving	1.0	110	8%
cream of brown rice/prepared	1 cup	1.0	170	5%
oat bran w/toasted wheat germ	1 oz	2.0	115	16%

Food and Description	Amount	Fat Grams	Total Calories	% Fat Calories
oatmeal/instant dry				
apple cinnamon	1 pkg	2.0	130	14%
apple raisin	1 pkg	2.0	140	13%
dates & walnuts	1 pkg	2.5	130	17%
maple spice	1 pkg	2.0	130	14%
raisins dates & nuts	1 pkg	2.5	130	17%
w/added oat bran	1 pkg	3.0	125	22%
(Fantastic Foods) cereal cup/dry				
banana nut barley	1.6 oz	2.5	170	13%
hearty grains w/apricots	2.3 oz	2.5	240	9%
maple raisin 3 grain	1.8 oz	1.0	180	5%
oatmeal				
apple cinnamon	1.7 oz	2.0	170	11%
cranberry orange	1.7 oz	2.0	180	10%
wheat n' berries	1.7 oz	1.0	170	5%
(General Mills) Wheat Hearts/dry	¼ cup	1.0	130	7%
generic				
farina				
cooked	½ cup	–	57	–
	1 cup	–	116	–
dry	3 tbs	<1.0	105	1%
oatmeal/regular				
cooked	4 oz	1.0	70	13%
	1 cup	2.0	145	12%
dry	1 oz	1.8	109	15%
(Highspire)				
Maltex	⅓ cup	0.5	170	3%
Wheatena	⅓ cup	1.0	150	6%
(H-O) oatmeal				
instant/dry				
apple cinnamon	1 pkg	2.0	130	14%
maple & brown sugar	1 pkg	2.0	160	11%
oats 'n fiber				
apple & bran	1 pkg	2.0	130	14%
plain	1 pkg	2.0	110	16%
raisin & bran	1 pkg	2.0	150	12%
plain	1 pkg	2.0	110	16%
raisins & spice	1 pkg	2.0	150	12%
sweet 'n mellow	1 pkg	2.0	150	12%
regular				
gourmet	⅓ cup	2.0	100	18%
quick	½ cup	2.0	130	14%
(Holden Foods) farina	3 Tbs	–	100	–
(Krusteaz)/dry				
Grain Gourmet Cracked Wheat Bulgur	¼ cup	0.5	150	3%
Zoom	⅓ cup	0.5	120	4%
(Lundberg Family)				
hot 'n creamy rice cereal/prepared				
plain	1 serving	1.0	110	8%
w/almonds & nuts	1 serving	1.0	110	8%

Food and Description	Amount	Fat Grams	Total Calories	% Fat Calories
(Malt-O-Meal)				
maple brown sugar	1 serving	–	100	–
plain or chocolate	1 serving	–	120	–
plus 40% oat bran	1 serving	2.0	130	14%
(Maypo)				
instant maple	½ cup	2.0	190	9%
Vermont style	⅓ cup	2.0	150	12%
(Mother's)				
multigrain/dry	½ cup	1.5	130	10%
oat bran/dry	½ cup	3.0	150	18%
oatmeal/instant/dry	½ cup	3.0	150	18%
whole wheat hot natural cereal	1 serving	1.0	130	7%
(Nabisco)				
Cream of Rice/instant/dry	¼ cup	–	170	–
Cream of Wheat/dry				
Cook & Eat				
1-minute	3 Tbs	–	120	–
2-minute	3 Tbs	–	120	–
10-minute	3 Tbs	–	120	–
instant	¼ cup	1.5	150	3%
	1 pkg	–	100	–
Mix & Eat/prepared				
apple cinnamon	1 serving	–	130	–
banana nut	1 serving	1.5	150	9%
blueberry	1 serving	1.0	140	6%
brown sugar/cinnamon	1 serving	–	130	–
maple/brown sugar	1 serving	–	130	–
original	1 serving	–	100	–
raspberry	1 serving	1.5	140	10%
quick	3 Tbs	–	120	–
regular	3 Tbs	–	120	–
(Nature's Path) Dry				
apple cinnamon	1 pkg	2.0	190	9%
apple cranberry	1 pkg	1.0	190	9%
flax'n oats	1 pkg	4.0	200	18%
heritage raspberry	1 pkg	1.4	190	7%
maple nut	1 pkg	4.0	200	18%
multigrain raisin spice	1 pkg	1.3	180	7%
(Pritikin) hearty hot cereal				
apple raisin spice	1 pkg	3.0	170	16%
multigrain	1 pkg	2.0	160	11%
(Quaker)				
oat bran	½ cup	3.0	150	18%
oatmeal				
instant				
apple & cinnamon	1 pkg	1.5	130	8%
bananas & cream	1 pkg	2.5	140	16%
blueberries & cream	1 pkg	2.5	140	16%
chocolate chip cookie	1 pkg	2.5	160	14%
cinnamon & spice	1 pkg	2.0	170	11%

Food and Description	Amount	Fat Grams	Total Calories	% Fat Calories
cookies'n cream	1 pkg	3.0	160	17%
dinosaur eggs-brown sugar cinnamon	1 pkg	4.0	200	18%
maple & brown sugar	1 pkg	2.0	160	12%
peaches & cream	1 pkg	2.5	140	16%
regular	1 pkg	2.0	100	18%
raisins, dates, & walnuts	1 pkg	2.5	140	16%
s'mores	1 pkg	2.5	160	14%
strawberries & cream	1 pkg	2.5	140	16%
Quick 'N Hearty Microwave				
apple spice	1 pkg	2.0	170	11%
brown sugar cinnamon	1 pkg	2.0	150	12%
cinnamon double raisin	1 pkg	2.0	170	11%
honey bran	1 pkg	2.0	150	12%
regular	1 pkg	2.0	110	16%
oats				
old-fashioned	½ cup	3.0	150	18%
quick-cooking	½ cup	3.0	150	18%
steel cut	¼ cup	2.5	150	15%
multigrain	½ cup	1.5	130	10%
Whole Wheat Natural Cereal	½ cup	1.0	130	7%
(Ralston) 100% milled wheat cereal	½ cup	1.0	150	6%
(Roman Meal) Dry				
cream of rye	⅓ cup	1.0	110	8%
granola	½ cup	8.0	240	30%
oatmeal/instant				
hearty				
apple cinnamon	⅓ cup	1.0	120	8%
raisins, dates, & almonds	⅓ cup	2.0	130	14%
original	⅓ cup	1.0	110	8%
(Skinners) oat bran	1 serving	2.0	110	16%
(Stone-Buhr)				
4 grain cereal mates	⅓ cup	2.0	140	13%
7-grain cereal	⅓ cup	2.0	140	13%
oat bran	⅓ cup	2.0	90	20%
oats				
rolled old fashion	¼ cup	3.0	150	16%
Scotch	¼ cup	4.0	150	24%
CEREAL BAR (See GRANOLA/GRANOLA-TYPE BAR)				
CERVELAT (See SAUSAGE)				
CHAMPAGNE (See WINE)				
CHARD				
fresh				
cooked	½ cup	–	18	–
raw/chopped	½ cup	–	3	–
frozen				
(C&W) Swiss	3.3 oz	–	20	–
CHARLOTTE RUSSE				
w/lady fingers & whipped cream filling	4 oz	16.6	326	46%

Food and Description	Amount	Fat Grams	Total Calories	% Fat Calories
CHAYOTE /fresh				
boiled	½ cup	–	19	–
raw/whole	1 medium	–	56	–
CHEESE (*See also* CHEESE ALTERNATIVE/IMITATION; CHEESE SPREAD; COTTAGE CHEESE; CREAM CHEESE)				
■ **(Alouette)**				
Baby Brie				
plain	1 oz	9.0	110	74%
w/herbs	1 oz	9.0	110	74%
Baby Swiss				
light	1 oz	6.0	90	60%
regular	1 oz	8.0	110	65%
smoked	1 oz	8.0	110	65%
Montrachet	1 oz	6.0	70	77%
New Holland	1 oz	7.0	90	70%
Saladena				
blue cheese crumbles	¼ cup	9.0	100	81%
feta				
Mediterranean	¼ cup	6.0	90	60%
plain	¼ cup	7.0	90	70%
southwestern crumbles	¼ cup	7.0	90	70%
goat				
plain	¼ cup	6.0	80	68%
Provencal	¼ cup	6.0	80	68%
■ **(Alpine Lace)**				
American/white & yellow				
fat-free	1 oz	–	45	–
reduced-fat	1 oz	6.0	80	68%
cheddar				
fat-free	1 oz	–	45	–
reduced fat	1 oz	4.5	70	58%
Colby/reduced fat	1 oz	5.0	80	56%
Feta/reduced-fat				
plain	1 oz	3.0	50	54%
w/sundried tomato & basil	1 oz	3.0	50	54%
garlic & herb/fat-free	1 oz	–	40	–
goat/reduced-fat	1 oz	3.0	40	68%
Havarti/reduced fat	1 oz	8.0	90	80%
hot pepper/reduced-fat	1 oz	6.0	80	68%
Mexican nacho/fat-free	1 oz	–	40	–
Monterey Jack/reduced fat	1 oz	4.5	70	58%
mozzarella				
fat-free	1 oz	–	45	–
reduced-fat	1 oz	3.0	70	39%
Muenster/reduced sodium	1 oz	9.0	100	81%
Parmesan/fat-free	2 tsp	–	10	–
provolone/reduced fat	1 oz	5.0	70	64%
Swiss/reduced fat				
baby	1 oz	6.0	90	60%
regular	1 oz	6.0	90	60%

Food and Description	Amount	Fat Grams	Total Calories	% Fat Calories
■ (Athenos)				
feta/crumbled				
basil & tomato	1 oz	6.0	80	68%
traditional	1 oz	6.0	80	68%
■ BONBEL (See (Laughing Cow) in this section)				
■ (Borden)				
processed				
American				
original				
fat-free	⅔ oz	–	25	–
low-fat/light	⅔ oz	1.0	30	30%
regular	1 oz	9.0	110	74%
loaf	1 oz	9.0	110	74%
singles	1 oz	7.0	90	70%
sliced	1 slice	5.0	60	75%
salad blend/shredded	1 oz	8.0	100	72%
sharp				
fat-free	⅔ oz	–	25	–
regular	1 oz	8.0	100	72%
very sharp	1 oz	9.0	110	74%
cheddar				
Lite Line	1 oz	2.0	50	36%
sharp/block	1 oz	9.0	100	74%
mozzarella/Lite Line	1 oz	2.0	50	36%
Swiss				
cheese food	⅔ oz	5.0	70	64%
fat-free	⅔ oz	–	25	–
Lite Line	1 oz	2.0	50	36%
sliced	1 oz	8.0	100	72%
■ (Churny)				
Maybud				
Edam/reduced fat	1 oz	5.0	80	56%
farmers	1 oz	8.0	100	72%
Gouda/reduced fat	1 oz	5.0	80	56%
Lite Line	1 oz	2.0	50	36%
regular				
cheddar/diet snack	1 oz	3.0	70	39%
port wine/diet snack	1 oz	3.0	70	39%
■ (Cornville)				
Brie	1 oz	7.0	90	70%
Camembert	1 oz	7.0	90	70%
■ (County Line)				
Crackerbackers				
Colby-jack	1 oz	9.0	110	74%
mild cheddar	1 oz	9.0	110	74%
Monterey Jack	1 oz	9.0	110	74%
regular				
American/sliced	1 slice	5.0	70	64%
cheddar				
extra sharp	1 oz	10.0	120	75%

Food and Description	Amount	Fat Grams	Total Calories	% Fat Calories
finely shredded	¼ cup	10.0	120	75%
medium sharp	1 oz	10.0	120	75%
mild	1 oz	10.0	120	75%
sharp				
chunk	1 oz	10.0	120	75%
shredded	¼ cup	10.0	120	75%
Colby				
jack	1 oz	9.0	110	74%
medium sharp	1 oz	10.0	120	75%
mild				
chunk	1 oz	10.0	120	75%
sliced	1 slice	9.0	110	74%
sharp	1 oz	10.0	120	75%
Garden Jack	1 oz	9.0	110	74%
Monterey Jack	1 oz	9.0	110	74%
mozzarella				
part skim/low-moisture/finely shredded	¼ cup	5.0	80	56%
regular/chunk	1 oz	5.0	80	56%
string	1 oz	5.0	80	56%
Muenster	1 oz	9.0	110	74%
Swiss, Old World	1 oz	8.0	110	65%
taco/shredded	¼ cup	10.0	120	75%

■ **CRACKER BARREL** (*See* (Kraft) in this section)
■ **CRACKERBACKERS** (*See* (County Line) in this section)

Food and Description	Amount	Fat Grams	Total Calories	% Fat Calories
(Crystal Farms)				
American/slices	.66 oz	4.0	60	60%
cheddar				
medium super chunk	1 oz	10.0	120	75%
mild brick	1 oz	10.0	120	75%
natural cheese waves	1 oz	9.0	110	74%
shredded				
natural	1 oz	9.0	110	74%
reduced-fat	1 oz	5.0	80	56%
marble Jack/shredded natural	1 oz	9.0	110	74%
mozzarella				
shredded/natural	1 oz	6.0	80	68%
string/low-moisture part-skim	1 oz	5.0	80	56%
Parmesan/grated	2 tsp	1.5	25	54%
Swiss/slices	.66 oz	6.0	70	77%
(Di Giorno)				
Parmesan				
chunk	2 tsp	2.0	25	72%
grated	2 tsp	2.0	20	90%
shredded	2 tsp	2.0	20	90%
Romano				
chunk	2 tsp	2.0	25	72%
grated	2 tsp	2.0	25	90%
shredded	2 tsp	2.0	20	90%

Food and Description	Amount	Fat Grams	Total Calories	% Fat Calories
■ **(Dorman's)**				
natural				
blue				
Castello/70%	1 oz	12.0	135	80%
Danablu				
40%	1 oz	8.0	100	72%
60%	1 oz	10.0	110	82%
brick	1 oz	9.0	110	74%
Brie	1 oz	6.5	80	73%
Camembert/50%	1 oz	7.0	90	70%
Cheda-Jack				
reduced fat/low-sodium	1 oz	5.0	80	56%
regular	1 oz	7.0	90	70%
cheddar				
reduced fat/low sodium	1 oz	5.0	80	56%
regular	1 oz	9.0	110	74%
Colby	1 oz	9.0	110	74%
Edam	1 oz	8.0	100	72%
feta/45%	1 oz	7.0	90	70%
Gouda	1 oz	8.0	100	72%
Havarti				
45%	1 oz	7.0	90	70%
60%	1 oz	11.0	120	83%
Monterey Jack				
reduced fat/low sodium	1 oz	5.0	80	56%
regular	1 oz	8.0	100	72%
mozzarella				
part skim/low-sodium	1 oz	5.0	80	56%
reduced fat/low-sodium	1 oz	4.0	80	45%
regular	1 oz	6.0	90	60%
Muenster				
low-sodium	1 oz	9.0	110	74%
reduced fat/low-sodium	1 oz	5.0	80	56%
regular	1 oz	9.0	100	81%
Parmesan	1 oz	9.0	130	62%
provolone				
reduced fat/low-sodium	1 oz	4.0	80	45%
regular	1 oz	7.0	100	63%
Romano	1 oz	7.0	100	63%
Slim Jack	1 oz	7.0	90	70%
Swiss				
no salt added	1 oz	8.0	100	72%
reduced fat/low-sodium	1 oz	5.0	90	50%
regular	1 oz	8.0	100	72%
tybo/45%	1 oz	7.5	100	68%
■ **(Friendship)**				
farmer	2 Tbs	3.0	50	54%
hoop	2 Tbs	2.0	20	90%
■ **(Frigo)**				
natural				
asiago	1 oz	9.0	110	74%

Food and Description	Amount	Fat Grams	Total Calories	% Fat Calories
blue	1 oz	8.0	100	72%
cheddar	1 oz	9.0	110	74%
lite	1 oz	5.0	80	56%
string	1 oz	5.0	70	64%
feta	1 oz	8.0	100	72%
mozzarella				
all natural/shredded	¼ cup	6.0	80	45%
part skim/low-moisture	1 oz	5.0	80	56%
string				
light	1 oz	2.0	60	30%
regular	1 oz	6.0	80	45%
whole milk				
lite	1 oz	2.0	60	30%
regular	1 oz	7.0	90	70%
Parmazest	1 oz	7.0	120	53%
Parmesan				
chunk	1 oz	7.0	110	57%
grated	1 oz	7.0	110	57%
Parmesan & Romano				
grated	1 oz	7.0	110	57%
grated/dry	1 oz	9.0	130	62%
pizza/shredded	1 oz	3.0	65	42%
provolone/lite	1 oz	4.0	70	51%
ricotta/low-fat				
low-salt	1 oz	1.0	30	30%
part skim	1 oz	3.0	40	68%
whole milk	1 oz	5.0	60	75%
Romano				
grated	1 oz	8.0	110	65%
grated/dry	1 oz	9.0	130	62%
whole	1 oz	8.0	110	65%
Swiss	1 oz	8.0	110	65%
taco/shredded	¼ cup	9.0	110	74%
■ GENERIC				
American				
chunk	1 oz	7.0	95	66%
sliced	1 oz	7.0	95	66%
blue	1 oz	8.0	100	72%
	1 cup	38.8	477	73%
Brie	1 oz	7.9	95	74%
Camembert	1 oz	7.0	85	74%
caraway	1 oz	8.0	107	67%
cheddar				
reduced fat	1.5 oz	6.0	105	51%
shredded	1 cup	37.0	455	73%
smoky/sharp	1 oz	9.0	110	74%
Cheshire				
reduced fat	1.5 oz	6.0	110	49%
regular	1 oz	9.0	110	74%
Colby	1 oz	9.0	110	74%

Food and Description	Amount	Fat Grams	Total Calories	% Fat Calories
Edam				
reduced-fat	1.5 oz	6.0	110	49%
regular	1 oz	8.0	100	72%
feta	1 oz	6.0	75	72%
fontina	1 oz	9.0	110	74%
Gjetost	1 oz	8 0	130	55%
goat				
hard	1 oz	10.0	130	69%
semisoft	1 oz	8.0	105	69%
soft	1 oz	6.0	75	72%
Gouda	1 oz	9.0	110	74%
Gruyère	1 oz	9.0	120	68%
Havarti	1 oz	10.6	121	79%
Lancashire	1.5 oz	12.0	150	72%
Limburger	1 oz	8.0	95	76%
Monterey	1 oz	8.5	105	73%
Monterey Jack	1 oz	9.0	110	74%
mozzarella				
low-moisture	1 oz	7.0	90	70%
part skim	1 oz	5.0	80	56%
Muenster	1 oz	8.5	105	73%
Neutchatel	1 oz	7.0	80	79%
Parmesan				
grated	1 Tbs	1.5	23	59%
	1 oz	8.5	129	59%
hard	1 oz	7.0	110	57%
Port du Salut	1 oz	8.0	100	72%
provolone	1 oz	7.5	100	68%
ricotta/part skim	1 oz	3.0	42	64%
	½ cup	9.8	171	52%
Romano	1 oz	7.5	110	61%
Roquefort	1 oz	8.7	105	75%
Stilton				
blue	1.5 oz	15.0	175	77%
white	1.5 oz	14.0	155	81%
Swiss	1 oz	7.8	110	64%
Tilsit	1 oz	7.0	96	66%
yogurt	1 oz	–	20	–
■ (Healthy Choice)				
American				
white singles	¾ oz	1.0	40	23%
yellow singles	¾ oz	1.0	40	23%
	¾ oz	–	30	–
cheddar/shredded/94% fat-free	¼ cup	1.5	50	27%
Colby-Jack/94% fat-free	1 oz	1.5	50	27%
garlic & herbs/shredded 94% fat-free	¼ cup	1.5	50	27%
Italian/shredded 94% fat-free	¼ cup	1.5	50	27%
jalapeño singles/94% fat-free	¾ oz	1.0	40	23%
Mexican/shredded/shredded/94% fat-free	¼ cup	1.5	50	27%

Food and Description	Amount	Fat Grams	Total Calories	% Fat Calories
mozzarella				
shredded/94% fat-free	1 oz	1.5	50	27%
string/94% fat-free	1 oz	1.5	50	27%
pizza/94% fat-free				
shredded	1 oz	1.5	50	27%
string	1 oz	1.5	50	27%
process cheese loaf	1" cube	–	35	–
Swiss singles/94% fat-free	1 oz	1.0	40	23%
■ (Heluva Good Cheese)				
cheese food/cold pack				
cheddar				
sharp	2 Tbs	7.0	90	70%
w/bacon	2 Tbs	7.0	90	70%
w/horseradish	2 Tbs	7.0	90	70%
w/jalapeños	2 Tbs	7.0	90	70%
w/port wine	2 Tbs	7.0	90	70%
natural cheese				
cheddar				
curds snack	1 oz	9.0	115	39%
extra sharp/white or yellow	1 oz	9.0	110	74%
mild				
reduced fat/yellow	1 oz	6.0	80	68%
regular/white	1 oz	9.0	110	74%
sharp/white or yellow	1 oz	9.0	110	74%
shredded/white or yellow	¼ cup	9.0	110	74%
very low sodium/white or yellow	1 oz	9.0	110	74%
Colby	1 oz	9.0	110	74%
Colby Jack	1 oz	9.0	110	74%
curd/washed	1 oz	9.0	110	74%
Monterey Jack				
shredded	¼ cup	8.0	100	72%
w/jalapeños	1 oz	8.0	100	72%
mozzarella				
part skim/shredded	¼ cup	5.0	80	56%
whole milk	1 oz	6.0	80	68%
Swiss	1 oz	8.0	110	65%
■ (Hickory Farms)				
Neufchatel				
chocolate	1 oz	8.0	110	65%
orange	1 oz	8.0	100	72%
peach	1 oz	8.0	90	80%
pineapple	1 oz	8.0	90	80%
rum date nut	1 oz	8.0	100	72%
strawberry	1 oz	8.0	90	80%
■ (Hoffman)				
processed cheese food				
hot pepper	1 oz	7.0	90	70%
smoky sharp	1 oz	9.0	110	74%
super sharp	1 oz	9.0	110	74%

Food and Description	Amount	Fat Grams	Total Calories	% Fat Calories
■ **(Kaukauna)**				
cheese ball w/almonds & hazelnuts/cheddar				
port wine	1 oz	7.0	100	63%
sharp	1 oz	7.0	100	63%
w/bacon	1 oz	7.0	100	63%
w/green onion	1 oz	7.0	100	63%
cheese log w/almonds				
cheddar				
port wine	1 oz	7.0	100	63%
sharp				
white				
hickory smoke flavored	1 oz	7.0	100	63%
w/green onion	1 oz	7.0	100	63%
yellow	1 oz	7.0	100	63%
smoky bacon	1 oz	7.0	100	63%
Swiss	1 oz	7.0	100	63%
garden vegetable	2 Tbs	12.0	130	83%
garlic & herb	2 Tbs	12.0	130	83%
ranch	2 Tbs	12.0	130	83%
Edam	1 oz	8.0	100	72%
Gouda				
caraway seeds	1 oz	8.0	100	72%
hickory smoke	1 oz	8.0	100	72%
plain	1 oz	8.0	100	72%
Monterey Jack	1 oz	9.0	110	74%
Muenster	1 oz	9.0	110	74%
Neutchatel				
garlic & herb	1 oz	7.0	80	79%
garden vegetable	1 oz	7.0	80	79%
■ **(Kraft)**				
NATURAL CHEESES				
cheddar				
Cracker Barrel/sharp				
extra sharp	1 oz	10.0	120	75%
marbled	1 oz	9.0	110	74%
New York aged reserve	1 oz	10.0	120	75%
Reduced-fat/2% milk				
chunk/extra sharp	1 oz	6.0	90	60%
chunk/sharp	1 oz	6.0	90	60%
chunk/Vermont sharp	1 oz	6.0	90	60%
shredded	¼ cup	5.0	80	56%
regular				
sharp	1 oz	10.0	120	75%
Vermont sharp	1 oz	9.0	110	74%
extra sharp/chunk	1 oz	10.0	120	75%
Kraft Free/shredded	¼ cup	–	40	–
medium				
chunk	1 oz	9.0	110	74%
finely shredded	¼ cup	8.0	90	80%
Off The Block/chunk	1 oz	9.0	110	74%

Food and Description	Amount	Fat Grams	Total Calories	% Fat Calories
shredded	¼ cup	10.0	120	75%
mild				
marbled	1 oz	9.0	110	74%
Off The Block/chunk	1 oz	9.0	110	74%
mild/2% milk reduced-fat				
chunk	1 oz	6.0	90	60%
shredded				
finely	⅓ cup	7.0	100	63%
regular	¼ cup	6.0	80	68%
slices	1 oz	9.0	110	74%
sharp				
Off The Block/chunk	1 oz	10.0	120	75%
shredded				
finely	⅓ cup	10.0	120	75%
regular	¼ cup	9.0	110	74%
2% milk reduced-fat/shredded				
finely	⅓ cup	7.0	100	63%
regular	¼ cup	6.0	80	68%
Colby				
chunk				
⅓ less fat	1 oz	5.0	80	56%
regular	1 oz	9.0	110	74%
shredded	¼ cup	10.0	120	75%
Colby & Monterey Jack				
Off The Block/chunk	1 oz	9.0	110	74%
regular	1 oz	9.0	110	74%
shredded				
finely shredded	⅓ cup	9.0	110	74%
regular	¼ cup	8.0	100	72%
slices	1.6 oz	14.0	180	70%
2% milk reduced-fat/shredded	¼ cup	5.0	80	56%
Italian blend/grated	2 tsp	1.5	25	54%
Italian style finely shredded				
classic garlic	⅓ cup	8.0	100	72%
hearty Italian	⅓ cup	8.0	100	72%
mozzarella & Parmesan	⅓ cup	8.0	100	72%
marbled blends				
cheddar & Monterey Jack	1 oz	9.0	110	74%
cheddar & whole milk mozzarella	1 oz	8.0	100	72%
colby & Monterey Jack	1 oz	9.0	110	74%
Mexican style shredded cheeses				
cheddar and Monterey Jack				
regular	⅓ cup	10.0	120	75%
w/jalapeño peppers	⅓ cup	10.0	120	75%
four cheese	⅓ cup	10.0	120	75%
taco cheese	⅓ cup	10.0	120	75%
Monterey Jack				
Off The Block/chunk	1 oz	9.0	110	74%
plain				
⅓ less fat	1 oz	5.0	80	56%

Food and Description	Amount	Fat Grams	Total Calories	% Fat Calories
regular				
chunk	1 oz	9.0	110	74%
shredded	¼ cup	8.0	100	72%
w/jalapeño peppers	1 oz	9.0	110	74%
mozzarella				
Deli-Thin Slices	1 slice	5.0	80	56%
Kraft Free	¼ cup	–	45	–
Low-moisture/part skim				
chunk	1 oz	5.0	80	56%
finely shredded	¼ cup	4.5	70	58%
shredded	¼ cup	6.0	90	60%
slices	1.6 oz	8.0	130	55%
	1.5 oz	8.0	120	60%
string	1 stick	6.0	80	68%
Off The Block/chunk	1 oz	5.0	80	56%
2% milk/shredded	⅓ cup	5.0	80	56%
whole milk/shredded	⅓ cup	8.0	100	72%
Muenster	1 oz	9.0	110	74%
Parmesan				
Plus! Seasoning blend				
garlic herb	2 tsp	–	15	–
zesty red pepper	2 tsp	–	15	–
regular/100% Parmesan				
grated	2 tsp	1.5	20	68%
shredded	2 tsp	1.5	20	68%
Parmesan & Romano/grated	2 tsp	1.5	25	54%
pizza cheese/shredded				
mild cheddar & whole milk/				
low-moisture mozzarella	¼ cup	7.0	90	70%
four cheese	¼ cup	7.0	90	70%
low-moisture mozzarella				
& cheddar	⅓ cup	9.0	120	68%
low-moisture mozzarella &				
provolone, w/smoke flavor	¼ cup	7.0	90	70%
2% milk/shredded	⅓ cup	6.0	90	60%
provolone w/smoke flavor added/slices	1 oz	7.0	100	63%
	1.5 oz	11.0	150	66%
Romano/grated	2 tsp	1.5	20	68%
Swiss				
chunk	1 oz	9.0	110	74%
Cracker Barrel/baby Swiss chunk	1 oz	9.0	110	74%
Deli-Thin Slices				
aged	1 slice	7.0	90	70%
regular	1 slice	7.0	90	70%
shredded				
finely	⅓ cup	8.0	100	72%
regular	⅓ cup	8.0	110	65%
slices	¾ oz	7.0	90	70%
	1.35 oz	12.0	150	72%
	1.5 oz	13.0	170	69%
	1.6 oz	14.0	180	70%

Food and Description	Amount	Fat Grams	Total Calories	% Fat Calories
slices/aged Swiss	1.5 oz	13.0	170	69%
Topping/grated fat-free	2 tsp	–	15	–
PROCESSED CHEESE FOODS & PRODUCTS				
American				
deluxe/white or yellow				
loaf	1 oz	9.0	100	81%
sliced	⅔ oz	6.0	70	77%
	¾ oz	7.0	80	79%
	1 oz	9.0	110	74%
Light N' Lively processed cheese product/lower fat				
white	¾ oz	2.5	45	50%
yellow	¾ oz	2.5	45	50%
Old English				
loaf	1 oz	9.0	100	81%
slice	1 oz	9.0	110	74%
shredded	¼ cup	9.0	110	74%
singles/sliced				
white				
Kraft Free	⅔ oz	–	30	–
	¾ oz	–	30	–
reduced-fat	¾ oz	3.0	50	54%
regular	⅔ oz	4.5	60	68%
yellow/singles				
Kraft Free	⅔ oz	–	30	–
	¾ oz	–	30	–
reduced-fat	¾ oz	3.0	50	54%
regular	⅔ oz	4.5	60	68%
	¾ oz	5.0	70	64%
	1.2 oz	8.0	110	65%
25% less fat	¾ oz	5.0	70	64%
cheddar				
Cheddary Melts cheese foods				
loaf or chunk				
medium	1 oz	9.0	110	74%
mild	1 oz	9.0	110	74%
Shreds				
medium	¼ cup	9.0	120	68%
mild	¼ cup	9.0	120	68%
sharp/singles				
Kraft Free	¾ oz	–	30	–
⅓ less fat	¾ oz	3.0	50	54%
regular	¾ oz	6.0	70	77%
cheese food				
w/garlic	1 oz	7.0	90	70%
w/jalapeño peppers	1 oz	7.0	90	70%
Cheese Whiz (See CHEESE SPREAD (Kraft)				
Mexican style/mild slices	¾ oz	5.0	70	64%
Monterey/singles	¾ oz	5.0	70	64%
mozzarella string/Handi-Snacks	1 stick	6.0	80	68%
pimiento/sliced				
Deluxe singles	¾ oz	5.0	70	64%

Food and Description	Amount	Fat Grams	Total Calories	% Fat Calories
Singles slices	⅔ oz	4.5	60	68%
	1 oz	8.0	100	72%
Swiss				
shredded				
regular	¾ oz	5.0	70	64%
⅓ less fat	¾ oz	2.5	50	45%
singles				
Deluxe	¾ oz	6.0	70	64%
	1 oz	7.0	90	70%
Kraft Free	¾ oz	–	30	–
sliced	¾ oz	5.0	70	64%
Velveeta cheese product				
loaf				
hot Mexican	1 oz	6.0	90	60%
mild Mexican	1 oz	6.0	90	60%
plain	1 oz	6.0	90	60%
Mexican /mild shredded	¼ cup	9.0	120	68%
light	1 oz	3.0	60	45%
regular				
shredded	¼ cup	9.0	130	62%
sliced	¾ oz	4.5	60	68%
	⅘ oz	4.5	70	58%
	1.2 oz	7.0	100	63%
■ (Lake To Lake)				
American				
loaf	1 oz	9.0	110	74%
slices	1 oz	9.0	110	74%
cheddar				
extra sharp	1 oz	9.0	110	74%
medium	1 oz	9.0	110	74%
mild	1 oz	9.0	110	74%
sharp	1 oz	9.0	110	74%
cheddarella	1 oz	8.0	110	65%
Colby	1 oz	9.0	110	74%
Monterey Jack	1 oz	8.0	110	65%
mozzarella	1 oz	6.0	80	68%
Snack'N Cheeese To-Go				
cheddar				
medium	¾ oz	7.0	80	79%
mild	¾ oz	7.0	80	79%
chedarella	¾ oz	6.0	70	77%
Monterey Jack	¾ oz	7.0	80	79%
■ (Land O'Lakes)				
natural cheese				
brick	1 oz	8.0	100	72%
cheddar				
Chedarella	1 oz	8.0	100	72%
regular	1 oz	9.0	110	74%
white	1 oz	9.0	110	74%
Colby	1 oz	9.0	110	74%

Food and Description	Amount	Fat Grams	Total Calories	% Fat Calories
Monterey Jack				
hot pepper	1 oz	8.0	110	65%
plain	1 oz	8.0	110	65%
mozzarella/part skim/low-moisture	1 oz	6.0	80	68%
Muenster	1 oz	7.0	100	63%
Parmesan/grated	1 Tbs	2.5	35	64%
provolone	1 oz	8.0	100	72%
Swiss				
baby wheel				
light	1 oz	4.0	80	45%
loaf/wheel	1 oz	8.0	110	65%
regular	1 oz	8.0	110	65%
processed cheese food				
American/white & yellow				
regular	1 oz	9.0	110	74%
Sharp	1 oz	9.0	100	81%
Singles	¾ oz	4.5	60	68%
American & Swiss	1 oz	8.0	100	72%
cheddar				
& bacon	1 oz	9.0	110	74%
extra sharp	1 oz	9.0	100	81%
La Chedda	1 oz	7.0	90	70%
Italian herb	1 oz	7.0	90	70%
jalapeño	1 oz	7.0	90	70%
jalapeño jack onion	1 oz	8.0	90	80%
pepperoni	1 oz	7.0	90	70%
salami	1 oz	7.0	90	70%
■ (Laughing Cow)				
natural cheese				
Babybel				
mini	1 piece	6.0	70	77%
mini light	1 piece	3.0	45	60%
regular	1 oz	7.0	90	70%
Bonbel				
mini	1 piece	6.0	70	77%
regular	1 oz	8.0	100	72%
Bonbino	1 oz	9.0	100	81%
Edam	1 oz	8.0	100	72%
Gouda				
mini	1 piece	6.0	80	68%
regular	1 oz	9.0	110	74%
processed cheese food				
cheesebits	6 pieces	6.0	70	77%
wedges				
assorted	1 oz	6.0	70	77%
light	1 oz	3.0	50	54%
original	1 oz	6.0	70	77%
■ (Lifetime)				
Fat-Free				
cheddar	1 oz	–	40	–
garden vegetable	1 oz	–	40	–

Food and Description	Amount	Fat Grams	Total Calories	% Fat Calories
Mexican/mild	1 oz	–	40	–
Monterey Jack	1 oz	–	40	–
mozzarella	1 oz	–	40	–
Swiss	1 oz	–	40	–
■ LIGHT N' LIVELY (See (Kraft) in this section)				
■ (Montrachet)				
goatcheese				
bulk	1 oz	6.0	70	77%
chive	1 oz	6.0	70	77%
classic	1 oz	6.0	70	77%
herb	1 oz	6.0	70	77%
herbs & garlic	1 oz	6.0	70	77%
in oil/drained	1 oz	6.0	70	77%
plain	1 oz	6.0	70	77%
w/ash	1 oz	6.0	70	77%
■ MOOTOWN SNACKERS (See (Sargento/String) in this section)				
■ (Nikos)				
Feta Cheese-crumbled/tub				
plain	1 oz	6.0	80	68%
w/tomato & basil	1 oz	8.0	100	72%
■ OLD ENGLISH (See (Kraft) in this section)				
■ (Polly-O) Processed Cheese				
mozzarella				
bite-size balls	1.5 oz	10.0	120	75%
cherry-size balls	1 oz	7.0	80	79%
shredded				
fat-free	¼ cup	–	45	–
lite	¼ cup	3.0	60	45%
part skim	¼ cup	5.0	80	56%
whole milk	¼ cup	7.0	90	70%
mozzarella w/parmesan So-Quick/ finely shredded	¼ cup	8.0	100	72%
Parmesan/grated	2 tsp	1.5	20	27%
Parmesan & Romano/grated	2 tsp	1.5	20	27%
ricotta				
fat-free	¼ cup	–	50	–
lite	¼ cup	3.0	70	39%
part skim	¼ cup	6.0	90	60%
whole milk	¼ cup	8.0	110	65%
string cheese				
mozzarella	1.oz	6.0	80	68%
w/pizza dipping sauce	1.15 oz	4.5	70	58%
Twistarellas				
regular	1.13 oz	7.0	100	63%
	¾ oz	4.0	60	60%
super long	1.5 oz	9.0	120	60%
■ (Precious)				
mozzarella/part skim	1 oz	6.0	80	68%
ricotta				
part-skim				
fat-free	¼ cup		40	–

Food and Description	Amount	Fat Grams	Total Calories	% Fat Calories
low-fat	¼ cup	3.0	60	45%
original	¼ cup	6.0	100	54%
whole milk	¼ cup	8.0	110	65%
string/part skim	1 oz	6.0	80	68%
■ (Quaker)				
pimiento loaf	2 Tbs	8.0	80	90%
relish loaf	2 Tbs	8.0	80	90%
scallion loaf	2 Tbs	9.0	90	90%
■ (Sargento)				
American/Deli-style	6.7 oz slice	6.0	70	77%
blue cheese/crumbled	¼ cup	8.0	100	72%
cheddar				
Chef Style/shredded				
mild	¼ cup	9.0	110	74%
sharp	¼ cup	9.0	110	74%
Deli-style slices				
medium	¾ oz slice	7.0	90	70%
sharp	¾ oz slice	7.0	90	70%
Fancy supreme/shredded				
Mild				
Light	¼ cup	4.5	70	58%
regular	¼ cup	9.0	110	74%
sharp	¼ cup	9.0	110	74%
sliced/regular				
medium	1 oz slice	9.0	110	74%
mild	1 oz slice	9.0	110	74%
sharp	1 oz slice	9.0	110	74%
Colby/Deli-style slices	¾ oz slice	7.0	90	70%
Colby-Jack/Fancy-shredded	¼ cup	9.0	110	74%
Homestyle Creamy Melt/4-cheese	¼ cup	9.0	110	74%
Jarlsberg/Celi-style slices	¾ oz slice	6.0	80	68%
Monterey Jack				
Deli-style/slices	¾ oz slice	6.0	80	68%
Fancy/shredded	¼ cup	9.0	110	65%
MooTown Snackers (See String in this section)				
mozzarella				
Chef Style/shredded				
low moisture part-skim	¼ cup	6.0	80	68%
whole milk	¼ cup	8.0	100	72%
Deli-style slices				
light	1 oz slice	3.5	70	45%
regular	¾ oz slice	4.0	60	60%
Fancy/shredded				
regular	¼ cup	6.0	80	68%
light	¼ cup	3.0	70	39%
whole milk/sliced	1.5 oz slice	9.0	130	62%
Muenster/sliced				
Deli-style	¾ oz slice	6.0	80	68%
regular	1 oz slice	9.0	100	81%
nacho & taco/shredded	¼ cup	9.0	110	74%

Food and Description	Amount	Fat Grams	Total Calories	% Fat Calories
Parmesan				
grated	1 Tbs	1.5	25	54%
shredded	¼ cup	7.0	110	57%
Parmesan & Romano/grated	1 Tbs	1.5	25	54%
	¼ cup	7.0	110	57%
pizza cheese/shredded				
double cheese	¼ cup	6.0	90	60%
Sicilian 5 cheese	¼ cup	7.0	100	63%
provolone/sliced				
deli style				
light	1 slice	3.0	50	54%
light/smoke flavor	1 slice	5.0	70	64%
regular	1 slice	8.0	100	72%
recipe blend				
4 cheese Mexican				
light	¼ cup	4.5	70	58%
regular	¼ cup	9.0	110	74%
6 cheese Italian				
light	¼ cup	3.5	70	45%
regular	¼ cup	7.0	90	70%
ricotta				
light	¼ cup	2.5	60	38%
old fashioned	¼ cup	6.0	90	60%
part skim	¼ cup	5.0	80	56%
Romano/shredded	¼ cup	7.0	110	57%
Salad Creations				
Angel Hair/shredded blend	¼ cup	7.0	100	63%
cheddar & Monterey Jack/diced & shredded	¼ cup	9.0	110	74%
Southwestern pepper Jack/shredded	¼ cup	9.0	110	74%
String/Mootown Snackers				
Colby-Jack	1 piece	7.0	80	79%
light				
mild cheddar	1 piece	4.0	60	60%
mozzarella	1 piece	2.5	50	45%
regular	1 piece	4.5	70	58%
twirls	1 piece	4.0	60	60%
Swiss				
preferred light/sliced	1 slice	4.0	80	45%
regular				
Deli-style				
light	1 slice	4.0	80	45%
regular	1 slice	8.0	110	65%
shredded/fancy	¼ cup	8.0	110	65%
sliced	1 slice	6.0	80	68%
wafer-thin slices	2 slices	9.0	110	74%
taco/shredded				
preferred light	¼ cup	4.5	70	58%
regular	¼ cup	9.0	110	74%

Food and Description	Amount	Fat Grams	Total Calories	% Fat Calories
■ (Smart Beat)				
processed cheese food/sliced				
American	1 slice	2.0	35	51%
low-sodium	1 slice	2.0	35	51%
sharp	1 slice	2.0	35	51%
■ VELVEETA (See (Kraft) in this section)				
■ (Weight Watchers)				
fat-free				
American/white or yellow Fat-Free				
reduced sodium	¾ oz	–	30	–
regular	¾ oz	–	30	–
cheddar				
fat-free				
sharp	¾ oz	–	30	–
white or yellow/sliced	¾ oz	–	30	–
low-fat				
mild				
low-sodium	1 oz	5.0	80	56%
regular	1 oz	5.0	80	56%
sharp	1 oz	5.0	80	56%
Parmesan/fat-free/grated	1 Tbs	–	15	–
Swiss/fat-free/sliced	¾ oz	–	30	–
■ (WisPride)				
cheese ball				
sharp cheddar w/almonds & hazelnuts	1 oz	6.0	90	60%
Swiss	1 oz	8.0	110	60%
chunk/cheddar	1 oz	8.0	110	65%
CHEESE, COTTAGE (See COTTAGE CHEESE)				
CHEESE, CREAM (See CREAM CHEESE)				
CHEESE ALTERNATIVE/IMITATION				
(Borden)				
American	⅔ oz	5.0	60	75%
	1 oz	7.0	90	70%
cheddar/shredded	1 oz	8.0	100	72%
Cheeztwo	1 oz	7.0	90	70%
Monterey Jack bland	1 oz	7.0	90	70%
mozzarella				
shredded	1 oz	7.0	90	70%
sliced	1 oz	8.0	100	72%
sandwich mate	⅔ oz	5.0	60	75%
Swiss	⅔ oz	5.0	60	75%
Taco Mate	1 oz	7.0	100	63%
(CEMAC) Nu Tofu				
fat-free				
cheddar	1 oz	–	40	–
Monterey Jack	1 oz	–	40	–
mozzarella	1 oz	–	40	–
regular				
cheddar	1 oz	4.0	40	90%
Monterey Jack	1 oz	4.0	40	90%

Food and Description	Amount	Fat Grams	Total Calories	% Fat Calories
mozzarella	1 oz	4.0	40	90%
(Dorman's) Lo-Chol				
cheddar	1 oz	7.0	100	63%
Colby	1 oz	7.0	100	63%
mozzarella	1 oz	6.0	90	60%
Muenster	1 oz	7.0	100	63%
Swiss	1 oz	7.0	100	63%
(Formagg)				
American/sliced				
Classic	1 oz	3.0	60	45%
white	.67 oz slice	4.0	60	60%
yellow	.67 oz slice	4.0	60	60%
zesty jalapeño	1 oz	3.0	60	45%
cheddar				
shredded	1 oz	3.0	60	45%
sliced	.67 oz slice	4.0	60	60%
Parmesan/grated	2 tsp	1.0	15	60%
provolone/Vintage	1 oz	3.0	60	45%
mozzarella/shredded	1 oz	3.0	60	45%
ricotta/fat-free	½ cup	–	40	–
Swiss/sliced	1 oz	3.0	60	45%
(Frigo)				
cheddar	1 oz	7.0	90	70%
mozzarella	1 oz	7.0	90	70%
(Harvest Moon) shredded				
American	¼ cup	9.0	120	68%
cheddar	¼ cup	9.0	120	68%
mozzarella	¼ cup	8.0	110	65%
(Sargento)				
cheddar/Fancy shredded	¼ cup	7.0	90	70%
mozzarella/Classic shredded	¼ cup	6.0	80	68%
(Soya Kaas) tofu				
American cheddar/mild	1 oz	5.0	70	64%
garlic & herb	1 oz	5.0	70	64%
hickory smoked cheddar	1 oz	5.0	80	56%
mozzarella				
fat-free	1 oz	–	40	–
regular	1 oz	5.0	70	64%
(Soyco) tofu				
American/sliced				
mozzarella	1 slice	3.0	50	54%
Swiss				
regular	1 slice	3.0	50	54%
veggie	1 slice	2.0	40	45%
yellow				
regular	1 slice	3.0	50	54%
veggie	1 slice	2.0	40	45%
Caesar's Italian/grated	2 tsp	0.5	15	30%
Cajun/grated	2 tsp	0.5	15	30%
Cheddar				
baked potato/grated	2 tsp	0.5	15	30%

Food and Description	Amount	Fat Grams	Total Calories	% Fat Calories
fat-free	1 oz	–	30	–
low-fat	1 oz	3.0	60	45%
jalapeño				
fat-free	1 oz	–	30	–
low-fat	1 oz	3.0	60	45%
Monterey/low-fat	1 oz	3.0	60	45%
mozzarella				
fat-free	1 oz	–	30	–
low-fat	1 oz	3.0	60	45%
veggie/sliced	1 slice	2.0	40	45%
Parmesan/grated	2 tsp	0.5	15	30%
pepper jack/veggie/sliced	1 slice	2.0	40	45%
provolone/veggie/sliced	1 slice	2.0	40	45%
Romano/grated	2 tsp	0.5	15	30%
(Soymage) tofu				
American/yellow/sliced	1 slice	–	20	–
cheddar	1 oz	–	40	–
grated cheese	2 tsp	0.5	15	30%
herb	1 oz	–	40	–
jalapeño	1 oz	–	40	–
mozzarella				
chunk	1 oz	–	40	–
sliced	1 slice	–	20	–
(Totufti) Better Than Cream Cheese				
French onion	2 Tbs	8.0	80	90%
garden vegetable	2 Tbs	8.0	80	90%
garlic & herb	2 Tbs	8.0	80	90%
ginseng & dill	2 Tbs	8.0	80	90%
herbs & chives	2 Tbs	8.0	80	90%
jalapeño	2 Tbs	8.0	80	90%
plain	2 Tbs	8.0	80	90%
smoked salmon	2 Tbs	8.0	80	90%
wildberry	2 Tbs	8.0	80	90%
(White Wave) Soy A Melt				
American/singles	1 slice	4.0	60	60%
cheddar				
fat-free	1 oz	–	40	–
regular	1 oz	5.0	80	56%
garlic	1 oz	5.0	80	56%
jalapeño Jack	1 oz	5.0	80	56%
Monterey Jack	1 oz	5.0	80	56%
mozzarella				
chunk	1 oz	5.0	80	56%
singles	¾ oz slice	4.0	60	60%

CHEESE DISH (*See* CHEESE SOUFFLÉ; FROZEN ENTRÉE/DINNER; VEGETARIAN FOODS; WELSH RAREBIT)
CHEESE SAUCE (*See* SAUCE)
CHEESE SEASONING (*See* SEASONINGS)
CHEESE SNACK (*See* SNACKS)

Food and Description	Amount	Fat Grams	Total Calories	% Fat Calories
CHEESE SOUFFLÉ				
Homemade/USDA Standard Home Recipe				
8" square	~4 oz	19.0	240	71%
CHEESE SOUP (*See* SOUP)				
CHEESE SPREAD (*See* CHEESE ALTERNATIVE/IMITATION; CREAM CHEESE)				
(Alouette)				
creme de brie				
herb	2 Tbs	8.0	90	80%
original	2 Tbs	8.0	90	80%
crème fraiche	2 Tbs	11.0	100	100%
cream cheese spread				
light				
herbs & garlic	2 Tbs	4.0	50	72%
spring vegetable	2 Tbs	4.0	50	72%
regular/Deli				
French onion melange	2 Tbs	7.0	80	79%
garlic & herbs	2 Tbs	7.0	70	90%
spinach Florentine	2 Tbs	6.0	60	90%
sundried tomato	2 Tbs	7.0	70	90%
vegetable Jardin	2 Tbs	6.0	60	90%
Elegante				
roasted peppers & olive Tapenade	2 Tbs	9.0	90	100%
sundried tomatoes & garlic	2 Tbs	9.0	100	90%
(Alpine Lace) cream cheese spread				
garden vegetable	2 Tbs	–	40	–
garlic & herb	2 Tbs	–	40	–
(Chavrie) goat cheese spread				
basil & roasted garlic	2 Tbs	4.0	50	72%
original	2 Tbs	4.0	50	72%
Cheez Whiz (*See* (Kraft) in this section)				
(Fleur de Lait)				
Light				
crunchy garden vegetable	2 Tbs	4.5	60	68%
Mediterranean Olive	2 Tbs	4.5	60	68%
nacho chipotle	2 Tbs	4.5	60	68%
red ripe strawberry	2 Tbs	4.5	70	58%
Vidalia sweet onion	2 Tbs	4.5	60	68%
Neufchatel spread				
Bermuda onion	2 Tbs	8.0	90	80%
date nut rum	2 Tbs	8.0	90	80%
garden vegetable	2 Tbs	8.0	80	90%
garlic & spice	2 Tbs	9.0	90	90%
herb & spice	2 Tbs	9.0	90	90%
lemon	2 Tbs	7.0	90	70%
lox/smoked salmon	2 Tbs	8.0	90	80%
mandarin orange	2 Tbs	7.0	90	70%
peach	2 Tbs	7.0	90	70%
pineapple	2 Tbs	8.0	90	80%
strawberry	2 Tbs	8.0	90	80%

Food and Description	Amount	Fat Grams	Total Calories	% Fat Calories
toasted onion	2 Tbs	9.0	90	90%
wildberry	2 Tbs	7.0	90	70%
generic				
American cheese spread	2 Tbs	6.0	80	68%
(Kaukauna)				
cheese spread log/ sharp cheddar w/almonds				
& hazelnuts	1 oz	7.0	100	63%
Cold Pack Cups				
lite 50				
port wine	2 Tbs	3.5	70	45%
sharp cheddar	2 Tbs	3.5	70	45%
smoky bacon	2 Tbs	3.5	70	45%
Swiss w/almonds	2 Tbs	3.5	70	45%
original				
cheddar	2 Tbs	7.0	90	70%
bacon & horseradish	2 Tbs	7.0	100	63%
port wine	2 Tbs	7.0	90	70%
sharp	2 Tbs	7.0	90	70%
smoky sharp	2 Tbs	7.0	90	70%
(Kraft)				
Cheez Whiz				
jarred				
light	2 Tbs	3.0	80	34%
original	2 Tbs	8.0	100	72%
sauce				
jalapeño pepper	2 Tbs	7.0	90	70%
mild salsa	2 Tbs	7.0	100	63%
plain	2 Tbs	7.0	90	70%
spread				
original	2 Tbs	7.0	90	70%
salsa				
hot	2 Tbs	7.0	90	70%
mild	2 Tbs	7.0	90	70%
w/jalapeño peppers	2 Tbs	8.0	90	80%
squeezable/plain	2 Tbs	8.0	100	72%
Cracker Barrel whipped spreadables/cheddar & cream cheese				
extra sharp cheddar	2 Tbs	8.0	80	90%
sharp cheddar	2 Tbs	8.0	80	90%
sharp cheddar w/herbs	2 Tbs	8.0	80	90%
Old English brand				
sharp spread	2 Tbs	8.0	90	80%
regular Kraft jarred spreads				
bacon	2 Tbs	8.0	90	80%
jalapeño pepper loaf	1 oz	6.0	80	68%
olive & pimiento	2 Tbs	6.0	70	77%
pimiento	2 Tbs	6.0	80	68%
pineapple	2 Tbs	5.0	70	64%
Roka/blue cheese spread	2 Tbs	7.0	80	79%
Velveeta spread/Mexican				
hot	1 oz	6.0	90	60%

Food and Description	Amount	Fat Grams	Total Calories	% Fat Calories
mild	1 oz	6.0	90	60%
original	1 oz	6.0	90	60%
(Land O'Lakes) Golden Velvet	1 oz	6.0	80	68%
(Laughing Cow) Spreadable cheeses				
Babybel/mini spreadable				
cheddar	1 oz	5.0	70	64%
original	1 oz	6.0	70	77%
Original spreadable				
light	1 oz	2.0	30	60%
regular	1 oz	4.0	50	72%
(Merkts)				
almond Swiss	2 Tbs	8.0	100	72%
garlic herb	2 Tbs	8.0	100	72%
port wine	2 Tbs	8.0	100	72%
cheddar/sharp	2 Tbs	8.0	100	72%
(Nabisco) Easy Cheese spread				
American	2 Tbs	7.0	100	63%
cheddar				
regular	2 Tbs	7.0	100	63%
sharp	2 Tbs	7.0	100	63%
cheddar 'n bacon	2 Tbs	7.0	100	63%
nacho	2 Tbs	7.0	100	63%
(New Holland)				
garlic	1 oz	7.0	90	70%
jalapeño	1 oz	6.0	80	68%
natural vegetable	1 oz	6.0	80	68%
plain	1 oz	7.0	90	70%
Roka (See (Kraft) in this section)				
(Rondele)				
Deli-cups				
garden vegetable	2 Tbs	9.0	90	90%
garlic & herb				
lite	2 Tbs	5.0	70	64%
original	2 Tbs	9.0	100	81%
roasted garlic & aritchoke	2 Tbs	10.0	100	90%
vidalia onion	2 Tbs	9.0	100	90%
Gourmet Wheel				
Four pepper	2 Tbs	9.0	90	90%
Mediterranean	2 Tbs	9.0	100	81%
Snack Pack garlic & herb	2 Tbs	9.0	100	81%
Velveeta (See (Kraft) in this section)				
(Wispride)				
cheese spread				
ball	1 oz	6.0	90	60%
log	1 oz	6.0	90	60%
port wine				
lite	2 Tbs	3.5	70	45%
regular	2 Tbs	7.0	90	70%
sharp cheddar				
lite	2 Tbs	3.5	70	45%
regular	2 Tbs	7.0	90	70%

Food and Description	Amount	Fat Grams	Total Calories	% Fat Calories
CHEESE SUBSTITUTE (*See* CHEESE ALTERNATIVE/IMITATION)				
CHERIMOYA				
raw/whole/medium	2 lbs	2.0	515	3%
CHERRY				
candied				
generic				
sweet	1 oz	<1.0	96	5%
whole	10 medium	<1.0	119	4%
(S&W)				
glacé cherries/green or red	5 pieces	–	80	–
canned or jarred				
(Del Monte)				
dark/pitted/in heavy syrup	½ cup	–	100	–
generic				
maraschino				
drained	1 large	–	10	–
	10 large	–	97	–
w/liquid	1 oz	–	33	–
sour red				
in extra heavy syrup	1 cup	<1.0	296	2%
in heavy syrup	1 cup	<1.0	232	2%
in light syrup	1 cup	<1.0	188	2%
in water	1 cup	<1.0	87	5%
sweet				
in extra heavy syrup	1 cup	<1.0	266	2%
in heavy syrup	1 cup	<1.0	213	2%
in juice	1 cup	<1.0	136	3%
in light syrup	1 cup	<1.0	170	3%
in water	1 cup	<1.0	114	4%
(S&W)				
dark sweet/pitted/in heavy syrup	½ cup	–	140	–
maraschino/green or red	1 cherry	–	10	–
royal Anne/light/sweet/pitted	½ cup	–	140	–
dried				
(Chukar)				
Bing	2 oz	1.0	160	6%
Rainier	2 oz	1.0	160	6%
tart	2 oz	–	170	–
tart 'n sweet	2 oz	–	180	–
(Traverse Bay) cherry snax/red tart	1 oz	–	100	–
fresh				
sour red	1 cup	<1.0	51	9%
sweet	10 medium	0.7	49	13%
	1 cup	1.0	103	9%
(Dole)	1 cup	1.0	90	10%
frozen				
(Big Valley) dark sweet	½ cup	–	60	–
generic				
sour red				
sweetened	1 cup	0.7	224	3%

Food and Description	Amount	Fat Grams	Total Calories	% Fat Calories
unsweetened	3.5 oz	<1.0	50	3%
	1 cup	0.7	72	9%
sweet				
sweetened	1 cup	<1.0	232	2%
unsweetened	3.5 oz	<1.0	60	8%
CHERRY DRINK (*See also* FRUIT PUNCH; SOFT DRINK MIX)				
bottled				
(Betty Crocker) Squeezit/ Chucklin Cherry	6.76 fl oz	–	110	–
frozen				
(Welch's) Welchade	8 fl oz	–	130	–
CHERRY JUICE/JUICE BLEND/JUICE DRINK				
bottled, boxed, or canned				
(Capri Sun) wild cherry	6.75 fl oz	–	110	–
(Dole) mountain cherry	8 fl oz	–	120	–
(Hi-C)				
drink box	8.45 fl oz	–	140	–
pet	8 fl oz	–	130	–
(Libby's) Juicy Juice	8 fl oz	–	140	–
frozen/prepared				
(Dole) mountain cherry	8 fl oz	–	140	–
	10 fl oz	–	150	–
CHERVIL				
dried	1 tsp	–	1	
raw	4 oz	–	65	
CHESTNUT				
Chinese				
boiled or steamed	1 oz	–	44	–
dried	1 oz	0.5	103	4%
roasted	1 oz	–	68	–
European				
boiled or steamed	1 oz	–	37	–
dried	1 oz	1.0	106	8%
roasted	1 oz	0.6	70	8%
Japanese				
boiled or steamed	1 oz	–	16	–
dried	1 oz	–	102	–
roasted	1 oz	–	57	–
CHESTNUT FLOUR (*See* FLOUR)				
CHEWING GUM (*See* GUM)				
CHICKEN (*See* LUNCHEON MEAT; VEGETARIAN FOODS)				
■ CHICKEN & CHICKEN PARTS/FRESH				
broiler/fryer				
dark meat				
meat & skin				
batter-dipped & fried	~9.5 oz	51.8	828	56%
flour-coated & fried	~6.5 oz	31.0	523	53%
roasted	~6 oz	26.0	423	55%
stewed	~6.5 oz	27.0	428	57%
meat only				
fried	~5 oz	16.0	334	43%

Food and Description	Amount	Fat Grams	Total Calories	% Fat Calories
roasted	~5 oz	13.6	286	43%
stewed	~5 oz	12.6	269	42%
giblets/organs				
giblets/chopped or diced				
flour-coated & fried	1 cup	19.5	402	44%
simmered	1 cup	6.9	228	27%
gizzard/simmered	1 oz	1.0	43	21%
	1 cup	5.0	222	20%
heart/simmered	3 oz	5.0	158	29%
	1 cup	11.5	268	39%
liver/simmered	~5 oz	7.6	219	31%
	1 cup	7.6	220	31%
half/meat & skin				
batter-dipped & fried	~1 lb	80.8	1347	54%
flour-coated & fried	~¾ lb	46.8	844	50%
roasted	~¾ lb	40.7	715	51%
stewed	~¾ lb	42.0	730	52%
light meat				
meat & skin				
batter-dipped & fried	~7 oz	29.0	520	50%
flour-coated & fried	~5 oz	15.7	320	44%
roasted	~5 oz	14.0	293	43%
stewed	~5 oz	15.0	302	45%
meat only				
fried	~5 oz	7.8	268	26%
roasted	~5 oz	6.0	242	22%
stewed	~5 oz	5.6	223	23%
parts				
backs				
meat & skin				
batter-dipped & fried	~4 oz	26.0	397	59%
flour-coated & fried	~2.5 oz	14.9	238	56%
roasted	~2 oz	11.0	159	62%
stewed	~2 oz	11.0	158	63%
meat only				
fried	~2 oz	8.9	167	48%
roasted	~1.5 oz	5.0	96	47%
stewed	~1.5 oz	4.7	88	48%
breast				
meat & skin				
batter-dipped & fried	~5 oz	18.5	364	46%
flour-coated & fried	~3.5 oz	8.7	218	36%
roasted	~3.5 oz	7.6	193	35%
stewed	~4 oz	8.0	202	36%
meat only				
fried	~3 oz	4.0	161	22%
roasted	~3 oz	3.0	142	19%
stewed	~3 oz	2.9	144	18%
drumstick				
meat & skin				
batter-dipped & fried	~2.5 oz	11.0	193	51%

Food and Description	Amount	Fat Grams	Total Calories	% Fat Calories
flour-coated & fried	~2 oz	6.7	120	50%
roasted	~2 oz	5.8	112	47%
stewed	~2 oz	6.0	116	47%
meat only				
fried	~1.5 oz	3.0	82	33%
roasted	~1.5 oz	2.0	76	24%
stewed	~1.5 oz	2.6	78	30%
leg				
meat & skin				
batter-dipped & fried	~5.5 oz	25.6	431	53%
flour-coated & fried	~4 oz	16.0	285	51%
roasted	~4 oz	15.0	265	51%
stewed	~4 oz	16.0	275	52%
meat only				
fried	~3 oz	8.8	195	40%
roasted	~3 oz	8.0	182	40%
stewed	~3.5 oz	8.0	187	39%
thigh				
meat & skin				
batter-dipped & fried	~3 oz	14.0	238	53%
flour-coated & fried	~2 oz	9.0	162	50%
roasted	~2 oz	9.6	153	56%
stewed	~2 oz	10.0	158	57%
meat only				
fried	~2 oz	5.0	113	40%
roasted	~2 oz	5.7	109	47%
stewed	~2 oz	5.0	107	42%
wing				
meat & skin				
batter-dipped & fried	~2 oz	10.7	159	61%
flour-coated & fried	~1 oz	7.0	103	61%
roasted	~1.5 oz	6.6	99	60%
stewed	~1.5 oz	6.7	100	60%
meat only				
fried	~1 oz	1.8	42	39%
roasted	~1 oz	1.7	43	36%
stewed	~1 oz	1.7	43	36%
whole/including meat, skin, giblets, & neck				
batter-dipped & fried	~2¼ lb	180.0	2987	54%
flour-coated & fried	~1½ lb	108.0	1928	50%
roasted	~1½ lb	90.0	1598	51%
stewed	~1½ lb	92.9	1625	52%
roaster/roasted				
dark meat/meat only				
chopped or diced	1 cup	12.3	250	44%
sliced	4 oz	10.0	205	44%
half/w/bones	1 lb	64.0	1070	53%
light meat/meat only				
chopped or diced	1 cup	5.7	214	24%
sliced	4 oz	4.6	175	24%
whole/meat & skin	4 oz	15.0	253	53%

Food and Description	Amount	Fat Grams	Total Calories	% Fat Calories
stewing chicken/stewed				
whole				
meat & skin	~9 oz	49.0	744	59%
meat only				
chopped or diced	1 cup	16.6	335	45%
sliced	4 oz	13.5	270	45%
meat, skin, & giblets	1½ lbs	107.0	1636	59%
dark meat/meat only				
chopped or diced	1 cup	21.0	360	53%
sliced	4 oz	17.0	295	52%
light meat/meat only				
chopped/diced	1 cup	11.2	300	34%
sliced	4 oz	9.0	240	34%
■ CHICKEN & CHICKEN PARTS/FRESH, FROZEN, OR CANNED/BRAND NAME				
(Butterball) fresh/raw				
best of the fryer	4 oz	14.0	200	63%
breast				
fillet				
seasoned				
Italian style	1 fillet	2.0	120	15%
lemon butter	1 fillet	1.0	120	8%
mesquite	1 fillet	1.0	120	8%
teriyaki	1 fillet	1.0	120	8%
thin	1 fillet	0.5	110	4%
unseasoned	1 fillet	0.5	110	4%
split				
family pack	1 breast	18.0	300	54%
skinless	1 breast	0.5	110	4%
tenders	3 tenders	–	70	–
ground	4 oz	13.0	200	59%
roasting broiler	4 oz	16.0	220	65%
thighs/family pack	1 thigh	15.0	210	64%
wings				
drummettes	3 pieces	10.0	150	60%
regular	2 wings	16.0	210	69%
(Hormel) chunk chicken				
breast of chicken				
no salt	2 oz	1.5	60	23%
regular	2 oz	1.5	60	23%
(Perdue)				
Deli/Rotisserie Heat'n Eat chicken products				
fully cooked				
breast				
nuggets, golden brown	5 nuggets	15.0	240	56%
tenderloins	3 oz piece	7.0	170	37%
nuggets, dino shaped	3 nuggets	13.0	210	56%
Kick'n Chicken				
breaded breast strips				
barbecue	3 oz	1.0	120	8%
hot & spicy	3 oz	1.0	110	8%

Food and Description	Amount	Fat Grams	Total Calories	% Fat Calories
original	3 oz	1.0	120	8%
wings				
barbecue	3 oz	12.0	200	54%
herb roasted	3 oz	13.0	190	62%
hot & spicy	3 oz	13.0	190	62%
roasted	3 oz	13.0	190	62%
teriyaki	3 oz	13.0	200	54%
Rotisserie whole fryers/roasted				
barbecue seasoned				
dark	3 oz	13.0	180	65%
white	3 oz	7.0	140	45%
Italian style				
dark	3 oz	13.0	180	65%
white	3 oz	7.0	140	45%
lemon pepper				
dark	3 oz	13.0	180	65%
white	3 oz	7.0	140	45%
plain				
dark	3 oz	13.0	180	65%
white	3 oz	7.0	140	45%
Fresh Fit'N Easy/ground chicken				
Breast				
cooked	3 oz	0.5	80	6%
raw	4 oz	0.5	100	5%
burgers				
cooked	3 oz	10.0	160	56%
raw	4 oz	11.0	170	58%
dark & white meat				
cooked	3 oz	11.0	170	58%
raw	4 oz	12.0	180	60%
Short Cuts/fully cooked				
carved breast				
honey roasted	½ cup	2.0	100	18%
Italian style	½ cup	2.5	100	23%
Lemon pepper	½ cup	2.5	100	23%
original roasted	½ cup	2.0	100	18%
southwestern seasoned	½ cup	2.5	100	23%
carved thighs/3 pepper blend	½ cup	9.0	130	62%
(Swanson) canned				
Premium chunk chicken breast	2 oz	1.0	60	15%
Mixin Chicken in broth	¼ cup	8.0	110	65%
(TastyBird Foods) frozen/raw/ready to cook				
breast fillet patty				
hoagie-shaped	3.5 oz	10.8	211	46%
regular	3.5 oz	14.0	229	55%
breast quarter/breaded	3.5 oz	11.0	192	52%
breast strip	1 oz	2.8	54	47%
breast tenderloin				
regular	3.5 oz	8.7	189	41%
spicy	3.5 oz	7.0	170	37%

Food and Description	Amount	Fat Grams	Total Calories	% Fat Calories
chicken delites	3.5 oz	19.0	252	68%
hi-pro patty	3.5 oz	19.0	252	68%
leg quarter/breaded	3.5 oz	11.7	199	53%
nuggets	3.5 oz	13.8	215	58%
(Tyson)				
FULLY-COOKED				
breast				
breaded				
chunks	6 pieces	14.0	220	57%
fillet	2 pieces	8.0	180	40%
nuggets	4 pieces	14.0	240	53%
patty	1 patty	12.0	190	57%
mesquite	1 patty	6.0	110	49%
patty tenders	3 pieces	–	100	–
tenders	5 pieces	15.0	220	61%
honey-battered	5 pieces	11.0	200	50%
microwave sandwich	1 piece	15.0	320	42%
southern fried				
fillets	2 pieces	11.0	210	47%
patty	1 piece	12.0	180	60%
strips	3 oz	1.0	90	10%
white meat chicken roll	2 oz	6.0	90	60%
Chick'n Quick Chick'n Cheddar	1 patty	14.0	220	57%
Drumsticks/hot bbq style	2 pieces	7.0	160	39%
grilled				
lemon pepper fillets	1 fillet	3.5	100	32%
chicken sandwich	1 piece	6.0	210	26%
kits				
fried rice	1 serving	6.0	440	8%
stir fry	1 serving	4.5	430	9%
Time Trimmers				
fully-cooked chicken breast				
diced	3 oz	1.0	90	10%
strips				
regular	3 oz	1.0	90	10%
Southwestern	3 oz	3.0	110	25%
Thick'n crispy patty	1 piece	14.0	200	63%
wings				
BBQ	3 pieces	13.0	200	59%
Tabasco sections	3 pieces	10.0	170	53%
teriyaki style	4 pieces	12.0	190	57%
wings on fire	3 pieces	15.0	220	61%
READY-TO-COOK				
breaded				
chicken breast tenderloins	2 pieces	9.0	180	10%
broth marinated				
boneless, skinless breast fillet	1 piece	3.5	140	23%
chicken breast fillet	1 piece	4.0	140	26%
breast tenderloin	4 pieces	1.0	110	8%
chicken drums	2 pieces	7.0	140	45%

Food and Description	Amount	Fat Grams	Total Calories	% Fat Calories
chicken thighs	1 piece	34.0	380	81%
chicken wing sections	4 pieces	18.0	240	68%
cornish game hens	4 oz	12.0	180	60%
half breast	1 piece	12.0	230	47%
nuggets	6 pieces	15.0	250	54%
(Valley Fresh) canned				
premium white	2 oz	1.0	70	13%
white & dark	2 oz	2.0	80	23%

CHICKEN ENTRÉE/DINNER (See also ASIAN FOOD; FROZEN ENTRÉE/DINNER; MEXICAN FOOD; PASTA ENTRÉE/DINNER; RICE DISH)

Food and Description	Amount	Fat Grams	Total Calories	% Fat Calories
(Banquet) frozen				
bone-in				
breast/fried	4.45 oz	26.0	410	57%
drums & thighs/fried	3 oz	18.0	260	62%
fried chicken				
country fried	3 oz	18.0	270	60%
hot & spicy	3 oz	18.0	260	62%
original	3 oz	18.0	280	58%
skinless				
honey BBQ	3 oz	13.0	230	51%
regular	3 oz	13.0	220	53%
Southern	3 oz	18.0	280	58%
Wings				
Firehouse Big	2 pieces	14.0	190	66%
honey bbq	4 pieces	28.0	380	66%
hot & spicy	4 pieces	20.0	290	62%
Smokehouse Big	2 pieces	14.0	200	63%
boneless				
nuggets				
hot 'n spicy	2.5 oz	17.0	230	67%
mozzarella cheese	6 pieces	18.0	280	58%
original	7 pieces	20.0	280	64%
Southern	5 pieces	18.0	270	60%
sweet & sour	6 pieces	18.0	320	51%
w/cheddar	2.86 oz	19.0	280	61%
patties				
fat-free breast	1 patty	4.0	100	36%
grilled honey bbq breast	1 patty	5.0	110	41%
grilled honey mustard breast	1 patty	5.0	120	38%
original	1 patty	14.0	190	66%
Southern	1 patty	13.0	190	62%
Tenders, breast				
fat-free	3 tenders	–	120	–
original	3 tenders	15.0	250	54%
Southern	3 tenders	16.0	260	55%
(Betty Crocker) Box mix				
Chicken Helper/prepared				
cheddar & broccoli	1 cup	9.0	310	26%
chicken fried rice	1 cup	8.0	260	28%
chicken & herb rice	1 cup	7.0	260	24%

Food and Description	Amount	Fat Grams	Total Calories	% Fat Calories
chicken potato au gratin	1 cup	8.0	280	26%
chicken & stuffing	1 cup	9.0	290	28%
fettuccini alfredo	1 cup	8.0	290	25%
roasted garlic	1 cup	8.0	290	25%
Skillet Chicken Helper/prepared				
Stir-fried chicken	1 cup	9.0	270	30%
(Butterball) frozen				
Breasts				
crispy baked				
Italian style	1 piece	6.0	190	19%
lemon	1 piece	7.0	200	32%
original	1 piece	6.0	180	30%
Parmesan	1 piece	7.0	200	32%
Southwestern	1 piece	6.0	170	32%
Tenders				
baked breast	3 pieces	6.0	170	32%
grilled w/sauce				
hickory smoked	4 pieces	5.0	160	28%
oriental	4 pieces	5.0	160	28%
(Country Pride) frozen				
chunks				
regular	3 oz	15.0	238	57%
Southern-fried	3 oz	20.0	276	65%
patties				
regular	3 oz	16.0	245	59%
Southern-fried	3 oz	15.0	232	58%
sticks	3 oz	14.0	233	54%
(Country Skillet) frozen				
bites	5 bites	16.0	270	53%
chunks				
original	5 pieces	18.0	270	60%
Southern-fried	5 pieces	18.0	270	60%
Fried chicken	3 oz	18.0	270	60%
nuggets	10 pieces	17.0	280	55%
patties				
original	2.5 oz	11.0	190	52%
Southern-fried	2.5 oz	12.0	190	57%
tenders, breast	3 tenders	14.0	240	53%
(Dinty Moore)				
canned/chicken stew	1 cup	11.0	220	45%
microwaveable				
American classics				
chicken & noodles	1 bowl	8.0	270	27%
chicken w/mashed potatoes	1 bowl	4.0	240	15%
microwave cup				
chicken & dumpling	1 cup	6.0	200	32%
chicken stew	1 cup	8.0	180	40%
generic/canned				
chicken à la king	~5 oz	11.7	182	58%

Food and Description	Amount	Fat Grams	Total Calories	% Fat Calories
homemade/USDA Standard Home Recipe				
chicken à la king	1 cup	34.0	468	65%
chicken cacciatore	1 cup	32.0	525	55%
chicken cordon bleu	8 oz	13.0	335	35%
chicken fricassee	1 cup	22.0	386	51%
chicken hash	1 cup	11.0	239	41%
chicken pot pie/9" dia	⅓ pie	31.0	545	51%
chicken salad	½ cup	8.0	121	60%
chicken w/noodles	1 cup	18.0	365	44%
creamed chicken	½ cup	12.0	208	52%
creole chicken/wo rice	¾ cup	3.0	137	20%
(Hormel) refrigerated				
Chicken By George				
Cajun	~4 oz	4.0	130	28%
Caribbean grill	~4 oz	4.0	150	24%
garlic & herb	~4 oz	2.5	120	19%
Italian blue cheese	~4 oz	5.0	130	35%
lemon herb	~4 oz	3.0	120	23%
lemon oregano	~4 oz	4.0	130	28%
mesquite barbeque	~4 oz	3.0	130	21%
mustard dill	~4 oz	5.0	140	32%
teriyaki	~4 oz	3.0	130	21%
tomato herb w/basil	~4 oz	5.0	140	32%
(Ozark Valley) frozen				
Mr. Dandy				
chix patty	1 patty	11.0	210	47%
nuggets	4 pieces	10.0	210	43%
tender	3 pieces	10.0	210	43%
regular				
nuggets	4 pieces	10.0	210	43%
patties	1 patty	11.0	210	47%
pie	7 oz	19.0	330	52%
(Passport Cuisine) frozen				
yakitori-skewered	3 oz	5.0	100	45%
(Schwan's) chicken/frozen/partially or fully cooked unless stated otherwise				
chicken breast				
fillet				
breaded	1 fillet	11.0	260	38%
broccoli & cheese	1 piece	15.0	240	56%
halves/roasted				
w/skin	1 piece	9.0	220	37%
w/o skin	1 piece	2.5	150	15
lemon-pepper	1 fillet	10.0	180	50%
Southern-style	1 fillet	13.0	230	51%
Diced chicken meat	3 oz	7.0	140	45%
drumstick/roasted				
w/skin	2 sticks	5.0	140	32%
w/o skin	2 sticks	3.5	110	29%
Dummies	3 pieces	17.0	240	64%

Food and Description	Amount	Fat Grams	Total Calories	% Fat Calories
meat for fajitas	½ cup	3.0	100	27%
nuggets, breaded	6 nuggets	15.0	230	59%
patties/breaded	1 patty	14.0	220	60%
strips/breaded	3 pieces	1.0	180	5%
stuffed w/asparagus & cheese	1 piece	12.0	260	42%
tenderloin/Southern-style	2 tenders	9.0	210	39%
tenders/breaded baked	2 tenders	8.0	170	42%
wings				
bar-b-que	4 pieces	11.0	170	58%
Hot	4 pieces	10.0	170	53%
(Swanson)				
Chicken/canned				
chicken & dumplings	7.5 oz	11.0	220	45%
chicken ala king	5.25 oz	11.0	220	45%
chicken stew	7.62 oz	7.0	160	39%
Chicken/frozen				
fried breast portion	4.5 oz	20.0	360	50%
nibbles	3.25 oz	19.0	300	57%
nuggets	3 oz	14.0	230	55%
pre-fried chicken parts	3.25 oz	16.0	270	53%
thighs & drumsticks	3.25 oz	18.0	290	56%
(Tyson) ready-to-cook				
chicken broccoli & cheese	1 piece	16.0	320	45%
chicken kiev	1 piece	32.0	460	63%
cordon bleu	1 piece	17.0	350	44%
stuffed chicken w/wild rice				
and mushrooms	1 piece	12.0	300	36%
(Weaver) frozen/boneless				
assorted parts				
batter-dipped	3.6 oz	18.0	290	56%
Crispy Dutch Frye	3.6 oz	18.0	290	56%
breast				
batter-dipped	4.4 oz	20.0	310	58%
Crispy Dutch Frye	4.5 oz	22.0	350	57%
breast fillet strips	3.3 oz	10.0	200	45%
breast fillets	4.5 oz	13.0	270	43%
breast patties	3 oz	11.0	205	48%
crispy light skinless chicken	2.9 oz	9.0	170	48%
croquettes				
w/½ cup gravy	½ cup	18.0	306	53%
w/o gravy	2 pieces	16.0	280	51%
drums & thighs				
batter-dipped	3 oz	14.0	210	60%
Crispy Dutch Frye	3.5 oz	19.0	290	59%
mini drums				
crispy	3 oz	12.0	210	51%
herb & spice	3 oz	11.0	200	50%
nuggets	2.6 oz	12.0	190	57%

Food and Description	Amount	Fat Grams	Total Calories	% Fat Calories
rondelet				
cheese	2.6 oz	11.0	190	52%
Italian	2.6 oz	11.0	190	52%
original	3 oz	10.0	190	47%
tenders				
honey batter	3 oz	12.0	220	49%
premium	3 oz	9.0	170	48%
wings				
batter-dipped	4 oz	28.0	400	63%
Crispy Dutch Frye	4 oz	28.0	400	63%
hot	2.7 oz	11.0	170	48%
CHICKEN SALAD (See CHICKEN ENTRÉE/DINNER)				
CHICKEN SEASONING (See SEASONINGS)				
CHICKEN SOUP (See SOUP)				
CHICKEN SUBSTITUTES (See also VEGETARIAN FOODS)				
(Harvest Direct)				
TVP Poultry				
chunks	3.5 oz	1.0	280	3%
ground	3.5 oz	1.0	280	3%
CHICKPEA/GARBANZO BEAN				
canned				
(Bush's Best)	½ cup	–	80	–
(Eden) garbanzo	½ cup	1.5	120	11%
generic	½ cup	1.0	143	6%
(Goya) Spanish style	7.5 oz	2.0	150	12%
(Green Giant)	½ cup	1.5	110	12%
(Hain)	½ cup	2.5	120	19%
(Joan of Arc)	½ cup	1.5	110	12%
(Nutradiet)	½ cup	1.0	100	9%
(Old El Paso)	½ cup	<1.0	190	2%
(Progresso)				
chickpeas	½ cup	2.5	120	19%
garbanzo beans	½ cup	1.5	110	12%
(ShariAnn's) whole	½ cup	2.0	110	16%
(S&W)				
lite/50% less salt	½ cup	1.0	110	8%
marinated	½ cup	1.0	120	8%
premium	½ cup	1.0	110	8%
(Seneca) garbanzo beans	½ cup	0.5	110	4%
dry				
boiled	½ cup	1.0	134	13%
raw	½ cup	6.0	364	15%
(Arrowhead Mills)	¼ cup	2.0	170	11%
(Bean Cuisine)	½ cup	1.0	115	8%
CHICORY /raw	8 oz	–	15	–
CHILI/CHILI BEANS (See MEXICAN FOOD)				
CHILI SAUCE (See SAUCE)				
CHINESE FOOD (See ASIAN FOOD)				

Food and Description	Amount	Fat Grams	Total Calories	% Fat Calories
CHINESE PARSLEY (*See* CILANTRO)				
CHIVES				
freeze-dried	1 Tbs	–	1	–
raw	1 Tbs	–	1	–
	¼ cup	–	2	–
CHOCOLATE (*See* BAKING BITS, CHIPS, CHUNKS, & PIECES; CANDY)				
CHOCOLATE SYRUP (*See* ICE CREAM TOPPING; MILK MIX)				
CHUB (*See* CISCO)				
CHUTNEY				
generic				
apple	1 Tbs	–	30	–
apple-cranberry	1 Tbs	–	20	–
tomato	1 Tbs	–	23	–
(Major Grey's) mango	1 Tbs	–	60	–
CIDER				
bottled or boxed				
(Alpenglow) apple/sparkling				
mulled	8 fl oz	–	110	–
regular	8 fl oz	–	110	–
generic/apple/sweet	8 fl oz	–	124	–
(Indian Summer)				
apple	8 fl oz	–	110	–
apple-cherry	8 fl oz	–	130	–
apple-cinnamon	8 fl oz	–	100	–
apple-cranberry	8 fl oz	–	130	–
apple-raspberry	8 fl oz	–	100	–
cranberry	8 fl oz	–	130	–
(Knudsen) Thirst Quencher				
cherry	8 fl oz	–	130	–
cider & spice	8 fl oz	–	120	–
(Musselman's) apple				
Lucky Leaf	6 fl oz	–	90	–
(S. Martinelli) apple/sparkling	6 fl oz	–	100	–
(TreeTop) apple	8 fl oz	–	120	–
mix				
(Alpine) apple cider drink/prepared				
original	8 fl oz	–	80	–
spiced	8 fl oz	–	80	–
sugar-free	8 fl oz	–	15	–
CILANTRO/CHINESE PARSLEY/CORIANDER LEAF				
dried	1 tsp	–	2	–
	1 Tbs	–	5	–
fresh	1 tsp	–	2	–
	1 Tbs	–	5	–
CINNAMON/ground	1 tsp	–	10	–
CISCO/CHUB				
meat only				
raw	3 oz	1.5	85	16%
smoked	2 oz	6.5	100	59%

Food and Description	Amount	Fat Grams	Total Calories	% Fat Calories
CITRON/candied				
generic	1 oz	–	89	–
(S&W)	39 pieces	–	90	–
CITRUS JUICE/JUICE DRINK (*See also* FRUIT PUNCH)				
bottled, boxed, or canned				
(Season's Best) citrus medley	8 fl oz	–	120	–
frozen or refrigerated/prepared				
(Chiquita) Citrus Twist	8 fl oz	–	120	–
CLAM (*See also* SEAFOOD ENTRÉE/DINNER)				
canned				
(Chicken of the Sea)				
chopped	2 oz	–	30	–
minced	2 oz	–	30	–
whole	2 oz	–	30	–
(Crown Prince) baby	⅓ cup	2.0	60	30%
(Doxsee) solids & liquid				
chopped	6.5 oz	0.5	100	5%
minced	6.5 oz	0.5	100	5%
(Empress) baby/whole	4 oz	1.0	60	15%
(Geisha)				
baby/whole	1.96 oz	0.5	50	9%
chopped	2.25 oz	–	30	–
minced	2.25 oz	–	30	–
generic	3 oz	1.7	125	12%
(Gorton's)				
chopped	¼ cup	–	20	–
(Progresso) minced	¼ cup	–	25	–
(S&W)				
baby				
smoked	2 oz	10.0	130	69%
whole	¼ cup	1.5	50	27%
regular				
chopped	¼ cup	–	20	–
minced	¼ cup	–	20	–
(Snow's)				
minced	6.5 oz	–	90	–
fresh				
breaded & fried	3 oz	9.0	171	47%
	20 small	21.0	380	50%
raw	3 oz	0.8	63	11%
steamed	3oz	1.7	126	12%
	20 small	1.8	133	12%
	1 cup	3.0	235	12%
frozen				
(Matlaw's) stuffed	1 clam	5.0	120	38%
(Mrs. Paul's) fried	18 pieces	12.0	250	43%
(Sea Pak) strips	5 oz	23.0	410	50%
(Singleton) strips	5 oz	13.0	300	39%
(Van De Kamp's) fried	18 pieces	12.0	250	43%

Food and Description	Amount	Fat Grams	Total Calories	% Fat Calories
CLAM CHOWDER (*See* SOUP)				
CLAM JUICE				
(Doxsee)	3 fl oz	–	4	–
(Mott's) Clamato	6 fl oz	–	90	–
CLAM SAUCE (*See* SAUCE)				
CLOVES /ground	1 tsp	–	7	–
CLUB SODA (*See* COCKTAIL MIXER; SOFT DRINK)				
COBBLER (*See* PIE & COBBLER)				
COCKTAIL SAUCE (*See* SAUCE)				
COCKTAIL (*See also* LIQUEUR; LIQUOR, DISTILLED; WINE)				
general				
Alexander	2.5 fl oz	1.8	179	9%
Bacardi	2.5 fl oz	–	118	–
black Russian	3 fl oz	–	255	–
bloody Mary	5 fl oz	–	116	–
bourbon & soda	4 fl oz	–	105	–
brandy	1 fl oz	–	75	–
daiquiri	2 fl oz	–	111	–
Gibson	2.5 fl oz	–	158	–
gimlet	2.5 fl oz	–	132	–
gin rickey	7 fl oz	–	114	–
gin & tonic	7.5 fl oz	–	171	–
gold Cadillac	4.5 fl oz	3.6	394	8%
grasshopper	2.25 fl oz	3.6	164	20%
highball	8 fl oz	–	165	–
mai tai	4.5 fl oz	–	310	–
Manhattan	2.5 fl oz	–	128	–
margarita	~3 fl oz	–	170	–
martini	2.5 fl oz	–	156	–
mini julep	10 fl oz	–	215	–
old fashioned	4 fl oz	–	180	–
piña colada				
canned	4.5 fl oz	11.0	347	29%
homemade/USDA Standard Home Recipe	4.5 fl oz	2.6	262	9%
rum/hot buttered	~9 fl oz	11.9	317	34%
screwdriver	7 fl oz	–	174	–
Singapore sling	8 fl oz	–	228	–
sloe gin fizz	8 fl oz	–	121	–
stinger	3 fl oz	–	282	–
tequila sunrise	5.5 fl oz	–	189	–
Tom Collins	7.5 fl oz	–	121	–
	10 fl oz	–	180	–
whiskey sour	3 fl oz	–	123	–
white Russian	3.5 fl oz	1.0	268	3%
COCKTAIL MIXER (*See also* SOFT DRINK; WATER; individual fruit juice listings)				
(Bacardi) frozen/prepared				
margarita	8 fl oz	–	100	–
piña colada	8 fl oz	6.0	190	28%

Food and Description	Amount	Fat Grams	Total Calories	% Fat Calories
rum runner	8 fl oz	–	140	–
strawberry daiquiri	8 fl oz	–	140	–
(Canada Dry)				
club soda				
regular	8 fl oz	–	–	–
sodium-free	8 fl oz	–	–	–
Collins	8 fl oz	–	100	–
Gingerale				
Cherry				
diet	8 fl oz	–	–	–
regular	8 fl oz	–	90	–
cranberry				
diet	8 fl oz	–	–	–
regular	8 fl oz	–	90	–
golden				
diet	8 fl oz	–	–	–
regular	8 fl oz	–	90	–
plain				
diet	8 fl oz	–	–	–
regular	8 fl oz	–	100	–
half & half	8 fl oz	–	100	–
hi-spot	8 fl oz	–	110	–
island lime	8 fl oz	–	120	–
Jamaica cola	8 fl oz	–	100	–
lemon sour	8 fl oz	–	100	–
seltzer/sparkling water	8 fl oz	–	–	–
sour mixer	8 fl oz	–	80	–
sunripe orange	8 fl oz	–	110	–
tonic water				
plain				
diet	8 fl oz	–	–	–
regular	8 fl oz	–	100	–
w/twist of lime				
diet	8 fl oz	–	–	–
regular	8 fl oz	–	100	–
vanilla cream brown	8 fl oz	–	110	–
Vichy water	8 fl oz	–	–	–
Wild cherry	8 fl oz	–	110	–
(Coco Lopez)				
cream of coconut	2 Tbs	5.0	110	41%
piña colada				
canned	3 fl oz	4.0	120	30%
jarred	3 fl oz	5.0	160	28%
generic				
grenadine	1 fl oz	–	64	–
quinine water	12 fl oz	–	142	–
Tom Collins/bottled	1 fl oz	–	42	–
whisky sour				
bottled				
mix only	2 fl oz	–	55	–

Food and Description	Amount	Fat Grams	Total Calories	% Fat Calories
prepared	3.5 fl oz	–	158	–
dry mix/mix only	1 pkg	–	64	–
(Health Valley) ginger ale	12 fl oz	1.0	153	6%
(Holland House)				
bloody Mary/bottled				
regular	4.5 fl oz	–	20	–
smooth n' spicy	1 fl oz	–	3	–
daiquiri				
raspberry/bottled	1 fl oz	–	30	–
regular/dry mix	1 pkg	–	65	–
strawberry/bottled	1 fl oz	–	31	–
mai tai				
bottled	1 fl oz	–	32	–
dry mix	1 pkg	–	64	–
Manhattan/bottled	1 fl oz	–	28	–
margarita				
regular				
bottled	1 fl oz	–	27	–
dry mix	1 pkg	–	57	–
strawberry				
bottled	1 fl oz	–	31	–
dry mix	1 pkg	–	66	–
old fashioned/bottled	1 fl oz	–	33	–
piña colada				
bottled	1 fl oz	–	33	–
dry mix	1 pkg	–	82	–
sweet & sour	1 fl oz	–	34	–
Tom Collins				
bottled	1 fl oz	–	47	–
dry mix	1 pkg	–	65	–
whisky sour				
bottled	1 fl oz	–	37	–
dry mix	1 pkg	–	64	–
(Mr. & Mrs. T) bottled				
bloody Mary				
regular	4.5 fl oz	–	20	–
rich & spicy	4.5 fl oz	–	30	–
margarita				
regular	3 fl oz	–	80	–
strawberry	3.5 fl oz	–	100	–
piña colada	4 fl oz	<1.0	150	3%
sweet & sour	3 fl oz	–	70	–
(Nehi) ginger ale	8 fl oz	–	90	–
(Roses) grenadine syrup	1 fl oz	–	65	–
(Schweppes)				
bitter lemon	8 fl oz	–	110	–
club soda				
regular	8 fl oz	–	–	–
sodium-free	8 fl oz	–	–	–
collins mixer	8 fl oz	–	90	–

Food and Description	Amount	Fat Grams	Total Calories	% Fat Calories
ginger ale				
diet	8 fl oz	–	–	–
dry grape	8 fl oz	–	90	
regular	8 fl oz	–	80	–
lemon sour	8 fl oz	–	100	–
seltzer/sparkling water	8 fl oz	–	–	–
tonic water				
citrus	8 fl oz	–	80	–
cranberry	8 fl oz	–	80	–
plain				
diet	8 fl oz	–	–	–
regular	8 fl oz	–	90	–
(Tabasco) bloody Mary	8 fl oz	–	60	–
COCOA (See also MILK MIX)				
(Baker's)	3.5 oz	13.0	220	53%
generic	⅓ cup	4.0	120	30%
	½ cup	5.0	173	26%
(Ghirardelli)				
hot chocolate mixes/prepared w/2% milk				
double chocolate	1 cup	6.0	210	36%
hazelnut	1 cup	6.0	210	36%
mocha	1 cup	6.0	210	36%
white mocha	1 cup	5.0	210	21%
sweet ground chocolate & cocoa	2.5 Tbs	1.5	80	17%
unsweetened	1 Tbs	1.5	20	68%
(Hershey)				
European	1 Tbs	0.5	20	23%
	½ cup	3.0	90	30%
Original	1 Tbs	0.5	20	23%
	⅓ cup	3.0	110	25%
(Nestlé)	1 Tbs	1.0	15	60%
(Wonderslim) low-fat	1¼ tsp	–	15	–
COCONUT				
(Baker's) Angel Flake				
canned	2 Tbs	6.0	70	77%
packaged	2 Tbs	5.0	70	64%
premium shred	2 Tbs	5.0	70	64%
(Durkee) shredded	2 Tbs	6.0	80	68%
generic				
dried				
flaked/sweetened				
canned	4 oz	36.0	505	64%
packaged	1 cup	23.8	351	61%
	4 oz	36.1	539	61%
shredded				
sweetened	4 oz	40.0	570	63%
unsweetened	1 oz	18.0	187	87%
raw/shredded	½ cup	13.4	141	86%
toasted	1 oz	13.0	168	70%

Food and Description	Amount	Fat Grams	Total Calories	% Fat Calories
COCONUT CREAM				
canned/sweetened				
(Coco Lopez)	2 Tbs	5.0	110	41%
generic	1 Tbs	3.0	36	75%
	1 cup	52.0	568	82%
raw	1 Tbs	5.0	50	18%
	1 cup	83.0	795	94%
COCONUT MILK				
canned				
(A Taste of Thai) unsweetened				
lite	¼ cup	3.0	36	75%
original	¼ cup	11.0	110	90%
generic	1 Tbs	3.0	30	90%
	1 cup	48.0	445	97%
frozen	1 Tbs	3.0	30	90%
	1 cup	50.0	486	93%
raw	1 Tbs	3.6	35	92 %
	1 cup	57.0	552	93%
COCONUT WATER	1 Tbs	–	3	–
	1 cup	0.5	46	10%
COD (*See also* COD ROE; SEAFOOD ENTRÉE/DINNER)				
Atlantic & Pacific				
breaded & fried	3 oz	9.0	175	46%
canned	3 oz	0.7	89	7%
cooked-dry heat	3 oz	0.7	89	7%
dried	3 oz	2.0	246	7%
raw	3 oz	0.6	70	7%
COD ROE	3 oz	1.7	111	14%
COFFEE/COFFEE-LIKE BEVERAGE				
bottled				
(Maxwell House) iced cappuccino				
Coffee Cappio	8 fl oz	2.5	130	17%
Mocha Cappio	8 fl oz	2.5	140	16%
Vanilla Cappio	8 fl oz	2.5	140	16%
(Starbucks) Frappuccino	9.5 fl oz	3.0	190	14%
brewed				
decaffeinated				
(Brim)	6 fl oz	–	2	–
generic	6 fl oz	–	4	–
(Maxwell House)	6 fl oz	–	2	–
(Sanka)	6 fl oz	–	2	–
(Yuban)	6 fl oz	–	2	–
espresso	2 fl oz	–	1	–
regular				
generic	6 fl oz	–	4	–
(Yuban)	6 fl oz	–	2	–
Turkish	4 fl oz	–	45	
ground (Folger's)				
decaffeinated	1 Tbs	–	17	
regular	1 Tbs	–	16	

Food and Description	Amount	Fat Grams	Total Calories	% Fat Calories
instant				
flavored				
generic/mix only				
w/cappuccino	2 round tsp	2.0	62	29%
w/chicory	1 round tsp	–	6	–
w/French flavor	2 round tsp	3.0	57	47%
(General Foods) International Coffees/				
prepared				
Cafe Francais	1 cup	3.5	60	53%
Cafe Vienna	1 cup	2.5	70	32%
French vanilla cafe				
fat-free	1 cup	–	25	–
regular	1 cup	2.5	60	38%
sugar-free	1 cup	–	25	–
hazelnut Belgian cafe	1 cup	2.0	70	26%
Irish cream cafe	1 cup	1.5	60	23%
Italian cappuccino	1 cup	2.0	60	30%
kahlua cafe	1 cup	2.0	60	30%
orange cappuccino				
regular	1 cup	2.0	70	26%
sugar-free	1 cup	1.5	30	45%
Suisse Mocha				
decaffeinated	1 cup	2.0	60	30%
fat-free	1 cup	–	25	–
regular	1 cup	2.0	60	30%
sugar-free	1 cup	–	25	–
Viennese chocolate cafe	1 cup	1.5	50	27%
(Hills Bros) prepared				
Bavarian mint mocha				
regular	6 fl oz	1.0	50	18%
sugar-free	6 fl oz	1.0	35	26%
Cafe Vienna	6 fl oz	2.0	60	30%
Dutch Chocolate	6 fl oz	2.0	60	30%
Orange Capri	6 fl oz	2.0	60	30%
Swiss Mocha				
regular	6 fl oz	2.0	60	30%
sugar free	6 fl oz	2.0	40	45%
(Maxwell House) cappuccino/prepared				
amaretto	1 cup	1.0	90	10%
Irish cream	1 cup	1.0	90	10%
mocha				
decaffeinated	1 cup	2.5	100	23%
regular	1 cup	2.5	100	23%
sugar-free	1 cup	3.0	60	45%
vanilla				
decaffeinated	1 cup	1.0	90	10%
regular	1 cup	1.0	90	10%
sugar-free	1 cup	3.0	60	45%
(MJB) prepared				
banana nut mocha/sugar-free	6 fl oz	2.0	40	45%

Food and Description	Amount	Fat Grams	Total Calories	% Fat Calories
cafe mocha	6 fl oz	1.0	50	18%
cherry mocha	6 fl oz	1.0	50	18%
fudge mocha/sugar-free	6 fl oz	2.0	40	45%
mint mocha				
regular	6 fl oz	1.0	50	18%
sugar-free	6 fl oz	1.0	35	26%
vanilla mocha/sugar-free	6 fl oz	2.0	40	45%
nonflavored				
(Brim) prepared	6 fl oz	–	4	–
(Kava) mix only	1 tsp	–	2	–
(Maxwell House) prepared	6 fl oz	–	2	–
(Nescafé) prepared				
Brava	6 fl oz	–	4	–
classic	6 fl oz	–	4	–
decaf	6 fl oz	–	4	–
Silka	6 fl oz	–	4	–
(Pero) hot beverage drink w/malt &				
barley/no caffeine/prepared	6 fl oz	–	4	–
(Postum) coffee-flavored grain beverage				
prepared w/water	8 fl oz	–	10	–
(Sanka) prepared	6 fl oz	–	2	–
(Taster's Choice) prepared				
decaffeinated	6 fl oz	–	4	–
regular	6 fl oz	–	4	–
(Worthington) Natural Touch				
Kaffree Roma/mix only	1 tsp	–	10	–
(Yuban) prepared	6 fl oz	–	4	–

COFFEE CREAMER (See CREAM; CREAMER, NONDAIRY)
COLD CUTS (See LUNCHEON MEAT)
COLESLAW (See CABBAGE DISH)
COLLARDS

canned				
(Glory Foods) collard greens	½ cup	1.0	50	18%
(Luck's) chopped greens	½ cup	3.0	60	45%
seasoned w/pork				
fresh				
cooked	½ cup	–	13	–
raw/chopped	½ cup	–	18	–
frozen				
generic/cooked	½ cup	–	31	–
(Pictsweet)	3.3 oz	–	25	–

CONDIMENTS (See ASIAN FOOD; MEXICAN FOOD; SAUCE; SEASONINGS; individual listings)
COOKIE (See also BROWNIE/BLONDIE; CRACKER; CAKE; SNACK)
■ **(Andre Prost)**

Olof ginger snaps	7 cookies	4.0	120	30%

■ **(Archway)**

apple bar/fat-free	1 bar	–	60	–
apple 'n raisin	1 cookie	4.0	110	33%
apple-filled oatmeal	1 cookie	3.0	100	27%

Food and Description	Amount	Fat Grams	Total Calories	% Fat Calories
apricot-filled oatmeal	1 cookie	3.5	100	29%
Aunt Bea's pound cake	1 cookie	4.0	100	36%
black walnut ice box	1 cookie	6.0	120	45%
blueberry filled	1 cookie	4.0	110	33%
carrot cake	1 cookie	5.0	120	38%
cashew nougat	1 cookie	10.0	160	56%
cherry filled	1 cookie	4.0	110	33%
chocolate/fat-free	1 cookie	–	90	–
chocolate chip				
bag	1 cookie	7.0	130	48%
drop	1 cookie	3.5	100	32%
ice box	1 cookie	6.0	120	45%
semi-sweet	1 cookie	6.0	130	42%
sugar-free	1 cookie	5.0	110	41%
walnut	1 cookie	7.0	140	45%
chocolate chip & toffee	1 cookie	6.0	130	42%
cinnamon honey hearts/fat-free	3 cookies	–	100	–
cinnamon snap	5 cookies	7.0	150	42%
coconut macaroon	1 cookie	6.0	100	54%
cookie jar hermits	1 cookie	2.5	90	25%
dark molasses	1 cookie	3.5	120	26%
devil's food/fat-free	1 cookie	–	70	–
Dutch cocoa	1 cookie	3.0	100	27%
frosty				
lemon	1 cookie	4.5	110	37%
orange	1 cookie	4.5	110	37%
fruit & honey bar	1 bar	3.5	100	32%
honey harts/fat-free	3 cookies	–	110	–
ginger snap				
iced	4 cookies	4.0	120	30%
original	5 cookies	5.0	150	30%
reduced fat	5 cookies	3.5	140	23%
iced molasses	1 cookie	4.0	110	30%
iced oatmeal	1 cookie	5.0	120	38%
lemon				
drop	1 cookie	3.5	90	35%
snaps	5 cookies	7.0	150	42%
sugar-free	1 cookie	5.0	110	41%
molasses				
old-fashioned	1 cookie	3.0	100	27%
oatmeal				
chocolate chip	1 cookie	4.5	120	34%
date-filled	1 cookie	3.0	100	27%
pecan	1 cookie	5.0	120	38%
raisin				
fat-free	1 cookie	–	110	–
original/packaged	1 cookie	3.5	110	29%
raspberry/fat-free	1 cookie	–	100	–
sugar-free	1 cookie	5.0	110	41%
peanut butter				
chocolate	1 cookie	7.0	150	42%

Food and Description	Amount	Fat Grams	Total Calories	% Fat Calories
old-fashioned	1 cookie	5.0	100	45%
sugar-free	1 cookie	6.0	110	49%
peanut jumble	1 cookie	6.0	110	49%
pecan crunch	1 cookie	8.0	150	48%
pecan ice box	1 cookie	6.0	120	45%
raspberry filled	1 cookie	4.0	110	33%
rocky road/sugar-free	1 cookie	5.0	100	45%
Ruth's golden oatmeal	1 cookie	5.0	120	38%
Shortbread/fat-free	1 cookie	5.0	110	41%
soft sugar drop	1 cookie	3.0	90	30%
strawberry-filled	1 cookie	3.5	100	32%
sugar	1 cookie	3.0	100	27%
vanilla wafer	5 cookies	4.0	130	28%
windmill/old-fashioned	1 cookie	3.5	90	35%
■ (Arrowhead Mills)				
Mixes/prepared				
chocolate chip	1 cookie	1.5	80	17%
espresso chip	1 cookie	1.5	80	17%
oatmeal raisin	1 cookie	–	70	–
■ (Austin)				
peanut butter chocolate stix	1 bar	8.0	130	55%
seanimals	10 cookies	5.0	140	32%
vanilla creme	1.8 oz	11.0	260	38%
zoo animal cracker	17 cookies	2.0	120	15%
■ (Bakery Wagon)				
cobbler/fat-free				
apple	1 cookie	–	70	–
boysenberry	1 cookie	–	70	–
cranberry apple	1 cookie	–	70	–
mixed fruit	1 cookie	–	70	–
peach/apricot	1 cookie	–	70	–
raspberry	1 cookie	–	70	–
strawberry	1 cookie	–	70	–
cookie/low-fat				
apple-filled oat	1 cookie	1.5	90	15%
date-filled oat	1 cookie	1.5	90	15%
iced molasses				
mini	3 cookies	2.0	130	14%
regular	1 cookie	2.0	90	20%
raspberry filled oat	1 cookie	1.5	90	15%
soft oatmeal				
iced	1 cookie	1.5	100	5%
plain	1 cookie	1.5	90	15%
ginger snap	5 cookies	7.0	160	37%
■ (Barbara's Bakery)				
Animal cookies/vanilla	8 cookies	5.0	130	35%
Crisp cookies				
chocolate chip	1 cookie	4.0	80	45%
double Dutch chocolate	1 cookie	4.0	80	45%
old fashioned oatmeal	1 cookie	3.0	70	39%

Food and Description	Amount	Fat Grams	Total Calories	% Fat Calories
traditional shortbread	1 cookie	4.0	80	45%
Dipped desserts				
coconut almond	1 bar	4.5	120	34%
espresso bean	1 bar	3.0	120	23%
lemon yogurt	1 bar	3.5	120	26%
roasted peanut	1 bar	4.5	130	31%
Fig bars				
fat-free				
fig	1 bar	–	60	–
raspberry	1 bar	–	60	–
whole wheat fig	1 bar	–	60	–
whole wheat apple	1 bar	–	60	–
low-fat traditional				
blueberry	1 bar	1.0	60	15%
fig	1 bar	1.0	60	15%
Snackimals				
chocolate chip	8 cookies	5.0	120	38%
oatmeal/wheat-free	8 cookies	5.0	120	38%
vanilla	8 cookies	5.0	120	38%
■ (Betty Crocker)				
mix/prepared				
bar & cookie mixes				
chocolate peanut butter	1 bar	9.0	200	41%
easy layer dessert bar	1 bar	6.0	140	39%
Hershey cookie bars	1 bar	6.0	150	34%
Sunkist lemon bar	1 bar	4.5	140	29%
cookie mixes				
chocolate chip	2 cookies	8.0	160	45%
chocolate peanut butter	2 cookies	7.0	150	42%
double chocolate chunk	2 cookies	6.0	150	34%
oatmeal chocolate chip	2 cookies	7.0	150	42%
peanut butter	2 cookies	8.0	160	45%
sugar cookie	2 cookies	8.0	160	45%
■ (Break Cake)				
brownie creme/2-oz cookie	1 cookie	8.0	240	30%
chips & creme	1 cookie	6.0	140	39%
chocolate chip	1 oz	6.0	140	39%
chocolate sugar wafer	4 cookies	9.0	200	41%
coconut macaroon/2-oz cookie	2 cookies	14.0	270	47%
devil's food creme	1 cookie	5.0	130	35%
ginger snap	5 cookies	5.0	130	42%
hermit/2-oz cookie	1 cookie	7.0	230	27%
marshmallow pie				
banana	1.2 oz	5.0	150	30%
chocolate	1.2 oz	5.0	150	30%
devil's food	1.2 oz	4.0	140	26%
double decker chocolate	3 oz	11.0	360	28%
oatmeal	5 cookies	6.0	140	39%
peanut butter	1 cookie	7.0	140	45%
peanut butter wafer	1 cookie	9.0	180	45%

Food and Description	Amount	Fat Grams	Total Calories	% Fat Calories
raisin creme	1 cookie	5.0	140	32%
shortbread	5 cookies	6.0	140	39%
strawberry wafer	4 cookies	11.0	220	45%
striper wafer	1 cookie	10.0	190	47%
vanilla sugar wafer	4 wafers	11.0	220	45%
■ **BRETON** (*See* (Dare) in this section)				
■ **(Burns & Ricker)**				
biscotti/~2 per oz				
almond	1 oz	4.5	130	31%
chocolate almond	1 oz	5.0	130	35%
■ **CAMEO** (*See* (Nabisco) in this section)				
■ **(Carr's)**				
biscuits for tea				
dark chocolate	2 biscuits	6.0	130	41%
milk chocolate	2 biscuits	6.0	130	41%
plain	2 biscuits	6.0	140	39%
Chococcines	2 cookies	9.0	150	54%
Imperials				
dark chocolate	2 cookies	7.0	150	42%
milk chocolate	2 cookies	7.0	140	45%
ginger lemon cremes	2 cookies	7.0	140	45%
Hob-Nobs	2 cookies	6.0	140	39%
Petits Bijoux	4 cookies	5.0	140	32%
■ **CHIPS AHOY** (*See* (Nabisco); (Pillsbury) in this section)				
■ **CHIPS DELUXE** (*See* (Keebler) in this section)				
■ **(Dare)**				
Breton				
Belmont				
Black Forest	1 cookie	3.0	81	33%
mallow	1 cookie	2.4	78	28%
strawberry	1 cookie	3.0	81	33%
Breaktime				
chocolate chip	1 cookie	1.7	37	41%
coconut	1 cookie	1.4	35	36%
ginger	1 cookie	1.1	34	29%
oatmeal	1 cookie	1.3	29	40%
sprinkle	1 cookie	1.6	36	40%
butter creme	1 cookie	3.9	85	41%
butter shortbread	1 cookie	3.7	63	53%
chocolate chip	1 cookie	4.1	77	48%
chocolate fudge	1 cookie	4.8	97	45%
chocolate galore	1 cookie	4.0	80	45%
cinnamon Danish	1 cookie	1.6	47	31%
cinnamon snap	1 cookie	0.7	31	20%
coconut creme	1 cookie	5.2	99	47%
digestive	1 cookie	2.0	45	40%
Encore/low-fat	1 cookie	0.6	28	19%
French creme	1 cookie	5.3	80	60%
golden caramel	1 cookie	3.3	73	41%
graham/low-fat	1 cookie	0.8	31	23%

Food and Description	Amount	Fat Grams	Total Calories	% Fat Calories
Harvest from the Rain Forest	1 cookie	4.0	68	53%
key lime creme	1 cookie	4.0	86	42%
lemon creme	1 cookie	4.5	95	43%
maple leaf creme	1 cookie	3.8	83	41%
maple walnut fudge	1 cookie	5.0	99	45%
midnight mint	1 cookie	4.0	75	48%
milk chocolate fudge	1 cookie	4.8	99	44%
oatmeal raisin	1 cookie	2.8	59	43%
Oats Up!	1 cookie	2.9	66	40%
Peanut Butter Delite	1 cookie	4.0	72	50%
social tea	1 cookie	1.0	26	35%
sugar	1 cookie	1.4	39	32%
Sun Maid				
chocolate & raisins	1 cookie	3.0	56	48%
raisin	1 cookie	2.5	52	43%
vanilla water	1 cookie	0.6	17	32%
■ (Cookie Lover's)				
classic shortbread	1 cookie	7.0	110	57%
Dutch chocolate chip	1 cookie	4.0	90	40%
fancy peanut butter	1 cookie	6.0	100	54%
grahams				
cinnamon honey	2 pieces	2.0	100	18%
honey	2 pieces	1.0	110	8%
old time raisin	1 cookie	3.0	90	30%
■ (Delicious)				
almond windmill	3 cookies	5.0	130	35%
animal crackers	9 cookies	5.0	130	35%
butter thins	10 cookies	5.0	110	41%
Chiquita Bananarama	2 cookies	4.0	120	30%
chocolate chip	2 cookies	8.0	140	51%
chocolate chip thins	10 cookies	5.0	110	41%
coconut bar	3 cookies	7.0	140	45%
fig bar	1 cookie	1.0	70	13%
	2 cookies	2.0	130	14%
ginger snap	4 cookies	3.0	130	21%
Heath English toffee crunch	3 cookies	10.0	170	53%
honey graham				
cinnamon	2 whole	5.0	130	35%
plain	2 whole	3.5	120	26%
iced oatmeal	2 cookies	6.0	130	42%
jelly top	47 pieces	8.0	260	28%
Heath				
English toffee	3 cookies	10.0	170	53%
striped toffee delights	2 cookies	8.0	140	51%
macaroon	2 cookies	6.0	130	42%
maple leaf creme	2 cookies	5.0	120	38%
Nestlé				
Butterfinger	3 cookies	6.0	130	42%
Raisinets oatmeal	3 cookies	4.5	140	29%

Food and Description	Amount	Fat Grams	Total Calories	% Fat Calories
oatmeal				
iced	2 cookies	5.0	120	38%
plain	2 cookies	5.0	130	35%
w/Raisinets	3 cookies	4.5	140	29%
sandwich cookies				
assorted	3 cookies	6.0	150	36%
assorted creme	3 cookies	6.0	150	36%
banana creme	3 cookies	6.0	150	36%
chocolate creme	3 cookies	6.0	150	36%
duplex	3 cookies	5.0	140	32%
duplex creme	3 cookies	6.0	150	36%
lemon	3 cookies	5.0	140	32%
lemon creme	3 cookies	6.0	150	36%
peanut butter creme	3 cookies	6.0	150	36%
	2 cookies	5.0	150	30%
strawberry creme	3 cookies	6.0	150	36%
vanilla	3 coolies	5.0	140	32%
vanilla creme	3 cookies	6.0	150	36%
	2 cookies	5.0	150	30%
shortbread	4 cookies	6.0	140	39%
Skippy peanut butter	3 cookies	10.0	150	60%
sugar cookie	2 cookies	5.0	130	35%
sugar wafer				
assorted				
regular	4 wafers	6.0	140	39%
sugar-free	3 wafers	10.0	150	60%
chocolate				
regular	3 wafers	9.0	150	54%
sugar-free	6 wafers	11.0	170	58%
chocolate/strawberry	1 cookie	2.0	35	26%
lemon	1 cookie	2.0	35	26%
mini creme	1 cookie	1.5	25	54%
strawberry				
regular	3 wafers	9.0	150	54%
sugar-free	6 wafers	11.0	170	58%
strawberry/vanilla	1 cookie	2.0	35	26%
vanilla				
regular	3 wafers	9.0	150	54%
sugar-free	6 wafers	11.0	170	58%
vanilla wafers				
fat-free	8 cookies	–	110	–
original	8 cookies	4.5	130	31%
■ (Drake's)				
chocolate chocolate chip	2 cookies	5.0	130	35%
coconut	2 cookies	5.0	130	35%
coconut macaroon	1 cookie	7.0	135	47%
hermit	1 cookie	7.0	230	27%
oatmeal	2 cookies	5.0	120	38%
oatmeal creme	1 cookie	9.0	240	34%
peanut butter wafer	1 cookie	16.0	325	44%

Food and Description	Amount	Fat Grams	Total Calories	% Fat Calories
■ (Duncan Hines)				
mix				
chocolate chip				
mix only	⅟₂₄ pkg	5.0	140	32%
prepared	2 cookies	8.0	170	42%
fudge brownie cookie				
mix only	⅟₂₄ pkg	4.0	120	30%
prepared	2 cookies	7.0	140	45%
golden sugar				
mix only	⅟₂₄ pkg	3.0	110	25%
prepared	2 cookies	7.0	150	42%
peanut butter				
mix only	⅟₂₄ pkg	5.0	120	38%
prepared	2 cookies	8.0	140	51%
■ (Dunkin' Donuts)				
chocolate chocolate chunk	1 cookie	11.0	210	47%
chocolate chunk				
plain	1 cookie	11.0	220	45%
w/nuts	1 cookie	12.0	230	47%
chocolate white chocolate chunk	1 cookie	12.0	230	47%
oatmeal raisin pecan	1 cookie	10.0	220	41%
peanut butter chocolate chunk	1 cookie	14.0	240	53%
■ ELFIN DELIGHTS (See (Keebler) in this section)				
■ (Entenmann's) Soft Baked				
chocolate brownie/fat-free	2 cookies	–	80	–
chocolate chip				
little bites/pouch	1.75 oz	10.0	190	47%
milk chocolate	3 cookies	5.0	100	45%
original recipe	3 cookies	7.0	150	42%
reduced-fat/50% less fat	2 cookies	3.5	130	24%
oatmeal chocolate chip/fat-free	2 cookies	–	100	–
oatmeal raisin/fat-free	2 cookies	–	100	–
■ (Estee)				
chocolate chip				
original	4 cookies	7.0	150	42%
sugar-free	3 cookies	3.5	110	29%
chocolate sandwich	3 cookies	6.0	160	34%
chocolate walnut/sugar-free	3 cookies	3.5	110	29%
coconut				
original	4 cookies	6.0	140	39%
sugar-free	3 cookies	3.5	110	29%
fig bar/low-fat	2 bars	1.0	100	9%
fudge	4 cookies	7.0	150	42%
lemon				
sugar-free	3 cookies	3.0	110	25%
thins	4 cookies	6.0	140	39%
oatmeal raisin	4 cookies	5.0	130	35%
original sandwich	3 cookies	6.0	160	34%
peanut butter sandwich	3 cookies	7.0	160	39%
shortbread	4 cookies	4.0	130	28%

Food and Description	Amount	Fat Grams	Total Calories	% Fat Calories
sugar wafer				
chocolate creme	7 cookies	8.0	160	45%
double decker lemon creme	5 cookies	8.0	170	42%
triple decker banana, chocolate, strawberry creme	3 cookies	7.0	140	45%
vanilla creme	7 cookies	7.0	160	37%
vanilla & strawberry creme	5 cookies	8.0	170	42%
vanilla sandwich	3 cookies	5.0	160	28%
vanilla thins	4 cookies	6.0	140	39%
■ **(Featherweight)**				
chocolate chip	4 cookies	5.0	140	32%
creme wafer				
chocolate	7 cookies	8.0	160	45%
vanilla	7 cookies	7.0	160	39%
double chocolate chip	4 cookies	5.0	140	32%
lemon	4 cookies	5.0	140	32%
oatmeal raisin	4 cookies	5.0	140	32%
peanut butter	4 cookies	5.0	140	32%
vanilla	4 cookies	5.0	140	32%
■ **(Formagg)**				
chocolate chip cheesecake	1 cookie	2.0	49	37%
■ **(Frookie)**				
animal frackers crackers	10 cookies	5.0	130	35%
apple cinnamon oat bran	3 cookies	5.0	130	35%
chocolate chip				
organic wheat	3 cookies	7.0	150	42%
wheat & glutent free	3 cookies	4.5	140	29%
chocolate chunk/fructose-sweetened	3 cookies	6.0	150	36%
double chocolate				
organic wheat	3 cookies	6.0	140	39%
wheat & gluten free	3 cookies	4.0	130	28%
Dream Cream				
strawberry	4 cookies	8.0	140	51%
vanilla	2 cookies	4.0	70	51%
Frookwich				
chocolate	3 cookies	6.0	150	36%
chocolate & vanilla duplex				
fructose-sweetened	2 cookies	0.5	110	4%
regular	3 cookies	6.0	150	36%
lemon				
fructose-sweetened	2 cookies	0.5	110	4%
regular	3 cookies	6.0	150	36%
peanut butter	3 cookies	6.0	150	36%
vanilla				
fructose-sweetened	2 cookies	0.5	110	4%
regular	3 cookies	6.0	150	36%
vanilla power	2 cookies	6.0	140	39%
Funky Monkey				
chocolate	12 cookies	4.0	120	30%
vanilla	12 cookies	4.0	120	30%

Food and Description	Amount	Fat Grams	Total Calories	% Fat Calories
ginger snaps, old fashioned	8 cookies	2.0	120	15%
graham				
cinnamon	2 cookies	3.0	100	27%
honey	2 cookies	3.0	100	27%
lemon cookies, iced	3 cookies	6.0	165	33%
oatmeal raisin				
fat-free	2 cookies	–	90	–
fructose-sweetened	3 cookies	2.0	140	13%
original	3 cookies	5.0	130	35%
peanut butter/fructose-sweetened	3 cookies	6.0	140	39%
peanut butter chunk	3 cookies	5.0	140	32%
shortbread	5 cookies	5.0	130	35%
wafers/fat-free				
lemon	8 cookies	–	110	–
vanilla wafer	8 cookies	–	110	–
■ GENERIC				
animal crackers	1 cookie	<1.0	11	30%
	11 cookies	4.0	126	30%
arrowroot	1 cookie	1.0	25	36%
butter	1 cookie	1.0	23	39%
chocolate chip				
refrigerated dough				
¼" thick/2¼" dia	4 cookies	11.0	225	44%
soft style	1 cookie	4.0	70	51%
chocolate w/creme filling	1 cookie	5.0	80	56%
chocolate sandwich/1¾" dia	4 cookies	8.0	195	37%
chocolate wafer	1 cookie	1.0	25	36%
coconut bar	1 bar	5.0	110	41%
coconut macaroon	2 cookies	5.0	100	45%
fig bar	4 bars	4.0	210	17%
fortune	1 cookie	–	30	–
fudge	1 cookie	1.0	75	13%
ginger snap	1 cookie	1.0	30	30%
lady finger	1 cookie	1.0	40	23%
marshmallow/chocolate-coated	1 cookie	2.0	55	33%
marshmallow pie/chocolate-coated	1 cookie	7.0	165	38%
molasses	1 cookie	2.0	65	28%
oatmeal				
refrigerated	1 cookie	3.0	60	45%
soft style	1 cookie	2.0	60	30%
traditional	1 cookie	4.0	70	51%
oatmeal raisin	1 cookie	3.0	80	34%
peanut butter				
refrigerated	1 cookie	3.0	60	45%
soft style	1 cookie	4.0	70	51%
peanut butter sandwich	1 cookie	3.0	70	39%
shortbread	1 cookie	2.0	40	45%
shortbread pecan	1 cookie	5.0	80	56%
sugar/refrigerated dough				
¼" thick/2½" dia	1 cookie	3.0	60	45%

Food and Description	Amount	Fat Grams	Total Calories	% Fat Calories
sugar wafer w/creme filling	1 cookie	1.0	20	45%
vanilla sandwich/1¾" dia	4 cookies	8.0	190	37%
vanilla wafer/1¾" dia	10 cookies	7.0	185	34%
zwieback	1 oz	1.0	107	8%
■ (Girl Scout)				
Chalet cremes/sugar-free	4 cookies	6.0	150	36%
Do-si-dos	3 cookies	8.0	170	42%
Samoas	2 cookies	9.0	160	51%
Snaps	7 cookies	2.0	130	14%
striped chocolate chip	3 cookies	10.0	180	50%
Tagalongs	2 cookies	10.0	150	60%
Thin Mints	4 cookies	8.0	140	51%
Trefoils	5 cookies	8.0	160	45%
■ (Grandma's)				
big cookies/homestyle				
chocolate chip	1 cookie	9.0	190	43%
fudge chocolate chip	1 cookie	7.0	170	37%
molasses	1 cookie	4.0	160	23%
oatmeal raisin	1 cookie	6.0	160	34%
peanut butter	1 cookie	9.0	190	43%
peanut butter chocolate chip	1 cookie	9.0	190	43%
mini cookies				
fudge	9 cookies	7.0	150	42%
peanut butter	9 cookies	7.0	150	42%
vanilla	9 cookies	7.0	150	42%
regular cookies				
chocolate fudge bar	1 bar	7.0	190	33%
peanut butter sandwich	5 cookies	10.0	210	43%
rich n' chewy	1 pkg	12.0	270	40%
sugar wafers				
strawberry	3 wafers	7.0	160	34%
vanilla	3 wafers	7.0	160	34%
vanilla sandwich				
regular	5 cookies	10.0	210	43%
tiny bites				
animal crackers	11 cookies	9.0	260	31%
chocolate chip	12 cookies	12.0	280	39%
oatmeal raisin	12 cookies	12.0	280	39%
sugar	12 cookies	13.0	280	42%
value line				
fudge sandwich	3 cookies	5.0	180	25%
fudge vanilla sandwich	3 cookies	4.0	120	30%
vanilla sandwich	3 cookies	5.0	180	25%
■ (Hain)				
animal graham				
chocolate	15 cookies	3.0	120	23%
original	15 cookies	3.0	80	34%
graham cracker				
chocolate	2 cookies	3.0	120	23%
cinnamon	2 cookies	3.0	80	34%

Food and Description	Amount	Fat Grams	Total Calories	% Fat Calories
honey	2 cookies	3.0	80	34%
■ **(Health Valley)**				
Fat-free cookies				
fruit bake				
apple spice	3 cookies	–	75	–
apricot delight	3 cookies	–	75	–
banana spice	3 cookies	–	75	–
date delight	3 cookies	–	75	–
Hawaiian fruit	3 cookies	–	75	–
jumbos				
apple raisin	1 cookie	–	70	–
raisin raisin	1 cookie	–	70	–
raspberry	1 cookie	–	70	–
Traditional cookies				
amaranth	1 cookie	3.0	70	39%
fancy fruit chunks				
apricot almond	2 cookies	4.0	90	40%
date pecan	2 cookies	4.0	90	40%
raisin oat bran	2 cookies	2.0	70	26%
tropical fruit	2 cookies	3.0	90	30%
fancy peanut chunks	2 cookies	3.0	90	30%
fiber jumbos				
blueberry nut	1 cookie	3.0	100	27%
chunky pecan	1 cookie	3.0	100	27%
raisin nut	1 cookie	3.0	100	27%
fruit jumbos				
almond date	1 cookie	3.0	70	39%
oat bran	1 cookie	3.0	70	39%
raisin nut	1 cookie	3.0	70	39%
tropical fruit	1 cookie	3.0	70	39%
grahams				
Amaranth	7 pieces	3.0	110	25%
honey crisp cinnamon	7 pieces	4.0	100	36%
honey jumbos				
crisp cinnamon	1 cookie	2.0	70	26%
crisp peanut butter	1 cookie	4.0	70	51%
fancy oat bran	2 cookies	4.0	130	28%
oat bran				
animal cookies	7 cookies	4.0	110	33%
fruit & nut	2 cookies	4.0	110	33%
The Great Tofu Cookie	2 cookies	3.0	90	30%
The Great Wheat-Free Cookie	2 cookies	3.0	80	34%
■ **HOMEMADE**				
USDA Standard Home Recipe (Note: All homemade cookies were made with margarine.)				
chocolate chip/2⅓" dia	4 cookies	12.0	206	52%
macaroons/¼" thick/2¾" dia	2 cookies	8.8	181	44%
oatmeal				
traditional	1 cookie	3.0	65	42%
w/raisins/¼" thick/2⅝" dia	4 cookies	10.0	245	37%

Food and Description	Amount	Fat Grams	Total Calories	% Fat Calories
oatmeal chocolate chip	1 cookie	3.0	60	45%
peanut butter/2⅝" dia	4 cookies	14.0	245	51%
pumpkin bar	1.5 oz	11.0	190	52%
shortbread	1 cookie	4.0	60	60%
sugar/¼" thick/2½" dia	1 cookie	3.0	90	30%
■ **HONEY MAID** (*See* (Nabisco) in this section)				
■ **(Kashi)**				
graham cracker				
amaranth graham	8 cookies	–	100	–
oat bran honey	6 cookies	3.0	110	25%
great tofu cookie	2 cookies	3.0	90	30%
oat bran fruit & nut	2-3 cookies	4.0	110	33%
■ **(Keebler)**				
Chips Deluxe				
chocolate chip				
bite-size	8 cookies	9.0	160	51%
regular	1 cookie	4.5	80	51%
chocolate lovers	1 cookie	5.0	90	50%
coconut	1 cookie	5.0	80	56%
crunchy walnut	1 cookie	6.0	90	60%
peanut butter chips	1 cookie	4.5	80	51%
rainbow				
bite-size	7 cookies	7.0	140	45%
regular	1 cookie	4.0	80	45%
soft & chewy	1 cookie	3.5	80	39%
Classic Collection				
chocolate fudge sandwich	1 cookie	3.5	80	39%
French vanilla creme	1 cookie	3.5	80	39%
oatmeal	2 cookies	8.0	150	48%
Cookie Stix				
chocolate chip cookie stix	5 cookies	6.0	140	39%
rainbow cookie stix	5 cookies	5.0	140	32%
E.L. Fudge sandwich cookies				
butter flavored w/fudge creme filling	2 cookies	6.0	120	45%
chocolate w/peanut butter creme filling	2 cookies	6.0	120	45%
fudge w/fudge creme filling	2 cookies	6.0	120	45%
Fudge Shoppe cookies				
fudge-covered grahams/deluxe	3 pieces	7.0	140	45%
fudge'n caramel/double	3 cookies	7.0	140	45%
fudge sticks				
peanut butter	3 cookies	8.0	160	45%
regular	3 cookies	8.0	150	48%
fudge stripes				
original	3 cookies	8.0	160	45%
25% reduced-fat	3 cookies	5.0	140	32%
Grasshopper	4 cookies	8.0	160	45%
S'mores	3 cookies	8.0	160	45%
Golden Fruit biscuits				
cranberry	1 cookie	2.0	80	23%

Food and Description	Amount	Fat Grams	Total Calories	% Fat Calories
raisin	1 cookie	1.5	80	17%
Grahams				
chocolate	8 crackers	4.0	140	26%
cinnamon crisp				
low-fat	8 crackers	1.5	110	12%
regular	8 crackers	3.0	130	21%
honey graham				
low-fat	9 crackers	1.5	120	11%
regular	8 cookies	4.0	140	26%
original	8 cookies	3.5	130	24%
Snackin'				
chocolate	12 crackers	3.5	120	26%
cinnamon	12 crackers	3.0	120	23%
Iced Animals				
chocolate chip/lightly frosted	7 cookies	4.5	130	31%
frosted/11oz & 16oz pkg	6 cookies	6.0	130	42%
lightly frosted	6 cookies	5.0	150	30%
lightly frosted w/sprinkles	6 cookies	4.5	150	27%
Keebler original cookies				
animal crackers	10 pieces	4.0	130	28%
butter cookies/artificially flavored	5 cookies	6.0	150	36%
country style oatmeal	2 cookies	6.0	120	45%
Danish wedding	4 cookies	5.0	120	38%
Droxies	3 cookies	6.0	140	39%
ginger snaps	5 cookies	6.0	150	36%
Krisp Kreem sugar wafer	5 pieces	7.0	140	45%
Lemon coolers	5 cookies	5.0	140	32%
vanilla wafers				
original	8 cookies	7.0	150	42%
rainbow	8 cookies	5.0	130	35%
reduced-fat (30%)	8 cookies	3.5	130	24%
Sandies				
original				
w/almonds	1 cookie	5.0	80	56%
w/pecans	1 cookie	5.0	80	56%
simply shortbread	1 cookie	4.5	80	51%
25% reduced fat w/pecans	1 cookie	3.0	80	34%
Snack Size/Single Serve				
Animal Crackers				
frosted	1 package	14.0	290	43%
plain	1 package	9.0	250	32%
Chips Deluxe				
chocolate lover's	1 package	15.0	280	48%
plain	1 package	16.0	300	48%
rainbow	1 package	16.0	290	50%
Elf Grahams				
cinnamon	16 crackers	4.5	140	29%
honey	16 crackers	4.0	140	26%
Elfin crackers	23 pieces	2.0	130	14%
Fudge Stripes/mini	1 package	14.0	280	45%

Food and Description	Amount	Fat Grams	Total Calories	% Fat Calories
Sandies w/pecans	1 package	17.0	300	51%
Soft Batch cookies				
chocolate chip	1 cookie	3.5	80	45%
chocolate chunk/homestyle				
double	1 cookie	7.0	130	48%
regular	1 cookie	7.0	130	48%
oatmeal raisin				
homestyle	1 cookie	4.5	130	31%
original	1 cookie	3.0	70	34%
Sugar Wafers				
peanut butter	4 wafers	9.0	160	51%
vanilla	3 wafers	6.0	130	42%
Vienna Fingers				
lemon	2 cookies	6.0	140	39%
original	2 cookies	6.0	140	39%
reduced-fat (25%)	2 cookies	4.5	130	32%
■ (Lance)				
chocolate chip mini cookies/2 oz package	½ pkg	4.0	130	28%
sugar wafers/creme-filled				
chocolate	4 wafers	8.0	150	48%
peanut butter				
1½ oz package	1 pkg	12.0	220	49%
2 oz package	½ piece	9.0	150	42%
strawberry	4 wafers	8.0	150	48%
vanilla	4 wafers	8.0	150	48%
■ (Little Debbie)				
bars				
caramel cookie bar	1 bar	8.0	160	45%
marshmallow crispy bars	1 bar	3.5	140	23%
nutty bar				
big & Hungry	2.1 oz	20.0	320	56%
boxed	1 pkg	17.0	260	59%
individual pkg	2.5 oz	19.0	350	49%
peanut butter bar				
boxed	1 pkg	15.0	270	50%
individual pkg	1 pkg	14.0	250	50%
creme pies				
jelly	1 cookie	7.0	150	42%
oatmeal				
boxed	1 pkg	7.0	170	29%
individual pkg	2.5 oz	12.0	300	36%
	3 oz	14.0	360	35%
raisin				
boxed	1 pkg	5.0	140	32%
individual pkg	1 pkg	11.0	260	38%
cookies				
animal cookie	1 pkg	5.0	190	24%
apple flips	1 pkg	6.0	150	36%
cherry cordials	2 cookie	8.0	170	42%
chocolate chip cookie/individual pkg	1 cookie	9.0	180	45%

Food and Description	Amount	Fat Grams	Total Calories	% Fat Calories
coconut round	1 pkg	7.0	150	42%
cookie wreaths	1 pkg	6.0	100	54%
Easter puffs	1 pkg	6.0	150	36%
Figaroos				
fat-free/individual pkg	1 pkg	–	180	–
regular	1 pkg	3.5	150	21%
fudge delights	1 cookie	2.0	110	16%
fudge round				
boxed	1 pkg	6.0	140	39%
individual pkg	2.5 oz	12.0	310	35%
	3 oz	14.0	380	33%
German chocolate cookie ring	1 cookie	7.0	140	45%
Ginger	1 pkg	3.0	90	30%
lemon creme wafer	1 pkg	5.0	100	45%
marshmallow supreme	1 pkg	6.0	130	42%
oatmeal delights	1 cookie	2.0	110	16%
oatmeal lights snack	1 pkg	2.5	130	17%
oatmeal raisin/individual pkg	1 cookie	6.0	160	34%
peanut cluster	1 pkg	11.0	190	52%
pumpkin delight	1 pkg	5.0	140	32%
star crunch snack/individual pkg	1 pkg	12.0	280	39%
	1 oz	5.0	140	32%
strawberry fruit/fat-free	1 pkg	–	130	–
Yo-Yo's	1 cookie	5.0	130	35%
marshmallow pies				
banana				
boxed	1 pkg	8.0	240	30%
individual pkg	2.5 oz	11.0	320	31%
	1.5 oz	5.0	160	28%
chocolate				
boxed	1 pkg	5.0	160	28%
individual pkg	1 pkg	11.0	320	31%
■ (LU)				
Aloha	1 cookie	5.0	75	60%
barre chocolat	1 cookie	3.0	65	42%
chips chocolat				
fudge	1 cookie	4.0	75	48%
regular	1 cookie	5.0	85	53%
chocolatiers	3 cookies	11.0	170	58%
craquelin	1 cookie	3.0	55	49%
crokine	2 cookies	–	20	–
Euphrates	2 cookies	2.0	40	45%
fondant	4 cookies	8.0	170	37%
gaufrettes	2 cookies	4.0	85	42%
Marie LU				
mini	12 cookies	5.0	130	35%
original	3 cookies	6.0	170	32%
whole wheat	3 cookies	4.0	140	26%
milk lunch	4 cookies	4.0	140	26%
palmito	1 cookie	3.0	50	54%

Food and Description	Amount	Fat Grams	Total Calories	% Fat Calories
petit-beurre	4 cookies	4.0	150	26%
petit-ecolier/little schoolboy				
dark chocolat	2 cookies	7.0	130	48%
milk chocolat	2 cookies	7.0	130	48%
pims				
orange	2 cookies	4.0	100	35%
raspberry	2 cookies	3.0	100	27%
truffe	4 cookies	11.0	180	55%
■ (M&M * Mars)				
Twix cookie bars				
caramel				
family size	1 cookie	7.0	140	45%
single size	2 cookies	14.0	280	45%
■ (Manischewitz)				
chocolate chip	3 cookies	7.0	150	42%
macaroon				
almond	2 cookies	5.0	100	45%
banana split	2 cookies	4.0	110	33%
cappuccion chip	2 cookies	5.0	100	45%
chocolate				
almond	2 cookies	5.0	110	41%
chip	2 cookies	5.0	100	45%
chunk cherry	2 cookies	4.0	110	33%
plain	2 cookies	4.0	90	40%
coconut	2 cookies	6.0	100	54%
cookies'n cream	2 cookies	5.0	100	45%
fudgey nut brownie	2 cookies	5.0	100	45%
honey nut	2 cookies	5.0	100	45%
rocky road	2 cookies	5.0	100	45%
toffee crunch	2 cookies	5.0	100	45%
■ (Mother's)				
almond shortbread	3 cookies	11.0	180	55%
ABC				
cinnamon grahams	12 cookies	6.0	140	39%
sugar cookies	12 cookies	6.0	140	39%
butter-flavored	5 cookies	6.0	140	39%
checkerboard wafer	8 cookies	8.0	150	48%
chocolate chip				
angel	3 cookies	9.0	180	45%
bag	5 cookies	5.0	140	32%
package	2 cookies	8.0	160	45%
parade	4 cookies	5.0	130	35%
circus animal	6 cookies	7.0	140	45%
classic assortment	2 cookies	7.0	140	45%
cocadas coconut	5 cookies	7.0	150	42%
cookie parade	4 cookies	7.0	140	45%
Dinosaur Grrrahams	2 cookies	3.0	130	21%
double fudge sandwich	2 cookies	9.0	180	45%
duplex sandwich/reduced fat	3 cookies	5.0	160	28%
English tea sandwich	2 cookies	7.0	180	35%

Food and Description	Amount	Fat Grams	Total Calories	% Fat Calories
fig bar				
regular				
fat-free	1 bar	–	70	–
regular	1 bar	2.0	80	23%
whole wheat				
fat-free	1 bar	–	70	–
regular	1 bar	3.0	80	34%
Flaky Flix fudge wafer	2 cookies	7.0	140	45%
Flaky Flix vanilla wafer	2 cookies	8.0	140	51%
Gaucho peanut butter sandwich	2 cookies	10.0	190	47%
iced oatmeal				
bag	4 cookies	4.0	120	30%
package	2 cookies	4.0	130	28%
iced raisin	2 cookies	8.0	180	40%
macaroon	2 cookies	8.0	150	48%
Marias	3 cookies	6.0	170	32%
oatmeal				
chocolate chip	2 cookies	5.0	120	38%
original	2 cookies	5.0	110	41%
raisin	5 cookies	7.0	150	42%
walnut chocolate chip	2 cookies	6.0	130	28%
rainbow wafer	8 wafers	8.0	150	48%
striped shortbread	3 cookies	8.0	170	42%
sugar	2 cookies	6.0	140	39%
taffy sandwich	2 cookies	8.0	180	40%
triplet assortment	2 cookies	7.0	140	45%
vanilla wafer	6 cookies	6.0	150	36%
Wallops				
boysenberry	1 cookie	1.5	80	17%
honey graham fig	1 cookie	2.0	80	23%
peach/apricot	1 cookie	1.5	80	17%
raspberry	1 cookie	1.5	80	17%
strawberry	1 cookie	1.5	80	17%
walnut fudge	2 cookies	7.0	130	48%
Zoo Pals	14 cookies	5.0	140	32%
■ (Murray)				
assortment	5 cookies	5.0	120	38%
butter pecan	4 cookies	6.0	160	34%
choco chips	6 cookies	5.0	140	32%
chocolate chip	2 cookies	6.0	130	42%
chocolate creme	3 cookies	6.0	150	36%
coconut	2 cookies	6.0	130	42%
creme/assorted	3 cookies	5.0	150	30%
creme wafer/sugar-free				
strawberry	6 cookies	8.0	160	45%
vanilla	6 cookies	9.0	160	51%
duplex creme	3 cookies	5.0	150	30%
fig bar	2 cookies	2.0	90	20%
ginger snap/old-fashioned	6 cookies	2.5	130	17%
lemon creme	3 cookies	6.0	150	36%

Food and Description	Amount	Fat Grams	Total Calories	% Fat Calories
oatmeal				
frosted	2 cookies	4.0	120	30%
plain	2 cookies	4.0	120	30%
peanut butter creme	3 cookies	6.0	150	36%
6 in 1 assortment	5 cookies	6.0	140	39%
sugar wafer/duplex	5 cookies	10.0	150	60%
vanilla creme	3 cookies	6.0	150	36%
vanilla wafer	8 cookies	3.0	120	23%
windmill	3 cookies	5.0	150	30%
■ (Nabisco)				
brown edge wafer	5 cookies	6.0	140	39%
Cafe Creams/sandwich				
cappuccino	1 serving	8.0	160	45%
vanilla	1 serving	7.0	160	39%
vanilla fudge	1 serving	10.0	200	45%
Cameo creme sandwich	2 cookies	5.0	130	35%
Chips Ahoy				
chunky	1 cookie	4.0	80	45%
double chocolate fudge	1 cookie	7.0	160	39%
milk chocolate	1.5 oz bag	11.0	220	45%
mini chocolate chip				
1.5 oz bag	1 bag	11.0	220	45%
16 oz bag	1 serving	7.0	150	42%
real chocolate chip	3 cookies	8.0	160	45%
1.4 oz. package	1 pkg	9.0	200	41%
reduced fat	1 cookie	5.0	140	32%
soft	1 cookie	7.0	160	39%
sprinkled	3 cookies	8.0	170	42%
w/pecans	1 cookie	9.0	150	54%
Family Favorites				
Fudge-covered grahams	3 cookies	7.0	140	45%
oatmeal				
iced	1 cookie	3.0	80	34%
regular	1 cookie	3.0	80	34%
vanilla sandwich	1 cookie	3.0	160	17%
ginger snap/old-fashioned	4 cookies	2.5	120	19%
grahams				
fudge-covered grahams	1 serving	7.0	140	45%
original	8 cookies	3.0	120	23%
Honey Maid Grahams				
chocolate	8 cookies	3.0	120	23%
cinnamon	8 cookies	3.0	140	19%
low-fat	8 cookies	1.5	110	12%
oatmeal crunch	8 cookies	2.5	120	19%
original	8 cookies	2.5	120	17%
low-fat	8 cookies	1.5	120	11%
Heyday bar	1 bar	5.0	110	41%
Lorna Doone shortbread	4 cookies	7.0	140	45%
Mallomars chocolate cakes	2 cookies	5.0	120	38%
marshmallow puffs	1 cookie	4.0	90	40%

Food and Description	Amount	Fat Grams	Total Calories	% Fat Calories
marshmallow twirls	1 piece	6.0	130	42%
Mystic Mint sandwich	1 cookie	4.5	90	45%
Nabisco				
Barnum's animal crackers	12 cookies	4.0	140	26%
Biscos sugar wafer	8 cookies	6.0	140	39%
Biscos waffle creme	4 cookies	9.0	180	45%
National arrowroot biscuit	1 cookie	0.5	20	23%
Newtons				
Cobblers				
apple	2 cookies	–	90	–
apple cinnamon	2 cookies	–	70	–
fig				
fat-free	2 cookies	–	90	–
regular	2 cookies	2.5	110	20%
	2 oz pkg	4.5	210	19%
cranberry	2 cookies	–	100	–
peach apricot	2 cookies	–	70	–
raspberry	2 cookies	–	100	–
strawberry	2 cookies	–	100	–
tropical strawberry kiwi/low-fat	2 cookies	1.5	90	15%
Nilla vanilla wafer				
chocolate reduced-fat	1 oz	2.0	110	16%
original	8 cookies	5.0	140	32%
reduced-fat	1 oz	2.0	120	15%
Nutter Butter				
chocolate peanut butter sandwich	2 cookies	5.0	130	35%
1.9 oz package	1 pkg	10.0	250	36%
peanut butter creme patty	5 cookies	9.0	160	51%
peanut butter sandwich	2 cookies	6.0	150	34%
soft peanut butter cookie	1 cookie	8.0	170	42%
Oreo				
brownie bar	1.3 oz pkg	7.0	160	39%
crunchies	1 oz	2.5	50	45%
double stuff	2 cookies	7.0	140	45%
fudge covered	1 cookie	6.0	110	50%
Halloween treats	2 cookies	7.0	140	45%
mini bite-size	1.5 oz	9.0	200	41%
Magic Dunkers	3 cookies	7.0	160	39%
munch madness	3 cookies	7.0	140	45%
original	3 cookies	7.0	160	39%
	2 oz pkg	12.0	270	40%
reduced fat	3 cookies	3.5	130	24%
white fudge-covered	1 cookie	6.0	110	49%
SnackWell's				
fat-free				
devil's food cookie cakes	1 cookie	–	50	–
reduced fat				
caramel delights	2 cookies	2.0	70	26%
chocolate chip				
bite-size	13 cookies	4.0	130	28%

Food and Description	Amount	Fat Grams	Total Calories	% Fat Calories
regular	1 oz	4.0	130	28%
chocolate sandwich w/chocolate	2 cookies	3.0	110	25%
coconut creme	2 cookies	4.0	110	33%
creme	1.7 oz pkg	3.0	110	25%
50% less fat	2 cookies	2.5	110	20%
golden devil's food	1 cookie	0.5	50	9%
mint creme	2 cookies	3.5	110	29%
oatmeal raisin	2 cookies	3.0	110	25%
peanut butter/bite-size	13 cookies	4.0	120	30%
Social Tea biscuits	6 cookies	4.0	120	30%
Teddy Grahams				
chocolate	24 pieces	4.5	130	31%
Dizzy Grizzlies				
chocolate-honey w/sprinkles	24 pieces	5.0	150	30%
chocolatey chip	24 pieces	4.5	130	31%
cinnamon				
Dizzy Grizzle\ies				
vanilla-frosted w/sprinkles	24 pieces	5.0	130	35%
regular	24 pieces	4.0	130	27%
honey	24 pieces	4.0	130	27%
zwieback	1 piece	1.0	35	26%
■ (Nature's Warehouse)				
almond butter	2 cookies	4.0	120	30%
banana/wheat-free	1 oz	1.0	90	10%
caramel crisp/wheat-free	1 oz	1.0	90	10%
cherry/wheat-free	1 oz	1.0	90	10%
chocolate chocolate chip	2 cookies	6.0	140	39%
cinnamon graham	1 cookie	3.5	115	27%
fig bar				
wheat-free				
apple cinnamon	1 oz	2.0	100	18%
original	1 oz	2.0	100	–
raspberry	1 oz	2.0	100	18%
whole wheat	1 oz	2.0	100	18%
oat bran/wheat-free	2 cookies	6.0	130	42%
oat bran chocolate chip	2 cookies	6.0	140	39%
peanut butter chocolate chip	2 cookies	8.5	140	55%
raspberry/wheat-free	1 oz	1.0	90	10%
■ (Nestlé) Toll House				
refrigerated/ready-to-bake				
Break & Bake				
chocolate chip	1 cookie	5.0	110	41%
chocolate chip white fudge	1 cookie	6.0	150	36%
chocolate chunk	1 cookie	6.0	150	36%
peanut butter	1 cookie	7.0	150	42%
sugar	1 cookie	5.0	110	41%
rolled cookies				
chocolate chip				
original	1 cookie	6.0	150	36%
reduced-fat	1 cookie	3.5	130	24%

Food and Description	Amount	Fat Grams	Total Calories	% Fat Calories
sugar	1 cookie	5.0	120	38%
■ **OREO** (*See* (Nabisco) in this section)				
■ **(Otis Spunkmeyer)**				
Sweet Discovery/1.3 oz medium size				
Butter sugar	1 cookie	8.0	160	45%
Carnival	1 cookie	7.0	160	39%
Chocolate chip				
double	1 cookie	9.0	180	45%
milk chocolate chunk	1 cookie	8.0	170	42%
regular	1 cookie	8.0	170	42%
w/pecans	1 cookie	9.0	170	48%
w/walnuts	1 cookie	9.0	180	45%
Oatmeal raisin	1 cookie	7.0	160	39%
Peanut butter	1 cookie	10.0	180	50%
Rocky road	1 cookie	8.0	160	45%
Triple chocolate	1 cookie	8.0	170	42%
Turtle	1 cookie	9.0	170	48%
White chocolate macadamia nut	1 cookie	10.0	180	50%
Sweet Discovery/2 oz old fashion size				
Butter sugar	1 cookie	12.0	250	43%
Carnival	1 cookie	11.0	250	45%
Chocolate chip				
regular	1 cookie	14.0	250	50%
milk chocolate chunk	1 cookie	13.0	250	47%
Oatmeal raisin	1 cookie	10.0	240	38%
Peanut butter				
peanut butter chocolate chunk	1 cookie	11.0	240	41%
regular	1 cookie	15.0	270	50%
Rocky road	1 cookie	11.0	240	41%
Triple chocolate	1 cookie	12.0	250	43%
Turtle	1 cookie	13.0	250	47%
White chocolate macadamia nut	1 cookie	15.0	280	48%
Sweet Discovery/4 oz cookies				
Butter sugar	1 cookie	22.0	490	40%
Carnival	1 cookie	22.0	490	40%
Chocolate chip				
double	1 cookie	25.0	500	45%
regular	1 cookie	23.0	490	42%
Oatmeal raisin	1 cookie	22.0	480	41%
Peanut butter	1 cookie	28.0	520	48%
White chocolate macadamia nut	1 cookie	27.0	520	47%
Traditional Recipe/2.5 oz cookies				
Carnival	1 cookie	14.0	310	41%
Chocolate chip				
double	1 cookie	15.0	310	44%
regular	1 cookie	14.0	310	41%
Oatmeal raisin	1 cookie	13.0	300	39%
Peanut butter	1 cookie	18.0	320	51%
Ranger	1 cookie	16.0	310	46%
Sugar	1 cookie	14.0	310	41%

Food and Description	Amount	Fat Grams	Total Calories	% Fat Calories
White chocolate macadamia nut	1 cookie	16.0	320	45%
■ (Pamela's)				
Wheat-Free				
Oatmeal				
date coconut	1 cookie	6.0	110	49%
raisin walnut	1 cookie	6.0	110	49%
Wheat & Gluten-Free				
biscotti				
almond anise	2 biscotti	6.0	170	32%
chocolate walnut	2 biscotti	6.0	170	32%
lemon almond	2 biscotti	7.0	170	37%
butter shortbread	1 cookie	7.0	130	48%
carob hazelnut	1 cookie	7.0	120	53%
chocolate chip				
double chip	1 cookie	5.0	110	41%
pecan shortbread	1 cookie	7.0	130	48%
walnut	1 cookie	8.0	130	55%
chunky chocolate chip	1 cookie	6.0	120	45%
ginger	1 cookie	5.0	110	41%
lemon shortbread	1 cookie	6.0	120	45%
peanut butter	1 cookie	5.0	90	50%
pecan shortbread	1 cookie	8.0	130	55%
shortbread swirl	1 cookie	7.0	120	53%
simply chololate shorbread	1 cookie	5.0	120	38%
■ (Peak Frean)				
arrowroot	4 biscuits	4.0	150	40%
coffee creme	2 biscuits	7.0	150	42%
fruit creme	2 biscuits	5.0	130	35%
fruit shortcake	3 cookies	7.0	170	37%
■ (Pepperidge Farm)				
American Collection				
Beacon Hill brownie nut	1 cookie	7.0	130	48%
Charleston milk chocolate toffee	1 cookie	7.0	130	48%
Chesapeake chocolate chunk pecan	1 cookie	8.0	140	51%
Entertaining/9 varieties	1 cookie	7.0	140	45%
Golden orchard	1 cookie	6.0	140	39%
Nantucket chocolate chunk				
bite size	1 oz	8.0	150	48%
	1.75 oz	13.0	260	45%
regular/big	1 cookie	7.0	140	45%
Santa Fe oatmeal raisin	1 cookie	4.5	120	34%
Sausalito milk chocolate macadamia				
bite size	1 oz	9.0	160	51%
regular/big	1 cookie	8.0	140	51%
soft baked	1 cookie	7.0	130	48%
Tahoe white chunk macadamia	1 cookie	7.0	130	48%
biscotti				
almond				
chocolate-dipped				
3.5" cookie	1 cookie	4.0	110	33%

Food and Description	Amount	Fat Grams	Total Calories	% Fat Calories
5.5" cookie	1 cookie	10.0	210	43%
plain				
3.5" cookie	1 cookie	3.5	90	35%
5.5" cookie	1 cookie	6.0	160	34%
anise	1 cookie	3.0	90	30%
chocolate hazelnut				
3.5" cookie	1 cookie	5.0	90	50%
5.5" cookie	1 cookie	9.0	160	51%
cinnamon chip				
3.5" cookie	1 cookie	3.5	90	35%
5.5" cookie	1 cookie	6.0	160	34%
cranberry pistachio				
3.5" cookie	1 cookie	3.0	90	30%
5.5" cookie	1 cookie	6.0	160	34%
orange/chocolate-dipped				
3.5" cookie	1 cookie	4.5	110	37%
5.5" cookie	1 cookie	8.0	200	36%
Distinctive Assortment				
cafe favorites	4 cookies	7.0	140	45%
chocolate laced pirouettes	5 cookies	10.0	180	50%
dessert favorites	3 cookies	9.0	170	48%
party favorites	3 cookies	8.0	170	42%
personal favorites	4 cookies	9.0	170	48%
toy chest butter assortment	3 cookies	5.0	120	38%
Distinctive cookies				
Bordeaux				
milk chocolate	3 cookies	9.0	160	51%
original	4 cookies	5.0	130	35%
Brussels				
individual pkg	2 cookies	4.0	100	36%
regular pkg	3 cookies	7.0	150	42%
Brussels mint	3 cookies	10.0	190	47%
butter chessmen				
individual pkg	3 cookies	4.0	100	36%
regular pkg	3 cookies	5.0	120	38%
Chantilly hazelnut	1 cookie	3.0	80	34%
Geneva	3 cookies	9.0	160	51%
Lido	1 cookie	4.5	90	45%
Linzer				
original	1 cookie	4.0	100	36%
raspberry-filled	1 cookie	4.0	100	36%
Milano				
double chocolate	2 cookies	8.0	140	51%
milk chocolate	3 cookies	10.0	180	50%
mint	2 cookies	7.0	130	48%
orange	2 cookies	8.0	140	51%
original				
individual pkg	2 cookies	6.0	110	49%
regular pkg	3 cookies	10.0	180	50%
Nantucket/individual pkg	2 cookies	11.0	220	45%

Food and Description	Amount	Fat Grams	Total Calories	% Fat Calories
Verona strawberry	1 cookie	5.0	140	32%
Goldfish cookies				
chocolate	19 pieces	5.0	140	53%
chocolate chunk	19 pieces	7.0	150	42%
cinnamon graham	19 pieces	7.0	150	42%
goldfish cookies on the go	1 pouch	7.0	200	32%
graham goldfish	19 pieces	7.0	150	42%
vanilla	19 pieces	7.0	150	42%
International Collection				
Biarritz	6 cookies	8.0	160	45%
chocolat a l'orange	2 cookies	6.0	150	36%
deli choc dark chocolate	2 cookies	4.0	110	33%
espirit blanc	1 cookie	4.5	80	51%
espirits-noir/dark chocolate	1 cookie	5.0	90	50%
Highland shortbread	2 cookies	7.0	140	45%
madallon au beurre	4 cookies	5.0	150	30%
selection de choix	5 cookies	7.0	150	42%
large cookies				
brownie	2 cookies	13.0	260	45%
chocolate chip	2 cookies	11.0	240	41%
chocolate chocolate chip	2 cookies	12.0	250	43%
cinnamon chip	2 cookies	10.0	230	39%
oatmeal	2 cookies	9.0	240	34%
sugar	2 cookies	10.0	240	38%
mini cookies				
almond shortbread	9 cookies	17.0	300	51%
chocolate chip	9 cookies	14.0	260	48%
lemon nut	9 cookies	18.0	300	54%
oatmeal raisin	9 cookies	10.0	270	33%
peanut butter milk chocolate	9 cookies	15.0	280	48%
pecan Scotties	9 cookies	17.0	300	51%
toffee milk chocolate chunk	9 cookies	14.0	260	48%
old-fashioned cookies				
brownie chocolate nut	3 cookies	9.0	160	51%
butterscotch oatmeal	3 cookies	9.0	170	48%
chocolate chip	3 cookies	7.0	140	45%
ginger man				
individual pkg	3 cookies	3.0	90	30%
regular pkg	4 cookies	4.0	120	30%
hazelnut	3 cookies	8.0	160	45%
Irish oatmeal	3 cookies	6.0	130	42%
lemon nut crunch	3 cookies	9.0	170	48%
molasses crisp	5 cookies	6.0	150	36%
oatmeal raisin	3 cookies	6.0	160	34%
pecan shortbread	2 cookies	9.0	140	58%
shorthread	2 cookies	7.0	140	45%
sugar	3 cookies	6.0	140	39%
reduced-fat cookies				
chocolate chunk	1 cookie	4.5	120	34%
oatmeal raisin	1 cookie	3.0	110	25%

Food and Description	Amount	Fat Grams	Total Calories	% Fat Calories
vanilla creme Chantilly	1 cookie	2.0	70	26%
soft-baked cookies				
caramel pecan	1 cookie	7.0	130	37%
chocolate chocolate walnut	1 cookie	6.0	130	42%
chocolate chunk	1 cookie	6.0	130	42%
milk chocolate macadamia	1 cookie	6.0	130	42%
oatmeal raisin	1 cookie	4.0	110	33%
Wholesome Choice				
vanilla raspberry tart	2 cookies	3.0	120	23%
■ (Pillsbury)				
One-Step/prepared				
chocolate chip	1 cookie	7.0	150	42%
Refrigerated				
bat/hearts	2 cookies	7.0	130	48%
bunny/birthday balloon/candy cane/doughboy/				
flag/holiday tree/pumpkin/Rudolph/				
shamrock/tulip/valentine	2 cookies	7.0	130	48%
chocolate chip				
original	1 oz	7.0	140	35%
reduced fat	1 oz	3.0	110	25%
w/walnuts	1 oz	7.0	130	48%
chocolate chunk	1 oz	7.0	140	35%
double chocolate	1 oz	7.0	140	35%
gingerbread	1 oz	7.0	140	35%
holiday shapes	2 cookies	7.0	130	48%
M&M's	1 oz	6.0	130	42%
oatmeal chocolate chip	1 oz	6.0	120	45%
peanut butter	1 oz	6.0	130	42%
sugar	2 cookies	5.0	130	35%
white chocolate chunk	1 oz	6.0	130	42%
■ (Rippin'Good)				
carousel	6 cookies	6.0	140	39%
chocolate chip creme	2 cookies	6.0	160	34%
cookie jar	3 cookies	6.0	150	36%
creme wafers/assorted	3 cookies	7.0	140	45%
duplex creme	2 cookies	4.0	100	36%
fudge stripe oatmeal	2 cookies	8.0	140	51%
ginger snap	5 cookies	4.0	130	26%
granola & peanut butter sandwich	2 cookies	6.0	140	39%
iced oatmeal	2 cookies	2.0	90	30%
iced spice	3 cookies	3.0	130	21%
lemon crisp	3 cookies	8.0	160	45%
macaroon cremes	2 cookies	8.0	160	45%
marshmallow blossoms	2 cookies	2.0	90	30%
marshmallow daisies	2 cookies	2.0	90	30%
marshmallow fudge stripes	2 cookies	4.0	100	36%
peanut butter	2 cookies	4.0	100	36%
Rippie Cremes vanilla sandwich	3 cookies	6.0	160	34%
spice wafer	3 cookies	4.0	140	26%
striped dainties	1 cookie	3.0	50	54%

Food and Description	Amount	Fat Grams	Total Calories	% Fat Calories
■ **SNACKWELL's** (*See* (Nabisco) in this section)				
■ **(Spaans Cookie Co.)**				
banana/low-fat	2 cookies	3.0	100	27%
butter melt	2 cookies	6.0	130	42%
cherry crisp/sugar-free	4 cookies	5.0	110	41%
chocolate chip				
low-fat	2 cookies	3.0	110	25%
plain	2 cookies	6.0	120	45%
swirls/sugar-free	6 cookies	5.0	110	41%
w/walnuts	1 cookie	7.0	130	48%
cinnamon bears	1 cookie	4.0	100	36%
cocoa bears	1 cookie	4.0	100	36%
coconut krispies	2 cookies	5.0	120	38%
crunchy vanilla/sugar-free	4 cookies	5.0	120	38%
date oatmeal	2 cookies	4.5	120	34%
Dutch chocolate/sugar-free	3 cookies	5.0	110	41%
fruit 'n honey	2 cookies	3.5	110	29%
fudge brownie	2 cookies	4.5	120	34%
fudge 'n chips				
low-fat	2 cookies	2.5	100	23%
w/walnuts	1 cookie	6.0	120	45%
harvest	2 cookies	6.0	130	42%
holiday	2 cookies	7.0	130	48%
lemon coconut/sugar-free	3 cookies	6.0	120	45%
oat bran 'n chips/low-fat	2 cookies	3.0	100	27%
oat bran 'n raisin				
fat-free	2 cookies	–	80	–
low-fat	2 cookies	3.0	100	27%
regular	1 cookie	4.5	110	37%
peanut butter				
regular	2 cookies	7.0	130	48%
sugar-free	4 cookies	6.0	120	45%
shortbread	2 cookies	5.0	120	38%
soft oatmeal	2 cookies	3.5	110	29%
speculaas/windmills	2 cookies	6.0	130	42%
spiced windmill/sugar-free	2 cookies	5.0	110	41%
sugar bear	1 cookie	4.0	100	36%
toasted almond	2 cookies	7.0	130	48%
■ **(Stella D'Oro)**				
almond toast	2 pieces	2.5	110	20%
angel bars	2 cookies	9.0	140	13%
angel wings	1 cookie	5.0	70	64%
Angelica goodies	1 cookie	4.0	110	33%
anginetti	4 cookies	4.0	140	26%
anisette sponge	2 cookies	1.0	90	10%
anisette toast				
jumbo	1 cookie	1.0	110	8%
regular	3 cookies	1.0	130	7%
apple pastry	1 piece	3.0	80	34%

Food and Description	Amount	Fat Grams	Total Calories	% Fat Calories
biscotti				
almond fudge dipped	1 oz	4.0	120	30%
chocolate chunk	¾ oz	2.5	90	25%
chocolate chunk fudge dipped	1 oz	4.5	120	33%
French vanilla dipped	1 oz	4.0	120	30%
biscottini cashews	1 cookie	6.0	110	4%
castelets				
chocolate	1 piece	3.0	60	45%
vanilla	1 piece	3.0	70	39%
Chinese dessert	1 cookie	9.0	170	48%
coconut macaroon	1 cookie	3.0	60	45%
Como delight	1 cookie	7.0	150	42%
deep night fudge	1 cookie	4.0	65	55%
Dutch apple bar	1 piece	3.0	110	25%
fruit delight				
apple-cinnamon/fat-free	1 cookie	–	70	–
peach-apricot/fat-free	1 cookie	–	70	–
fruit slice				
fat-free	1 cookie	–	50	–
original	1 cookie	2.0	60	30%
golden bar	1 cookie	4.0	110	33%
hostess assortment	1 cookie	2.0	40	45%
kichel/low-sodium	21 pieces	9.0	150	54%
Lady Stella assortment	1 cookie	2.0	40	45%
Margherite				
chocolate	2 cookies	6.0	140	39%
vanilla	2 cookies	5.0	140	32%
peach-apricot pastry	1 piece	3.0	80	34%
pfeffernusse/spice drops	1 cookie	1.0	40	23%
prune pastry	1 piece	3.0	90	30%
royal nugget	1 piece	–	2	–
sesame Regina	1 piece	2.0	50	36%
Swiss fudge	2 pieces	7.0	130	48%
Viennese cinnamon breakfast treats	¾ oz	2.5	100	23%
■ (Tastykake)				
bars				
chocolate chip	1 bar	12.0	270	40%
chunky peanut butter	1 bar	11.0	240	41%
fudge	1 bar	10.0	250	36%
oatmeal raisin	1 bar	10.0	260	35%
strawberry	1 bar	10.0	260	35%
cookies				
boxed				
chocolate chip	3 cookies	6.0	130	42%
oatmeal raisin	3 cookies	6.0	130	42%
sugar	3 cookies	6.0	120	45%
chocolate chip/soft & chewy	1 cookie	7.0	180	35%
chocolate fudge/iced	1 cookie	7.0	170	37%
oatmeal raisin/soft & chewy/iced	1 cookie	6.0	170	32%

Food and Description	Amount	Fat Grams	Total Calories	% Fat Calories
■ **(Tofutti)** non-dairy				
chocolate chip	1 cookie	6.0	139	39%
fig bars	1 cookie	2.0	100	18%
oatmeal raisin	1 cookie	4.0	118	31%
peanut butter	1 cookie	7.0	137	46%
■ **TOLL HOUSE** (*See* (Nestlé) in this section)				
■ **(Tree Of Life)**				
Fat-Free				
classic carrot cake	1 cookie	–	60	–
devil's food chocolate	1 cookie	–	70	–
Fruit bars				
fig	1 cookie	–	70	–
peach-apricot	1 cookie	–	70	–
wildberry	1 cookie	–	70	–
golden oatmeal raisin	1 cookie	–	70	–
harvest fruit & nut	1 cookie	–	70	–
toasted almond butter	1 cookie	–	70	–
Regular				
creme supremes				
mint	2 cookies	5.0	120	38%
original	2 cookies	5.0	120	38%
fruit bars				
apple spice	2 cookies	3.0	120	23%
fig	2 cookies	3.0	120	23%
peach-apricot	2 cookies	3.0	120	23%
honey-sweet				
colossal carrot cake	1 cookie	5.0	110	41%
lemon burst	1 cookie	5.0	110	41%
oh-so-oatmeal	1 cookie	5.0	110	41%
pecans-a-plenty	1 cookie	7.0	125	39%
monster fat-free				
gingerbread	¼ cookie	–	80	–
maple pecan	¼ cookie	–	90	–
royal vanilla	2 cookies	5.0	120	38%
small world				
animal grahams	7 pieces	3.0	120	23%
chocolate chip	7 cookies	4.0	120	30%
soft-baked				
chocolate chip	1 cookie	7.0	125	50%
double fudge	1 cookie	5.0	110	41%
maui macaroon	1 cookie	10.0	135	67%
oatmeal	1 cookie	5.0	115	39%
peanut butter	1 cookie	7.0	125	50%
wheat-free				
American oatmeal	1 cookie	5.0	90	50%
California carob	1 cookie	5.0	105	43%
Georgia peanut butter	1 cookie	6.0	95	57%
Mountain maple walnut	1 cookie	6.0	100	54%
■ **TWIX** (*See* (M&M *Mars) in this section)				

Food and Description	Amount	Fat Grams	Total Calories	% Fat Calories
■ (Umeya)				
fortune cookie	4 cookies	<1.0	120	4%
■ (Voortman)				
almonette	1 cookie	5.0	90	50%
chocolate chip	1 cookie	5.0	100	45%
chocolate wafer	3 cookies	9.0	160	51%
coconut delight	1 cookie	5.0	90	50%
Dutch creme	1 cookie	5.0	110	41%
Maple leaf sandwich	1 cookie	4.0	100	36%
oatmeal apple	1 cookie	3.0	80	34%
shortbread swirl	2 cookies	6.0	110	49%
strawberry wafer	3 cookies	9.0	170	43%
vanilla wafer	3 cookies	9.0	170	43%
■ (Weight Watchers)				
apple raisin bar	1 cookie	2.0	70	26%
chocolate sandwich	2 cookies	4.0	140	26%
oatmeal raisin	2 cookies	2.0	120	15%
vanilla sandwich	2 cookies	3.0	140	19%
■ (Westbrae)				
Cookie Jar Classics				
Dutch apple cinnamon	1 cookie	4.0	110	32%
honey almond	1 cookie	4.0	110	32%
raspberry vanilla	1 cookie	4.0	110	32%
regular cookies				
crispy chocolate chip	1 cookie	4.0	110	32%
Dinosnaps animal oatmeal raisin	8 cookies	5.0	130	35%
soft chocolate chip				
coconut	1 cookie	4.5	110	37%
pecan	1 cookie	4.5	110	37%
walnut	1 cookie	5.0	110	41%
soft chocolate chocolate chip	1 cookie	3.0	90	30%
rice malt cookies				
ginger snap	3 cookies	5.0	130	35%
oatmeal	3 cookies	6.0	140	39%
COOKIE CRUMBS (See also CRACKER CRUMBS & MEAL)				
(Nabisco)				
Honey Maid graham cracker	2.5 Tbs	1.5	70	19%
Oreo	2 Tbs	4.0	90	40%
COOKING SPRAY				
(Mazola)	2-sec spray	0.8	6	100%
(Pam)				
butter flavor	⅓ of 10" skillet	<1.0	2	100%
olive oil	⅓ of 10" skillet	<1.0	2	100%
original	¼-sec spray	<1.0	7	100%
(Tryson House) flavor spray				
buttery delite	1-sec spray	0.8	8	100%
garlic mist	1-sec spray	0.8	8	100%
Italian mist	1-sec spray	0.8	8	100%
mesquite mist	1-sec spray	0.8	8	100%
olive mist	1-sec spray	0.8	8	100%

Food and Description	Amount	Fat Grams	Total Calories	% Fat Calories
Oriental mist (Weight Watchers)	1-sec spray	0.8	8	100%
butter	0.28 gm	–	–	–
cooking	0.33 gm	–	–	–
(Wesson)	0.27 gm	<1.0	<1	100%
CORIANDER LEAF (See CILANTRO)				
CORIANDER SEED				
whole	1 tsp	<1.0	5	53%
	1 Tbs	0.9	15	53%
	1 oz	5.0	85	53%
CORN				
canned				
(Bristol) baby corn on cob	4 ears	–	12	–
(Del Monte)				
cream style				
golden				
no salt added	½ cup	0.5	90	5%
regular	½ cup	0.5	90	5%
supersweet	½ cup	0.5	60	8%
white	½ cup	1.0	100	9%
whole kernel				
fiesta	½ cup	1.0	50	18%
golden				
regular	½ cup	1.0	90	10%
supersweet				
no salt added	½ cup	1.0	60	15%
no sugar added	½ cup	1.0	60	15%
vacuum packed	½ cup	1.0	70	13%
white	½ cup	1.0	60	15%
(Fancifood) baby	6 pieces	–	25	–
(Freshlike)				
cream style/golden				
no salt added	½ cup	1.0	100	9%
regular	½ cup	1.0	100	9%
crisp 'n sweet	½ cup	1.0	80	11%
whole kernel				
vacuum packed	½ cup	1.0	100	9%
water packed				
no salt added	½ cup	1.0	80	11%
no sugar or salt added	½ cup	1.0	80	11%
generic/cream style	½ cup	0.5	93	5%
(Green Giant)				
cream style	½ cup	0.5	100	5%
Mexicorn	⅓ cup	–	60	–
Niblets				
white shoepeg	⅓ cup	1.0	80	11%
yellow				
extra sweet	⅓ cup	0.5	50	9%
50% less sodium	⅓ cup	–	60	–
no salt or sugar added	⅓ cup	–	60	–

Food and Description	Amount	Fat Grams	Total Calories	% Fat Calories
regular	⅓ cup	–	70	–
whole kernel/sweet				
50% less sodium	½ cup	1.0	80	11%
regular	½ cup	1.0	80	11%
(S&W)				
cream style				
regular	½ cup	1.0	100	9%
w/starch	½ cup	1.0	100	9%
whole kernel				
regular	½ cup	1.0	90	10%
sweet 'n crisp	⅓ cup	1.5	70	19%
(Seneca)				
cream style	½ cup	–	80	–
whole kernel	½ cup	0.5	80	6%
(Stokely)				
cream style				
golden	½ cup	1.0	100	9%
white	½ cup	1.0	100	9%
whole kernel				
golden	½ cup	–	80	–
white	½ cup	–	80	–
(Veg-All) golden				
cream style	½ cup	1.0	110	8%
whole kernel				
regular	½ cup	1.0	80	11%
vacuum packed	½ cup	1.0	100	9%
fresh/sweet/white or yellow				
kernels/cooked	½ cup	1.0	89	10%
whole ear	1 medium	1.0	89	10%
frozen				
(Birds Eye)				
baby gold & white	⅔ cup	0.5	60	8%
baby white	⅔ cup	0.5	60	8%
big ears	1 ear	1.0	160	6%
cut kernels	⅓ cup	0.5	70	6%
little ears	2 ears	1.0	120	8%
sweet corn on cob	2 ears	1.0	110	8%
tendersweet, deluxe	½ cup	0.5	100	5%
tendersweet, deluxe, baby whole	½ cup	0.5	100	5%
(C&W) early harvest petite				
petite white	⅔ cup	1.0	80	11%
petite white and golden	⅔ cup	1.0	80	11%
sweet corn	⅔ cup	1.0	80	11%
generic				
corn on the cob	1 ear	1.0	150	6%
cream style	½ cup	0.6	120	5%
kernels/white shoepeg	½ cup	1.0	70	13%
(Green Giant)				
corn on the cob				
extra sweet	1 ear	2.0	120	15%

Food and Description	Amount	Fat Grams	Total Calories	% Fat Calories
Nibblers/6-ear pkg	1 ear	0.5	70	6%
Niblets/4-ear pkg	1 ear	1.0	150	6%
kernels				
Harvest Fresh				
white shoepeg	½ cup	0.5	70	6%
yellow	⅔ cup	0.5	80	6%
Niblets				
extra sweet	⅔ cup	1.0	70	13%
regular	⅔ cup	0.5	80	6%
regular/white				
extra sweet	⅔ cup	0.5	50	9%
shoepeg	¾ cup	1.0	100	9%
(Ore-Ida) corn on the cob				
mini gold	1 ear	1.0	80	11%
regular	1 ear	1.5	140	10%
(Pictsweet)				
corn on the cob				
3" ear	1 ear	<1.0	50	8%
6" ear	1 ear	1.0	110	8%
kernels/cut	½ cup	1.0	80	11%
(Seneca)				
corn on the cob	1 ear	–	140	–
kernels	⅔ cup	0.5	90	5%
CORN CAKE (*See* RICE CAKES)				
CORN CHIPS (*See* TORTILLA CHIPS)				
CORN CHOWDER (*See* SOUP)				
CORN DISH (*See also* FROZEN ENTRÉE/DINNER; VEGETABLES, MIXED)				
canned				
(Green Giant) corn relish	1 Tbs	–	20	–
frozen				
(Green Giant)				
cream style corn in cheese & cream sauce	½ cup	1.0	110	8%
Niblets in butter sauce	⅔ cup	1.5	110	12%
white shoepeg in butter sauce	¾ cup	2.0	110	16%
(Mrs. Paul's) corn fritter	1 fritter	6.0	130	42%
homemade/USDA Standard Home Recipe				
corn fritter	1 oz	2.0	62	29%
corn pudding	½ cup	6.6	136	44%
scalloped corn	½ cup	7.0	250	25%
CORN FLAKE CRUMBS				
(Kellogg's)	2 Tbs	–	40	
CORN GRITS				
(Albers) quick hominy	¼ cup	0.5	140	3%
(Arrowhead Mills) dry				
white	¼ cup	–	140	–
yellow	¼ cup	–	130	–
generic				
canned				
white	1 cup	1.5	115	11%

Food and Description	Amount	Fat Grams	Total Calories	% Fat Calories
yellow	1 cup	1.5	115	11%
dry				
cooked	4 oz	<1.0	68	3%
	1 cup	0.5	146	3%
uncooked	1 Tbs	<1.0	36	3%
	1 oz	<1.0	105	3%
	1 cup	1.8	579	3%
(Quaker) dry				
instant				
bacon cheddar cheese	1 pkt	1.5	100	5%
original	1 pkt	–	100	–
real butter flavor	1 pkt	1.5	100	14%
white hominy	1 pkt	–	80	–
w/cheese & sausage	1 pkt	1.5	100	5%
w/country bacon bits	1 pkt	0.5	100	5%
w/real cheddar cheese	1 pkt	1.5	100	14%
zesty cheddar	1 pkt	1.5	100	14%
quick				
golden grits	¼ cup	0.5	120	4%
white hominy	¼ cup	0.5	130	3%
regular-old fashion/white hominy	¼ cup	0.5	140	4%
CORN NUT (See SNACKS)				
CORN PONE (See BREAD)				
CORN PUDDING (See PUDDING & MOUSSE)				
CORN SYRUP (See also PANCAKE/WAFFLE SYRUP)				
generic	1 Tbs	–	59	–
(Karo)				
dark	2 Tbs	–	120	–
	½ cup	–	495	–
light	2 Tbs	–	120	–
	½ cup	–	500	–
CORNBREAD (See BREAD)				
CORNED BEEF (See also BEEF; LUNCHEON MEAT)				
generic				
canned	1 oz	4.0	71	51%
jellied loaf	1 oz	1.9	46	37%
(Mary Kitchen) canned				
Individual serving	1 cup	22.0	350	57%
(Morton's) fresh	4 oz	8.0	150	48%
CORNED BEEF HASH (See BEEF DISH/ENTRÉE)				
CORNISH GAME HEN				
fresh & frozen				
(Perdue) whole				
dark meat	3 oz	15.0	210	64%
white meat	3 oz	10.0	170	53%
(Tyson) w/giblets	4 oz	12.0	180	60%
fully cooked				
(Perdue) oven roasted				
dark meat	3 oz	9.0	140	58%
white meat	3 oz	7.0	130	48%

Food and Description	Amount	Fat Grams	Total Calories	% Fat Calories
CORNMEAL				
(Albers) yellow or white	3 Tbs	–	110	–
(Arrowhead Mills) blue	2 oz	3.0	210	13%
(Aunt Jemima) self-rising white/enriched				
bolted	3 Tbs	0.5	90	5%
degermed	3 Tbs	0.5	90	5%
CORNMEAL MIX (*See also* BAKE & FRY MIX)				
(Aunt Jemima) self-rising				
buttermilk white	3 Tbs	0.5	80	6%
white/bolted	3 Tbs	0.5	80	6%
yellow	3 Tbs	0.5	80	6%
(Miracle Maize) Prepared				
complete	2"x2" piece	3.0	195	14%
country style	2"x2" piece	5.0	230	20%
sweet	2"x2" piece	5.0	235	19%
CORNSTARCH	1 Tbs	–	30	–
	1 cup	–	463	–
COTTAGE CHEESE (*See also* CHEESE)				
(Borden)				
creamed				
4% fat	½ cup	5.0	120	38%
2% fat	½ cup	2.0	90	20%
dry curd/5% fat	½ cup	1.0	80	11%
(Breakstone)				
creamed				
4% fat				
large curd	½ cup	5.0	120	38%
small curd	½ cup	5.0	120	38%
snack size	4 oz	5.0	110	41%
2% fat				
large curd	½ cup	2.5	90	25%
small curd	½ cup	2.5	90	25%
snack size	4 oz	2.0	90	20%
dry curd/<0.5% fat	¼ cup	–	45	–
ricotta	¼ cup	–	45	–
(Carnation)				
creamed				
4% fat				
large curd	½ cup	5.0	115	38%
small curd	½ cup	5.0	115	38%
w/pineapple	½ cup	5.0	130	35%
1.5% fat/Slender	½ cup	2.0	90	20%
(Crowley) creamed				
4% fat				
plain	½ cup	5.0	120	38%
w/peaches	½ cup	3.0	140	19%
w/pineapple	½ cup	4.0	140	26%
1% fat				
calcium-fortified	½ cup	1.0	90	10%

Food and Description	Amount	Fat Grams	Total Calories	% Fat Calories
plain	½ cup	1.0	90	10%
w/pineapple	½ cup	1.0	110	8%
(Darigold) creamed				
4% fat	½ cup	5.0	120	38%
2% fat/trim	½ cup	2.5	100	23%
(Friendship) creamed				
4% fat				
California style	½ cup	4.0	120	30%
w/pineapple	½ cup	4.0	140	26%
1% fat				
plain	½ cup	1.0	90	10%
lactose reduced	½ cup	1.0	90	10%
no salt added	½ cup	1.0	90	10%
w/pineapple	½ cup	1.0	110	8%
2% fat/large curd pot-style	½ cup	2.5	100	23%
generic				
creamed				
4% fat				
large curd	½ cup	5.0	117	39%
small curd	½ cup	5.0	117	39%
1% fat	½ cup	1.0	80	11%
2% fat	½ cup	2.5	100	23%
dry curd				
large curd	½ cup	0.5	95	5%
small curd	½ cup	0.5	95	5%
(Hood)				
1% Fat				
chive & onion	½ cup	2.0	90	20%
no salt added	½ cup	2.0	90	20%
pepper & herb	½ cup	2.0	90	20%
pineapple cherry	½ cup	1.0	110	8%
plain	½ cup	2.0	90	20%
4% Fat				
chive	½ cup	4.0	130	28%
pineapple				
non-fat	½ cup	–	110	–
regular	½ cup	4.0	130	28%
non-fat	½ cup	–	80	–
plain	½ cup	4.0	120	30%
(Kemps)				
creamed				
nonfat	4 oz	–	80	–
1% fat/lite	4 oz	1.0	90	10%
2% fat/low-fat	4 oz	2.5	100	23%
whole milk	4 oz	5.0	120	38%
dry curd	4 oz	1.0	80	11%
(Knudsen) creamed				
4% fat				
large curd	½ cup	5.0	130	35%
small curd	½ cup	5.0	120	38%

Food and Description	Amount	Fat Grams	Total Calories	% Fat Calories
nonfat/free				
On The Go!	4 oz	–	70	–
reguar	½ cup	–	80	
snack size	4 oz	–	70	–
1.5% fat "On The Go"				
peach	½ cup	1.5	110	12%
pineapple	½ cup	2.0	120	15%
strawberry	½ cup	1.5	110	12%
tropical fruit	½ cup	2.0	110	18%
2% fat/small curd	½ cup	2.5	100	23%
(Land O'Lakes) creamed				
4% fat	½ cup	5.0	120	38%
1% fat	½ cup	1.0	90	10%
2% fat	½ cup	2.0	100	18%
(Light N' Lively) creamed				
1% fat				
plain	½ cup	1.0	80	11%
w/garden salad	½ cup	1.5	80	17%
w/peach & pineapple	½ cup	1.0	110	8%
nonfat	½ cup	–	80	–
(Sealtest) creamed				
4% fat				
large curd	½ cup	5.0	120	38%
small curd	½ cup	5.0	120	38%
2% fat/small curd	½ cup	2.5	90	25%
(Weight Watchers) creamed				
1% fat	½ cup	1.0	90	10%
2% fat	½ cup	2.0	90	20%
COUSCOUS (See also PASTA, SOUP/DEHYDRATED)				
(Casbah) Mix only				
almond chicken vegetarian	1 pkg	2.0	160	11%
asparagus au gratin organic	1 pkg	2.0	150	12%
cheddar broccoli	1 pkg	2.0	130	14%
hearty harvest	1 pkg	1.0	180	5%
(Kitchen Del Sol) Mix/prepared				
Aegean citrus	½ cup	3.0	110	25%
Moroccan ginger	½ cup	3.0	120	23%
spicy vegetable	½ cup	3.0	120	23%
tomato & olive	½ cup	4.0	120	30%
(Melting Pot) Mix/prepared				
calypso cranberry	1 cup	–	200	–
lucky seven	1 cup	1.0	190	5%
roasted garlic	1 cup	–	170	–
sesame ginger	1 cup	1.0	180	5%
sun-dried tomatoes	1 cup	1.0	190	5%
wild mushroom	1 cup	–	190	–
(Near East) Mix/prepared				
broccoli	1 cup	2.5	210	11%
herbed chicken	1 cup	3.5	220	14%
Mediterranean curry	1 cup	3.5	220	14%

Food and Description	Amount	Fat Grams	Total Calories	% Fat Calories
Parmesan	1 cup	3.0	220	12%
roasted garlic & olive oil	1 cup	4.5	230	18%
toasted pine nut	1 cup	6.0	230	23%
tomato lentil	1 cup	3.5	220	14%
COWPEA (*See* BLACK-EYED PEA)				
CRAB (*See also* CRAB, IMITATION; CRAB DISH; SEAFOOD ENTRÉE/DINNER)				
canned/meat only				
(Chicken of the Sea) drained				
fancy	2 oz	0.5	40	11%
jumbo lump	2 oz	0.5	35	13%
lump	2 oz	0.5	35	13%
white	2 oz	–	30	–
(Crown Prince) drained	½ cup	–	50	–
(Geisha)				
lump	2.21 oz	0.5	45	10%
snow	1.96 oz	–	35	–
generic/blue	3 oz	1.0	84	11%
(S&W) Dungeness	⅓ cup	1.0	80	11%
fresh/meat only				
Alaska/Alaskan king				
cooked-moist heat	3 oz	1.0	82	11%
	1 leg	2.0	129	14%
raw	3 oz	1.0	71	13%
	1 leg	1.0	145	6%
blue				
cooked-moist heat	3 oz	1.5	90	15%
raw	3 oz	1.0	75	12%
Dungeness				
cooked-moist heat	3 oz	1.0	95	9%
raw	3 oz	1.0	75	12%
queen/raw	3 oz	1.0	76	12%
soft shell				
cooked-moist heat	3 oz	1.5	90	15%
fried	1 medium	13.0	213	55%
frozen				
(Wakefield) snow	3 oz	1.0	60	15%
CRAB, IMITATION				
generic/from surimi	3 oz	1.0	87	10%
(Icicle Seafood)	⅔ cup	–	90	–
(Louis Kemp) crab delights				
chunk style	½ cup	–	80	–
flake style	½ cup	–	80	–
leg style	½ cup	–	80	–
CRAB DISH (*See also* SEAFOOD ENTRÉE/DINNER)				
frozen				
(Carnival) crab cake/low-fat	1 cake	1.0	110	8%
(King & Prince)				
crab crisp	4 oz	19.0	310	55%
crab del ray	3 oz	9.0	155	52%
(Mrs. Paul's)				
cheese & crab poppers	4 poppers	16.0	320	45%

Food and Description	Amount	Fat Grams	Total Calories	% Fat Calories
deviled crab cake				
miniatures	6 pieces	12.0	220	49%
regular	1 cake	10.0	180	50%
(Nancy's) Seafood Crab Cakes	6 oz package	20.0	350	51%
(Van De Kamp's)				
cheese & crab poppers	4 poppers	16.0	320	45%
crab cakes	1 cake	9.0	170	48%
homemade/USDA Standard Home Recipe				
crab cake/fried	4 oz	8.5	180	43%
crab salad	5.5 oz	10.7	205	47%
CRAB SOUP (See SOUP)				
CRABAPPLE				
canned				
(Lucky Leaf) spiced	½ cup	–	110	–
fresh/raw/w/skin				
sliced	½ cup	–	40	–
whole	3 oz	–	60	–
CRACKER (See also COOKIE; SNACKS)				
■ (Adrienne's)				
Appeleazers				
double cheddar	1 oz	5.0	130	35%
garlic & herb	1 oz	4.0	130	28%
original	1 oz	4.0	130	28%
Courtney's English Water Crackers				
classic	4 crackers	1.0	60	15%
cracked pepper	4 crackers	1.0	60	15%
savory herb	4 crackers	1.0	60	15%
sundried tomato	4 crackers	1.0	60	15%
Darcia's Crostini				
aged cheddar	8 pieces	3.5	90	35%
cheddar	8 pieces	3.5	90	35%
fennel	8 pieces	3.5	90	35%
onion	8 pieces	3.5	90	35%
original	8 pieces	3.5	90	35%
rosemary	8 pieces	3.5	90	35%
Gourmet Lavosh Hawaii flatbread				
caraway & rye	1 oz	3.0	115	23%
classic island	1 oz	3.0	120	23%
peppercorn	1 oz	3.0	115	23%
rosemary-garlic	1 oz	3.0	125	22%
slightly onion	1 oz	3.0	120	23%
ten grain	1 oz	3.0	110	25%
■ (Ak-Mak)				
100% whole wheat	5 crackers	2.0	116	16%
Cracker Bread				
Armenian				
regular	1 sheet	2.0	100	18%
whole wheat	1 sheet	2.0	116	16%
round				
no seeds	1 cracker	1.0	100	9%

Food and Description	Amount	Fat Grams	Total Calories	% Fat Calories
seeded	1 cracker	2.0	100	18%
whole wheat	1 cracker	2.0	116	16%
■ (Andre Prost)				
Olof crispbread/Sweden crisp				
four grain	2 pieces	2.0	90	29%
whole-grain	2 pieces	1.5	60	23%
■ (Austin)				
snack pack				
cheese Dolphins & Friends	28 crackers	2.5	60	38%
	43 crackers	4.0	100	36%
	60 crackers	6.0	140	39%
	114 crackers	11.0	260	38%
cheese 'n peanut butter				
50% more	6 crackers	12.0	230	47%
regular	4 crackers	8.0	140	51%
	6 crackers	11.0	200	50%
cheese on cheese	4 crackers	8.0	140	51%
	6 crackers	11.0	200	50%
crispy crackers sandwiches				
w/cream cheese'n chives	6 sdw	10.0	190	47%
w/cheddar cheese	6 sdw	11.0	200	50%
w/peanut butter	6 sdw	10.0	190	47%
reduced-fat crackers				
w/cheese filling	6 crackers	7.0	170	42%
w/peanut butter	6 crackers	7.0	170	42%
toast crackers				
reduced-fat				
w/peanut butter	6 crackers	7.0	170	42%
	4 crackers	4.5	120	34%
regular				
w/cheese filling	6 crackers	11.0	200	50%
w/peanut butter	4 crackers	7.0	140	49%
	6 crackers	10.0	190	47%
toasty crackers				
w/salsa filling	6 crackers	10.0	190	47%
wafers				
w/cheddar cheese filling	6 crackers	11.0	200	50%
w/creme cheese filling	6 crackers	10.0	190	47%
w/honey roasted peanut butter filling	6 crackers	11.0	230	43%
wheat crackers				
reduced fat/w/cheese	6 crackers	7.0	170	37%
regular/w/cheese filling	4 crackers	8.0	140	51%
	6 crackers	11.0	200	50%
Zoo animal crackers				
Dinosaur graham	20 crackers	5.0	140	32%
mini	57 crackers	2.0	130	14%
regular	16 crackers	2.0	130	14%
■ (Barbara's Bakery)				
Cheese Bites	26 crackers	1.5	120	11%

Food and Description	Amount	Fat Grams	Total Calories	% Fat Calories
Rite Lite Rounds	5 crackers	<1.0	55	8%
Wafer Crisps				
French onion	3 wafers	1.0	60	30%
roasted garlic & herb	3 wafers	1.0	60	30%
sundried tomato & basil	3 wafers	1.0	60	30%
toasted sesame	3 wafers	1.0	60	30%
Wheatines/all natural				
cracked pepper	4 crackers	1.5	50	27%
lightly salted tops	4 crackers	1.5	50	27%
original	4 crackers	1.5	50	27%
sesame	4 crackers	1.5	50	27%
unsalted tops	4 crackers	1.5	50	27%
■ BRETON (See (Dare) in this section)				
■ (Burns & Ricker)				
Crispini				
fat-free	½ cup	–	110	–
seeds & spice	5 pieces	3.0	110	25%
sesame	5 pieces	3.0	110	25%
sesame garlic	5 pieces	3.0	110	25%
S.F. stone-ground wheat	5 pieces	<0.5	110	4%
Pita Crisps/~5 per oz				
pesto	1 oz	5.0	130	35%
tomato & onion	1 oz	6.0	130	42%
Tuscany toast				
pesto	10 pieces	5.0	120	38%
tomato & onion	10 pieces	6.0	130	42%
■ (Campbell's)				
soup & oyster	32 pieces	3.0	70	39%
■ (Carr's)				
Cocktail Crackers				
Cocktail Cheddars	22 pieces	8.0	150	48%
Cocktail Croissant				
original golden	22 crackers	3.0	140	19%
sesame & spring vegetable	22 crackers	3.5	140	23%
Assortments				
biscuits for cheese	3 biscuits	2.5	83	27%
distinctive flavour assortment	3 crackers	2.5	70	32%
Entertainers				
cheddar crackers	3 crackers	4.0	80	45%
croissant crackers	3 crackers	3.0	70	39%
poppy & sesame crackers	4 crackers	5.0	80	56%
wheatolo English biscuits	1 biscuit	3.0	70	39%
whole wheat crackers	2 crackers	3.5	80	39%
Monterey Crackers				
hearty wheat	3 crackers	2.0	60	30%
roasted vegetable	3 crackers	2.0	60	30%
savory wheat	3 crackers	2.5	70	32%
Table Water Crackers				
plain	5 crackers	1.5	70	19%
w/cracked pepper	5 crackers	1.5	70	19%

Food and Description	Amount	Fat Grams	Total Calories	% Fat Calories
w/roasted garlic & herbs	5 crackers	1.5	70	19%
w/toasted sesame seeds	5 crackers	1.5	70	19%

■ **CHRISTIE BROWN** (*See* (Nabisco) in this section)
■ **COMBOS** (*See* (M&M* Mars) in this section)
■ **CRISPINI** (*See* (Burns & Ricker) in this section)
■ **(Dare)**
Breton

Food and Description	Amount	Fat Grams	Total Calories	% Fat Calories
50% less salt	1 cracker	1.0	22	41%
	4 crackers	4.0	84	43%
garden vegetable	1 cracker	0.9	20	41%
light	1 cracker	0.6	20	27%
	4 crackers	2.4	80	27%
minis				
cheddar cheese	20 crackers	3.7	87	38%
garden vegetable	20 crackers	3.9	87	40%
original	20 crackers	4.1	89	41%
original	1 cracker	1.0	21	41%
	4 crackers	3.6	84	39%
sesame	1 cracker	1.1	22	45%
	4 crackers	4.4	88	45%
Cabaret	1 cracker	1.1	23	43%
	4 crackers	4.4	92	43%
	4 crackers	2.4	80	27%
Vinta	1 cracker	1.3	30	39%
Vivant Italian	1 cracker	0.9	22	37%
	4 crackers	4.0	84	43%

■ **(Delicious)**
cheddar cheese

Food and Description	Amount	Fat Grams	Total Calories	% Fat Calories
low-fat	22 crackers	1.5	110	12%
original	24 crackers	4.5	140	29%
snack	28 crackers	7.0	150	42%
chicken flavored snack	10 crackers	9.0	160	51%
cracked pepper/fat-free	17 crackers	–	110	–
crispy bacon	11 crackers	7.0	150	42%
garden vegetable				
low-fat	14 crackers	1.5	120	11%
original	13 crackers	7.0	150	42%
graham crackers				
chocolate	2 crackers	3.0	130	21%
cinnamon	2 crackers	3.5	130	24%
honey	2 crackers	3.0	130	21%
hearty wheat snack	13 crackers	6.0	140	39%
saltines				
original	5 crackers	1.5	60	27%
unsalted tops	5 crackers	1.5	60	27%
savory ranch	10 crackers	8.0	160	45%
sesame wheat	13 crackers	7.0	150	42%
snack crackers	9 crackers	8.0	150	48%
soup & chili crackers	37 crackers	1.5	60	23%
sour cream & chive snack	9 crackers	9.0	160	51%

Food and Description	Amount	Fat Grams	Total Calories	% Fat Calories
tangy onion snack	11 crackers	6.0	140	39%
■ (Devonsheer)				
Melba Rounds				
garlic	½ oz	1.0	60	15%
honey bran	½ oz	1.0	50	18%
onion	½ oz	1.0	50	18%
plain				
regular	½ oz	1.0	50	18%
unsalted	½ oz	1.0	50	18%
rye	½ oz	1.0	50	18%
sesame				
regular	½ oz	2.0	60	30%
unsalted	½ oz	2.0	60	30%
twelve grain	½ oz	1.0	50	18%
vegetable	½ oz	1.0	50	18%
wheat				
regular	½ oz	1.0	50	18%
unsalted	½ oz	1.0	50	18%
■ (Estee) Sugar-Free				
Classic				
cracked pepper	18 crackers	2.0	120	15%
golden	10 crackers	2.0	130	14%
wheat	17 crackers	1.5	100	14%
Grahams				
chocolate	2 crackers	2.0	110	
cinnamon	2 crackers	2.0	90	20%
old fashion	2 crackers	2.0	90	20%
■ (Finn)				
crispbread/dark				
plain	2 pieces	–	40	–
w/caraway seeds	2 pieces	–	40	–
■ (Frito Lay)				
Cheetos				
bacon cheddar	1 pkg	9.0	190	43%
cheddar cheese	1 pkg	11.0	210	47%
golden toast & cheddar	1 pkg	14.0	240	53%
Doritos				
jalapeño & cheddar	1 pkg	13.0	230	51%
nacho cheesier	1 pkg	14.0	240	53%
Peanut Pan				
cheese peanut butter	1 pkg	10.0	210	43%
toast peanut butter	1 pkg	11.0	210	47%
■ (Frookie)				
Frookwich crackers				
cracked pepper	8 crackers	–	130	–
garlic & herb	8 crackers	–	130	–
water	8 crackers	–	70	–
whole wheat	4 crackers	–	35	–
Graham crackers				
cinnamon	2 crackers	3.0	100	27%

Food and Description	Amount	Fat Grams	Total Calories	% Fat Calories
honey	2 crackers	3.0	110	25%
Snack				
garden vegetable	13 crackers	4.0	120	30%
snack & party	10 crackers	5.0	140	32%
wheat & onion	12 crackers	4.0	120	30%
wheat & rye	13 crackers	4.0	120	30%
■ GENERIC				
cracker				
cheese				
plain	1 cracker	<1.0	5	51%
	14 crackers	4.0	70	51%
w/peanut butter	1 cracker	2.0	35	51%
oyster	10 crackers	1.0	44	21%
peanut butter sandwich	1 cracker	2.0	35	51%
rye				
wafers				
plain	8 crackers	2.0	90	20%
seasoned	8 crackers	2.0	90	20%
w/cheese	1 cracker	2.0	35	51%
saltine square	1 square	<1.0	13	18%
	4 squares	1.0	50	18%
soup	1 cracker	–	4	–
wafer/plain	13 crackers	3.0	130	21%
water biscuit	3 pieces	3.0	90	30%
wheat				
thin	2 crackers	<1.0	10	39%
	7 crackers	3.0	70	39%
w/cheese filling	1 cracker	2.0	35	51%
w/peanut butter filling	1 cracker	2.0	35	51%
whole wheat	1 cracker	1.0	20	45%
crispbread				
plain	3 pieces	2.0	60	30%
rusk/½" thick/3⅜" dia	1 piece	0.8	38	19
rye	3 pieces	1.0	75	12%
■ (Goodman's) Matzo crackers				
Passover				
egg	1 matzo	1.0	130	7%
plain	1 matzo	–	130	–
■ (Hain)				
cheese	1 oz	6.0	130	42%
onion				
no salt added	1 oz	6.0	130	42%
regular	1 oz	6.0	130	42%
rich				
no salted added	1 oz	5.0	130	35%
regular	1 oz	5.0	130	35%
rye				
no salt added	1 oz	4.0	120	30%
regular	1 oz	4.0	120	30%
sesame				
no salt added	1 oz	7.0	140	45%

Food and Description	Amount	Fat Grams	Total Calories	% Fat Calories
regular	1 oz	7.0	140	45%
sour cream & chive				
no salt added	1 oz	6.0	130	42%
regular	1 oz	6.0	130	42%
sourdough				
low-salt	1 oz	5.0	130	35%
regular	1 oz	6.0	130	42%
vegetable				
no salt added	1 oz	5.0	130	35%
regular	1oz	5.0	130	35%
■ (Health Valley)				
herb stoned wheat				
no salt	13 crackers	2.0	55	33%
regular	13 crackers	2.0	55	33%
rice bran	7 crackers	4.0	130	28%
sesame stoned wheat				
no salt added	13 crackers	2.0	55	33%
regular	13 crackers	2.0	55	33%
seven grain vegetable stoned wheat				
no salt added	13 crackers	2.0	55	33%
regular	13 crackers	2.0	55	33%
stoned wheat				
no salt added	13 crackers	2.0	55	33%
regular	13 crackers	2.0	55	33%
■ (Hopi)				
seaweed wrap	18 pieces	–	110	–
sesame bits	½ cup	–	120	–
■ (Ideal)				
crispbread				
extra thins	3 slices	–	48	–
fiber thins	2 slices	–	40	–
oat bran thins	2 slices	–	50	–
flatbread				
fiber w/sesame seeds	2 slices	–	40	–
whole grain/no salt	2 slices	–	43	–
■ (J.J. Flats)				
Breadflats				
caraway	1 piece	1.0	50	18%
caraway & salt	1 piece	1.0	50	18%
cinnamon	1 piece	1.0	50	18%
flavorall	1 piece	1.0	50	18%
garlic	1 piece	1.0	50	18%
oat bran	1 piece	1.0	50	18%
onion	1 piece	1.0	50	18%
plain	1 piece	1.0	50	18%
poppy	1 piece	1.0	50	18%
sesame	1 piece	1.0	50	18%
■ (Kavli)				
Norwegian crispbread				
crispy thin	2 slices	<1.0	15	10%

Food and Description	Amount	Fat Grams	Total Calories	% Fat Calories
hearty thick	1 slice	<1.0	35	10%
rye-bran	2 slices	–	30	–
■ (Keebler)				
cracker sandwiches				
cheese & peanut butter	1 pkg	9.0	190	43%
Club & cheddar	1 pkg	11.0	190	52%
toast & peanut butter	1 pkg	9.0	190	43%
wheat & cheddar	1 pkg	10.0	180	50%
Munch 'Ems				
cheddar	30 crackers	4.0	140	39%
original/seasoned	41 crackers	5.0	140	32%
ranch	40 crackers	5.0	140	32%
sour cream & onion	39 crackers	5.0	140	32%
regular crackers				
Club partners				
50% reduced sodium	4 crackers	3.0	70	39%
33% reduced fat	5 crackers	2.0	70	36%
original	4 crackers	3.0	70	39%
Export soda crackers	3 crackers	2.0	60	30%
garlic bread flavored	4 crackers	3.0	70	39%
original	4 crackers	3.0	70	39%
onion toast	9 crackers	6.0	140	39%
Toasteds				
buttercrisp	5 crackers	3.5	80	39%
onion	5 crackers	3.0	80	34%
sesame	5 crackers	4.0	80	45%
wheat				
original	5 crackers	3.5	80	39%
reduced-fat	5 crackers	2.0	60	30%
touch of cheddar	4 crackers	2.5	70	32%
Town House				
original	5 crackers	4.5	80	51%
reduced fat/50%	6 crackers	2.0	70	39%
reduced sodium/50%	5 crackers	4.5	80	51%
wheat	5 crackers	4.0	80	45%
Wheatables				
honey wheat	12 crackers	6.0	140	39%
original/savory				
reduced fat	29 crackers	3.5	130	24%
reduced sodium	25 crackers	7.0	150	42%
seven grain	12 crackers	6.0	140	39%
Zesta saltines				
fat-free	5 crackers	–	50	–
original	5 crackers	2.0	60	30%
reduced sodium	5 crackers	2.0	70	26%
soup & oyster	45 crackers	3.0	70	39%
unsalted tops	5 crackers	2.0	70	26%
Snack stix				
hearty wheat	20 crackers	5.0	130	35%
seasoned original	21 crackers	5.0	130	35%

Food and Description	Amount	Fat Grams	Total Calories	% Fat Calories
zesty cheddar	20 crackers	5.0	120	38%
■ **(Lance)**				
snack crackers				
Gold-N-Cheese	½ cup	7.0	140	45%
	¾ cup	8.0	170	42%
	.96 oz pkg	6.0	110	49%
snack mix	1¾ pkg	17.0	290	53%
■ **(Little Debbie)**				
cream cheese & chive	1 pkg	7.0	140	45%
toasty crackers w/peanut butter				
boxed	1 pkg	8.0	140	51%
individual pkg	1.39 oz pkg	11.0	200	50%
wheat crackers w/cheddar cheese	1 pkg	8.0	140	51%
■ **(M&M* Mars)**				
Combos snack crackers/Singles				
cheddar cheese	1.7 oz pkg	11.0	240	41%
cheddar cheese pretzel	1.82 oz pkg	8.0	240	30%
nacho cheese pretzel	1.82 oz pkg	8.0	230	55%
peanut butter/family	1 oz	8.0	140	51%
pepperoni pizza	1.7 oz pkg	11.0	240	41%
pizzeria pretzel	1.82 oz pkg	8.0	230	55%
■ **(Manischewitz)**				
Matzo				
apple cinnamon	1 matzo	–	110	–
egg & onion	1 matzo	1.0	100	9%
everything				
matzo	1 matzo	0.5	110	4%
matzo crackers	12 crackers	0.5	110	4%
saltine				
original	1 matzo	2.0	110	16%
unsalted	1 matzo	–	110	–
savory garlic	1 matzo	–	100	–
thin				
original	1 matzo	–	100	–
tea	1 matzo	–	100	–
unsalted				
matzo	1 matzo	–	90	–
matzo crackers	12 crackers	0.5	110	4%
Tam Tams				
everything	10 pieces	5.0	130	35%
garlic	10 pieces	4.0	130	28%
no salt	10 pieces	4.0	130	28%
onion	10 pieces	5.0	140	32%
original	10 pieces	4.0	130	28%
■ **MUNCH 'EMS** (*See* (Keebler) in this section)				
■ **(Nabisco)**				
Christie Brown & Co.				
Today's Choice/reduced fat				
classic wheat	4 crackers	1.5	70	19%
cracked pepper	4 crackers	1.5	70	19%
garden vegetable	4 crackers	1.5	70	19%

Food and Description	Amount	Fat Grams	Total Calories	% Fat Calories
Red Oval Farms				
club	3½ crackers	4.6	117	35%
mini				
lemon pepper	20 crackers	3.0	130	21%
roast garlic	27 crackers	3.0	130	21%
some of each	3 crackers	2.5	60	38%
wheat thins/low-salt	2 crackers	1.5	60	23%
Nabisco				
Barnum's animals	1 serving	4.0	140	26%
Better Cheddars				
low-sodium	22 crackers	7.0	150	42%
reduced fat	24 crackers	6.0	140	39%
regular	22 crackers	8.0	150	48%
Cheese Nips				
Air Crisps	1.75 oz bag	7.0	220	29%
Cat Dog	1 oz	6.0	140	39%
mini	1 oz	6.0	150	36%
no cholesterol	29 crackers	6.0	150	36%
reduced fat	1 oz	3.5	130	24%
regular	29 crackers	6.0	150	36%
	1.65 oz	10.0	230	39%
Flavor Crisps				
bacon-flavored thins	15 crackers	8.0	160	45%
baked				
sociables/savory	1 oz	4.0	80	45%
swiss cheese	1 oz	7.0	140	45%
vegetable thins	1 oz	9.0	160	51%
Twigs/sesame & cheese	1 oz	7.0	150	42%
Cheese Tid-Bits	32 crackers	8.0	150	48%
Chicken In a Biskit	14 crackers	9.0	160	51%
Crown Pilot	1 cracker	1.5	70	19%
Garden Crisps	15 pieces	3.5	130	24%
Grahams (See COOKIE, Nabisco)				
Honey Maid (See COOKIE, Nabisco)				
Nut Thins				
almond	1 oz	4.5	140	29%
hazelnut	1 oz	4.0	120	30%
pecan	1 oz	5.0	130	35%
Oat thins	18 crackers	6.0	140	39%
Oysterettes soup & oyster	19 crackers	2.5	60	38%
Premium saltine				
bits	34 crackers	7.0	150	42%
fat-free	5 crackers	–	50	–
low-sodium	5 crackers	1.5	60	23%
multi-grain	5 crackers	1.5	60	23%
original	5 crackers	1.5	60	23%
soup & oyster	23 crackers	1.5	60	23%
unsalted tops	5 crackers	1.5	60	23%
Ritz				
Air crisps				
original	24 crackers	5.0	140	32%

Food and Description	Amount	Fat Grams	Total Calories	% Fat Calories
sour cream & onion	24 crackers	5.0	140	32%
baseball shaped	1 serving	4.0	80	45%
bits				
original	1.1 oz	10.0	170	53%
w/real cheese	1.75 oz pkg	16.0	270	53%
low sodium	5 crackers	1.5	60	23%
multigrain	5 crackers	1.5	60	23%
peanut butter	1.1 oz	8.0	150	48%
	1.75 oz bag	13.0	260	45%
reduced fat	5 crackers	2.0	70	26%
regular	54 crackers	4.0	80	45%
Toast Crackers				
w/cheddar cheese	1.38 oz pkg	10.0	200	45%
w/peanut butter	1.38 oz pkg	10.0	190	47%
Triscuit				
garden herb	6 crackers	7.0	130	48%
low-sodium	7 crackers	5.0	140	32%
original	7 crackers	5.0	140	32%
reduced fat	5 crackers	2.0	120	15%
Thin Crisps				
French onion	1 oz	4.5	130	10%
Original	1 oz	4.5	130	10%
wheat 'n bran	7 crackers	5.0	140	32%
Waverly	5 crackers	3.0	70	39%
Wheat thin				
Air Crisps				
crispy	1 oz	4.5	130	31%
ranch	1.75 oz bag	8.0	230	31%
low-salt	16 crackers	6.0	140	39%
multigrain	17 crackers	4.5	130	31%
original	16 crackers	6.0	140	39%
	1.75 oz bag	10.0	250	36%
reduced fat	18 crackers	4.0	120	30%
Wheatsworth	5 crackers	3.5	80	39%
Zwieback toast	1 piece	1.0	35	26%
SnackWell's				
fat-free				
cracked pepper	7 crackers	–	60	–
wheat	5 crackers	–	60	–
reduced fat				
classic golden	6 crackers	1.0	60	15%
cracked pepper	6 crackers	1.5	60	23%
French onion snack	1 oz	3.0	130	21%
wheat	.5 oz	1.5	70	19%
zesty cheese snack	1 oz	3.0	130	21%
■ (North Castle) Jarlsberg Cheese Crisps				
cheese pizza	11 pieces	6.0	140	39%
cheese & garlic	11 pieces	7.0	150	42%
■ (Old London)				
Melba Toast				
pumpernickel	½ oz	1.0	54	17%

Food and Description	Amount	Fat Grams	Total Calories	% Fat Calories
rye	½ oz	1.0	52	17%
sesame				
regular	½ oz	2.0	55	33%
unsalted	½ oz	2.0	55	33%
wheat	½ oz	1.0	51	18%
white				
regular	½ oz	1.0	51	18%
unsalted	½ oz	1.0	51	18%
whole grain				
regular	½ oz	1.0	53	17%
unsalted	½ oz	1.0	53	17%
Melba Rounds				
bacon	½ oz	1.0	53	17%
garlic	½ oz	1.0	56	16%
onion	½ oz	1.0	52	17%
rye	½ oz	1.0	52	17%
sesame	½ oz	2.0	56	32%
white	½ oz	1.0	48	19%
whole grain	½ oz	1.0	54	17%
■ (O.T.C.)				
chowder & oyster	3 pieces	2.0	70	26%
wine	11 pieces	3.0	130	21%
■ (Pacific Grain)				
No Fries/fat-free				
potato crackers				
BBQ	30 pieces	–	110	–
au gratin	30 pieces	–	110	–
tortilla crackers				
cheddar	30 pieces	–	110	–
ranch	30 pieces	–	110	–
salsa	30 pieces	–	110	–
sour cream	30 pieces	–	110	–
■ (Pepperidge Farm)				
International Collection				
cracked pepper water biscuit	5 crackers	1.0	60	15%
original water biscuit	5 crackers	1.0	60	15%
Distinctive crackers				
butter thins	4 crackers	3.0	70	39%
cracked wheat	4 crackers	2.5	70	32%
English water biscuits	4 crackers	1.5	70	19%
hearty wheat	3 crackers	3.5	80	39%
quartet assortment	3 crackers	2.5	70	32%
sesame	3 crackers	2.5	70	32%
three-cracker assortment	3 crackers	2.5	60	38%
Goldfish/tiny				
cheddar cheese				
blasted				
extra cheddar	1 oz	6.0	140	39%
wild white cheddar	1 oz	6.0	140	39%
cinnamon	1 oz	6.0	150	36%

Food and Description	Amount	Fat Grams	Total Calories	% Fat Calories
honey	1 oz	6.0	150	36%
low-salt	55 pieces	6.0	140	39%
reduced sodium	60 pieces	6.0	150	36%
regular				
on-the-go or variety pack	1 pouch	5.0	130	35%
regular pkg	55 pieces	6.0	140	39%
team fun				
baseball shapes	1 oz	6.0	140	39%
racing car shapes	1 oz	6.0	140	39%
white cheddar	1 oz	7.0	150	42%
Halloween pack	1 pouch	2.5	70	32%
original				
on-the-go or variety pack	1 pouch	6.0	130	42%
regular or warehouse club pkg	55 pieces	6.0	140	39%
Parmesan cheese	60 pieces	5.0	140	32%
pizza-flavored	55 pieces	6.0	140	39%
pretzel				
on-the-go or variety pack	1 pouch	2.5	110	20%
regular or warehouse club pkg	45 pieces	2.5	120	19%
Snack Sticks/three cheese crunchy	1.1 oz	6.0	150	36%
Water crackers	.5 oz	1.0	60	15%
■ (Planters)				
cracker sandwich				
cheese peanut butter	1 pkg	10.0	190	47%
toast peanut butter	1 pkg	10.0	190	47%
RED OVAL FARMS (*See* (Nabisco) in this section)				
RITZ (*See* (Nabisco) in this section)				
■ (Ry-Krisp)				
fat-free	2 crackers	–	60	–
fiber plus	1 slice	1.0	35	–
golden rye	1 slice	–	30	–
hearty rye	1 slice	–	50	–
lite rye	2 slices	–	50	–
natural	2 crackers	–	40	–
seasoned	2 crackers	1.0	45	20%
sesame	2 crackers	2.0	50	36%
■ (Ryvita)				
crispbread				
dark	2 pieces	–	38	–
dark rye				
plain	2 pieces	1.0	50	18%
w/caraway seeds	2 pieces	1.0	50	18%
high-fiber	2 pieces	1.0	45	20%
light rye/high-fiber	2 pieces	1.0	50	18%
original wheat	2 pieces	1.0	45	20%
toasted sesame rye	2 pieces	1.0	60	15%
■ (Sesmark)				
brown rice	15 pieces	2.0	120	15%
cheese thins	15 pieces	3.0	130	21%
rice thins				
original	15 pieces	3.0	130	21%

Food and Description	Amount	Fat Grams	Total Calories	% Fat Calories
teriyaki-flavored	15 pieces	3.0	130	21%
savory thins	15 pieces	2.0	125	14%
sesame thins				
cheddar	9 pieces	8.0	150	48%
garlic	9 pieces	8.0	150	48%
original	9 pieces	8.0	150	48%
unsalted	11 pieces	8.0	150	48%
■ SNACKWELL'S (*See* (Nabisco) in this section)				
■ (Sunshine)				
Cheez-It				
Big				
original	13 crackers	8.0	150	48%
reduced fat	15 crackers	4.5	140	29%
single serve	2 oz package	16.0	290	50%
8 count	1 pkg	12.0	220	49%
chip its	29 crackers	5.0	130	35%
Heads & Tails	37 crackers	6.0	140	39%
Single serve	1 pkg	9.0	210	39%
hot & spicy	26 crackers	8.0	150	48%
low-sodium	27 crackers	8.0	160	39%
nacho	28 crackers	7.0	150	42%
original				
reduced fat	29 crackers	4.5	140	29%
regular	27 crackers	8.0	160	45%
white cheddar	26 crackers	7.0	150	42%
single serve/8 count	1 pkg	11.0	220	45%
Hi-Ho				
butter-flavored	9 crackers	9.0	160	51%
cracked pepper	9 crackers	9.0	160	51%
multigrain	9 crackers	9.0	160	51%
original	4 crackers	4.0	70	51%
reduced fat	5 crackers	2.5	70	32%
whole wheat	9 crackers	8.0	150	48%
Krispy saltine				
fat-free	5 crackers	–	50	–
mild cheddar	5 crackers	2.0	60	30%
original	5 crackers	1.5	60	23%
soup & oyster	17 crackers	1.5	60	23%
unsalted tops	5 crackers	1.5	60	23%
whole wheat	5 crackers	1.5	60	23%
■ TRISCUIT (*See* (Nabisco) in this section)				
■ TUSCANY TOAST (*See* (Burns & Ricker) in this section)				
■ (Valley Lahvosh)				
cracker bread				
hearts	9 crackers	1.0	110	8%
rounds				
15" dia	1.8 oz	2.0	190	9%
5" dia	1 cracker	0.5	70	6%
3" dia	4 crackers	1.0	110	8%
2" dia	7 crackers	1.0	110	8%

Food and Description	Amount	Fat Grams	Total Calories	% Fat Calories
wheat rounds				
15" dia	1.8 oz	2.0	190	9%
5" dia	1 cracker	0.5	60	8%
3" dia	4 crackers	1.0	110	8%
sweetheart crispies	7 crackers	2.0	120	15%
■ (Venus)				
bran wafers	5 crackers	1.0	60	15%
cracked wheat wafers	5 crackers	1.0	60	15%
cracker bread				
Armenian thin	2 pieces	1.0	100	9%
original	5 pieces	1.0	60	15%
Hors D'oeuvre	3 pieces	2.0	60	30%
oat bran wafers				
regular	5 crackers	1.0	60	15%
salt free	5 crackers	1.0	60	15%
Old Brussells Waferettes				
cheddar	5 pieces	5.0	80	56%
jalapeño	5 pieces	5.0	80	56%
rye wafers/low-salt	5 pieces	1.0	60	15%
stoned wheat wafers/bite-size	7 crackers	1.0	60	15%
water crackers/fat-free	5 crackers	–	55	–
wheat wafers/low-salt	5 crackers	2.0	60	30%
■ (Wasa)				
Crispbread				
Cinnamon toast	1 slice	1.0	60	15%
fiber rye	1 slice	1.0	30	30%
gluten & wheat-free corn	1 slice	1.0	40	23%
hearty rye	1 slice	–	45	–
light rye	1 slice	–	25	–
multigrain	1 slice	–	45	–
organic rye	1 slice	–	25	–
sodium-free rye	1 slice	–	30	–
sourdough rye	1 slice	–	35	–
toasted wheat	1 slice	2.0	50	36%
whole wheat	1 slice	1.0	50	18%
Crisp'N Light				
sourdough rye	3 pieces	–	60	–
wheat	2 pieces	–	50	–
■ (Westbrae)				
wafers				
5-piece	4½ crackers	–	40	–
no salt	4½ crackers	–	40	–
onion garlic	4½ crackers	–	40	–
sesame	4½ crackers	–	40	–
CRACKER CRUMBS/MEAL (See also MATZO MEAL & MIX)				
(Golden Dipt) cracker meal/no salt				
extra fine	¼ cup	0.9	145	5%
fine	¼ cup	0.9	145	5%
medium	¼ cup	0.7	143	4%
Modern Maid matzah meal	¼ cup	0.9	145	5%

Food and Description	Amount	Fat Grams	Total Calories	% Fat Calories
(Keebler)	1 cup	3.0	100	27%
(Nabisco) crumbs				
Honey Maid graham	1 serving	1.5	70	19%
Premium/fat-free	¼ cup	–	100	–
Ritz	⅓ cup	7.0	140	45%
CRANBERRY				
dried				
(Ocean Spray) Craisins	⅓ cup	–	130	–
(Traverse Bay)	⅓ cup	0.5	140	3%
fresh				
chopped	½ cup	–	27	–
	1 cup	–	54	–
(Ocean Spray)	1 cup	–	50	–
whole/w/o stems	½ cup	–	23	–
	1 cup	–	46	–
CRANBERRY BEAN				
canned/generic				
w/liquid	½ cup	<1.0	110	4%
dried				
(Bean Cuisine)	½ cup	1.0	115	8%
fresh				
boiled	½ cup	<1.0	120	4%
raw	½ cup	1.0	330	3%
CRANBERRY JUICE/JUICE BLEND/JUICE BLEND DRINK				
bottled, boxed, or canned				
(Chiquita) cranberry seabreeze	8 fl oz	–	120	–
(Hain) concentrate	1 oz	–	40	–
(Knudsen) Thirst Quencher				
Cape Cod cranberry	8 fl oz	–	100	–
cranberry nectar	8 fl oz	–	150	–
Just Cranberry	8 fl oz	–	60	–
(Ocean Spray)				
Lightstyle				
cranberry juice cocktail	8 fl oz	–	40	–
crangrape	8 fl oz	–	40	–
cranmango	8 fl oz	–	40	–
cranraspberry	8 fl oz	–	40	–
Reduced Calorie				
cranapple	8 fl oz	–	50	–
cranberry juice cocktail	8 fl oz	–	50	–
cranraspberry	8 fl oz	–	50	–
Regular				
cranapple	8 fl oz	–	160	–
cranberry juice cocktail	8 fl oz	–	140	–
cranicot	8 fl oz	–	160	–
cranblueberry	8 fl oz	–	160	–
crancherry	8 fl oz	–	160	–
crancurrant	8 fl oz	–	140	–
crangrape	8 fl oz	–	170	–
cranmango	8 fl oz	–	130	–

Food and Description	Amount	Fat Grams	Total Calories	% Fat Calories
cranraspberry	8 fl oz	–	140	–
cranstrawberry	8 fl oz	–	140	–
crantangerine	8 fl oz	–	130	–
Wellfleet Farms				
cranberry	8 fl oz	–	130	–
cranberry & Georgia peach	8 fl oz	–	140	–
cranberry & Granny Smith apple	8 fl oz	–	130	–
cranberry & key lime	8 fl oz	–	140	–
(Smucker's)	8 fl oz	–	130	–
(Snapple)				
cranberry apple	12 fl oz	–	200	–
	11.5 oz can	–	190	–
cranberry raspberry				
diet	8 fl oz	–	10	–
regular	8 fl oz	–	120	–
cranberry raspberry winter whipper	10 fl oz	–	150	–
(Tropicana) Twister/cranberry, raspberry, strawberry				
light	8 fl oz	–	45	–
	10 fl oz	–	60	–
regular	8 fl oz	–	120	–
	10 fl oz	–	160	–
(Welch's)				
juice	8 fl oz	–	140	–
juice cocktail	5.5 fl oz	–	100	–
JuiceMakers				
cranberry apple juice cocktail	8 fl oz	–	160	–
frozen/prepared				
(Seneca) juice cocktail				
cranberry	8 fl oz	–	140	–
cranberry-apple	8 fl oz	–	140	–
(Welch's) juice cocktail				
cranberry				
light	8 fl oz	–	50	–
regular	8 fl oz	–	140	–
cranberry-apple	8 fl oz	–	160	–
cranberry-cherry	8 fl oz	–	150	–
cranberry-orange	8 fl oz	–	140	–
cranberry-raspberry				
light	8 fl oz	–	50	–
regular	8 fl oz	–	150	–
CRANBERRY SAUCE /canned				
generic/sweetened	½ cup	–	210	–
(Ocean Spray) canned				
Cran-Fruit cranberry crushed fruit				
orange	¼ cup	–	120	–
raspberry	¼ cup	–	120	–
strawberry	¼ cup	–	120	–
jellied	¼ cup	–	110	–
whole berry	¼ cup	–	110	–

Food and Description	Amount	Fat Grams	Total Calories	% Fat Calories
(S&W)				
jellied	¼ cup	–	100	–
whole berry	¼ cup	–	100	–
CRANBERRY-ORANGE RELISH				
canned	½ cup	–	246	–
uncooked	½ cup	–	245	–
CRAYFISH/mixed species				
cooked-moist heat	3 oz	1.0	97	9%
raw	3 medium	<1.0	24	19%
	3 oz	0.9	76	11%
CREAM (*See also* CREAMER, NONDAIRY; SOUR CREAM; SOUR CREAM SUBSTITUTE; WHIPPED TOPPING)				
(Farmland)				
half & half	2 Tbs	3.0	40	68%
light cream	2 Tbs	3.0	30	90%
generic				
coffee/table cream				
light	1 Tbs	3.0	30	90%
	1 cup	46.0	470	88%
medium/25% fat	1 Tbs	4.0	40	90%
	1 cup	60.0	585	92%
half & half	1 Tbs	2.0	20	90%
	1 cup	28.0	315	80%
whipping cream				
heavy				
unwhipped	1 cup	88.0	820	96%
whipped	2 cups	88.0	820	97%
light				
unwhipped	1 cup	74.0	700	95%
whipped	2 cups	74.0	700	95%
(Land O'Lakes)				
half & half	1 Tbs	2.0	20	90%
whipping cream				
heavy/gourmet				
unwhipped	1 Tbs	6.0	60	90%
whipped	1 cup	73.9	704	94%
regular				
unwhipped	1 Tbs	5.0	45	90%
whipped	2 cups	73.9	704	94%
CREAM CHEESE (*See also* CHEESE ALTERNATIVE/IMITATION; CHEESE SPREAD)				
(Breakstone) Temp-Tee/whipped	3 Tbs	8.0	80	90%
(Darigold)	2 Tbs	10.0	100	90%
(Dorman's)				
70% fat	2 Tbs	10.0	100	90%
65% fat	2 Tbs	8.0	90	80%
(Fleur de Lait) light				
blueberries & cream	2 Tbs	4.0	70	51%
chive & onion	2 Tbs	4.0	60	60%
fresh garden delight	2 Tbs	6.0	60	90%
garden vegetable	2 Tbs	4.0	50	72%

Food and Description	Amount	Fat Grams	Total Calories	% Fat Calories
garlic	2 Tbs	4.0	60	60%
nacho	2 Tbs	4.0	60	60%
salsa	2 Tbs	4.0	60	60%
strawberry	2 Tbs	4.0	60	60%
(Formagg)				
fat-free	2 Tbs	–	25	–
original	2 Tbs	7.0	80	79%
(Fresh Cut)				
bacon & horseradish	2 Tbs	9.0	90	90%
bermuda onion & chives	2 Tbs	8.0	90	80%
date nut & rum	2 Tbs	8.0	90	80%
garlic & spice	2 Tbs	9.0	90	90%
herb & spice	2 Tbs	9.0	90	90%
lox	2 Tbs	8.0	90	80%
peaches & cream	2 Tbs	7.0	90	70%
strawberry	2 Tbs	8.0	90	80%
(Friendship)				
New York style/reduced fat	2 Tbs	3.0	50	54%
soft	2 Tbs	10.0	100	90%
(Healthy Choice) fat-free				
herbs & garlic	2 Tbs	–	25	–
plain	2 Tbs	–	25	–
strawberry	2 Tbs	–	35	–
(Heluva Good Cheese)	2 Tbs	10.0	100	90%
(Kraft)				
Philadelphia brand				
brick				
fat-free	1 oz	–	30	–
Neufchatel	1 oz	6.0	70	77%
regular	1 oz	10.0	100	90%
with chives	1 oz	6.0	90	60%
regular/soft				
fat free				
plain	2 Tbs	–	30	–
w/garden vegetables	2 Tbs	–	30	–
w/strawberries	2 Tbs	–	30	–
light	2 Tbs	5.0	70	64%
original	2 Tbs	10.0	100	90%
whipped				
plain	2 Tbs	7.0	70	90%
w/chives	2 Tbs	6.0	70	77%
w/smoked salmon	2 Tbs	6.0	70	77%
Philly Flavors/regular soft				
apple cinnamon	2 Tbs	8.0	100	63%
cheesecake	2 Tbs	9.0	110	74%
chives & onion	2 Tbs	10.0	110	82%
garden vegetable	2 Tbs	11.0	110	90%
honey nut	2 Tbs	10.0	110	82%
pineapple	2 Tbs	9.0	100	81%
smoked salmon	2 Tbs	9.0	100	81%

Food and Description	Amount	Fat Grams	Total Calories	% Fat Calories
strawberries	2 Tbs	9.0	110	74%
Philly Flavors/lower fat soft				
jalapeño	2 Tbs	5.0	60	75%
raspberry	2 Tbs	4.5	70	58%
roasted garlic	2 Tbs	5.0	70	64%
(Weight Watchers) light	2 Tbs	3.0	40	68%
CREAM OF TARTAR	1 tsp	–	7	–
	1 Tbs	–	23	–
CREAMER, NONDAIRY (*See also* CREAM)				
liquid				
(Carnation) Coffee-mate				
amaretto	1 Tbs	2.0	40	45%
cafe mocha	1 Tbs	2.0	40	45%
fat-free	1 Tbs	–	25	–
cinnamon vanilla	1 Tbs	2.0	40	45%
French vanilla	1 Tbs	2.0	40	45%
fat-free	1 Tbs	–	25	–
hazelnut	1 Tbs	2.0	40	45%
Irish creme	1 Tbs	2.0	40	45%
original				
fat-free	1 Tbs	–	10	–
light	1 Tbs	0.5	10	45%
regular	1 Tbs	1.0	20	45%
toasted almond	1 Tbs	2.0	40	45%
(Coffee Delight)	1 Tbs	2.0	20	90%
(International Delight)				
amaretto				
fat-free	1 Tbs	–	30	–
original	1 Tbs	2.0	45	40%
cinnamon	1 Tbs	2.0	45	40%
French vanilla royal				
fat-free	1 Tbs	–	30	–
original	1 Tbs	2.0	45	40%
Hawaiian macadamia/fat-free	1 Tbs	–	30	–
hazelnut	1 Tbs	2.0	45	40%
Irish creme				
fat-free	1 Tbs	–	30	–
original	1 Tbs	2.0	45	40%
Suisse chocolate mocha	1 Tbs	2.0	45	40%
(Land O'Lakes) Half & Half				
fat-free	1 Tbs	–	20	–
original	1 Tbs	3.0	40	68%
(Mocha Mix)				
fat-free	1 Tbs	–	10	–
lite	1 Tbs	<0.5	10	45%
original	1 Tbs	2.0	20	90%
Signature flavors				
French vanilla	1 Tbs	–	35	–
Irish creme	1 Tbs	–	35	–
kahlua	1 Tbs	–	35	–

Food and Description	Amount	Fat Grams	Total Calories	% Fat Calories
mauna loa macadamia nut	1 Tbs	–	35	–
amaretto	1 Tbs	1.0	35	20%
Irish creme	1 Tbs	1.0	35	20%
Kahlua/fat-free	1 Tbs	–	35	–
original				
lite/fat-free	1 Tbs	–	10	–
regular	1 Tbs	2.0	20	90%
(Real) half & half				
almond roca	2 Tbs	1.0	80	11%
French vanilla	2 Tbs	2.0	80	23%
Irish cream	2 Tbs	3.5	80	39%
(Rich's) frozen				
Coffee Rich				
light	1 Tbs	1.0	10	90%
original	1 Tbs	1.5	25	54%
Farm Rich				
fat-free	1 Tbs	–	10	–
light	1 Tbs	1.0	10	90%
original	1 Tbs	1.5	20	68%
Poly Rich	1 Tbs	1.0	20	68%
powdered				
(Borden) Cremora				
fat-free	1 tsp	–	10	–
lite	1 tsp	–	10	–
original	1 tsp	1.0	10	90%
(Carnation) Coffee-mate				
amaretto	1⅓ Tbs	3.0	60	45%
cinnamon creme	1⅓ Tbs	3.0	60	45%
French vanilla	1⅓ Tbs	3.0	60	45%
fat-free	1⅓ Tbs	–	50	–
hazelnut	1⅓ Tbs	3.0	60	45%
fat-free	1⅓ Tbs	–	50	–
Irish creme	1⅓ Tbs	3.0	60	45%
mocha almond	1⅓ Tbs	3.0	60	45%
original				
fat-free	1 tsp	–	10	–
lite	1 tsp	–	10	–
regular	1 tsp	0.5	10	45%
Swiss chocolate	1⅓ Tbs	1.0	50	18%
fat-free	1⅓ Tbs	–	50	–
(Hershey) Great American Cafe				
chocolate amaretto	1⅓ Tbs	2.5	60	38%
French vanilla	1⅓ Tbs	2.5	60	38%
CREPE				
frozen				
(Chef Francois)	1 crepe	3.0	80	34%
mix				
(Krusteaz)				
mix only	2 Tbs	1.0	80	11%
prepared	2 crepes	3.0	100	27%

Food and Description	Amount	Fat Grams	Total Calories	% Fat Calories
ready to serve				
(Table de France) 9" dia	1 crepe	1.0	45	20%
CRISPBREAD (*See* CRACKER)				
CROAKER				
breaded & fried	3 oz	10.0	188	48%
raw	3 oz	2.7	89	27%
CROISSANT				
frozen				
(Chef Pierre) prebaked/all-butter				
1-oz croissant	1 croissant	5.0	110	41%
2-oz croissant	1 croissant	9.0	210	39%
3-oz croissant	1 croissant	22.0	360	55%
(Sara Lee) all-butter/petite	2 croissants	11.0	230	43%
generic				
apple	2 oz croissant	5.0	145	31%
cheese	2 oz croissant	12.0	235	46%
plain				
2 oz	1 croissant	12.0	230	47%
1 oz	1 croissant	6.0	115	47%
homemade/USDA Standard Home Recipe				
~2-oz croissant	1 croissant	12.0	235	46%
ready to serve				
(Awrey's)				
butter	2 oz	11.0	200	50%
	3 oz	17.0	300	51%
margarine	1.25 oz	7.0	120	53%
	2.5 oz	14.0	250	50%
wheat	2.5 oz	14.0	240	53%
(Dunkin' Donuts)				
almond	1 croissant	21.0	360	53%
cheese	1 croissant	15.0	240	56%
chocolate	1 croissant	23.0	370	56%
plain	1 croissant	17.0	270	57%
(Pepperidge Farm) all-butter				
petite/all butter	1 croissant	6.0	120	45%
sandwich	1 croissant	7.0	170	37%
(Sara Lee)				
food service				
1⅛-oz croissant	1 croissant	6.0	130	42%
1½-oz croissant	1 croissant	8.0	170	43%
2-oz croissant	1 croissant	10.0	220	41%
3-oz sandwich croissant	1 croissant	15.0	320	42%
sandwich croissant/sliced	1 croissant	11.0	220	45%
retail				
broccoli and cheese	1 croissant	13.0	280	42%
ham & swiss cheese	1 croissant	16.0	300	48%
petite	2 croissants	11.0	230	43%
plain	1 croissant	8.0	170	42%
CROUTONS				
(Arnold) crispy				
cheddar romano	½ oz	3.0	64	42%

Food and Description	Amount	Fat Grams	Total Calories	% Fat Calories
cheese garlic	½ oz	2.0	60	30%
fine herbs	½ oz	1.0	50	18%
Italian	½ oz	3.0	60	45%
onion & garlic	½ oz	2.0	60	30%
seasoned	½ oz	3.0	60	45%
(Brownberry)				
Caesar salad	½ oz	3.0	62	44%
cheddar cheese	½ oz	3.0	63	43%
onion & garlic	½ oz	2.0	60	30%
seasoned	½ oz	2.0	59	31%
toasted	½ oz	1.0	56	16%
(Chatam Village)				
bread crisps				
cinnamon & raisin	3 crisps	3.0	70	39%
garlic & butter	3 crisps	3.0	70	39%
sesame seed	3 crisps	4.0	80	45%
Fat-free				
garlic & onion	2 Tbs	–	25	–
sundried tomato	2 Tbs	–	30	–
Regular				
Caesar	2 Tbs	1.5	35	39%
cheese & garlic	2 Tbs	2.5	40	56%
garden herb	2 Tbs	1.5	35	39%
garlic & butter	2 Tbs	1.5	35	39%
(Marzetti)				
bread crisps				
cinnamon & raisin	3 crisps	3.0	70	39%
garlic & butter	3 crisps	3.0	70	39%
sesame seed	3 crisps	4.0	80	45%
Fat-free				
garlic & onion	2 Tbs	–	25	–
sundried tomato	2 Tbs	–	30	–
Regular				
Caesar	2 Tbs	1.5	35	39%
cheese & garlic	2 Tbs	2.5	40	56%
garden herb	2 Tbs	1.5	35	39%
garlic & butter	2 Tbs	1.5	35	39%
(Mrs. Cubberson's) restaurant style				
Caesar salad	5 croutons	1.0	30	30%
cheese & garlic	5 croutons	1.0	30	30%
fat-free	5 croutons	–	30	–
onion & garlic	5 croutons	1.0	30	30%
ranch	5 croutons	1.0	30	30%
seasoned	5 croutons	1.0	30	30%
(Old London) restaurant style				
garlic	2 Tbs	1.5	30	39%
Italian	2 Tbs	1.5	30	39%
sourdough	2 Tbs	1.5	30	39%
(Pepperidge Farm)				
cheddar & romano cheese	½ oz	2.0	60	30%

Food and Description	Amount	Fat Grams	Total Calories	% Fat Calories
cheese & garlic	½ oz	3.0	70	39%
onion & garlic	½ oz	3.0	70	39%
seasoned	½ oz	3.0	70	39%
sour cream & chive	½ oz	3.0	70	39%
CROWDER PEA/canned				
(Luck's) seasoned w/pork	7.5 oz	7.0	200	32%
CRUMPET				
(Wolferman's)				
blueberry	1 crumpet	–	90	–
brown sugar-cinnamon	1 crumpet	–	80	–
lemon-poppy seed	1 crumpet	0.5	90	5%
original	1 crumpet	0.5	90	5%
raspberry	1 crumpet	1.0	90	10%
CUCUMBER (See also PICKLE)				
raw				
sliced	½ cup	–	7	–
whole	1 medium	–	29	–
CUCUMBER DISH (See also PICKLE; PICKLE RELISH)				
(Rosoff's) cucumber salad	1 oz	–	12	–
(Schorr's) cucumber garden salad	1 oz	–	12	–
CUMIN SEED/whole	1 tsp	0.5	8	56%
CUPCAKE (See CAKE, SNACK)				
CURRANT				
black				
dried	½ cup	–	204	–
raw	½ cup	–	36	–
	½ lb	–	140	–
red or white/raw	½ cup	–	31	–
	½ lb	–	125	–
Zante/dried				
(Del Monte) dried	½ cup	–	200	–
(S&W) canned	¼ cup	–	130	–
(Sun Maid)	½ cup	–	210	–
CURRANT JUICE/black	8 fl oz	–	138	–
CURRY POWDER/ground	1 tsp	–	6	–
CURRY SAUCE (See SAUCE)				
CUSK				
raw	3 oz	1.0	74	12%
steamed	1 oz	<1.0	30	15%
	1 lb	3.0	481	6%
CUSTARD (See also BABY FOOD; PUDDING & MOUSSE)				
Homemade/USDA Standard Home Recipe				
baked	1 cup	14.6	305	43%
boiled	½ cup	7.0	164	38%
zabaglione	¼ cup	4.0	80	45%
mix (Note: 1 serving of mix = the amount in ½ cup prepared)				
(Goya) flan/prepared	½ cup	0.5	60	8%
(Jell-O)				
custard dessert				
mix only	1 serving	–	80	–

Food and Description	Amount	Fat Grams	Total Calories	% Fat Calories
prepared w/2% milk	½ cup	2.5	140	16%
flan				
mix only	1 serving	–	80	–
prepared w/2% milk	½ cup	2.5	140	16%
(Knorr) Alsa international dessert				
creme caramel flan/mix only	¼ pkg	–	110	–
(Royal) flan-caramel custard/	½ cup	–	60	–
prepared				
CUTTLEFISH /				
cooked-moist heat	3 oz	1.0	135	6%
raw	3 oz	0.6	67	8%

D

Food and Description	Amount	Fat Grams	Total Calories	% Fat Calories
DANDELION GREENS /fresh				
cooked	½ cup	–	17	–
raw/chopped	½ cup	–	13	–
DANISH (See PASTRY)				
DATE				
(Del Monte)				
chopped	¼ cup	–	120	–
pitted	5-6 medium	–	120	–
(Dole)				
chopped	1 oz	–	120	–
dried/ground	1 oz	–	110	–
pitted	5-6 cates	–	120	–
(Dromedary)				
chopped	¼ cup	–	130	–
whole/pitted	5 medium	–	100	–
generic				
chopped	1 cup	0.8	489	2%
natural/dried	10 medium	–	228	–
(Sun Giant)				
chopped	1 cup	1.0	490	2%
whole/pitted	10 medium	1.0	220	4%
DATE FILLING (Solo)	2 Tbs	1.0	100	9%
DEER (See VENISON)				
DESSERT TOPPING (See CREAM; ICE CREAM TOPPING; WHIPPED TOPPING)				

Food and Description	Amount	Fat Grams	Total Calories	% Fat Calories
DIETING AID (*See* BREAKFAST DRINK; GRANOLA/GRANOLA-TYPE BAR; NUTRITIONAL SUPPLEMENT)				
DILL LEAVES/fresh	1 cup	–	5	–
DILL SAUCE (*See* SAUCE)				
DILL SEED				
dried	1 tsp	–	3	–
whole	1 tsp	–	6	–
DINNER (*See* ASIAN FOOD; BEEF DISH/ENTRÉE; EGG DISH/MEAL; FAST FOOD; FROZEN ENTRÉE/DINNER; MEXICAN FOOD; PASTA ENTRÉE/DINNER; PIZZA; PORK ENTRÉE/DINNER; RICE DISH; SEAFOOD ENTRÉE/DINNER; VEGETARIAN FOODS; individual listings)				
DIP (*See also* SALAD DRESSING; SAUCE; SEASONINGS)				
■ **FROZEN**				
(AVO King) Southwestern guacamole	2 Tbs	5.0	57	79%
(Calavo) Mexican-style avocado guacamole	2 Tbs	4.5	50	81%
■ **MIX**				
(Note: Unless otherwise stated, data are for dry mix only)				
(Casbah) hummus	2 oz	10.0	220	41%
(Fantastic Foods) hummus	2 Tbs	2.0	60	30%
(Golden Dipt)				
clam seafood	½ tsp	–	5	–
dill seafood	½ tsp	–	5	–
horseradish	½ tsp	–	–	–
Louis	1 tsp	–	10	–
pesto	1 tsp	–	10	–
(Hain)				
hot bean	4 Tbs	1.0	70	13%
Mexican bean	4 Tbs	1.0	60	15%
(Hidden Valley)				
(Note: 1 serving of mix = the amount in 2 Tbs prepared.)				
Fiesta				
mix only	1 serving	–	5	–
prepared	2 Tbs	6.0	70	77%
French onion				
mix only	1 serving	–	5	–
prepared	2 Tbs	6.0	70	77%
garden vegetable				
mix only	1 serving	–	5	–
prepared	2 Tbs	6.0	70	77%
original				
reduced calorie				
mix only	1 serving	–	5	–
prepared	2 Tbs	3.0	40	68%
regular recipe				
mix only	1 serving	–	5	–
prepared	2 Tbs	6.0	70	77%
(Knorr)				
black bean	⅟₁₆ pkg	–	10	–
chili caliente	⅟₂₀ pkg	–	5	–

Food and Description	Amount	Fat Grams	Total Calories	% Fat Calories
cracked pepper ranch	⅟₂₀ pkg	–	5	–
garden dill	⅟₂₀ pkg	–	2	–
Mexican bean	⅟₁₆ pkg	–	10	–
nacho cheese	⅟₁₅ pkg	–	10	–
onion chive	⅟₂₀ pkg	–	5	–
(McCormick/Schilling)				
Dip Classics				
country herb	1 tsp	–	10	–
French onion	¾ tsp	–	5	–
garlic & pepper	¾ tsp	–	5	–
ranch	¾ tsp	–	5	–
spring onion	½ tsp	–	5	–
vegetable	½ tsp	–	–	–
McCormick Collection				
black bean	1 Tbs	–	35	–
jalapeño bean	1 Tbs	–	40	–
pinto bean	1 Tbs	–	40	–
poppy seed	2 tsp	–	25	–
spinach	1 tsp	–	5	–
spring vegetable	2 tsp	–	10	–
toasted onion	1 tsp	–	5	–
(Produce Partners)				
garden vegetable	2 tsp	–	10	–
guacamole				
mild	2 tsp	–	15	–
spicy	2 tsp	–	15	–
■ READY TO SERVE				
(Athenos) Hummus				
3 pepper	2 Tbs	3.0	50	54%
original	2 Tbs	3.0	50	54%
(Breakstone) sour cream dip				
bacon & onion	2 Tbs	5.0	60	75%
Chesapeake clam	2 Tbs	4.0	50	72%
French onion	2 Tbs	4.5	50	81%
toasted onion	2 Tbs	3.0	50	54%
(Calavo) guacamole				
Mexican avocado	2 Tbs	3.0	45	60%
mild	2 Tbs	4.0	45	80%
original avocado	2 Tbs	3.0	45	60%
zesty	2 Tbs	4.0	45	80%
(Dean's)				
French onion				
fat-free	2 Tbs	–	30	–
original	2 Tbs	5.0	60	75%
w/bacon bits	2 Tbs	5.0	60	75%
ranch	2 Tbs	5.0	60	75%
(Enrico's) fat-free				
black				
mild	2 Tbs	–	30	–
spicy	2 Tbs	–	30	–

Food and Description	Amount	Fat Grams	Total Calories	% Fat Calories
nacho cheese				
mild	2 Tbs	–	20	–
spicy	2 Tbs	–	20	–
(Frito-Lay)				
bean	2 Tbs	1.0	40	23%
cheddar cheese/mild	2 Tbs	4.0	60	60%
French onion	2 Tbs	5.0	60	75%
hot bean	2 Tbs	1.0	40	23%
jalapeño & cheese	2 Tbs	4.0	50	72%
(Guiltless Gourmet) spicy				
black bean				
mild	2 Tbs	–	30	–
Spicy	2 Tbs	–	30	–
(Heluva Good Cheese)				
bacon horseradish	2 Tbs	5.0	60	75%
clam	2 Tbs	5.0	50	90%
French onion				
light	2 Tbs	2.0	35	51%
original	2 Tbs	5.0	50	90%
homestyle onion	2 Tbs	5.0	60	75%
jalapeño cheddar/light	2 Tbs	2.0	40	45%
ranch	2 Tbs	5.0	60	75%
(Knudsen)				
fat-free				
creamy ranch	2 Tbs	–	25	–
creamy salsa	2 Tbs	–	20	–
French onion	2 Tbs	–	25	–
(Kraft)				
avocado/guacamole	2 Tbs	4.0	60	60%
bacon horseradish				
premium	2 Tbs	5.0	60	75%
regular	2 Tbs	5.0	60	75%
bacon onion/premium	2 Tbs	5.0	60	60%
cheese				
blue/premium	2 Tbs	4.0	45	60%
jalapeño/premium	2 Tbs	5.0	60	75%
nacho/premium	2 Tbs	5.0	60	75%
clam				
premium	2 Tbs	4.0	50	72%
regular	2 Tbs	4.0	60	60%
creamy cucumber/premium	2 Tbs	4.0	50	72%
creamy onion/premium	2 Tbs	4.0	45	80%
creamy salsa/lower-fat	2 Tbs	–	20	–
French onion				
fat-free	2 Tbs	–	25	–
lower-fat	2 Tbs	–	25	–
premium	2 Tbs	4..0	45	80%
regular	2 Tbs	4.0	60	60%
green onion	2 Tbs	4.0	60	60%
jalapeño pepper	2 Tbs	4.0	60	60%

Food and Description	Amount	Fat Grams	Total Calories	% Fat Calories
ranch				
fat-free	2 Tbs	–	25	–
lower-fat	2 Tbs	–	25	–
premium	2 Tbs	4.0	50	72%
regular	2 Tbs	4.5	60	68%
salsa/fat-free	2 Tbs	–	20	–
(La Famous)				
mild bean	2 Tbs	–	25	–
spicy bean	2 Tbs	–	25	–
(Louise's) fat-free				
honey mustard	1 oz	–	40	–
sour cream & onion	1 oz	–	25	–
white cheese peppercorn	1 oz	–	25	–
(Marzetti)				
for fruit				
caramel apple				
fat-free	2 Tbs	–	110	–
original	2 Tbs	7.0	160	39%
reduced fat	2 Tbs	3.0	130	21%
chocolate-flavored				
fat-free	2 Tbs	–	100	–
original	2 Tbs	4.0	120	30%
peanut butter caramel	2 Tbs	6.0	150	36%
for vegetables				
bacon ranch	2 Tbs	12.0	120	90%
blue cheese	2 Tbs	19.0	180	95%
cheese veggie topping	2 Tbs	7.0	90	70%
dill				
fat-free	2 Tbs	–	35	–
regular	2 Tbs	14.0	140	90%
French onion	2 Tbs	13.0	130	90%
Guacamole	2 Tbs	12.0	120	90%
ranch				
fat-free	2 Tbs	–	35	–
light	2 Tbs	6.0	80	68%
original	2 Tbs	13.0	130	90%
Southwestern				
fat-free	2 Tbs	–	35	–
original	2 Tbs	14.0	140	90%
fat-free	2 Tbs	–	35	–
originals	2 Tbs	14.0	140	90%
Southwestern/fat-free	2 Tbs	–	30	–
veggie dill/fat-free	2 Tbs	–	30	–
(Mr. Hommus)				
garlic	2 Tbs	2.0	50	36%
garlic & chives	2 Tbs	2.0	50	36%
original	2 Tbs	2.0	50	36%
red pepper	2 Tbs	2.0	50	36%
(Nasoya) Vegi-Dip				
French onion	2 Tbs	3.0	50	54%

Food and Description	Amount	Fat Grams	Total Calories	% Fat Calories
garlic & herb	2 Tbs	2.0	50	36%
(Old El Paso)				
black bean	2 Tbs	–	20	–
cheese 'n salsa				
medium	2 Tbs	3.0	40	68%
mild	2 Tbs	3.0	40	68%
jalapeño	2 Tbs	1.0	30	30%
(Poore Brothers)				
bean	2 Tbs	1.5	40	34%
sour cream & onion	2 Tbs	5.0	60	75%
(Rod's)				
dip				
French onion				
regular	2 Tbs	6.0	70	77%
w/bacon	2 Tbs	6.0	70	77%
green onion	2 Tbs	6.0	70	77%
ranch	2 Tbs	6.0	70	77%
dip & dressing				
avocado	2 Tbs	11.0	110	90%
French onion/fat-free	2 Tbs	–	25	–
guacamole				
regular	2 Tbs	11.0	110	90%
zesty	2 Tbs	8.0	80	90%
ranch				
regular	2 Tbs	11.0	110	90%
fat-free	2 Tbs	–	25	–
w/bacon	2 Tbs	11.0	110	90%
(Smucker's) fat-free				
caramel fruit	2 Tbs	–	130	–
chocolate fruit	2 Tbs	–	130	–
(Snyder's)				
sour cream & onion	2 Tbs	5.0	60	75%
tangy honey mustard pretzel	2 Tbs	1.0	70	13%
(Taco Bell)				
wild black bean	2 Tbs	–	25	–
wild salsa	2 Tbs	–	15	–
(Thank You)				
creamy ranch	2 Tbs	5.0	60	75%
French onion	2 Tbs	5.0	60	75%
nacho cheese	2 Tbs	5.0	50	90%
DISTILLED LIQUOR (See LIQUOR, DISTILLED)				
DOCK				
cooked-drained	3 oz	0.5	17	26%
raw/chopped	3 oz	0.5	15	30%
DOGFISH (See also SHARK)				
raw	3 oz	8.0	135	53%
DOLPHIN FISH (See also MAHI MAHI)				
raw	3 oz	0.6	73	7%
DONUT (See also PASTRY)				
(Break Cake)				
chocolate	1 donut	8.0	130	55%

Food and Description	Amount	Fat Grams	Total Calories	% Fat Calories
cinnamon	1 donut	6.0	115	47%
powdered	1 donut	5.0	115	39%
(Dolly Madison)				
chocolate				
gems	4 gems	15.0	260	52%
iced/old-fashioned	1 donut	14.0	300	42%
cinnamon stix	1 stix	9.0	170	48%
cinnamon sugar				
gems	6 gems	17.0	360	43%
stix	2 stix	12.0	230	47%
crunch				
gems	6 gems	18.0	390	42%
regular	1 donut	6.0	140	39%
dunkin stix	2 stix	19.0	360	48%
frosted	1 donut	6.0	130	42%
glazed/old-fashioned	1 donut	14.0	300	42%
iced/jumbo	1 donut	12.0	230	47%
plain				
jumbo	1 donut	11.0	190	52%
regular	2 donuts	10.0	170	53%
powdered sugar/gems	6 gems	17.0	360	43%
sugar				
jumbo	1 donut	12.0	230	47%
regular	1 donut	6.0	130	42%
white iced/old-fashioned	1 donut	14.0	230	55%
yeast glazed	1 donut	8.0	180	40%
(Dunkin' Donuts)				
crullers/sticks				
chocolate	1 donut	15.0	280	48%
plain	1 donut	15.0	240	56%
powdered	1 donut	15.0	270	50%
sugar	1 donut	15.0	250	54%
chocolate/glazed	1 donut	24.0	410	53%
Dunkin' donut	1 donut	14.0	240	53%
glazed	1 donut	14.0	340	37%
jelly stick	1 donut	14.0	330	38%
plain	1 donut	14.0	260	48%
powdered	1 donut	15.0	290	47%
sugar	1 donut	14.0	270	47%
donuts				
cake				
blueberry	1 donut	16.0	290	50%
blueberry crumb	1 donut	10.0	240	38%
bow tie	1 donut	17.0	300	51%
butternut ring	1 donut	16.0	300	48%
cinnamon	1 donut	15.0	270	50%
coconut	1 donut	17.0	290	53%
glazed	1 donut	15.0	270	50%
old fashioned	1 donut	15.0	250	54%
powdered	1 donut	15.0	270	50%

Food and Description	Amount	Fat Grams	Total Calories	% Fat Calories
sugared	1 donut	15.0	250	54%
toasted coconut	1 donut	17.0	300	51%
chocolate				
double chocolate	1 donut	17.0	310	49%
glazed cake	1 donut	16.0	290	50%
regular	1 donut	14.0	210	60%
chocolate coconut	1 donut	19.0	300	57%
chocolate frosted				
cake	1 donut	16.0	300	48%
coffee roll	1 donut	15.0	290	47%
other				
Bismark chocolate iced	1 donut	15.0	340	40%
cinnamon bun	1 bun	15.0	510	26%
coffee roll				
maple-frosted	1 donut	14.0	290	43%
plain	1 donut	14.0	270	47%
Dunkin' Donut	1 donut	15.0	240	56%
Eclair donut	1 donut	11.0	270	37%
fritter				
apple	1 donut	14.0	300	42%
glazed	1 donut	14.0	260	48%
yeast				
apple crumb	1 donut	10.0	230	39%
apple n' spice	1 donut	8.0	200	36%
Bavarian kreme	1 donut	9.0	210	39%
black raspberry	1 donut	8.0	210	34%
Boston kreme	1 donut	9.0	240	34%
chocolate frosted	1 donut	9.0	200	41%
chocolate kreme filled	1 donut	13.0	270	43%
glazed	1 donut	7.0	160	39%
jelly filled	1 donut	8.0	210	34%
lemon	1 donut	9.0	200	41%
maple frosted	1 donut	9.0	210	39%
raised/sugar	1 donut	8.0	170	42%
strawberry	1 donut	8.0	210	34%
strawberry frosted	1 donut	9.0	210	39%
vanilla frosted				
donut	1 donut	9.0	210	39%
roll	1 roll	9.0	210	39%
vanilla kreme filled	1 donut	13.0	270	43%
whole wheat glazed	1 donut	19.0	310	55%
Munchkins				
cake				
butternut	3 Munchkins	11.0	200	50%
chocolate glazed	4 Munchkins	14.0	250	50%
cinnamon	4 Munchkins	14.0	250	50%
coconut				
regular	3 Munchkins	12.0	200	54%
toasted coconut	3 Munchkins	11.0	200	50%
glazed	3 Munchkins	10.0	200	45%

Food and Description	Amount	Fat Grams	Total Calories	% Fat Calories
plain	4 Munchkins	14.0	220	63%
powdered	4 Munchkins	14.0	250	50%
sugared	4 Munchkins	14.0	240	53%
yeast				
jelly-filled	5 Munchkins	9.0	210	39%
lemon	4 Munchkin	8.0	170	42%
raised				
glazed	5 Munchkins	9.0	200	41%
sugar	7 Munchkin	12.0	220	49%
(Earth Grains)				
cinnamon-apple	1 donut	17.0	310	49%
devil's food	1 donut	21.0	330	57%
glazed/old-fashioned	1 donut	18.0	310	52%
powdered/old-fashioned	1 donut	19.0	290	59%
(Entenmann's)				
donuts				
buttermilk/glazed	1 donut	13.0	270	43%
cinnamon sugar/variety donuts	1 donut	19.0	310	55%
devil's food, frosted	1 donut	19.0	290	59%
rich frosted	1 donut	19.0	310	55%
Softee variety	1 conut	13.0	230	51%
Popems				
glazed	4 pieces	15.0	260	52%
chocolate/glazed	4 pieces	12.0	240	45%
Popettes				
rich frosted	3 popettes	18.0	280	58%
softee powdered cinnamon	3 popettes	15.0	240	56%
(Hostess)				
Donettes bite-size donuts				
crumb	3 donettes	8.0	170	42%
frosted	3 donettes	12.0	200	54%
powdered	3 donettes	9.0	180	45%
donuts				
blueberry	1 donut	13.0	210	56%
frosted	1 donut	11.0	180	55%
glazed/old fashioned	1 donut	13.0	260	45%
plain	1 donut	7.0	140	45%
powdered	1 donut	8.0	150	48%
raspberry O's	1 donut	10.0	230	39%
(KrispyKreme)				
cake				
blueberry, old fashioned glazed	1 donut	15.0	300	45%
devil's food, old fashioned glazed	1 donut	13.0	240	49%
fudge-iced	1 donut	12.0	230	47%
powdered-sugar coated	1 donut	11.0	220	45%
sour cream, old fashioned	1 donut	11.0	230	43%
traditional	1 donut	11.0	200	50%
cinnamon bun	1 bun	11.0	220	45%
crullers				
fudge iced	1 donut	14.0	240	53%

Food and Description	Amount	Fat Grams	Total Calories	% Fat Calories
plain glazed	1 donut	14.0	220	57%
fudge iced glazed w/sprinkles	1 donut	10.0	220	41%
yeast				
cinnamon apple-filled sugar coated	1 donut	9.0	210	43%
blueberry-filled powder sugar coated	1 donut	9.0	200	41%
fudge iced glazed				
creme filled	1 donut	14.0	270	47%
custard filled	1 donut	9.0	250	32%
regular	1 donut	14.0	260	48%
creme-filled glazed	1 donut	14.0	270	47%
lemon-filled glazed	1 donut	10.0	210	43%
maple iced glazed	1 donut	9.0	200	41%
original glazed	1 donut	10.0	170	53%
raspberry-filled glazed	1 donut	10.0	210	43%
(Little Debbie) donut sticks				
box	1 pkg	12.0	210	51%
individual	1 pkg	13.0	220	53%
(Rich's) frozen/glazed	1 donut	7.0	130	48%
(Sara Lee) Food Service				
chocolate iced chocolate flavored chip	1 donut	13.0	280	42%
coconut glazed old fashion chocolate cake	1 donut	18.0	320	51%
crunchy peanut glazed cake	1 donut	13.0	270	43%
devil's food cake	1 donut	16.0	320	45%
glazed old fashion sour cream cake	1 donut	9.0	290	28%
powdered sugar cake	1 donut	13.0	290	40%
(TastyKake)				
Mini Donuts				
plain glaze	6 donuts	11.0	260	38%
powdered sugar	6 donuts	12.0	260	42%
rich frosted	6 donuts	22.0	370	54%
regular donuts				
assortment pkg				
cinnamon	1 donut	12.0	210	51%
plain	1 donut	11.0	180	55%
powdered sugar	1 donut	11.0	210	47%
dunkin stix	1 piece	11.0	190	52%
honey wheat	1 donut	10.0	230	39%
orange glazed	1 donut	9.0	220	37%
rich frosted	1 donut	16.0	270	53%
(Winchell's)				
cinnamon crumb	1 donut	11.0	240	41%
cinnamon roll	1 roll	21.0	360	53%
glazed				
jelly	1 donut	13.0	300	39%
round	1 donut	12.0	210	51%
twist	1 donut	11.0	210	51%
iced				
chocolate cake	1 donut	10.0	230	39%
chocolate devil's food	1 donut	12.0	240	45%

Food and Description	Amount	Fat Grams	Total Calories	% Fat Calories
chocolate French	1 donut	13.0	220	53%
raised	1 donut	10.0	210	43%
plain				
donut hole	1 piece	3.0	50	54%
regular	1 donut	11.0	200	50%

DRESSING (*See* MAYONNAISE/MAYONNAISE-TYPE DRESSING; SALAD DRESSING; STUFFING/DRESSING)

DRUM /freshwater

baked	3 oz	5.0	130	35%
raw	3 oz	4.0	100	36%

DUCK

domesticated

liver/raw	1.5 oz	2.0	60	30%
meat & skin/roasted	~¾ lb	108.0	1287	76%
meat only/roasted	8 oz	25.0	456	49%
wild/raw	3 oz	9.0	170	48%
breast meat only	3 oz	3.5	105	30%
meat & skin	9.5 oz	41.0	570	65%

DUMPLING (*See also* FROZEN ENTRÉE/DINNER; PASTRY)

Frozen

(Pepperidge Farm) Apple dumpling	1 dumpling	13.0	260	45%
Mix				
(Maggi)				
tiny Swiss style spaetzle mix	¼ cup	1.5	180	8 %
(Panni)				
Bavarian potato dumpling mix	½ pkg	–	80	–

Food and Description	Amount	Fat Grams	Total Calories	% Fat Calories
ECLAIR (*See* PASTRY)				
EEL				
cooked-dry heat	3 oz	12.7	200	57%
raw	3 oz	10.0	156	58%
smoked	~2 oz	16.0	188	77%

EGG (*See also* EGG SUBSTITUTE; VEGETARIAN FOODS)

chicken

boiled, hard or soft	1 medium	4.0	70	51%
	1 large	5.6	79	64%
fried in butter	1 large	7.0	95	66%

Food and Description	Amount	Fat Grams	Total Calories	% Fat Calories
pickled	1 large	5.0	80	56%
poached	1 large	5.6	79	64%
raw				
white only	1 medium	–	14	–
	1 large	–	16	–
	1 cup	–	120	–
whole	1 medium	4.0	70	51%
	1 large	5.6	79	64%
yolk only	1 medium	4.0	56	64%
	1 large	5.6	63	64%
duck/raw	1 egg	9.6	130	67%
goose/raw	1 egg	19.0	276	62%
quail/raw	1 egg	1.0	14	64%
turkey/raw	1 egg	9.0	135	60%
EGG DISH/MEAL (*See also* BREAKFAST SANDWICH; EGG; EGG SUBSTITUTE)				
frozen or refrigerated				
(Chef's Omelet)				
ham & cheese	½ pkg	12.0	180	60%
salsa & cheese	½ pkg	11.0	160	62%
sausage & cheese	½ pkg	18.0	240	68%
spinach & feta	½ pkg	10.0	160	56%
three cheese	½ pkg	16.0	230	63%
western style	½ pkg	9.0	150	54%
(Downeyflake)Scrambled eggs				
w/ham & hash browns	1 pkg	26.0	360	65%
w/ham & pecan twirl	1 pkg	28.0	470	54%
w/hash browns & sausage	1 pkg	34.0	420	73%
w/sausage & pecan twirl	1 pkg	33.0	510	58%
(La Terra Fina)				
broccoli-cheddar quiche	6 oz	15.0	292	46%
(Nancy's) quiche/microwaveable				
Petite appetizers				
assortment				
box of 12	6 quiche	23.0	390	53%
box of 48				
classic French	6 quiche	24.0	400	54%
florentine	6 quiche	21.0	370	51%
florentine puffs	12 pieces	21.0	400	47%
Santa Fe quiche tartlets	12 tartlets	40.0	650	55%
Single servings				
broccoli cheddar	1 quiche	26.0	430	54%
classic French	1 quiche	33.0	470	63%
Florentine	1 quiche	26.0	440	53%
Lorraine	1 quiche	29.0	490	53%
Monterey	1 quiche	29.0	470	56%
(Quelle) quiche				
broccoli	⅙ quiche	28.0	360	70%
Lorraine	⅙ quiche	28.0	360	70%
spinach	⅙ quiche	28.0	360	70%
(Swanson)				
Egg, sausage & cheese	1 pkg	28.0	460	55%

Food and Description	Amount	Fat Grams	Total Calories	% Fat Calories
Omelet w/cheese & ham	1 pkg	29.0	390	67%
Reduced Cholesterol Eggs w/mini oatbran muffin	1 pkg	12.0	250	43%
Scrambled eggs				
& bacon w/home fries	1 pkg	26.0	340	69%
& home fries	1 pkg	19.0	260	66%
& sausage w/hash browns	1 pkg	34.0	430	71%
w/cheese & cinnamon pancakes	1 pkg	23.0	290	71%
(Weight Watchers) Handy Omelet				
ham & cheese	4 oz	5.0	220	20%
homemade/USDA Standard Home Recipe				
deviled egg	2 halves	13.0	145	81%
egg foo young	~5 oz	10.0	150	60%
egg salad	⅓ cup	19.0	205	83%
omelet/made w/1 egg & 1 Tbs whole milk/cooked in butter	1 omelet	7.0	95	66%
quiche				
cheese	5 oz	33.0	470	63%
Lorraine/8" dia	⅛ quiche	48.0	600	72%
mushroom	5 oz	30.0	430	63%
spinach	5 oz	26.0	337	69%
scrambled egg/made w/whole milk/cooked in butter	1 egg	7.0	95	66%

EGG ROLL (*See* ASIAN FOOD; FROZEN ENTRÉE/DINNER; SEAFOOD ENTRÉE/DINNER)
EGG SALAD (*See* EGG DISH/MEAL)
EGG SUBSTITUTE
Generic

Food and Description	Amount	Fat Grams	Total Calories	% Fat Calories
frozen	¼ cup	6.7	96	64%
liquid	1½ oz	1.6	39	37%
powder	0.35 oz	1.0	44	21%
(Featherweight) Egg Magic	1 pouch	8.0	110	65%
(Fleischmann's) Egg Beaters				
cheese omelet mix	½ cup	5.0	110	41%
plain	¼ cup	–	25	–
(Healthy Choice)	¼ cup	–	25	–
(Just Whites) dried egg whites	2 tsp	–	14	–
(Morningstar Farms) frozen				
Better'n Eggs	¼ cup	–	20	–
Scramblers	¼ cup	–	35	–
(Nulaid) no cholesterol/no fat				
cheese	¼ cup	–	40	–
original	¼ cup	–	30	–
(Second Nature)				
No-Cholesterol	2 fl oz	2.0	60	30%
No-fat	2 fl oz	–	40	–
No-fat w/garden vegetables	2.5 fl oz	–	40	–
(Simply Eggs)	1.75 fl oz	1.0	35	26%
(Tofutti) Egg Watchers	¼ cup	–	30	–
(Wonderslim) fat & egg substitute	¼ cup	–	35	–

Food and Description	Amount	Fat Grams	Total Calories	% Fat Calories
EGGNOG				
canned				
(Borden)				
light	4 fl oz	2.0	130	14%
original	4 fl oz	9.0	160	51%
mix				
generic				
mix only	2 tsp	–	110	–
prepared				
w/skim milk	8 fl oz	1.0	200	5%
w/1% low-fat milk	8 fl oz	3.0	215	13%
w/2% low-fat milk	8 fl oz	5.0	230	20%
w/whole milk	8 fl oz	8.0	260	28%
(PDQ) prepared w/whole milk	8 fl oz	5.0	230	20%
refrigerated				
(Darigold)	8 fl oz	17.0	350	44%
classic	8 fl oz	17.0	390	39%
(Farm Rich) nondairy	8 fl oz	18.0	380	43%
generic				
light	4 fl oz	1.0	60	15%
regular	8 fl oz	19.0	342	50%
(Kemp's)				
Holly Nog	4 fl oz	2.0	110	16%
lite	4 fl oz	3.0	120	23%
original	4 fl oz	9.0	175	46%
premium	4 fl oz	9.0	180	45%
(Land O'Lakes)				
light	4 fl oz	3.0	130	21%
original	4 fl oz	8.0	170	42%
(Robert's)				
classic	8 oz	9.0	190	43%
home town holiday				
regular	8 oz	9.0	200	41%
w/vitamins A & D	8 oz	5.0	280	16%
EGGPLANT /fresh				
boiled	½ cup	–	13	–
raw/sliced	½ cup	–	11	–
EGGPLANT DISH (See also FROZEN ENTRÉE/DINNER)				
(Michael Angelo's) eggplant Parmesan/ frozen	1 cup	21.0	300	63%
(Mrs. Paul's) eggplant parmesan/frozen	½ cup	11.0	190	52%
(Progresso) appetizer	2 Tbs	2.0	25	72%
ELDERBERRY /raw	1 cup	0.8	105	7%
	½ lb	1.0	154	6%
ELK /meat only				
raw	1 oz	0.4	31	17%
	1 pound	6.6	504	12%
roasted	3 oz	1.6	124	12%

Food and Description	Amount	Fat Grams	Total Calories	% Fat Calories
ENCHILADA (*See* FROZEN ENTRÉE/DINNER; MEXICAN FOOD)				
ENCHILADA SAUCE (*See* MEXICAN FOOD; SAUCE)				
ENDIVE /raw	½ cup	–	4	–
ENGLISH MUFFIN (*See* MUFFIN)				
ESCARGOT (*See* SNAIL)				
ESCAROLE /raw	4 oz	–	20	–
ESCAROLE SOUP (*See* SOUP)				
EXTRACTS & FLAVORINGS				
(Durkee)				
almond extract	1 tsp	–	13	–
anise extract	1 tsp	–	16	–
banana flavor	1 tsp	–	15	–
black walnut flavor	1 tsp	–	4	–
brandy flavor	1 tsp	–	15	–
butter flavor	1 tsp	–	3	–
cherry extract	1 tsp	–	3	–
chocolate flavor	1 tsp	–	7	–
coconut flavor	1 tsp	–	8	–
crème de menthe extract	1 tsp	–	9	–
lemon extract	1 tsp	–	17	–
maple extract	1 tsp	–	6	–
orange extract	1 tsp	–	14	–
peppermint extract	1 tsp	–	15	–
pineapple flavor	1 tsp	–	6	–
raspberry extract	1 tsp	–	10	–
rum flavor	1 tsp	–	14	–
strawberry extract	1 tsp	–	12	–
vanilla butter & nut extract	1 tsp	–	5	–
vanilla extract	1 tsp	–	8	–
vanilla flavor	1 tsp	–	3	–
(McCormick/Schilling)				
almond extract	1 tsp	–	10	–
anise extract	1 tsp	–	23	–
banana imitation extract	1 tsp	–	11	–
black walnut extract				
cold	1 tsp	–	12	–
heated	1 tsp	–	<1	–
brandy imitation extract	1 tsp	–	20	–
butter flavor	1 tsp	–	<1	–
chocolate extract				
cold	1 tsp	–	8	–
heated	1 tsp	–	2	–
coconut imitation extract	1 tsp	–	7	–
lemon extract				
cold	1 tsp	–	35	–
heated	1 tsp	–	<1	–
maple imitation flavor	1 tsp	–	8	–
mint & peppermint extract	1 tsp	–	20	–
orange extract	1 tsp	–	23	–

Food and Description	Amount	Fat Grams	Total Calories	% Fat Calories
pineapple imitation extract	1 tsp	–	12	–
root beer concentrate	1 tsp	–	13	–
rum imitation extract	1 tsp	–	19	–
sherry extract	1 tsp	–	14	–
strawberry imitation extract	1 tsp	–	7	–
vanilla				
cold	1 tsp	–	12	–
heated	1 tsp	–	<1	–

F

Food and Description	Amount	Fat Grams	Total Calories	% Fat Calories
FAJITA (*See* MEXICAN FOOD; FROZEN ENTRÉE/DINNER)				
FALAFEL				
homemade/USDA Standard Home Recipe				
pattied or balled	1 oz	6.0	115	47%
mix				
(Casbah) prepared	5 balls	3.0	130	21%
(Fantastic Foods) Fantastic Falafel				
mix only	½ cup	4.0	250	14%
prepared	1 cup	4.0	250	14%
(Near East) vegetarian patty mix				
broiled	1½ patties	1.5	110	12%
fried	5 patties	15.0	230	59%
FAST FOOD (*See* separate section at end of book)				
FAT (*See also* BEEF TALLOW; BUTTER; COOKING SPRAY; LARD; MARGARINE, MARGARINE SPREAD, & SPRAY; OIL; PORK FAT; SHORTENING)				
bacon fat	1 Tbs	14.0	126	100%
beef fat/separable/raw	1 Tbs	12.0	108	100%
chicken fat	1 Tbs	12.0	115	100%
duck fat	1 Tbs	12.0	115	100%
pork backfat/raw	2 oz	50.0	464	100%
FAT SUBSTITUTE (*See also* OIL; SHORTENING)				
(Wonderslim) fat & egg substitute	¼ cup	–	35	–
FAVA BEAN/canned				
(Progresso)	½ cup	0.5	110	4%
FENNEL LEAVES/raw	2 oz	–	15	–
FENNEL SEED	1 tsp	–	7	–
FENUGREEK SEED	1 tsp	–	12	–

Food and Description	Amount	Fat Grams	Total Calories	% Fat Calories
FIELD PEA				
(Allen's)				
fresh	½ cup	0.5	100	5%
tiny	½ cup	0.5	100	5%
w/snaps	½ cup	0.5	100	5%
(Bush's Best)	½ cup	–	80	–
(Glory Foods)	½ cup	0.5	120	4%
FIG				
canned				
generic/solids & liquid				
In extra heavy syrup	1 cup	–	280	–
In heavy syrup	1 cup	–	228	–
In light syrup	1 cup	–	175	–
In water	1 cup	–	130	–
(Oregon) Kadota in heavy syrup	½ cup	1.0	130	7%
(S&W) Kadota/in heavy syrup	5 pieces	1.0	140	6%
dried				
generic				
cooked	1 large	–	55	–
	½ cup	–	140	–
uncooked	½ cup	1.0	250	4%
(Mariani) Calimyrna	½ cup	2.0	250	7%
(Sun Maid)				
Calimyrna	¼ cup	–	110	–
Mission	¼ cup	–	110	–
fresh	1 medium	–	37	–
	1 large	–	47	–
FILBERT/HAZELNUT (*See also* HAZELNUT BUTTER/SPREAD)				
(Diamond)				
in the shell	1 oz	19.0	190	90%
shelled	1 oz	19.0	190	90%
generic				
dried				
blanched	1 oz	17.8	179	90%
unblanched	1 oz	18.5	190	88%
dry-roasted	1 oz	18.8	188	90%
oil-roasted	1 oz	18.0	187	87%
FISH (*See* GEFILTE FISH; SEAFOOD ENTRÉE/DINER; individual listings)				
FISH CHOWDER (*See* SOUP)				
FISH SEASONING (*See* SEASONINGS)				
FIVE SPICE SEASONING (*See* SEASONINGS)				
FLAN (*See* CUSTARD)				
FLATBREAD (*See* CRACKER)				
FLATFISH (*See also* FLOUNDER)				
cooked	3 oz	1.0	100	9%
raw	3 oz	1.0	80	11%
FLAVORINGS (*See* EXTRACTS & FLAVORINGS)				
FLAXSEED (Arrowhead Mills)	3 Tbs	10.0	140	64%

Food and Description	Amount	Fat Grams	Total Calories	% Fat Calories
FLOUNDER (*See also* SEAFOOD ENTRÉE/DINNER)				
baked				
w/butter	3 oz	7.0	171	37%
w/o butter	3 oz	1.0	80	11%
frozen				
breaded	5 oz	15.0	300	45%
(Van de Kamp's) raw	1 fillet	2.0	110	16%
FLOUR				
acorn	1 oz	9.0	142	57%
amaranth				
(Arrowhead Mills)	¼ cup	1.5	110	13%
generic	1 oz	<1.0	95	3%
	1 cup	2.0	698	3%
arrowroot	1 Tbs	–	29	–
barley				
(Arrowhead Mills)	¼ cup	0.5	75	6%
generic	1 Tbs	<1.0	28	16%
bread				
generic	1 cup	3.0	401	7%
(Gold Medal) Better for Bread	¼ cup	–	100	–
(Hodgson Mill) Best for Bread	¼ cup	–	100	–
(Pillsbury)	¼ cup	–	100	–
(Red Brand) Better for Bread	¼ cup	–	100	–
buckwheat				
(Arrowhead Mills)	¼ cup	1.0	100	9%
generic				
dark	1 cup	2.0	326	6%
light	1 cup	1.0	340	3%
whole-grain	1 cup	2.0	335	5%
(Hodgson Mill)	⅓ cup	1.0	160	6%
cake or pastry				
(Arrowhead Mills) soft pastry	¼ cup	0.5	100	5%
(Betty Crocker) Softasilk velvet cake	¼ cup	–	100	–
generic	1 cup	1.0	430	2%
(Swan's Down) cake	¼ cup	–	100	–
carob				
(St. John's Bread)	1 cup	3.0	420	6%
chestnut	4 oz	4.0	410	9%
corn	1 oz	0.7	102	6%
	1 cup	3.0	430	6%
cottonseed				
low-fat	1 oz	–	95	–
partially defatted	1 oz	–	40	–
	1 cup	6.0	335	16%
garbanzo/toasted				
(Arrowhead Mills)	¼ cup	1.0	90	10%
gluten				
(Arrowhead Mills) Vital wheat gluten	3 Tbs	–	35	–

Food and Description	Amount	Fat Grams	Total Calories	% Fat Calories
(La Pina) Supreme Hygluten	¼ cup	–	100	–
kamut				
(Arrowhead Mills)	¼ cup	0.5	110	4%
millet				
(Arrowhead Mills)	¼ cup	1.0	110	8%
multigrain				
(Arrowhead Mills) multi-blend	¼ cup	0.5	120	4%
oat				
(Arrowhead Mills)	⅓ cup	2.0	120	15%
(Hodgson Mill) oat bran blend	¼ cup	1.0	110	8%
peanut				
defatted	1 oz	–	92	–
	1 cup	–	200	–
low-fat	1 oz	6.0	120	45%
	1 cup	13.0	260	45%
pecan	1 oz	–	93	–
potato	1 cup	1.5	632	2%
quinoa				
(Quinoa) gluten-free, whole-grain	¼ cup	2.0	130	14%
rice				
(Arrowhead Mills)				
brown	¼ cup	1.0	120	8%
white	¼ cup	0.5	130	3%
generic				
brown	1 oz	<1.0	100	5%
white	1 oz	<1.0	100	2%
	1 cup	1.0	398	2%
(Tres Estrellas)	¼ cup	1.0	150	6%
rye				
(Arrowhead Mills)	¼ cup	1.0	100	9%
generic				
dark	1 cup	3.0	419	6%
light	1 cup	1.0	364	3%
(Hodgson Mill)	¼ cup	1.0	90	10%
(Krusteaz) medium	⅓ cup	0.5	110	4%
(Pillsbury)				
Bohemian style rye-wheat	¼ cup	–	100	–
medium	¼ cup	–	100	–
sesame				
high-fat	4 oz	42.0	595	64%
low-fat	1 cup	–	95	–
	4 oz	2.0	380	5%
partially defatted	4 oz	14.0	440	29%
soy				
(Arrowhead Mills)	½ cup	9.0	200	41%
generic				
defatted	1 cup	1.0	327	3%
full-fat				
not stirred	1 cup	17.6	358	44%
stirred	1 cup	14.0	295	43%

Food and Description	Amount	Fat Grams	Total Calories	% Fat Calories
gluten-free	½ cup	<1.0	180	3%
low-fat	1 cup	6.0	326	17%
spelt				
(Arrowhead Mills)	¼ cup	0.5	100	5%
sunflower seed	1 Tbs	<1.0	16	4%
	1 cup	1.3	261	4%
triticale	1 oz	0.5	95	5%
	1 cup	2.5	440	5%
white				
(Arrowhead Mills)				
semolina mix	½ cup	1.0	240	4%
unbleached	⅓ cup	0.5	160	3%
(Betty Crocker)				
All Trump	¼ cup	–	100	–
(Gold Medal)				
all-purpose	¼ cup	–	100	–
self-rising	¼ cup	–	100	–
unbleached	¼ cup	–	100	–
Wondra	¼ cup	–	100	–
(La Pina)	¼ cup	–	100	–
(Red Band)				
all-purpose	¼ cup	–	100	–
self-rising	¼ cup	–	100	–
Robin Hood				
all-purpose	¼ cup	–	100	–
self-rising	¼ cup	–	100	–
unbleached	¼ cup	–	100	–
(Hodgson Mill)				
regular	¼ cup	–	100	–
seasoned	¼ cup	–	90	–
(Pillsbury)				
all-purpose				
bleached	¼ cup	–	100	–
unbleached	¼ cup	–	100	–
self-rising				
bleached	¼ cup	–	100	–
unbleached	¼ cup	–	100	–
shake & blend	¼ cup	–	100	–
(Quaker) Aunt Jemima self-rising/ enriched	3 Tbs	–	90	–
whole wheat				
(Alma)				
coarse wheat	¼ cup	–	100	–
fine wheat	¼ cup	–	100	–
(Arrowhead Mills)				
stone-ground	¼ cup	0.5	130	3%
whole-grain	¼ cup	0.5	110	4%
(Gold Medal)				
whole wheat	¼ cup	0.5	90	5%
whole wheat blend	¼ cup	0.5	100	5%

Food and Description	Amount	Fat Grams	Total Calories	% Fat Calories
(Hodgson Mill)				
50/50	¼ cup	1.0	100	9%
whole wheat	¼ cup	1.0	100	9%
(Pillsbury)	¼ cup	1.0	120	8%
FRANKFURTER (*See also* FRANKFURTER, VEGETARIAN; SAUSAGE; VEGETARIAN FOODS; individual FAST FOOD listings)				
(Ball Park)				
beef				
bun size	2 oz	16.0	180	80%
regular	4 oz	32.0	340	85%
	3.25 oz	25.0	270	83%
	2.71 oz	21.0	230	82%
	2 oz	16.0	170	80%
	1.6 oz	13.0	140	84%
fat-free	1.78 oz	–	45	–
Fun Franks on a bun	1 pkg	10.0	180	50%
lite	1 frank	8.0	110	65%
meat				
beef & pork				
bun size	2 oz	16.0	180	80%
regular	4 oz	33.0	380	78%
	3.25 oz	26.0	280	84%
	2 oz	16.0	180	80%
	1.6 oz	13.0	140	84%
beef, pork, & turkey	3.25 oz	26.0	280	84%
(Butterball) turkey	1 frank	11.0	130	76%
(Denver Buffalo Co.) Buffalo Will's Western hot dogs w/buffalo & beef	1 frank	8.0	110	65%
(Eckrich) jumbo				
cheese	1 frank	17.0	180	85%
regular	1 frank	17.0	190	80%
generic				
Cheesefurter	1.5 oz	12.5	141	80%
(Health Valley)				
weiners				
regular	1 weiner	8.0	96	75%
turkey	1 weiner	8.0	96	75%
(Healthy Choice)				
beef	1 frank	1.5	60	23%
bun size	1 frank	1.5	70	20%
deli beef franks	1 frank	3.0	100	27%
regular	1 frank	1.5	50	27%
(Hebrew National)				
beef	1.7 oz	14.0	150	84%
beef franks in a blanket	4 pieces	28.0	340	74%
cocktail franks				
2-oz link/4 per pkg	4 links	16.0	180	80%
1.8-oz link/6 per pkg	1 link	15.0	160	84%
dinner franks/beef	4 oz	32.0	350	82%

Food and Description	Amount	Fat Grams	Total Calories	% Fat Calories
97% fat-free	1.75 oz	1.5	50	27%
reduced-fat beef	1.7 oz	10.0	120	75%
(Hillshire Farm)				
franks				
bun size				
all-beef super dogs	4 oz	34.0	350	87%
beef	2 oz	17.0	180	85%
cheese	2 oz	17.0	180	85%
regular	2 oz	17.0	180	85%
light & mild/jumbo	1 frank	8.0	110	65%
Lit'l Beef	2 oz	15.0	170	79%
Lit'l Smokies				
beef	6 pieces	15.0	170	79%
meat	6 pieces	16.0	180	80%
Wieners				
bun size	2 oz	17.0	180	85%
foot long	3.25 oz	26.0	280	84%
light & mild	1 wiener	8.0	90	80%
Lit'l wieners	6 pieces	16.0	170	85%
natural casing	2 oz	17.0	180	85%
(Hormel)				
cocktail franks				
smokies	5 smokies	16.0	180	80%
wieners	5 wieners	14.0	160	79%
corn dogs	2.75 oz	11.0	220	45%
franks				
beef/10 per pkg	1 frank	12.0	140	77%
Big 8	1 frank	17.0	180	85%
(Light & Lean 97)				
beef	1 frank	1.0	45	20%
jumbo	1 frank	1.5	60	23%
regular	1 frank	1.0	45	20%
meat/10 per pkg	1 frank	13.0	140	84%
(Wranglers)				
beef	1 frank	15.0	170	79%
cheese	1 frank	15.0	170	79%
smoked	1 frank	15.0	170	79%
(Kahn's)				
franks				
beef				
bun size	1 frank	16.0	180	80%
jumbo	2 oz	17.0	180	85%
regular	1 frank	14.0	150	84%
beef 'n cheddar	1 frank	16.0	180	80%
fat-free/jumbo	1 frank	–	40	–
pork & beef				
bun size	1 frank	17.0	190	81%
jumbo	2 oz	16.0	170	85%
smoky				
Big Red	1 frank	14.0	170	74%

Food and Description	Amount	Fat Grams	Total Calories	% Fat Calories
bun size	1 frank	15.0	180	75%
wieners				
bun size	2 oz	16.0	180	80%
cheese	1 wiener	13.0	150	78%
regular	1 wiener	13.0	140	84%
(Louis Rich)				
bun-length/8 per 16-oz pkg	1 frank	8.0	110	65%
cheese/10 per 16-oz pkg	1 frank	6.0	90	60%
turkey & chicken				
10 per 16-oz pkg	1 frank	6.0	80	68%
8 per 12-oz pkg	1 frank	6.0	80	68%
(Mr. Turkey)				
bun size	1 link	11.0	130	76%
cheese	1 link	12.0	140	77%
hot dog	1 link	9.0	110	74%
(Oscar Mayer)				
franks				
big & juicy/beef				
deli style	1 frank	22.0	230	86%
original	1 frank	22.0	240	83%
quarter pound	1 frank	33.0	350	85%
bun length	1 frank	17.0	180	85%
jumbo beef	1 frank	17.0	180	85%
light beef	1 frank	8.0	110	65%
regular				
beef	1 frank	13.0	140	77%
cheese	1 frank	13.0	140	77%
hot dogs				
cheese	1 link	13.0	140	84%
Free/fat-free				
beef	1 link	–	40	–
turkey & beef	1 link	–	35	–
wieners				
big & juicy				
hot 'n spicy	1 wiener	20.0	220	82%
original beef	1 wiener	22.0	240	83%
Smokie Links	1 wiener	19.0	220	78%
bun-length/pork & turkey	1 wiener	17.0	190	81%
jumbo	1 link	17.0	180	85%
Light/pork, turkey, & beef	1 wiener	8.0	110	65%
little/original	6 links	17.0	180	85%
regular/pork & turkey	1 wiener	13.0	150	78%
(Schwan's)				
franks/skinless	1 link	13.0	140	84%
Little Smokies w/BBQ Sauce	5 links	14.0	250	50%
(Shelton's)				
chicken bites	6 links	13.0	10	73%
regular franks	1 link	6.0	70	77%
(State Fair) beef corn dogs	1 corn dog	10.0	210	43%

Food and Description	Amount	Fat Grams	Total Calories	% Fat Calories
((Wampler Longacre)				
chicken				
1.6 oz	1 link	9.0	110	74%
2 oz	1 link	11.0	130	76%
turkey				
1.6 oz	1 link	9.0	110	74%
2 oz	1 link	11.0	130	76%
(Woody's) Corny Dogs	1 corn dog	11.0	210	47%
FRANKFURTER, VEGETARIAN (See also VEGETARIAN FOODS)				
(Loma Linda)				
Big Franks				
low-fat	1 link	3.0	80	34%
regular	1 link	7.0	110	57%
corn dogs	1 corn dog	4.0	150	54%
Linketts	1 link	4.5	70	58%
Little Links	2 links	6.0	90	69%
(Lightlife)				
Smart Dogs	1.5 oz	–	45	–
Tofu Pups	1.5 oz	2.5	60	38%
Wonderdogs	1.5 oz	1.0	55	16%
(Morningstar Farms) America's Original Veggie Dog	1 link	6.0	100	54%
(Worthington)				
Leanies/frozen	1.4 oz	7.0	100	63%
Super-Links	1.7 oz	8.0	110	65%
Veja-Links/canned	1.1 oz	3.0	50	54%
(Yves) Veggie Cuisine				
chili dogs	1 chili dog	–	70	–
tofu wieners	1 wiener	0.5	57	8%
veggie wieners	1 wiener	–	60	–
FRENCH FRIES (See FROZEN ENTRÉE/DINNER; POTATO; individual FAST FOOD listings)				
FRENCH ONION SOUP (See SOUP)				
FRENCH TOAST				
Frozen				
(Aunt Jemima)				
cinnamon swirl	4.5 oz	17.0	350	44%
original	4.5 oz	20.0	400	45%
(Downyflake)				
cinnamon swirl				
regular cut	1 slice	2.0	90	20%
thick cut	1 slice	2.5	110	20%
traditional				
regular cut	1 slice	1.0	90	20%
thick cut	2 slice	2.5	110	20%
(Farm Rich) sticks				
apple-cinnamon	1 serving	15.0	310	44%
blueberry	1 serving	14.0	310	41%
original	1 serving	15.0	300	45%
(Krusteaz)				
cinnamon swirl	2 slices	5.0	230	20%

Food and Description	Amount	Fat Grams	Total Calories	% Fat Calories
classic style	2 slices	5.0	230	20%
sourdough	1 slice	2.0	140	13%
(Pepperidge Farm)cinnamon swirl	⅛ pkg	7.0	200	32%
(Schwan's) apple-cinnamon sticks	5 sticks	21.0	390	48%
(Swanson)				
French stix w/syrup	1 meal	10.0	320	28%
Great Starts				
cinnamon swirl w/sausages	1 meal	26.0	410	57%
Kid's Breakfast Blast				
mini French stix w/syrup	1 meal	14.0	310	41%
Homemade/USDA Standard Home Recipe	1 slice	7.0	155	41%
Liquid Mix (Nulaid)	¼ cup	–	40	–
FRITTER (See also CORN DISHES; PASTRY)				
(Mrs. Paul's) Apple/frozen	2 fritters	11.0	240	41%
USDA Standard Home Recipe	1 fritter	7.5	132	51%
FROG/legs				
floured & fried	1 oz	4.8	70	61%
	3 oz	17.0	250	61%
raw	3 oz	<1.0	63	7%

FROSTING (See CAKE ICING/FROSTING)
FROZEN ENTRÉE/DINNER (See also ASIAN FOOD; BEEF DISH/ENTRÉE; CHICKEN ENTRÉE/DINNER; MEXICAN FOOD; PASTA DISH; PIZZA; POTATO DISH; RICE DISH; VEGETARIAN FOODS)
■ **(Armour)**
Classics

Food and Description	Amount	Fat Grams	Total Calories	% Fat Calories
chicken				
& noodles	1 meal	9.0	280	29%
mesquite	1 meal	13.0	280	42%
parmigiana	1 meal	18.0	360	45%
w/wine & mushrooms	1 meal	11.0	260	38%
glazed	1 meal	14.0	280	45%
meatloaf	1 meal	10.0	300	30%
Salisbury steak	1 meal	18.0	330	49%
Swedish meatballs	1 meal	17.0	300	51%
turkey & dressing	1 meal	7.0	270	23%
veal parmigiana	1 meal	22.0	400	50%

Classics Lite

Food and Description	Amount	Fat Grams	Total Calories	% Fat Calories
beef pepper	1 meal	4.0	210	17%
chicken burgundy	1 meal	5.0	210	21%
Salisbury steak	1 meal	7.0	260	24%
shrimp Creole	1 meal	1.0	220	4%
sweet & sour	1 meal	1.0	220	4%

■ **(Banquet)**
Bone-In Chicken

Food and Description	Amount	Fat Grams	Total Calories	% Fat Calories
firehouse big wings	2 pieces	14.0	190	67%
honey BBQ wings	4 pieces	26.0	380	62%
hot'n spicy fried chicken	3 oz	18.0	260	62%
original fried chicken/jumbo pack	3 oz	18.0	280	58%
skinless fried chicken	3 oz	13.0	220	53%
smokehouse big wings	2 pieces	14.0	200	63%

Food and Description	Amount	Fat Grams	Total Calories	% Fat Calories
Boneless Chicken & Misc.				
fat free baked breast tenders	3 tenders	–	120	–
grilled honey BBQ chicken breast patties	1 patty	5.0	110	41%
our original				
breast tenders	3 tenders	15.0	250	54%
chicken nuggets	6 nuggets	19.0	270	63%
chicken patties	1 patty	14.0	190	66%
southern				
breast tenders	3 tenders	16.0	260	55%
chicken nuggets	5 nuggets	18.0	270	60%
chicken patties	1 patty	13.0	190	62%
Extra Helping Dinners/Hearty Ones				
boneless				
pork riblet	1 meal	40.0	720	50%
white fried chicken	1 meal	48.0	690	63%
chicken fried beef steak	1 meal	50.0	820	55%
fried chicken	1 meal	55.0	910	54%
meat loaf	1 meal	40.0	610	59%
Salisbury steak	1 meal	54.0	740	66%
turkey & gravy w/Dressing	1 meal	32.0	620	46%
yankee pot roast	1 meal	20.0	410	44%
Family Size Entrée/Meals Made Easy				
brown gravy &				
Salisbury steaks	1 patty w/gravy	20.0	240	75%
sliced beef	2 slices w/gravy	8.0	140	51%
chicken & broccoli alfredo	1 cup	12.0	270	40%
creamy broccoli, chicken, cheese, & rice	1 cup	14.0	280	45%
country-style chicken & dumplings	1 cup	14.0	290	43%
egg noodles w/beef & brown gravy	1 cup	5.0	150	30%
hearty beef stew	1 cup	7.0	170	37%
hearty chicken pie	1 cup	29.0	460	57%
homestyle gravy & sliced turkey	2 slices w/gravy	10.0	140	64%
lasagna w/meat sauce	1 cup	10.0	270	33%
macaroni & cheese	1 cup	7.0	230	27%
mushroom gravy & 6 charbroiled beef patties	1 patty w/gravy	20.0	250	72%
potato, ham w/broccoli au gratin	⅔ cup	13.0	210	56%
savory gravy & meatloaf	1 patty w/gravy	13.0	190	62%
Hot Sandwich Toppers				
creamed chipped beef	1 bag	6.0	120	45%
gravy				
& Salisbury steak	1 bag	16.0	210	69%
& sliced beef	1 bag	2.0	70	26%
& sliced turkey	1 bag	11.0	160	62%

Food and Description	Amount	Fat Grams	Total Calories	% Fat Calories
Meals				
beef enchilada	1 meal	12.0	370	29%
beef enchilada & tamale combo	1 meal	20.0	450	40%
beef patty w/country style vegetables	1 meal	20.0	310	58%
boneless pork rib	1 meal	19.0	400	43%
cheese enchilada	1 meal	10.0	360	25%
chicken				
enchilada	1 meal	10.0	350	26%
fingers meal	1 meal	43.0	740	52%
fried beef steak	1 meal	23.0	420	49%
nuggets	1 meal	23.0	430	48%
parmigiana	1 meal	16.0	320	45%
pasta primavera	1 meal	12.0	320	34%
chimichanga meal	1 meal	24.0	500	43%
fettuccini alfredo	1 meal	16.0	350	41%
fish sticks	1 meal	13.0	290	40%
fried rice w/chicken & egg rolls	1 meal	9.0	330	25%
grilled chicken	1 meal	13.0	330	35%
homestyle noodles and chicken	1 meal	19.0	390	44%
honey roast turkey breast	1 meal	12.0	270	40%
lasagna w/meat sauce	1 meal	8.0	260	28%
macaroni & cheese	1 meal	14.0	240	53%
meat loaf	1 meal	16.0	280	51%
Mexican style enchilada combo	1 meal	11.0	360	28%
our original fried chicken	1 meal	27.0	470	52%
pepperoni pizza	1 meal	23.0	480	43%
pork cutlet meal	1 meal	25.0	420	54%
Salisbury steak	1 meal	24.0	380	57%
sliced beef	1 meal	10.0	270	33%
turkey (mostly white meat)	1 meal	11.0	270	37%
veal parmigiana	1 meal	14.0	330	38%
western style beef patty	1 meal	21.0	360	53%
white fried chicken/boneless	1 meal	34.0	540	57%
white meat fried chicken	1 meal	28.0	480	53%
yankee pot roast	1 meal	10.0	230	39%
Munchers				
cheese pizza snack	6 pieces	8.0	200	36%
pepperoni pizza snack	6 pieces	11.0	230	43%
pepperoni & sausage pizza snack	6 pieces	9.0	210	39%
Pot Pies				
Beef	1 pie	23.0	400	52%
cheesy potato & broccoli w/ham	1 pie	23.0	410	50%
chicken	1 pie	22.0	380	52%
chicken & broccoli	1 pie	20.0	350	51%
turkey	1 pie	20.0	370	49%
vegetable cheese	1 pie	17.0	340	45%
macaroni & cheese	1 pie	5.0	210	21%
■ **(Birds Eye)** Viola! All-In-One Meal/prepared				
Chicken				
alfredo	1 cup	8.0	230	31%

Food and Description	Amount	Fat Grams	Total Calories	% Fat Calories
garden herb	1 cup	15.0	310	44%
garlic/family size	1 cup	11.0	260	38%
Romano herb w/roasted potatoes	1 cup	7.0	210	30%
teriyaki	1 cup	9.0	240	34%
three cheese	1 cup	8.0	220	33%
three cheese/family size	1 cup	9.0	240	34%
Shrimp/garlic	1 cup	9.0	230	35%
Steak/beef sirloin & garlic potatoes	1 cup	9.0	240	34%
Turkey/homestyle w/roasted potatoes	1 cup	6.0	200	27%
■ **(Bob Evans Farms)**				
Bob Evans Homestyle				
beef & gravy w/noodles	1 meal	7.0	270	23%
beef pot roast	1 meal	5.0	230	20%
chicken & noodles	1 meal	33.0	670	44%
chicken pot pie	1 pie	28.0	510	49%
■ **(Boston Market)**				
Chicken				
oven roasted w/mashed potatoes & gravy	1 meal	19.0	450	38%
Garlic dill potatoes	9 oz serving	11.0	260	38%
Meatloaf w/gravy	1 meal	32.0	500	58%
■ **(Budget Gourmet)**				
Fettucini primavera	1 meal	8.0	280	26%
Swedish meatballs in cream sauce	1 meal	34.0	550	56%
Value Classics				
chicken in sauce w/rice-low fat	1 meal	7.0	250	25%
homestyle macaroni & cheese	1 meal	11.0	320	31%
■ **(Celentano)**				
Great Choice Entrées				
eggplant rollettes	10 oz	15.0	330	41%
lasagna	10 oz	2.5	260	9%
manicotti	10 oz	2.5	250	9%
ravioli	6.5 oz	9.0	400	20%
	4.2 oz	3.0	250	11%
stuffed shells	10 oz	2.5	400	6%
Non-Dairy Entrées/Vegetarian				
eggplant				
medallions w/garbanzo bean filling	10 oz	20.0	310	58%
parmigiana	10 oz	21.0	320	59%
rollettes	10 oz	13.0	220	53%
wraps w/three bean filling	10 oz	11.0	220	45%
lasagna primavera	10 oz	4.0	230	16%
porcini risotto w/roasted vegetables	10 oz	6.0	190	28%
risotto w/eggplant tofu & spinach	10 oz	19.0	340	50%
roasted vegetable lasagna	10 oz	12.0	290	37%
spinach & broccoli				
manicotti	10 oz	4.0	230	16%
stuffed shells	10 oz	4.0	210	17%
Regular Entrées				
broccoli stuffed shells	10 oz	6.0	300	18%

Food and Description	Amount	Fat Grams	Total Calories	% Fat Calories
eggplant parmigiana	10 oz	27.0	420	58%
eggplant rollettes	11 oz	14.0	320	39%
lasagna	10 oz	14.0	400	32%
manicotti	10 oz	21.0	450	42%
spinach tofu ravioli w/tomato sauce	10 oz	11.0	330	30%
stuffed shells	10 oz	20.0	400	45%
■ **(Chef America)** stuffed sandwiches				
Croissant pocket				
chicken, broccoli, & cheddar	1 sandwich	9.0	290	28%
eggs, sausage, & cheese	1 sandwich	15.0	340	40%
ham & cheddar	1 sandwich	12.0	320	34%
pepperoni pizza	1 sandwich	16.0	360	40%
Philly steak & cheese	1 sandwich	16.0	350	41%
supreme pizza	1 sandwich	20.0	390	46%
turkey, ham, & swiss	1 sandwich	10.0	390	23%
Hot Pockets				
barbecue	1 sandwich	11.0	330	30%
beef & cheddar	1 sandwich	16.0	350	41%
beef fajita	1 sandwich	14.0	340	37%
chicken & cheddar w/broccoli	1 sandwich	10.0	300	30%
ham'n cheese	1 sandwich	12.0	320	34%
meatballs w/mozzarella	1 sandwich	11.0	320	31%
pepperoni pizza	1 sandwich	15.0	350	39%
pepperoni & sausage	1 sandwich	14.0	330	38%
sausage pizza	1 sandwich	15.0	340	40%
turkey & ham w/cheese	1 sandwich	11.0	300	33%
Lean Pockets				
chicken broccoli supreme	1 sandwich	7.0	270	23%
chicken fajita	1 sandwich	7.0	270	23%
chicken parmesan	1 sandwich	7.0	280	23%
ham & cheddar	1 sandwich	7.0	270	23%
pepperoni pizza deluxe	1 sandwich	7.0	270	23%
Philly steak 7 cheese	1 sandwich	7.0	260	24%
turkey & ham w/cheddar	1 sandwich	7.0	270	23%
turkey, broccoli, & cheese	1 sandwich	7.0	250	25%
Pizza Mini's				
double cheese	1 serving	9.0	240	34%
pepperoni	1 serving	11.0	250	40%
pepperoni & sausage	1 serving	9.0	230	35%
sausage	1 serving	8.0	230	31%
Toaster Breaks				
Melts				
ham & cheese	1 melt	8.0	180	40%
Philly steak & cheese	1 melt	10.0	190	47%
Pizza				
double cheese	1 serving	9.0	190	43%
pepperoni	1 serving	10.0	200	45%
sausage & pepperoni	1 serving	8.0	180	40%
■ **(Chun King)** Munchers/Egg Rolls				
Chicken				
mini	3.1 oz	9.0	200	41%

Food and Description	Amount	Fat Grams	Total Calories	% Fat Calories
regular	½ pkg	9.0	190	43%
■ **(Delimex)**				
Nachos/beef stuffed	⅕ pkg	20.0	370	49%
Quesadillas				
cheeseburger	⅙ pkg	14.0	270	47%
chicken & cheese	⅙ pkg	9.0	220	37%
ham & cheese	⅙ pkg	13.0	260	45%
veggie pizza	⅙ pkg	9.0	220	37%
Taquitos				
beef	⅕ pkg	13.0	390	30%
chicken	⅕ pkg	15.0	370	36%
pepperoni	⅕ pkg	17.0	400	38%
seasoned beef & cheddar	⅕ pkg	16.0	360	40%
3-cheese	⅕ pkg	18.0	400	41%
■ **(Dinty Moore)** American Classics				
beef stew	1 meal	11.0	250	40%
chicken & noodles/97% fat free	1 meal	8.0	270	27%
chicken breast & gravy w/mashed potatoes	1 meal	4.0	240	15%
hearty lasagna w/meat	1 meal	16.0	340	42%
roast beef & gravy w/mashed potatoes	1 meal	5.0	240	19%
Salisbury steak w/sliced potatoes & gravy	1 meal	13.0	300	39%
■ **(Empire)** Blintzes				
apple	2 pieces	6.0	220	25%
blueberry	2 pieces	4.0	190	19%
cheese	2 pieces	6.0	200	27%
cherry	2 pieces	4.0	200	18%
potato	2 pieces	6.0	190	28%
■ **(Farm Rich)**				
Cheese Dippers/breaded sticks				
Italian 4 cheese	¼ pkg	8.0	140	51%
mozzarella	¼ pkg	10.0	190	47%
Fiesta Dippers				
cheddar cheese stuffed jalapeños	¼ pkg	7.0	140	45%
cream cheese stuffed jalapeños	¼ pkg	7.0	130	48%
Pizza Dippers/pizza crusts				
double cheese stuffed	1 serving	9.0	210	39%
pepperoni stuffed	1 serving	11.0	230	43%
■ **(Freezer Queen)**				
Cook-In-Pouch				
breaded veal parmigiana w/tomato sauce	1 pouch	9.0	190	43%
chicken a la king	1 pouch	1.5	70	19%
creamed chipped beef	1 pouch	5.0	100	45%
gravy				
& Salisbury steak	1 pouch	8.0	140	51%
& sliced beef	1 pouch	1.0	70	13%
& sliced chicken white meat	1 pouch	2.5	60	38%
& sliced turkey	1 pouch	1.5	70	19%
Deluxe Family Entrée				
breaded veal parmigiana	⅙ pkg	8.0	170	42%

Food and Description	Amount	Fat Grams	Total Calories	% Fat Calories
cheese ravioli & tomato sauce	⅓ pkg	5.0	280	16%
chicken & biscuits	1 serving	4.0	210	17%
chicken & vegetables in cheese sauce w/pasta	¼ pkg	6.0	220	25%
gravy & sliced beef	⅙ pkg	1.5	80	17%
lasagna in meat sauce	1 serving	8.0	270	27%
pasta & stroganoff sauce w/meatballs	1 serving	9.0	240	34%
pot roast w/gravy potatoes, carrots, & onions	1 serving	3.0	210	13%
turkey & gravy w/dressing	¼ pkg	3.5	160	20%
Family Entrée				
chicken nuggets	1 serving	15.0	250	54%
gravy				
& 6 breaded chicken croquettes	⅙ pkg	8.0	160	45%
& 6 breaded turkey croquettes	⅙ pkg	6.0	140	39%
& 6 Salisbury steaks	⅙ pkg	11.0	160	62%
& sliced turkey	⅙ pkg	2.0	60	30%
mushroom gravy & 6 charbroiled beef patties	⅙ pkg	12.0	180	60%
Homestyle Entrée				
macaroni & beef	1 meal	6.0	230	23%
macaroni & cheese	1 meal	11.0	350	28%
penne w/meat sauce	1 meal	6.0	250	22%
Salisbury steak & gravy w/whipped potatoes	1 meal	14.0	300	42%
sweet & sour chicken w/rice	1 meal	2.0	280	9%
turkey & gravy w/dressing & whipped potatoes	1 meal	5.0	210	21%
Other Meals				
char-broiled beef patty w/mashed potatoes, Peas, & carrots w/gravy	1 meal	11.0	230	43%
chicken fingers w/bbq sauce, mashed potatoes, & corn	1 meal	13.0	310	38%
chicken nuggets w/apple compote & potato puffs	1 meal	16.0	140	29%
chicken patty w/mashed potatoes & corn	1 meal	14.0	290	43%
fish sticks w/whipped potatoes & corn	1 meal	9.0	290	28%
gravy & sliced beef w/mashed potatoes & carrots	1 meal	2.0	140	13%
meatloaf w/tomato sauce & mashed potatoes	1 meal	15.0	310	44%
pot roast w/carrots and mashed potatoes	1 meal	2.5	140	16%
ravioli/cheese w/peas & carrots & brownie	1 meal	11.0	350	28%
Salisbury steak w/mashed potatoes, corn, & gravy	1 meal	14.0	260	48%
shells & cheese w/apple compote	1 meal	9.0	270	30%
turkey & gravy w/mashed potatoes	1 meal	4.5	220	18%

Food and Description	Amount	Fat Grams	Total Calories	% Fat Calories
veal parmigiana w/tomato sauce & peas	1 meal	9.0	320	25%
■ **(Golden) Blintzes**				
apple raisin	1 blintze	2.0	80	23%
blueberry	1 blintze	1.0	90	10%
cheese	1 blintze	2.0	80	23%
cherry	1 blintze	1.0	95	9%
potato	1 blintze	4.0	90	40%
■ **(Healthy Choice)**				
Bowls				
cheese & chicken tortellini	1 bowl	5.0	250	18%
chicken teriyaki w/rice	1 bowl	4.0	270	13%
chili & cornbread	1 bowl	8.0	350	21%
colonial chicken pie	1 bowl	7.0	310	20%
country chicken bake	1 bowl	8.0	230	31%
fiesta chicken	1 bowl	2.0	220	8%
garlic lemon chicken w/rice	1 bowl	4.0	300	12%
roasted potatoes w/ham	1 bowl	4.0	210	17%
southwestern chicken & pasta	1 bowl	4.0	320	11%
turkey divan	1 bowl	6.0	250	22%
Choice Meals To Go				
bread stuffs				
chicken & broccoli	1 meal	4.0	310	12%
ham & cheese w/broccoli	1 meal	5.0	320	14%
Italian style meatball	1 meal	5.0	330	14%
Philly beef steak	1 meal	5.0	310	15%
French bread pizza				
cheese	1 pizza	5.0	340	13%
pepperoni	1 pizza	5.0	340	13%
sausage	1 pizza	5.0	320	14%
supreme	1 pizza	5.0	330	14%
vegetable	1 pizza	4.0	280	14%
Dinner meals				
beef pot roast	1 meal	6.0	300	18%
beef stroganoff	1 meal	8.0	320	26%
beef tips portabella	1 meal	5.0	270	17%
charbroiled beef patty	1 meal	9.0	310	26%
chicken broccoli Alfredo	1 meal	7.0	300	21%
chicken Cantonese	1 meal	6.0	280	19%
chicken Dijon	1 meal	5.0	270	17%
chicken enchilada supreme	1 meal	7.0	300	21%
chicken Parmigiana	1 meal	8.0	330	22%
chicken teriyaki	1 meal	6.0	270	20%
country breaded chicken	1 meal	9.0	350	23%
country herb chicken	1 meal	8.0	320	23%
country inn roast turkey	1 meal	6.0	250	22%
herb baked fish	1 meal	7.0	340	19%
honey glazed chicken	1 meal	7.0	270	23%
lemon pepper fish	1 meal	7.0	320	20%
mesquite beef w/bbq sauce	1 meal	9.0	320	25%

Food and Description	Amount	Fat Grams	Total Calories	% Fat Calories
mesquite chicken BBQ	1 meal	5.0	310	15%
oriental style chicken & veg., stir fry	1 meal	6.0	360	15%
oven roasted beef	1 meal	8.0	280	26%
roasted chicken	1 meal	5.0	230	20%
sesame chicken	1 meal	7.0	360	18%
shrimp & vegetables	1 meal	6.0	270	20%
stuffed pasta shells	1 meal	6.0	370	15%
sweet & sour chicken	1 meal	7.0	360	18%
teriyaki chicken	1 meal	2.0	270	7%
traditional breast of turkey	1 meal	4.5	290	14%
traditional meat loaf	1 meal	7.0	330	19%
traditional Salisbury steak	1 meal	7.0	330	19%
Entrées & quick meals				
beef macaroni	1 meal	4.0	220	16%
beef pepper steak Oriental	1 meal	5.0	260	17%
beef tips Francais	1 meal	7.0	300	21%
breaded chicken breast strips w/ mac & cheeese	1 meal	5.0	270	17%
cheddar broccoli potatoes	1 meal	7.0	330	19%
cheese ravioli Parmigiana	1 meal	5.0	260	17%
chicken con queso burrito	1 meal	6.0	350	15%
chicken enchilada suiza	1 meal	6.0	280	19%
chicken fettuccini Alfredo	1 meal	7.0	280	23%
chicken & vegetables Marsala	1 meal	4.0	240	15%
country glazed chicken	1 meal	5.0	250	18%
country roast turkey w/mushrooms	1 meal	4.0	220	16%
fettuccini Alfredo	1 meal	5.0	240	19%
garlic chicken Sonoma	1 meal	4.0	230	16%
grilled chicken w/mashed potatoes	1 meal	4.0	180	20%
herb breaded pork patty	1 meal	6.0	280	19%
homestyle chicken & pasta	1 meal	6.0	270	20%
honey mustard chicken	1 meal	6.0	290	53%
lasagna Roma	1 meal	9.0	420	19%
macaroni & cheese	1 meal	5.0	240	19%
Mandarin chicken	1 meal	2.5	280	8%
manicotti w/3 cheeses	1 meal	9.0	300	27%
roast turkey breast	1 meal	5.0	220	20%
sesame chicken	1 meal	4.0	240	15%
spaghetti & sauce w/seasoned beef	1 meal	6.0	280	19%
tuna casserole	1 meal	5.0	240	23%
vegetable pasta Italiano	1 meal	1.0	220	4%
zucchini lasagna	1 meal	1.5	330	4%
■ **(Hormel)** (See also (Dinty Moore) in this section)				
Mrs. Patterson's Aussie Pie				
chicken				
5.57 oz	1 pie	25.0	460	49%
6.57 oz	1 pie	27.0	480	51%
potato top beef	1 pie	16.0	340	42%
potato top beef fajita	1 pie	17.0	350	44%
steak & mushroom	1 pie	24.0	420	51%

Food and Description	Amount	Fat Grams	Total Calories	% Fat Calories
turkey w/broccoli	1 pie	26.0	470	50%
quick meal				
BBQ beef sandwich	1 sandwich	16.0	360	40%
BBQ pork sandwich	1 sandwich	15.0	350	39%
cheesy Dog	1 "dog"	17.0	310	49%
chicken Sandwich	1 sandwich	12.0	340	32%
chili dog w/cheese	1 "dog"	20.0	350	51%
corn dog				
mini	5 "dogs"	15.0	250	54%
regular	1 "dog"	11.0	220	45%
fish fillet sandwich	1 sandwich	16.0	400	36%
grilled chicken sandwich	1 sandwich	9.0	300	27%
ham & Swiss	1 sandwich	8.0	330	22%
jumbo dog	1 "dog"	21.0	350	54%
pepperoni bagel	1 bagel	15.0	350	39%

■ **HOT POCKETS** (*See* (Chef America) in this section.)
■ **(Kid Cuisine)**

Food and Description	Amount	Fat Grams	Total Calories	% Fat Calories
Meals				
Big league hamburger pizza	1 meal	11.0	400	25%
Buckaroo beef patty sandwich w/cheese	1 meal	15.0	410	33%
Circus show corn dog	1 meal	20.0	490	37%
Cosmic chicken nuggets	1 meal	25.0	500	45%
Fantastic fish sticks	1 meal	16.0	410	35%
Game time taco roll up	1 meal	18.0	420	39%
High flying fried chicken	1 meal	20.0	440	41%
Magical macaroni & cheese	1 meal	13.0	440	26%
Parachuting pork ribettes	1 meal	19.0	390	44%
Pirate pizza w/cheese	1 meal	11.0	430	23%
Wave rider waffle sticks	1 meal	8.0	380	19%
Munchers				
Backpacking pizza snacks	6 pieces	11.0	230	43%
Mystical mini corn dogs	4 pieces	14.0	230	55%
Poolside pepperoni pizza	1 pizza	14.0	380	33%
Dino mite chicken nuggets	4 pieces	23.0	300	69%
Fire chief cheese pizza	1 pizza	10.0	340	26%

■ **(Lean Cuisine)**

Food and Description	Amount	Fat Grams	Total Calories	% Fat Calories
Cafe Classics baked chicken	1 meal	4.5	240	17%
baked fish	1 meal	6.0	290	19%
beef peppercorn	1 meal	7.0	260	24%
beef portabella	1 meal	7.0	220	29%
bow tie pasta & chicken	1 meal	4.0	220	16%
chicken				
a l'orange	1 meal	1.5	230	6%
& vegetables	1 meal	4.5	240	17%
carbonara	1 meal	7.0	280	23%
fiesta chicken	1 meal	5.0	270	17%
glazed	1 meal	6.0	240	23%
grilled	1 meal	5.0	250	18%
herb roasted	1 meal	3.5	190	17%

Food and Description	Amount	Fat Grams	Total Calories	% Fat Calories
honey mustard	1 meal	3.5	270	12%
honey roasted	1 meal	6.0	270	20%
in peanut sauce	1 meal	6.0	260	21%
in wine sauce	1 meal	5.0	220	20%
medallions w/creamy cheese sauce	1 meal	7.0	300	21%
Mediterranean	1 meal	4.0	260	14%
Parmesan	1 meal	6.0	300	18%
piccata	1 meal	9.0	300	27%
w/basil cream sauce	1 meal	7.0	260	24%
country vegetables & beef	1 meal	4.0	210	17%
glazed turkey tenderloins	1 meal	4.5	260	16%
honey roasted pork	1 meal	6.0	250	22%
meatloaf w/whipped potatoes	1 meal	7.0	260	24%
oriental beef	1 meal	3.5	210	15%
oven roasted beef	1 meal	8.0	260	28%
roasted turkey breast	1 meal	2.0	270	7%
Salisbury steak	1 meal	8.0	280	26%
shrimp & angel hair pasta	1 meal	4.5	240	17%
southern beef tips	1 meal	6.0	270	20%
Everyday Favorites				
Alfredo pasta primavera	1 meal	7.0	290	22%
angel hair pasta	1 meal	4.0	240	15%
cheddar potato, deluxe	1 meal	6.0	250	22%
cheese				
cannelloni	1 meal	4.0	230	16%
classic lasagna	1 meal	6.0	290	19%
five cheese lasagna/96 oz	1 serving	5.0	210	21%
lasagna casserole	1 meal	6.0	270	20%
ravioli	1 meal	7.0	260	24%
chicken				
chow mein	1 meal	3.5	240	13%
enchilada suiza	1 meal	5.0	280	16%
fettucini	1 meal	6.0	270	20%
florentine	1 meal	4.5	220	18%
lasagna				
10 oz	1 meal	7.0	280	23%
9.6 oz	1 serving	4.5	200	20%
Mandarin	1 meal	5.0	260	17%
pie	1 pie	8.0	300	24%
roasted	1 meal	7.0	260	24%
fettucini				
alfredo	1 meal	7.0	280	23%
primavera	1 meal	7.0	270	23%
homestyle turkey	1 meal	5.0	240	19%
hunan beef & broccoli	1 meal	3.5	240	13%
lasagna w/meat sauce	1 meal	8.0	300	24%
macaroni & beef	1 meal	4.0	270	13%
macaroni & cheese	1 meal	7.0	290	22%
oriental style dumplings	1 meal	6.0	300	18%
penne pasta	1 meal	3.5	260	12%

Food and Description	Amount	Fat Grams	Total Calories	% Fat Calories
roasted potatoes w/broccoli	1 meal	6.0	260	21%
Santa Fe rice & beans	1 meal	5.0	300	28%
Spaghetti				
w/meatballs	1 meal	7.0	290	22%
w/meat sauce	1 meal	5.0	290	16%
Swedish meatballs	1 meal	7.0	290	22%
teriyaki stir fry	1 meal	4.0	290	12%
three bean chili w/rice	1 meal	6.0	250	22%
vegetable eggroll	1 meal	5.0	300	15%
vegetable lasagna	1 meal	7.0	260	24%
French Bread Pizza				
cheese	1 pizza	7.0	320	20%
deluxe	1 pizza	6.0	290	19%
pepperoni	1 pizza	8.0	300	24%
sun dried tomatoes	1 pizza	8.0	3340	21%
Hearty Portions				
cheese & spinach manicotti	1 meal	8.0	370	19%
chicken				
& bbq sauce	1 meal	6.0	370	15%
fettucini w/broccoli	1 meal	9.0	390	21%
florentine	1 meal	7.0	380	17%
glazed	1 meal	8.0	330	22%
grilled w/penne pasta	1 meal	7.0	360	18%
oriental glazed	1 meal	2.0	370	5%
homestyle beef stroganoff	1 meal	9.0	350	21%
jumbo rigatoni w/meatballs	1 meal	9.0	440	18%
roasted chicken w/mushrooms	1 meal	5.0	330	14%
Salisbury steak	1 meal	6.0	300	18%
Skillet Sensations				
beef teriyaki & rice	½ pkg	3.0	280	10%
chicken				
Alfredo	½ pkg	6.0	280	19%
garlic	½ pkg	4.5	340	12%
herb w/roasted potatoes	½ pkg	5.0	270	17%
oriental	¼ pkg	3.0	280	10%
primavera	½ pkg	4.5	320	13%
three-cheese	½ pkg	10.0	370	24%
fiesta beef & rice	½ pkg	3.5	300	11%
roasted turkey	½ pkg	2.0	220	8%
savory beef & vegetables	½ pkg	7.0	290	22%
■ LEAN POCKETS (*See* (Chef America) in this section)				
■ LUIGINO'S (*See* (Michelina's) in this section)				
■ (Marie Callender's)				
Family Serve Entrées				
Chicken fried beef steak & gravy				
w/mashed potatoes	1 serving	42.0	650	58%
country fried chicken & gravy				
w/mashed potatoes	1 serving	30.0	550	49%
escalloped noodles & chicken	1 cup	17.0	280	55%
lasagna w/meat sauce	1 cup	17.0	350	44%

Food and Description	Amount	Fat Grams	Total Calories	% Fat Calories
macaroni & cheese	1 cup	9.0	300	27%
meatloaf & gravy w/mashed potatoes	1 serving	16.0	300	48%
turkey & gravy w/mashed potatoes	1 serving	16.0	310	46%
French Bread Pizza				
cheese	1 pizza	24.0	530	41%
pepperoni	1 pizza	28.0	570	44%
supreme	1 pizza	23.0	510	41%
Meals				
beef stroganoff w/noodles	1 meal	27.0	600	41%
beef tips in mushroom sauce	1 meal	19.0	430	40%
breaded chicken parmigiana	1 meal	32.0	660	44%
breaded fish w/mac & cheese	1 meal	28.0	550	46%
cheesy rice w/chicken & broccoli	1 meal	13.0	390	30%
cheese ravioli in marinara sacue	1 meal	29.0	750	35%
chicken & dumplings	1 meal	20.0	390	46%
chicken & noodles	1 meal	30.0	520	52%
chicken cordon bleu	1 meal	28.0	610	41%
chicken fried beef steak & gravy	1 meal	37.0	630	53%
chilli & cornbread	1 meal	21.0	560	34%
country fried chicken & gravy	1 meal	30.0	620	44%
country fried pork chop	1 meal	28.0	540	47%
escalloped noodles & chicken	1 meal	46.0	740	56%
extra cheese lasagna	1 mea.	27.0	590	41%
fettuccini Alfredo				
supreme	1 meal	27.0	450	54%
w/garlic bread	1 meal	55.0	920	54%
fettuccini primavera tortellini	1 meal	49.0	750	59%
fettuccini w/broccoli & chicken	1 meal	43.0	710	55%
glazed chicken	1 meal	25.0	490	46%
grilled chicken & mashed potatoes	1 meal	18.0	340	48%
grilled chicken & mushroom sauce	1 meal	15.0	480	28%
grilled chicken breast & rice pilaf	1 meal	14.0	360	35%
grilled turkey breast & rice pilaf	1 meal	10.0	310	29%
herb roasted chicken & mashed potatoes	1 meal	34.0	580	53%
homestyle tuna & noodles	1 meal	35.0	600	53%
honey roasted chicken	1 meal	17.0	440	35%
honey smoked ham steak w/mac & cheese	1 meal	13.0	490	24%
lasagna w/meat sauce	1 meal	31.0	630	44%
macaroni & cheese	1 meal	24.0	540	40%
meatloaf & gravy w/mashed potatoes	1 meal	30.0	540	50%
old-fashioned pot roast	1 meal	17.0	500	31%
roast beef	1 meal	19.0	390	44%
sirloin Salisbury steak & gravy	1 meal	25.0	550	41%
southwestern style chicken/grilled	1 meal	11.0	410	24%
spaghetti & meat sauce w/garlic bread	1 meal	25.0	670	34%
stuffed pasta trio	1 meal	18.0	380	43%
Swedish meatballs	1 meal	26.0	520	45%
sweet & sour chicken	1 meal	15.0	570	24%

Food and Description	Amount	Fat Grams	Total Calories	% Fat Calories
teriyaki chicken	1 meal	13.0	510	23%
turkey w/gravy & dressing	1 meal	19.0	500	34%
pot pies				
beef				
16.5 oz	1 cup	32.0	550	52%
9.5 oz	1 pie	42.0	660	57%
chicken				
16.5 oz	1 cup	40.0	590	61%
9.5 oz	1 pie	46.0	680	61%
chicken & broccoli				
16.5 oz	1 cup	45.0	620	65%
9.5 oz	1 pie	43.0	670	58%
chicken au gratin				
16.5 oz	1 cup	37.0	580	57%
9.5 oz	1 pie	46.0	690	60%
turkey				
16.5 oz	1 cup	40.0	590	61%
9.5 oz	1 pie	46.0	690	60%
Skillet Meals				
au gratin potatoes	⅔ cup	10.0	190	47%
beef stroganoff				
22 oz	½ pkg	11.0	310	32%
35 oz	¼ pkg	9.0	250	32%
beef pot roast	½ pkg	9.0	290	28%
chicken Alfredo				
23 oz	½ pkg	29.0	490	53%
37 oz	¼ pkg	24.0	400	54%
chicken & rice w/broccoli & cheese	½ pkg	14.0	440	29%
chicken teriyaki	½ pkg	6.0	260	21%
herb chicken	½ pkg	4.0	290	12%
penne pasta & meatballs	½ pkg	31.0	600	47%
rigatoni w/vegetables in cheese sauce	1 cup	12.0	290	37%
roast chicken & vegetables				
25 oz	½ pkg	6.0	260	21%
40 oz	¼ pkg	5.0	210	21%
white & wild rice w/broccoli in cheese sauce	1 cup	13.0	300	39%
■ (Michelina's)				
Low-fat				
black bean chili w/rice	1 pkg	5.0	400	11%
chicken				
& rice w/spicy sauce	1 pkg	2.5	240	9%
& vegetable stir fry	1 pkg	4.0	200	18%
glazed w/rice	1 pkg	4.0	250	14%
honey BBQ w/rice	1 pkg	3.0	290	9%
pesto w/penne	1 pkg	6.0	250	22%
primavera w/spirals	1 pkg	6.0	250	22%
fettuccini w/creamy pesto & vegetables	1 pkg	6.0	250	22%
lasagna				
layered	1 pkg	4.5	210	19%

Food and Description	Amount	Fat Grams	Total Calories	% Fat Calories
layered w/meat sauce	1 pkg	7.0	240	26%
macaroni				
& beef	1 pkg	5.0	250	18%
& cheese	1 pkg	6.0	270	20%
noodles Romanoff w/meatballs	1 pkg	6.0	300	18%
penne pasta w/mushrooms	1 pkg	6.0	250	22%
pepper steak w/rice	1 pkg	5.0	280	16%
rigatoni Pomodoro w/broccoli & olives	1 pkg	2.5	240	9%
spaghetti w/onions	1 pkg	5.0	270	17%
teriyaki chicken w/rice	1 pkg	2.5	290	8%
Regular				
beef burgundy w/garlic mashed potatoes	1 pkg	15.0	300	45%
beef pot roast	1 pkg	6.0	280	19%
black bean chili w/green tomatoes	1 pkg	4.0	310	12%
cheddar broccoli potatoes	1 pkg	19.0	380	45%
cheese ravioli				
jumbo	1 pkg	13.0	400	29%
w/Alfredo & broccoli	1 pkg	17.0	360	43%
chicken				
a la king	1 pkg	8.0	280	26%
breaded parmigiana	1 pkg	14.0	410	31%
cacciatore	1 pkg	7.0	270	23%
glazed w/rice	1 pkg	5.0	300	15%
grilled Alfredo w/broccoli	1 pkg	18.0	400	41%
herb roasted	1 pkg	5.0	260	17%
marsala w/garlic mashed potatoes	1 pkg	14.0	280	45%
piccata w/rice	1 pkg	12.0	330	33%
sorrentino w/linguini	1 pkg	9.0	310	26%
tetrazzini	1 pkg	12.0	320	34%
Italiano	1 pkg	7.0	240	26%
Chili-mac	1 pkg	9.0	290	28%
Cream sauce w/shaved cured beef	1 pkg	20.0	420	43%
egg noodles Alfredo	1 pkg	14.0	330	38%
eggplant parmigiano w/linguini	1 pkg	7.0	270	23%
fettuccine				
Alfredo	1 pkg	15.0	380	36%
Alfredo w/broccoli & chicken	1 pkg	10.0	310	29%
Carbonara	1 pkg	13.0	330	35%
primavera	1 pkg	9.0	270	30%
primavera w/chicken	1 pkg	9.0	280	29%
gravy w/turkey & dressing	1 pkg	14.0	260	48%
Italian meatballs in wine sauce	1 pkg	5.0	210	21%
lasagna				
Alfredo	1 pkg	16.0	360	40%
four cheese	1 pkg	7.0	290	22%
layered Pomodoro	1 pkg	10.0	260	35%
layered w/meat sauce	1 pkg	12.0	400	27%
layered w/white sauce	1 pkg	26.0	540	43%
pollo	1 pkg	9.0	280	29%

Food and Description	Amount	Fat Grams	Total Calories	% Fat Calories
primavera	1 pkg	10.0	270	33%
w/meat sauce	1 pkg	7.0	290	22%
w/vegetables	1 pkg	5.0	240	19%
linguini w/clams & sauce	1 pkg	3.0	290	9%
macaroni & beef	1 pkg	7.0	260	24%
macaroni & cheese				
regular	1 pkg	13.0	340	34%
w/ham	1 pkg	14.0	340	37%
macaroni & sharp cheddar	1 pkg	17.0	430	36%
mashed potatoes & meatballs	1 pkg	14.0	270	47%
meat ravioli w/Pomodoro sauce	1 pkg	10.0	290	31%
meatloaf & gravy				
w/mashed potatoes	1 pkg	23.0	340	61%
w/sour cream mashed potatoes	1 pkg	24.0	390	55%
noodles & Swedish meatballs	1 pkg	13.0	360	33%
noodles w/chicken	1 pkg	11.0	300	33%
noodles'n				
Alfredo	1 pkg	14.0	330	38%
Alfredo w/pepperoni	1 pkg	17.0	370	41%
cheese w/pepperoni	1 pkg	9.0	280	29%
chicken	1 pkg	9.0	290	28%
marinara	1 pkg	3.5	230	14%
red & green tomatoes	1 pkg	5.0	240	19%
vegetable Alfredo	1 pkg	12.0	320	34%
vegetables w/beef	1 pkg	3.0	220	12%
noodles stroganoff	1 pkg	15.0	350	39%
pasta w/tomato parmesan	1 pkg	4.5	250	16%
penne				
marinara w/Italian sausage	1 pkg	6.0	250	22%
pollo	1 pkg	8.0	290	25%
primavera	1 pkg	9.0	280	29%
w/mushroom sauce	1 pkg	8.0	280	26%
pepper steak w/rice	1 pkg	5.0	270	17%
rigatoni				
Pomodoro	1 pkg	2.5	220	10%
stuffed cheese	1 pkg	8.0	300	24%
risotto parmigiana	1 pkg	21.0	450	42%
roasted sirloin surpreme				
8.10 oz	1 pkg	6.0	240	23%
8.60 oz	1 pkg	9.0	270	30%
Salisbury steak & gravy w/mashed potatoes	1 pkg	21.0	330	57%
Salisbury w/shells & cheese	1 pkg	24.0	440	49%
shells & cheese w/jalapeños	1 pkg	12.0	360	30%
shrimp Alfredo w/fettuccine	1 pkg	12.0	310	35%
sirloin beef peppercorn	1 pkg	13.0	290	40%
spaghetti				
& meat balls	1 pkg	8.0	300	24%
bolognese	1 pkg	4.0	280	13%
marinara	1 pkg	2.5	240	9%

Food and Description	Amount	Fat Grams	Total Calories	% Fat Calories
w/tomato & basil sauce	1 pkg	3.0	250	11%
spicy tomato sauce w/spirals	1 pkg	1.5	210	6%
vegetable stir fry w/rice	1 pkg	4.0	240	15%
wheels & cheese	1 pkg	8.0	300	24%
■ **(Morton)**				
dinners				
breaded chicken patty	1 meal	17.0	290	53%
charbroiled beef patty w/gravy	1 meal	18.0	310	52%
chicken nuggets	1 meal	19.0	340	50%
chili gravy w/beef enchilada & tamale	1 meal	9.0	270	30%
fried chicken	1 meal	30.0	470	57%
macaroni & cheese	1 cup	8.0	240	30%
meat loaf w/tomato sauce	1 meal	13.0	250	47%
spaghetti w/meat sauce	1 meal	6.0	200	27%
turkey w/gravy & dressing	1 meal	10.0	240	38%
veal parmigiana w/tomato sauce	1 meal	15.0	290	47%
pot pies				
macaroni & cheese	1 container	5.0	210	21%
vegetable pie				
w/beef	1 pie	21.0	340	56%
w/chicken	1 pie	18.0	320	51%
w/turkey	1 pie	18.0	310	52%
■ **MRS. PATTERSON'S AUSSIE PIE** (*See* (Hormel) in this section)				
■ **(On-Cor)**				
BBQ rib patties	⅙ pkg	14.0	260	48%
beef patties	¼ pkg	18.0	270	60%
chicken parmigiana	⅙ pkg	11.0	260	38%
gravy & sliced turkey	⅙ pkg	4.0	70	51%
lasagna w/meat sauce	⅕ pkg	8.0	200	36%
macaroni & cheese	⅙ pkg	4.0	140	26%
mostaccioli pasta & meatballs	⅕ pkg	8.0	200	36%
Salisbury steaks w/gravy	⅙ pkg	13.0	200	59%
stuffed green peppers	¼ pkg	10.0	220	41%
Swedish meatballs & pasta	⅕ pkg	10.0	220	41%
veal parmigiana w/cheese & tomato sauce	⅙ pkg	8.0	210	34%
■ **(Patio)**				
Burritos				
bean & cheese burrito	1 burrito	9.0	300	27%
beef & bean				
hot	1 burrito	12.0	320	34%
medium	1 burrito	10.0	310	29%
mild	1 burrito	12.0	330	33%
red hot	1 burrito	12.0	320	34%
chicken	1 burrito	8.0	290	25%
Dinners				
beef enchilada	1 meal	12.0	370	29%
cheese enchilada	1 meal	12.0	370	29%
chicken enchilada	1 meal	12.0	400	27%
Fiesta	1 meal	11.0	350	28%

Food and Description	Amount	Fat Grams	Total Calories	% Fat Calories
Mexican	1 meal	19.0	470	36%
Ranchera	1 meal	22.0	470	42%
Extra large dinners				
beef enchiladas chili'n beans	1 meal	22.0	540	37%
beef & 2 cheese enchiladas chili'n beans	1 meal	30.0	670	40%
Family Entrées				
beef enchilada w/sauce	2 pieces	8.0	210	34%
cheese enchilada	2 pieces	7.0	210	30%
■ (Pepperidge Farm) Pot Pie				
chicken white meat	½ pkg	26.0	450	52%
turkey	½ pkg	26.0	420	56%
■ (Schwan's)				
Ethnic Foods				
apple flautas	1 flauta	4.5	150	27%
Barquito				
beef taco	1 taco	17.0	350	44%
meat-trio	1	21.0	380	50%
beef taquito	5 taquitos	12.0	340	32%
beef & bean burrito	1	12.0	290	37%
beef stuffed nachos	8 nachos	20.0	370	49%
chicken quesadilla	1 whole	9.0	220	37%
crab Rangoon	7 pieces	22.0	430	46%
egg rolls				
chicken	2 pieces	7.0	220	29%
pork	2 pieces	11.0	240	41%
vegetable	2 pieces	4.5	170	24%
5-cheese garlic French bread	1 piece	20.0	330	55%
tamales	1 tamale	10.0	210	43%
wonton rolls/pizza flavor	5 pieces	18.0	410	40%
Entrées				
beef casserole	1 cup	17.0	340	45%
beef pot roast/sliced				
w/noodles	1 cup	6.0	230	23%
beef shepherd's pie	1 cup	12.0	250	43%
beef & broccoli w/rice	1 cup	4.0	210	17%
Cheese				
ravioli	5 ravioli	12.0	370	29%
w/red sauce	1 serving	15.0	350	39%
tortellini	1 cup	6.0	240	23%
chicken				
Alfredo lasagna	1 cup	12.0	280	39%
Boston clam chowder	1 cup	8.0	190	38%
breaded cutlet	1 piece	15.0	260	52%
breast				
stirfry w/rice	1½ cup frozen	2.0	210	9%
tenderloin fajita	1 fajita	2.0	140	13%
casserole	1 cup	16.0	360	40%
cordon bleu	1 serving	12.0	270	40%

Food and Description	Amount	Fat Grams	Total Calories	% Fat Calories
fried rice stirfry	1½ cup frozen	3.0	240	11%
herb roasted breast dinner	1 meal	6.0	300	18%
Kiev	1 serving	24.0	370	58%
Marco Polo	1 serving	13.0	280	42%
ravioli	5 ravioli	11.0	310	32%
sweet & sour w/rice	1 cup	1.5	260	5%
tortellini	1 cup	4.0	230	16%
English style fish & chips	1 serving	27.0	480	51%
Express/chicken				
& broccoli	1 bowl	18.0	500	32%
teriyaki	1 bowl	3.5	360	9%
homestyle				
beef goulash	1 cup	13.0	280	42%
pot roast dinner	1 meal	8.0	320	23%
lasagna				
single serve				
traditional	1 tray	19.0	500	34%
vegetable	1 tray	18.0	420	39%
zesty	1 tray	28.0	580	60%
vegetable	1 cup	8.0	280	26%
w/beef sauce	1 cup	13.0	350	33%
lemon pepper fish dinner	1 meal	7.0	340	19%
macaroni & cheese	1 cup	20.0	340	53%
mostaccioli	1 cup	18.0	350	46%
stuffed pasta shells	3 shells	14.0	320	39%
w/red sauce	1 serving	20.0	440	41%
Personal Pouches				
chicken, broccoli & cheddar	1 piece	13.0	300	39%
ham & cheese	1 piece	12.0	300	36%
pepperoni	1 piece	14.0	320	39%
Philly steak & cheese	1 piece	11.0	290	34%
Sandwiches				
Bagel Dogs w/cheese	1 sandwich	18.0	360	45%
cheeseburger	1 sandwich	6.0	230	23%
corn dog	1 sandwich	11.0	180	55%
grilled chicken	1 sandwich	3.5	180	18%
Quick Graps reuben	1 sandwich	6.0	220	25%
Mini Pups	4 pieces	17.0	280	55%
roast beef	1 sandwich	6.0	220	25%
rotisserie chicken breast	1 sandwich	6.0	230	67%
Southwestern wrapped	1 wrap	10.0	400	23%
■ (Stouffer's)				
Entrées				
beef pie	1 pie	25.0	440	51%
broccoli au gratin	1 serving	5.0	100	45%
cheddar cheese and chicken bake	1 meal	21.0	450	42%
cheddar pasta	1 meal	24.0	500	54%
cheese manicotti	1 meal	16.0	360	40%
cheese ravioli	1 meal	15.0	450	30%

Food and Description	Amount	Fat Grams	Total Calories	% Fat Calories
cheesy spaghetti bake				
11.5 oz	1 meal	21.0	460	41%
40 oz	1 serving	17.0	370	41%
chicken à la king w/rice,	1 meal	11.0	370	27%
chicken				
broccoli pasta bake	1 serving	17.0	340	45%
enchilada & Mexican rice	1 serving	11.0	220	45%
lasagna	1 serving	15.0	310	44%
pie				
16-oz pkg	½ pkg	30.0	500	54%
10-oz pkg	1 pie	29.0	490	53%
chili w/beans	1 meal	11.0	290	34%
creamed chicken	1 meal	15.0	250	54%
creamed chipped beef	½ cup	10.0	160	56%
escalloped chicken & noodles	⅕ pkg	23.0	370	56%
fettucini Alfredo	1 meal	23.0	540	38%
fettucini primavera	1 meal	15.0	370	36%
five cheese lasagna	1 meal	13.0	360	33%
grandma's chicken & vegetable rice bake	¼ pkg	15.0	360	38%
green bean mushroom casserole	⅑ pkg	8.0	130	55%
green pepper steak w/rice	10.5 oz	9.0	330	25%
lasagna				
bake	1 meal	16.0	450	32%
lasagna w/meat sauce				
10-oz pkg	1 meal	14.0	370	34%
21 oz pkg	⅓ pkg	8.0	250	29%
40 oz pkg	⅕ pkg	10.0	270	33%
96 oz pkg	1/12 pkg	11.0	300	33%
w/tomato sauce & Italian sausage	1 meal	19.0	420	41%
macaroni & beef w/tomatoes	1 meal	15.0	380	36%
macaroni & cheese				
12-oz pkg	½ pkg	16.0	320	45%
20-oz pkg	⅛ pkg	18.0	340	48%
40 oz pkg	⅕ pkg	17.0	380	40%
76-oz pkg	⅑ pkg	17.0	360	43%
meatloaf in gravy	⅙ pkg	13.0	220	53%
noodles romanoff	1 meal	23.0	490	42%
pasta shells & American cheese	1 meal	9.0	280	29%
penne pasta & chicken bake	1 meal	14.0	340	37%
scalloped potatoes	⅛ pkg	5.0	140	32%
spaghetti				
w/meat sauce	1 meal	15.0	440	31%
w/meatballs in sauce	1 meal	13.0	390	30%
stuffed green peppers				
15.5 oz	½ pkg	7.0	180	35%
32 oz	¼ pkg	9.0	200	41%
single	1 meal	8.0	210	34%
Swedish meatballs	1 meal	25.0	520	43%

Food and Description	Amount	Fat Grams	Total Calories	% Fat Calories
Entrées & Side Dishes				
corn souffle	1 serving	7.0	170	37%
creamed spinach	½ pkg	11.0	160	62%
escalloped apples	½ pkg	3.0	180	15%
potatoes au gratin	1 serving	6.0	130	42%
scalloped potatoes	1 serving	9.0	170	48%
spinach soufflé	⅓ pkg	9.0	140	58%
tuna noodle casserole	1 meal	18.0	380	43%
turkey pie	1 pie	30.0	520	52%
turkey tetrazzini	1 meal	19.0	400	43%
vegetable & chicken pasta bake	1 meal	11.0	380	26%
vegetable lasagna				
96-oz pkg	1 cup	15.0	330	41%
10.5 pkg	1 meal	21.0	400	47%
French Bread Pizza				
cheese	½ pkg	16.0	370	39%
deluxe	½ pkg	19.0	420	41%
extra cheese	½ pkg	16.0	400	36%
five cheese	½ pkg	18.0	420	38%
grilled vegetable	½ pkg	12.0	350	31%
pepperoni	½ pkg	16.0	390	37%
pepperoni & mushroom	½ pkg	20.0	440	41%
sausage	½ pkg	18.0	420	39%
sausage & pepperoni	½ pkg	23.0	470	44%
three meat	½ pkg	22.0	460	43%
white	½ pkg	23.0	460	45%
Hearty Portions				
beef pot roast	1 meal	10.0	360	25%
chicken fettucini	1 meal	24.0	640	34%
chicken pot pie	½ pkg	37.0	590	56%
country fried beef steak	1 meal	25.0	560	40%
fried chicken breast	1 meal	17.0	500	31%
meatloaf w/mashed potatoes	1 meal	26.0	590	40%
pork & roasted potatoes	1 meal	13.0	510	23%
roast turkey breast	1 meal	16.0	460	31%
Salisbury steak w/pasta shells	1 meal	27.0	570	43%
veal parmigiana	1 meal	17.0	530	29%
Homestyle Dinners				
baked chicken breast	1 meal	11.0	260	38%
beef pot roast & browned potatoes	1 meal	8.0	250	29%
beef stroganoff	1 meal	15.0	350	39%
breaded pork cutlet	1 meal	19.0	370	46%
chicken & dumplings	1 meal	8.0	280	26%
chicken breast in BBQ sauce	1 meal	24.0	510	42%
chicken breast w/mushroom gray	1 meal	15.0	360	39%
chicken fettucini	1 meal	14.0	350	36%
chicken parmigiana	1 meal	16.0	460	31%
chunky beef & tomatoes	1 meal	9.0	290	28%
fish fillet w/mac & cheese	1 meal	21.0	430	44%
fried chicken breast	1 meal	16.0	360	40%

Food and Description	Amount	Fat Grams	Total Calories	% Fat Calories
green pepper steak	1 meal	6.0	270	20%
meatloaf	1 meal	21.0	390	48%
roast turkey	1 meal	13.0	310	38%
Salisbury steak	1 meal	17.0	360	43%
sliced beef briskit	1 meal	18.0	370	44%
veal parmigiana	1 meal	16.0	410	35%
Lean Cuisine (See (LEAN CUISINE) in this section)				
Skillet Sensations				
beef stroganoff	¼ pkg	12.0	340	32%
broccoli & beef	½ pkg	5.0	320	14%
cheddar beef	½ pkg	29.0	600	44%
chicken alfredo	½ pkg	16.0	450	32%
grilled chicken and vegetables	½ pkg	9.0	440	18%
homestyle beef	½ pkg	10.0	320	28%
savory chicken and rice	¼ pkg	4.0	300	12%
teriyaki chicken	½ pkg	3.0	340	8%
■ (Swanson)				
Homestyle				
chicken				
cacciatore	1 pkg	8.0	260	28%
fried	1 pkg	21.0	390	48%
nibbles	1 pkg	20.0	340	53%
fish & fries	1 pkg	16.0	340	42%
Salisbury steak	1 pkg	16.0	320	45%
scalloped potatoes & ham	1 pkg	13.0	300	39%
seafood creole w/rice	1 pkg	6.0	240	23%
sirloin tips in burgundy sauce	1 pkg	5.0	160	28%
turkey w/dressing & potatoes	1 pkg	11.0	290	34%
veal parmigiana	1 pkg	13.0	330	35%
Hungry Man				
boneless chicken	1 pkg	28.0	700	36%
chopped beef steak	1 pkg	37.0	640	52%
fried chicken				
dark	1 pkg	45.0	860	47%
white	1 pkg	46.0	870	48%
Salisbury steak	1 pkg	41.0	680	54%
sliced beef	1 pkg	12.0	450	24%
turkey	1 pkg	18.0	550	29%
veal parmigiana	1 pkg	26.0	590	40%
Regular				
beans & franks	1 pkg	19.0	440	39%
beef	1 pkg	6.0	310	17%
beef in BBQ sauce	1 pkg	17.0	460	33%
chopped sirloin beef	1 pkg	16.0	340	42%
fish'n'chips	1 pkg	21.0	500	38%
fried chicken				
dark meat	1 pkg	28.0	560	45%
white meat	1 pkg	25.0	550	41%
loin of pork	1 pkg	12.0	280	39%
macaroni & beef	1 pkg	15.0	370	36%

Food and Description	Amount	Fat Grams	Total Calories	% Fat Calories
meatloaf	1 pkg	15.0	360	38%
noodles & chicken	1 pkg	8.0	280	26%
Salisbury steak	1 pkg	17.0	400	38%
Swedish meatballs	1 pkg	20.0	360	50%
Swiss steak	1 pkg	11.0	350	28%
turkey	1 pkg	11.0	350	28%
veal parmigiana	1 pkg	20.0	430	42%
western style	1 pkg	19.0	430	40%
■ (Tyson)				
Chicken Pieces				
BBQ style				
drumsticks	2 pieces	7.0	160	39%
wings	3 pieces	13.0	200	59%
cordon bleu	1 breast	17.0	350	44%
hot'n spicy wings	4 pieces	15.0	220	61%
Tabasco flavored wings	3 pieces	10.0	170	53%
teriyaki style wings	4 pieces	12.0	190	57%
Dinners/Entrées				
Beef				
fajitas	1 meal	13.0	480	24%
stir fry	1 meal	5.0	430	10%
Chicken				
& BBQ sauce	1 meal	5.0	270	17%
blackened	1 meal	5.0	260	17%
divan w/candied carrots	1 meal	15.0	370	36%
fajitas	1 meal	11.0	460	22%
Francais w/sliced red potatoes	1 meal	10.0	260	35%
fried w/gravy	1 meal	15.0	360	38%
fried rice	1 meal	10.0	480	19%
garlic	1 meal	7.0	210	30%
grilled				
Italian style w/pasta	1 meal	3.5	190	17%
w/corn O'Brien and ranch beans	1 meal	4.0	230	16%
honey dijon	1 meal	6.0	350	15%
Kiev	1 meal	25.0	440	51%
Marsala	1 meal	5.0	180	25%
Mesquite w/au gratin potatoes	1 meal	7.0	310	20%
piccata	1 meal	5.0	180	25%
roasted w/garlic sauce & pasta	1 meal	7.0	210	30%
stir fry	1 meal	4.5	430	9%
w/BBQ sauce & potato, vegetable medley	1 meal	21.0	560	34%
w/broccoli & cheese sauce	1 meal	11.0	260	38%
w/mushroom sauce	1 meal	5.0	220	20%
w/Tabasco & BBQ sauce	1 meal	5.0	270	17%
■ (Ultra Slim-Fast)				
Beef pepper steak	1 meal	4.0	270	13%
Chicken				
& vegetables	1 meal	3.0	290	9%
fettuccini	1 meal	12.0	380	28%

Food and Description	Amount	Fat Grams	Total Calories	% Fat Calories
roasted in mushroom sauce	1 meal	6.0	280	13%
sweet & sour	1 meal	2.0	330	5%
Country style vegetables & beef tips	1 meal	5.0	230	20%
Shrimp				
creole	1 meal	4.0	240	15%
marinara	1 meal	3.0	290	9%
Turkey medallions in herb sauce	1 meal	6.0	280	19%
■ (Weight Watchers)				
Main Street Bistro				
fire-grilled chicken & vegetables	1 meal	5.0	280	52%
oven-roasted vegetable primavera	1 meal	8.0	300	24%
Smart Ones				
angel hair pasta	1 meal	2.0	180	10%
baked potato, broccoli & cheese	1 meal	6.0	250	22%
bowtie pasta	1 meal	7.0	200	32%
chicken				
chow mein	1 meal	2.0	200	9%
fiesta chicken	1 meal	2.0	220	8%
honey mustard chicken	1 meal	2.0	200	9%
Marsala	1 meal	2.0	150	12%
Mirabella	1 meal	2.0	170	11%
penne pollo	1 meal	6.0	290	19%
piccata/lemon herb	1 meal	2.0	210	9%
lasagna curls w/Italian vegetables	1 meal	2.0	170	11%
lasagna Florentine	1 meal	2.0	210	9%
ravioli Florentine	1 meal	2.0	200	9%
roast turkey medallions	1 meal	2.0	190	9%
Santa Fe rice & beans	1 meal	8.0	300	24%
shrimp marinara	1 meal	2.0	190	9%
■ (WolfGang Puck)				
Cannelloni				
chicken & spinach in marinara	1 meal	19.0	480	36%
ricotta	1 meal	21.0	420	45%
Lasagna				
four cheese w/sundried tomatoes	1 meal	22.0	480	41%
Italian vegetable	1 meal	16.0	410	35%
mushroom	1 meal	16.0	440	33%
spicy chicken	1 meal	21.0	470	40%
Other Meals/Entrées				
breaded chicken parmigiana	1 meal	21.0	540	35%
cheese & mushroom risotto	1 meal	18.0	520	31%
chicken bolognese & spaghetti	1 meal	22.0	480	41%
chicken pappardelle	1 meal	18.0	460	35%
eggplant parmesan	1 meal	28.0	370	68%
four cheese macaroni	1 meal	33.0	610	49%
meatloaf in port wine sauce	1 meal	32.0	560	51%
penne pasta w/beef ragout	1 meal	18.0	410	40%
radiatore pasta primavera	1 meal	10.0	310	29%
Pasta Wrap				
beef bolognese	1 meal	17.0	530	29%

Food and Description	Amount	Fat Grams	Total Calories	% Fat Calories
chicken & spinach	1 meal	11.0	460	22%
Italian sausage	1 meal	29.0	700	37%
vegetarian	1 meal	3.0	340	8%
Ravioli				
four cheese	1 meal	20.0	330	54%
mushroom & spinach w/wild mushroom sauce	1 meal	18.0	260	62%
sweet potato	1 meal	21.0	360	53%
Tortellini				
cheese w/red bell pepper sauce	1 meal	13.0	360	33%
mushroom w/white wine sauce	1 meal	18.0	430	38%
spicy chicken	1 meal	24.0	490	44%

■ **YU SING** (*See also* ASIAN FOOD)

FROZEN NONDAIRY DESSERT (*See* FRUIT ICES, BARS, & POPS; ICE CREAM & ICE CREAM-LIKE FROZEN DESSERTS; RICE FROZEN DESSERT; SHERBET; TOFU FROZEN DESSERT)
FRUCTOSE (*See* SUGAR SUBSTITUTE)
FRUIT (*See* FRUIT, MIXED; FRUIT COCKTAIL; individual listings)
FRUIT, MIXED (*See also* FRUIT COCKTAIL; SNACK MIX)

Food and Description	Amount	Fat Grams	Total Calories	% Fat Calories
candied				
(S&W) glaze cake mix/orange peel, grapefruit peel, cherries, pineapple, citron, lemon peel	2 Tbs	–	90	–
canned				
(Del Monte)				
chunky mixed				
in extra light syrup	½ cup	–	60	–
in heavy syrup	½ cup	–	100	–
naturals/in fruit juices	½ cup	–	60	–
fruit cups				
in extra light syrup	4¼ oz	–	60	–
in heavy syrup	4¼ oz	–	90	–
in light syrup	3½ oz	–	70	–
naturals/in fruit juices	4¼ oz	–	60	–
fruit pleasures/cherry mixed fruit in				
natural cherry-flavored light syrup	½ cup	–	90	–
Orchard Select				
California mixed in light syrup	½ cup	–	80	–
tropical fruit salad				
in light syrup	½ cup	–	80	–
in pineapple & passion fruit juices	½ cup	–	60	–
(Dole) tropical fruit salad/in light syrup	½ cup	–	80	–
generic				
fruit salad				
in extra heavy syrup	½ cup	<1.0	114	4%
in heavy syrup	½ cup	<1.0	94	15%
in juice	½ cup	<1.0	62	7%
in water	½ cup	<1.0	37	12%
tropical fruit	½ cup	–	110	–

Food and Description	Amount	Fat Grams	Total Calories	% Fat Calories
(Kraft)	½ cup	–	50	–
(S&W) natural style/chunky	½ cup	–	70	–
dried				
(Del Monte)	⅓ cup	–	110	–
(Mariani)				
fruit medley	¼ cup	1.0	150	5%
tropical	1 oz	1.0	90	10%
(Sun Giant)	1.5 oz	–	100	–
(Sun Maid)				
fruit bits	¼ cup	–	120	–
mixed fruit	¼ cup	–	110	–
frozen				
(Birds Eye)	½ cup	–	120	–
(C&W)				
berry medley	1 cup	–	60	–
mixed melon balls	⅔ cup	–	40	–
generic				
sweetened	1 cup	0.5	245	2%
unsweetened	3.5 oz	<1.0	45	10%
FRUIT & NUT MIX (*See* SNACKS)				
FRUIT COCKTAIL (*See also* FRUIT, MIXED)				
canned				
generic				
in extra heavy syrup	½ cup	–	115	–
in extra light syrup	½ cup	–	50	–
in heavy syrup	½ cup	–	80	–
in fruit juice	½ cup	–	50	–
in light syrup	½ cup	–	70	–
in water	½ cup	–	40	–
(Del Monte)				
Fruit Naturals in fruit juice	½ cup	–	60	–
Fruit Rageous				
Crazy cherry mixed in light syrup	½ cup	–	90	–
in heavy syrup	½ cup	–	100	–
in light/extra light syrup	½ cup	–	60	–
natural/in fruit juices	½ cup	–	50	–
Very cherry mixed	½ cup	–	90	–
(Hunt's)	½ cup	–	90	–
(Libby's) Lite	½ cup	–	50	–
(Nutradiet)	½ cup	–	40	–
(S&W)				
in heavy syrup	½ cup	–	90	–
natural style	½ cup	–	80	–
FRUIT DRINK (*See also* LEMONADE/LEMONADE-FLAVORED DRINK; TEA; FRUIT PUNCH; SOFT DRINK; SOFT DRINK MIX; individual listings)				
bottled, boxed, or canned				
(Fruitopia)				
Fruit Integration	8 fl oz	–	125	–
Tropical Consideration	8 fl oz	–	75	–
(Hi-C)				
Double Fruit Cooler	6 fl oz	–	90	–

Food and Description	Amount	Fat Grams	Total Calories	% Fat Calories
Ecto Cooler	6 fl oz	–	95	–
Hula	6 fl oz	–	95	–
(Libby's) Fruit Medley	8 fl oz	–	80	–
(Welch's)				
orange-pineapple-apple	8.45 fl oz	–	140	–
Sparkling Red Cocktail	8 fl oz	–	160	–
Sparkling White Cocktail	8 fl oz	–	160	–
Tropical punch drink	10 fl oz	–	160	–
Tropical Cocktail	11.5 fl oz	–	210	–
	11.5 fl oz	–	210	–
frozen/prepared				
(Mott's) Fruit Basket Tropical Blend	8 fl oz	–	120	–
(Welch's)				
orange-pineapple-apple	8 fl oz	–	140	–
Orchard juice cocktail				
Fruit Harvest punch	8 fl oz	–	140	–
Harvest Blend juice cocktail	8 fl oz	–	140	–
FRUIT ICES, BARS, & POPS (*See also* SHERBET)				
(Baskin-Robbins) Ices				
daiquiri	½ cup	–	110	–
	reg scoop	–	130	–
neon sour apple	½ cup	–	110	–
the mask	½ cup	–	120	–
watermelon	½ cup	–	110	–
(Chiquita) fruit & juice				
cherry	1 bar	–	50	–
raspberry	1 bar	–	50	–
strawberry	1 bar	–	50	–
strawberry-banana	1 bar	–	50	–
(Dole)				
Fruit Juice Bars				
grape				
no sugar added	1.75 oz	–	25	–
regular	1.75 oz	–	45	–
raspberry				
no sugar added	1.75 oz	–	25	–
regular	1.75 oz	–	45	–
strawberry				
no sugar added	1.75 oz	–	25	–
regular	1.75 oz	–	45	–
Fruit 'N Juice Bars				
lemonade	2.5 oz	–	70	–
raspberry	2.5 oz	–	70	–
strawberry	2.5 oz	–	70	–
(Dreyer's)				
Fruit Bars				
cranberry-apple	1 bar	–	90	–
lemonade	1 bar	–	80	–
lime	1 bar	–	80	–
peach	1 bar	–	90	–
raspberry-kiwi	1 bar	–	80	–

Food and Description	Amount	Fat Grams	Total Calories	% Fat Calories
strawberry	1 bar	–	80	–
wild berry	1 bar	–	80	–
Whole Fruit Sorbet				
boysenberry	½ cup	–	150	–
chocolate	½ cup	–	160	–
lemon	½ cup	–	140	–
mango	½ cup	–	130	–
peach	½ cup	–	130	–
raspberry	½ cup	–	130	–
strawberry	½ cup	–	120	–
(Edy's)				
Fruit Bars				
chocolate-dipped				
creamy banana	1 bar	9.0	210	39%
creamy strawberry	1 bar	9.0	170	48%
lemonade	1 bar	–	80	–
lime	1 bar	–	80	–
peach	1 bar	–	90	–
strawberry	1 bar	–	80	–
wild berry	1 bar	–	80	–
Whole Fruit Sorbet				
boysenberry	½ cup	–	150	–
chocolate	½ cup	–	160	–
lemon	½ cup	–	140	–
mango	½ cup	–	130	–
peach	½ cup	–	130	–
raspberry	½ cup	–	130	–
strawberry	½ cup	–	120	–
(Eskimo)				
Rainbow Twin Pops	1 pop	–	60	–
Welch's Double Dare pops				
double sours	1 pop	–	40	–
mega sours	1 pop	–	40	–
(Frookie) Cool Fruits				
Fruit Juice Freezers				
cranberry	2 pops	–	70	–
pink lemonade	2 pops	–	70	–
raspberry-apple	2 pops	–	70	–
strawberry-banana	2 pops	–	70	–
watermelon berry	2 pops	–	70	–
(Good Humor)				
Bubble Play Sports	1 bar	–	110	–
Cherry Torpedo	1 bar	–	35	–
Hyper Stripe	1 bar	–	80	–
Jumbo Jet Star	1 bar	–	80	–
Micro Pops	1 pop	–	80	–
Smile	1 bar	–	110	–
The Great White bar	1 bar	–	70	–
(Haagen-Dazs) Sorbet				
Ice Cream Shops				
Bar/raspberry & vanilla	1 bar	–	90	–

Food and Description	Amount	Fat Grams	Total Calories	% Fat Calories
Regular				
mango	½ cup	–	120	–
orange	½ cup	–	120	–
raspberry	½ cup	–	120	–
strawberry	½ cup	–	120	–
Zesty Lemon	½ cup	–	120	–
Soft serve/raspberry	½ cup	–	110	–
Retail stores				
Bars				
chocolate	1 bar		80	–
Pints				
chocolate	½ cup	–	120	–
mango	½ cup	–	120	–
orange	½ cup	–	120	–
orchard peach	½ cup	–	130	–
raspberry	½ cup	–	120	–
strawberry	½ cup	–	120	–
Zesty Lemon	½ cup	–	120	–
(Jell-O) gelatin pops				
all flavors/averaged data	1 bar	–	35	–
(Kemp)				
Pop Jr.'s				
banana	1 pop	–	180	–
cherry	1 pop	–	180	–
grape	1 pop	–	180	–
lime	1 pop	–	180	–
orange	1 pop	–	180	–
root beer	1 pop	–	180	–
Pop'N fudge				
cherry	1 pop	0.5	60	8%
grape	1 pop	0.5	60	8%
orange	1 pop	0.5	60	8%
Twin pops				
cherry	1 pop	–	60	–
grape	1 pop	–	60	–
orange	1 pop	–	60	–
(Kool-Aid) Kool-pops/all flavors	1 bar	–	40	–
orange	1 bar	–	80	–
strawberry	1 bar	–	80	–
(Luigi's) Real Italian Ice cups				
cherry	6 oz	–	120	–
lemon	6 oz	–	110	–
lemon & strawberry	6 oz	–	110	–
strawberry	6 oz	–	110	–
(Minute Maid) Fruit Juice Bars				
cherry	1 bar	–	60	–
grape	1 bar	–	60	–
orange	1 bar	–	60	–
(Nestlé USA) Ice screamers				
Ice Pops/all flavors				
Bug Pops	1 pop	–	90	–

Food and Description	Amount	Fat Grams	Total Calories	% Fat Calories
Galctic Pops	1 pop	–	70	–
Itzakadoozie	1 pop	–	90	–
Shock tarts/Willy Wonka variety	1 pop	–	45	–
Splash pops	1 pop	–	80	–
Sweetarts	1 pop	–	70	–
Tigger Tails orange & grape striped	1 pop	–	60	–
(Pet) Ice Pops				
assorted				
jr	1 pop	–	40	–
regular	1 pop	–	70	–
banana	1 pop	–	70	–
(Popsicle)				
Single-serve				
Big Bang	1 bar	1.0	100	9%
Big Stick				
cherry/pineapple	1 bar	–	60	–
Lick-A-Color	1 bar	–	90	–
rainbow	1 bar	–	90	–
Bubble gum swirl	1 bar	–	60	–
cotton candy Swirl	1 bar	–	60	–
Cups				
cherry	1 cup	–	240	–
lemon	1 cup	–	230	–
Firecracker Jr.	1 pop	–	40	–
Firecracker				
fire & ice	1 bar	–	80	–
root beer float	1 bar	–	80	–
LaFruit-A-Loca	1 bar	–	90	–
Red, White, & Blue Firecracker Bar	1 bar	–	80	–
Super Twin				
cello	1 bar	–	70	–
paper	1 bar	–	70	–
Supersicle				
Neon Traffic Signal	1 bar	–	80	–
Sour Tower	1 bar	–	80	–
Razzle Dazzle	1 bar	–	80	–
Towering Tornado	1 pop	1.5	90	15%
Variety Multipacks				
All natural/all flavors	1.75 oz	–	50	–
Big Stick/cherry pineapple swirl	3.5 oz	–	50	–
Fantastic Fruity	2 oz	–	60	–
Firecracker	1.6 oz	–	40	–
Fruit Juice w/calcium/all flavors	2.25 oz	–	60	–
Great White	1.75 oz	–	45	–
Juice Busters/all flavors	1.6 oz	–	70	–
La Fruta Loca juice pops	3.5 oz	–	90	–
Lick-A-Color	2 oz	–	50	–
Micro Pops	2.2 oz	–	40	–
Nickelodeon Green Slime	1.75 oz	–	70	–
Popsicle/all flavors	1.75 oz	–	45	–

Food and Description	Amount	Fat Grams	Total Calories	% Fat Calories
Pokemon	3 oz	–	80	–
Root Beer	1.75 oz	–	45	–
Scribblers	1.2 oz	–	60	–
Sherbet Cyclone	1.8 oz	0.5	50	9%
Sherbet Smile!/orange & lemon	1 bar	0.5	90	5%
Starship	2.3 oz	–	50	–
Sugar-free				
cherry	1.75 oz	–	15	–
grape	1.75 oz	–	15	–
orange	1.75 oz	–	15	–
Tropical Fruits	1.75 oz	–	15	–
Tingle Twister	1.75 oz	–	45	–
(Schwan's)				
Schwan's Pops	1 pop	–	15	–
Twin Pops/assorted	1 pop	–	60	–
specialty items				
Garfield	1 bar	–	90	–
Screwball Cup	1 cup	1.0	100	9%
Snow Cone	1 cone	–	60	–
Super Mario	1 bar	1.0	120	8%
The Great White Bar	1 bar	–	70	–
(Sunkist) bars				
lemonade	1 bar	–	90	–
orange juice	1 bar	–	100	–
wild berry fruit & juice	1 bar	–	140	–
(Trix) pops/all flavors	1 bar	–	40	–
(Welch's) fruit juice bars				
grape				
no sugar added	1 bar	–	25	–
regular				
1.75-oz bar	1 bar	–	45	–
3-oz bar	1 bar	–	80	–
orange-pineapple banana/1.75 oz	1 bar	–	45	–
pineapple/1.75 oz bar	1 bar	–	45	–
raspberry				
no sugar added	1 bar	–	25	–
regular	1 bar	–	45	–
strawberry				
no sugar added	1 bar	–	25	–
regular	1 bar	–	45	–
strawberry-banana				
1.75-oz bar	1 bar	–	45	–
3 oz-bar	1 bar	–	80	–
fruit punch	4 oz	–	157	–

FRUIT JUICE/JUICE DRINK, MIXED (*See also* FRUIT PUNCH; individual listings)
bottled, boxed, or canned
  (Capri Sun) juice drink

Mountain Cooler	6.75 fl oz	–	100	–
Pacific Cooler	6.75 fl oz	–	110	–
Surfer Cooler	6.75 fl oz	–	100	–

Food and Description	Amount	Fat Grams	Total Calories	% Fat Calories
(Chiquita)				
Caribbean Splash	8 fl oz	–	120	–
	8.45 fl oz	–	130	–
Hawaiian Sunrise	8 fl oz	–	120	–
Tropical Paradise	8 fl oz	–	120	–
	8.45 fl oz	–	130	–
(Knudsen)				
Morning Blend	8 fl oz	–	120	–
Natural Breakfast	8 fl oz	–	110	–
Thirst Quencher/Hibiscus Cooler	8 fl oz	–	90	–
(Libby's) Juicy Juice	8 fl oz	–	130	–
	8.45 fl oz	–	140	–
(Mott's) In-A-Minute unfrozen concentrate/tropical blend	2 fl oz	–	130	–
(Welch's) juice cocktail				
harvest blend	8 fl oz	–	150	–
orange, pineapple, apple	8 fl oz	–	140	–
Tropical Orange Passion	8 fl oz	–	140	–
frozen/prepared				
(Mott's) Fruit Basket juice cocktail/ tropical blend	8 fl oz	–	120	–
(Welch's) Orchard Harvest juice blend	8 fl oz	–	140	–
FRUIT PECTIN				
(Certo)	1 Tbs	–	2	–
(Sure-Jell)				
light	¼ tsp	–	5	–
sweetened	¼ tsp	–	5	–
FRUIT PROTECTOR (See also FRUIT PECTIN)				
(Ever-Fresh)	¼ tsp	–	5	–
FRUIT PUNCH (See also SOFT DRINK; SOFT DRINK MIX; SPORTS DRINK)				
bottled, boxed, or canned				
(Betty Crocker)				
Squeezit				
green	6.75 fl oz	–	110	–
rockin red puncher	6.76 fl oz	–	100	–
tropical	6.76 fl oz	–	110	–
Squeezit 100/Punch	6.76 fl oz	–	90	–
(Capri Sun)				
fruit	6.75 fl oz	–	100	–
Maui	6.75 fl oz	–	100	–
mountain cooler	6.75 fl oz	–	90	–
Pacific cooler	6.75 fl oz	–	100	–
safari	6.75 fl oz	–	100	–
super cooler	6.75 fl oz	–	100	–
(Hawaiian Punch)				
Fruit Juicy Red				
diet	8 fl oz	–	10	–
regular	8 fl oz	–	120	–
Island Fruit Cocktail	6 fl oz	–	90	–
Tropical Fruits	6 fl oz	–	90	–

Food and Description	Amount	Fat Grams	Total Calories	% Fat Calories
Very Berry	6 fl oz	–	90	–
Wild Fruit	6 fl oz	–	90	–
(Hi-C)				
fruit	8 fl oz	–	120	–
	8.45 fl oz	–	130	–
Hula	8 fl oz	–	110	–
	8.45 fl oz	–	120	–
(Knudsen) Rain Forest Punch	8 fl oz	–	120	–
(Kool Aid)				
Bursts/tropical	1 bottle	–	100	
Crystal Light/low-calorie	8 fl oz	–	5	–
Splash				
grape berry	8 fl oz	–	120	–
tropical	8 fl oz	–	120	–
(Libby's) Juicy Juice				
orange	4.23 fl oz	–	80	–
	8 fl oz	–	100	–
	8.45 fl oz	–	100	–
(Minute Maid)				
fruit	8 fl oz	–	113	–
(Mott's)				
In-A-Minute unfrozen concentrate	2 fl oz	–	140	–
ready to drink	8.45 fl oz	–	120	–
	10 fl oz	–	170	–
(Seneca) fruit				
100% Juice	8 fl oz	–	130	–
10% Juice	8 fl oz	–	120	–
(TreeTop)				
fruit punch				
100% Juice	8.45 fl oz	–	130	–
	10 fl oz	–	150	–
	11.5 fl oz	–	170	–
25% Juice	8 fl oz	–	130	–
	10 fl oz	–	160	–
	11.5 fl oz	–	180	–
Juice Rivers				
citrus	8.45 fl oz	–	130	–
fruit	8.45 fl oz	–	130	–
grape	8.45 fl oz	–	140	–
red	8.45 fl oz	–	130	–
(Tropicana)				
berry	8 fl oz	–	130	–
citrus	8 fl oz	–	140	–
	10 fl oz	–	180	–
cranberry	8 fl oz	–	140	–
	10 fl oz	–	170	–
	11.5 fl oz	–	200	–
fruit	8 fl oz	–	130	–
	10 fl oz	–	160	–
	11.5 fl oz	–	180	–

Food and Description	Amount	Fat Grams	Total Calories	% Fat Calories
pineapple	8 fl oz	–	130	–
	10 fl oz	–	160	–
(Welch's)				
fruit	11.5 fl oz	–	180	–
Fruit Harvest	8.45 fl oz	–	140	–
strawberry	8 fl oz	–	140	–
wild berry	8 fl oz	–	130	–
	10 fl oz	–	160	–
frozen or refrigerated/prepared				
(Minute Maid)				
berry	8 fl oz	–	120	–
citrus	8 fl oz	–	120	–
fruit	8 fl oz	–	120	–
grape	8 fl oz	–	120	–
tropical	8 fl oz	–	120	–
FRUIT SALAD (FRUIT, MIXED; FRUIT COCKTAIL)				
FRUIT SNACK (See also individual fruit listings)				
(Betty Crocker)				
Fruit-By-The-Foot				
berry tie dye	1 roll	1.5	80	17%
cherry	1 roll	1.5	80	17%
color by the foot	1 roll	1.5	80	17%
endless party	1 roll	1.5	80	17%
flavor wave	1 roll	1.5	80	17%
Pokemon	1 roll	1.5	80	17%
strawberry	1 roll	1.5	80	17%
watermelon	1 roll	1.5	80	17%
Fruit Roll-Ups				
cherry	1 roll	0.5	50	9%
Crazy Colors	1 roll	0.5	50	9%
Fun'n Games	1 roll	0.5	50	9%
Double Fruity	1 roll	0.5	50	9%
Galaxy Blast	1 roll	0.5	50	9%
Hot Colors	1 roll	0.5	50	9%
Peel'n Build	1 roll	0.5	50	9%
strawberry	1 roll	0.5	50	9%
XL Pouch				
Fun'n Games	2 rolls	1.5	130	10%
Peel'n Build	2 rolls	1.5	130	10%
strawberry	2 rolls	1.5	130	10%
Fruit String Thing				
Bugs Bunny	1 pouch	1.0	80	11%
Scooby Doo!	1 pouch	1.0	80	11%
sneaky stripes	1 pouch	1.0	80	11%
strawberry split	1 pouch	1.0	80	11%
Fruit Snacks				
Bugs Bunny	1 pouch	–	80	–
Hawaiian Punch	1 pouch	–	80	–
Lucky Charms	1 pouch	–	80	–
Pokemon	1 pouch	–	80	–

Food and Description	Amount	Fat Grams	Total Calories	% Fat Calories
Scooby Doo!	1 pouch	–	80	–
Shark Bites	1 pouch	–	80	–
Trix	1 pouch	–	80	–
XL Pouch				
Bugs Bunny	10 pieces	–	100	–
Scooby Doo!	10 pieces	–	100	–
Gushers				
Fruitomic Punch	1 pouch	1.0	90	10%
sour berry	1 pouch	1.0	90	10%
strawberry splash	1 pouch	1.0	90	10%
tropical punch	1 pouch	1.0	90	10%
watermelon blast	1 pouch	1.0	90	10%
wild cherry	1 pouch	1.0	90	10%
(Del Monte) yogurt raisins				
strawberry	0.9 oz	3.0	110	25%
vanilla	0.9 oz	3.0	110	25%
(Farley)				
Funnies/Trolls				
cherry	1 pouch	2.0	80	23%
strawberry	1 pouch	2.0	80	23%
turtles	1 pouch	–	80	–
Snacks				
cherry	1 pouch	–	80	–
Creepy Crawlers	1 pouch	–	80	–
dinosaurs	1 pouch	–	80	–
strawberry	1 pouch	–	80	–
Troll	1 pouch	–	80	–
The Roll/strawberry	1 pouch	2.0	80	23%
(Flavor Tree)				
Fruit Roll				
apple	1 roll	–	75	–
apricot	1 roll	0.5	75	6%
cherry	1 roll	–	75	–
grape	1 roll	–	75	–
raspberry	1 roll	–	75	–
strawberry	1 roll	–	75	–
(Sunkist) Fruit Roll/prepared				
apple/21-gm roll	1 roll	–	70	–
apricot/21-gm roll	1 roll	–	70	–
cherry				
14-gm roll	1 roll	–	50	–
21-gm roll	1 roll	–	70	–
fruit punch/21-gm roll	1 roll	–	70	–
grape				
14-gm roll	1 roll	–	50	–
21-gm roll	1 roll	–	80	–
raspberry				
14-gm roll	1 roll	–	45	–
21-gm roll	1 roll	–	70	–

Food and Description	Amount	Fat Grams	Total Calories	% Fat Calories
strawberry				
14-gm roll	1 roll	–	45	–
21-gm roll	1 roll	–	70	–
(Weight Watchers) fruit snack				
apple	0.5 oz	–	50	–
cinnamon	0.5 oz	–	50	–
peach	0.5 oz	–	50	–
strawberry	0.5 oz	–	50	–
FRUIT SPREAD (*See* JAM/JELLY/PRESERVES)				

G

Food and Description	Amount	Fat Grams	Total Calories	% Fat Calories
GARBANZO BEAN (*See* CHICKPEA)				
GARLIC (*See also* SEASONINGS)				
fresh/raw				
minced	1 clove	–	4	–
whole	1 clove	–	5	–
jar (Christopher Ranch) chopped	1 tsp	1.0	10	90%
powdered				
generic	1 tsp	–	9	–
(Spice Island)	1 tsp	–	5	–
GARLIC SALT (*See also* SEASONINGS)				
(Lawry's)	1 tsp	–	4	–
GAZPACHO (*See* SOUP)				
GEFILTE FISH				
(Manischewitz)				
Hemishe sweet	1 piece	1.0	60	15%
jelled				
14.5 oz jar	1 piece	3.0	70	39%
4 lb jar	1 piece	2.0	45	40%
non-jelled				
14.5 oz jar	1 piece	1.5	70	19%
24 oz jar	1 piece	1.5	70	19%
4 lb jar	1 piece	3.0	45	60%
Premium Gold				
14.5 oz jar	1 piece	5.0	110	41%
24 oz jar	1 piece	6.0	120	45%
4 lb jar	1 piece	3.0	70	39%

Food and Description	Amount	Fat Grams	Total Calories	% Fat Calories
sweet				
14.5 oz jar	1 piece	1.5	80	17%
24 oz jar	1 piece	2.0	90	20%
4 lb jar	1 piece	1.0	60	15%
(Mother's)				
old-fashioned				
12-oz jar	1 ball	1.0	55	16%
24-oz jar	1 ball	1.0	70	13%
Old World				
regular	1 ball	1.0	70	13%
sweet	1 ball	1.0	55	16%
unsalted	1 ball	1.0	45	20%
GELATIN				
■ DRINKING POWDER				
generic/1 packet + water	4 fl oz	–	67	–
(Knox) w/NutraSweet	1 envelope	–	39	–
■ DRY				
	1 pkt	–	23	–
■ MIX				
(Hain) SuperFruits dessert mix				
cherry				
mix only	2 Tbs	–	90	–
prepared	½ cup	–	90	–
kiwi-pineapple				
mix only	2 Tbs	–	90	–
prepared	½ cup	–	90	–
orange-pineapple				
mix only	2 Tbs	–	90	–
prepared	½ cup	–	90	–
strawberry				
mix only	2 Tbs	–	90	–
prepared	½ cup	–	90	–
tropical fruit punch				
mix only	2 Tbs	–	90	–
prepared	½ cup	–	90	–
(Jell-O) prepared				
Jell-O 1-2-3				
strawberry	⅔ cup	1.5	130	10%
Original				
apricot	½ cup	–	80	–
berry black	½ cup	–	80	
berry blue				
regular	½ cup	–	80	–
sugar-free	½ cup	–	10	–
black cherry	½ cup	–	80	–
cherry				
regular	½ cup	–	80	–
sugar-free	½ cup	–	10	–
cranberry				
regular	½ cup	–	80	–
sugar-free	½ cup	–	10	–

Food and Description	Amount	Fat Grams	Total Calories	% Fat Calories
cranberry raspberry	½ cup	–	80	–
cranberry strawberry	½ cup	–	80	–
grape	½ cup	–	80	–
lemon				
regular	½ cup	–	80	–
sugar-free	½ cup	–	10	–
lime				
regular	½ cup	–	80	–
sugar-free	½ cup	–	10	–
mango	½ cup	–	80	–
mixed fruit				
regular	½ cup	–	80	–
sugar-free	½ cup	–	10	–
orange				
regular	½ cup	–	80	–
sugar-free	½ cup	–	10	–
peach	½ cup	–	80	–
peach passion	½ cup	–	80	–
pineapple				
Hawaiian/sugar-free	½ cup	–	10	–
regular	½ cup	–	80	–
raspberry				
regular	½ cup	–	80	–
sugar-free	½ cup	–	10	–
sparkling white grape	½ cup	–	80	–
strawberry				
regular	½ cup	–	80	–
sugar-free	½ cup	–	10	–
strawberry-banana				
regular	½ cup	–	80	–
sugar-free	½ cup	–	10	–
strawberry-kiwi				
regular	½ cup	–	80	–
sugar-free	½ cup	–	10	–
triple berry/sugar-free	½ cup	–	10	–
tropical punch	½ cup	–	80	–
watermelon				
regular	½ cup	–	80	–
sugar-free	½ cup	–	10	–
wild strawberry	½ cup	–	80	–
(Jell-Well)				
cherry	½ cup	–	80	–
lemon	½ cup	–	80	–
lime	½ cup	–	80	–
mixed fruit	½ cup	–	80	–
orange				
regular	½ cup	–	80	–
sugar-free	½ cup	–	10	–
raspberry				
regular	½ cup	–	80	–

Food and Description	Amount	Fat Grams	Total Calories	% Fat Calories
sugar-free	½ cup	–	10	–
strawberry				
regular	½ cup	–	80	–
sugar-free	½ cup	–	10	–
strawberry-banana				
regular	½ cup	–	80	–
sugar-free	½ cup	–	10	–
(Royal)				
apple	½ cup	–	80	–
blackberry	½ cup	–	80	–
cherry				
regular	½ cup	–	80	–
sugar-free	½ cup	–	10	–
Concord grape	½ cup	–	80	–
lemon	½ cup	–	80	–
lemon-lime	½ cup	–	80	–
lime				
regular	½ cup	–	80	–
sugar-free	½ cup	–	10	–
mixed berry	½ cup	–	80	–
orange				
regular	½ cup	–	80	–
sugar-free	½ cup	–	10	–
peach	½ cup	–	80	–
pineapple	½ cup	–	80	–
raspberry				
regular	½ cup	–	80	–
sugar-free	½ cup	–	10	–
strawberry				
regular	½ cup	–	80	–
sugar-free	½ cup	–	10	–
strawberry-banana	½ cup	–	80	–
tropical fruit	½ cup	–	80	–
(SnackWell's)				
cherry	½ cup	–	80	–
lime	½ cup	–	80	–
orange	½ cup	–	80	–
strawberry	½ cup	–	80	–
■ READY TO SERVE				
(Del Monte) snack cups				
blueberry	3.5 oz cup	–	70	–
cherry	3.5 oz cup	–	70	–
grape	3.5 oz cup	–	70	–
strawberry	3.5 oz cup	–	70	–
(Jell-O)				
gelatin				
berry black	1 snack	–	70	–
berry blue	1 snack	–	70	–
cherry				
regular	1 snack	–	70	–

Food and Description	Amount	Fat Grams	Total Calories	% Fat Calories
sugar-free	1 snack	–	10	–
orange				
regular	1 snack	–	70	–
sugar-free	1 snack	–	10	–
orange-strawberry-banana	1 snack	–	70	–
raspberry				
regular	1 snack	–	70	–
sugar-free	1 snack	–	10	–
Rhymin' Lymon	1 snack	–	70	–
strawberry				
regular	1 snack	–	70	–
sugar-free	1 snack	–	10	–
strawberry-kiwi/sugar-free	1 snack	–	10	–
tropical berry/sugar-free	1 snack	–	10	–
tropical fruit punch	1 snack	–	70	–
wild watermelon	1 snack	–	70	–
(Kraft) Handi-Snacks				
blue raspberry	1 snack	–	80	–
cherry	1 snack	–	80	–
orange	1 snack	–	80	–
strawberry	1 snack	–	80	–
GIN (See LIQUOR, DISTILLED)				
GINGER ALE (See SOFT DRINK)				
GINGER ROOT				
candied	1 oz	–	95	–
fresh/raw/sliced	5 slices	–	8	–
	¼ cup	–	17	–
powdered-ground	1 tsp	–	6	–
GINGERBREAD (See BREAD; CAKE)				
GINKGO				
canned	1 oz	0.5	32	14%
dried	1 oz	0.6	99	5%
raw	1 oz	–	52	–
GIZZARD (See CHICKEN; GOOSE; TURKEY)				
GOAT /boneless				
raw	4 oz	3.0	125	22%
roasted	3 oz	3.0	122	22%
roasted/diced	1 cup	4.0	200	18%
GOOSE (See also PÂTÉ)				
domesticated/roasted				
gizzard, raw	3 oz	4.5	119	34%
liver				
raw	3 oz	3.6	114	28%
meat & skin	~2 lb	170.0	2362	65%
meat only	4 oz	14.5	270	48%
	1¼ lbs	75.0	1406	48%
GOOSEBERRY				
canned/in light syrup	½ cup	–	93	–
raw	1 cup	0.9	67	12%
GOULASH (See BEEF DISH/ENTRÉE; FROZEN ENTRÉE/DINNER)				

Food and Description	Amount	Fat Grams	Total Calories	% Fat Calories
GOURD				
dishcloth				
boiled-drained	½ cup	0.5	65	7%
boiled-drained/sliced	½ cup	0.3	50	5%
raw	~ 8.5 oz	0.5	40	11%
raw/sliced	½ cup	–	10	–
wax				
boiled-drained	½ cup	–	15	–
boiled-drained/chopped	½ cup	–	11	–
raw	~1 lb	<1.0	45	10%
raw/chopped	½ cup	–	8	–
white				
boiled-drained	½ cup	–	17	–
boiled-drained/chopped	½ cup	–	11	–
raw	~1 lb	<1.0	45	10%
raw/chopped	½ cup	–	8	–
GRAHAM CRACKER (See COOKIE; CRACKER)				
GRAHAM CRACKER CRUMBS (See CRACKER CRUMBS/MEAL)				
GRANADILLA (See PASSION FRUIT)				
GRANOLA (See CEREAL)				
GRANOLA/GRANOLA-TYPE BAR				
(Barbara's)				
Nature's Choice				
cereal bar				
fat-free				
apple	1 bar	–	110	–
blueberry	1 bar	–	110	–
cranberry	1 bar	–	110	–
peach	1 bar	–	110	–
raspberry	1 bar	–	110	–
strawberry	1 bar	–	110	–
low-fat				
very cherry	1 bar	2.0	130	14%
triple berry	1 bar	2.0	130	14%
granola bar				
carob chip	1 bar	2.0	80	23%
cinnamon & raisin	1 bar	2.0	80	23%
oats 'n honey	1 bar	2.0	80	23%
peanut butter	1 bar	3.0	80	34%
(Betty Crocker)				
Golden Grahams Treats				
marshmallow graham w/mini marshmallows	1 bar	2.0	90	20%
peanut butter chocolate	1 bar	3.5	90	35%
s'mores chocolate chunk				
king size	1 bar	5.0	190	24%
regular	1 bar	2.5	90	25%
(Glenny's) brown rice treat				
carob mint w/oat bran	1 bar	2.0	180	10%
cinnamon & raisin	1 bar	1.0	170	5%
peanut & raisin	1 bar	5.0	210	21%

Food and Description	Amount	Fat Grams	Total Calories	% Fat Calories
plain & fancy	1 bar	1.0	120	8%
raisin bran	1 bar	1.0	170	5%
toasted almond w/oat bran	1 bar	5.0	200	23%
(Grist Mill)				
chocolate granola bar snack				
chocolate chip	1 bar	10.0	180	50%
nutty fudge	1 bar	11.0	190	52%
granola bar				
chewy				
apple-cinnamon	1 bar	4.0	120	30%
chocolate chip	1 bar	4.0	130	28%
chunky nut & raisin	1 bar	6.0	130	42%
peanut butter	1 bar	5.0	130	35%
peanut butter chocolate	1 bar	4.0	130	28%
crunchy				
cinnamon	1 bar	5.0	110	41%
oats 'n honey	1 bar	5.0	110	41%
(Hain) Mini-Munchies bar/low-fat				
banana split	1 bar	1.5	90	15%
chewy caramel	1 bar	1.5	90	15%
double chocolate	1 bar	1.5	90	15%
peanut butter crunch	1 bar	1.5	90	15%
strawberry marshmallow	1 bar	1.5	90	15%
(Health Valley) fat-free				
Bakes				
apple	1 bar	–	70	–
date	1 bar	–	70	–
raisin	1 bar	–	70	–
chocolate flavor sandwich/healthy				
Bavarian creme	1 bar	–	150	–
caramel creme	1 bar	–	150	–
peanut creme	1 bar	–	150	–
vanilla creme	1 bar	–	150	–
crisp rice bar/healthy				
apple raisin	1 bar	–	110	–
orange date	1 bar	–	110	–
tropical fruit	1 bar	–	110	–
fruit bar				
apricot	1 bar	–	140	–
date fruit	1 bar	–	140	–
raisin	1 bar	–	140	–
granola bar				
blueberry apple	1 bar	–	140	–
chocolate flavor chip	1 bar	–	140	–
date almond	1 bar	–	140	–
raisin	1 bar	–	140	–
raspberry	1 bar	–	140	–
strawberry	1 bar	–	140	–
(Hostess) Cereal bars				
apple	1 bar	1.5	120	11%
banana nut	1 bar	2.0	120	20%

Food and Description	Amount	Fat Grams	Total Calories	% Fat Calories
blueberry	1 bar	1.5	120	11%
raspberry	1 bar	1.5	120	11%
strawberry	1 bar	1.5	120	11%
(Jack La Lanne) chewy fruit & nut bar				
apple	1 bar	2.0	90	20%
banana	1 bar	2.0	90	20%
date	1 bar	2.0	90	20%
orange	1 bar	3.0	100	27%
(Kellogg's)				
cereal bar				
chocolate chip Rice Krispies	1 bar	4.0	120	30%
Rice Krispies Treats squares	1 bar	2.0	90	20%
crunchy granola bar/low-fat				
almond & brown sugar	1 bar	1.5	80	17%
apple spice	1 bar	1.5	80	17%
cinnamon raisin	1 bar	1.5	80	17%
Nutri-Grain cereal bars				
Fruit-full Squares				
apple	1 bar	4.0	180	20%
banana	1 bar	4.5	190	21%
cinnamon	1 bar	4.0	180	20%
Original				
apple-cinnamon	1 bar	3.0	140	19%
blueberry	1 bar	3.0	140	19%
cherry	1 bar	3.0	140	19%
mixed-berry	1 bar	3.0	140	19%
peach	1 bar	3.0	140	19%
raspberry	1 bar	3.0	140	19%
strawberry	1 bar	3.0	140	19%
Rice Krispies Treats Squares				
cocoa	1 bar	2.0	90	20%
original	1 bar	2.0	90	20%
peanut butter chocolate	1 bar	4.0	110	33%
Twists				
apple cinnamon & brown sugar	1 bar	3.0	140	19%
banana & strawberry	1 bar	3.0	140	19%
strawberry & blueberry	1 bar	3.0	140	19%
strawberry & creme	1 bar	3.0	140	19%
(Kudos) whole-grain bar				
chocolate chip	1 bar	4.5	120	34%
chocolate fudge	1 bar	4.5	120	34%
M&M's milk chocolate mini's	1 bar	2.5	90	25%
peanut butter	1 bar	5.0	130	35%
Snickers Bar	1 bar	3.5	100	32%
(Nature Valley)				
granola bar				
chewy/low-fat				
chocolate chip	1 bar	2.5	120	19%
oatmeal raisin	1 bar	2.0	110	16%
crunchy				
cinnamon	1 bar	3.0	90	30%

Food and Description	Amount	Fat Grams	Total Calories	% Fat Calories
oats'n honey	1 bar	3.0	90	30%
peanut butter	1 bar	3.0	90	30%
Nature's Choice (*See* (Barbara's) in this section)				
(Nestlé) Sweet Success candy/snack bars				
chewy				
caramel, honey, & nougat	1 bar	3.5	100	32%
chocolate brownie	1 bar	4.0	120	30%
chocolate chip	1 bar	4.0	120	30%
chocolate peanut butter	1 bar	4.0	120	30%
peanut butter & caramel				
candy	1 bar	3.5	100	32%
snack	1 bar	3.0	100	27%
Nutri-Grain (*See* (Kellogg's) in this section)				
(Quaker)				
Cereal bars				
apple cinnamon	1 bar	3.0	140	19%
blueberry	1 bar	3.0	140	19%
cherry cobbler	1 bar	3.0	140	19%
strawberry	1 bar	3.0	140	19%
very berry	1 bar	3.0	140	19%
chewy granola bar				
apple berry/low-fat	1 bar	2.0	110	16%
chocolate chip	1 bar	4.0	120	30%
chocolate chip graham slam	1 bar	2.0	110	16%
cookies 'n cream/low-fat	1 bar	2.5	110	20%
oatmeal raisin	1 bar	2.0	220	16%
peanut butter & chocolate chunk	1 bar	3.0	120	23%
peanut butter graham slam	1 bar	2.0	110	16%
s'mores/low-fat	1 bar	2.0	110	16%
(Slim Fast/Ultra Slim Fast)				
Breakfast & lunch bars				
Dutch chocolate	1 bar	5.0	140	26%
peanut butter	1 bar	6.0	150	36%
Energy snack bars				
crispy peanut caramel	1 bar	4.0	120	30%
peanut butter crunch	1 bar	4.0	130	28%
rich chewy caramel	1 bar	4.0	120	30%
Meal On-The-Go bars				
apple cobbler	1 bar	5.0	220	20%
chocolate cookie dough	1 bar	5.0	220	20%
honey peanut	1 bar	5.0	220	20%
milk chocolate peanut	1 bar	5.0	220	20%
oatmeal raisin	1 bar	5.0	220	20%
rich chocolate brownie	1 bar	5.0	220	20%
toasted oats and spice	1 bar	5.0	220	20%
(Sunbelt)				
chewy granola bar				
almond				
1-oz bar	1 bar	7.0	130	48%
apple cinnamon/low-fat	1 bar	2.5	140	16%

Food and Description	Amount	Fat Grams	Total Calories	% Fat Calories
chocolate chip				
fudge-dipped/1.5-oz bar	1 bar	10.0	200	45%
regular				
1.2-oz bar	1 bar	7.0	160	37%
1.76-oz bar	1 bar	13.0	260	45%
dates & honey	1 bar	5.0	120	38%
macaroon/fudge-dipped				
1.37-oz bar	1 bar	10.0	190	47%
2-oz bar	1 bar	16.0	280	51%
oatmeal raisin/low-fat	1 bar	2.5	130	17%
oats & honey				
1-oz bar	1 bar	5.0	120	38%
1.69-oz bar	1 bar	9.0	210	39%
w/peanuts/fudge-dipped	1 bar	9.0	200	41%
Fruit Cereal bars				
apple	1.3 oz	2.5	130	17%
blueberry	1.3 oz	2.5	130	17%
raspberry	1.3 oz	2.5	130	17%
strawberry	1.3 oz	2.5	130	17%
(Sweet Rewards) Fat-free snack bars				
blueberry w/drizzle	1 bar	–	120	–
homestyle brownie	1 bar	–	100	–
double fudge supreme	1 bar	–	110	–
raspberry	1 bar	–	120	–
strawberry	1 bar	–	120	–
GRAPE				
canned				
generic/Thompson seedless				
in heavy syrup	½ cup	–	94	–
in water	½ cup	–	48	–
(S&W)				
fancy jubilee/in heavy syrup	½ cup	–	130	–
Thompson/in heavy syrup	½ cup	–	100	–
fresh/with or without seeds				
Concord	10 grapes	<1.0	15	15%
	½ cup	<1.0	30	15%
(Dole)	1⅓ cups	–	85	–
muscat	10 grapes	<1.0	40	8%
	½ cup	<1.0	55	8%
Thompson	10 grapes	<1.0	40	8%
	½ cup	<1.0	55	8%
Tokay	10 grapes	<1.0	40	8%
	½ cup	<1.0	55	8%
GRAPE JUICE/JUICE BLEND				
bottled, boxed, or canned				
generic/bottled				
purple grape	6 fl oz	–	120	–
white grape	6 fl oz	–	110	–
(R.W. Knudsen)				
concord	8 fl oz	–	160	

Food and Description	Amount	Fat Grams	Total Calories	% Fat Calories
(Libby's) Juicy Juice/grape	4.23 fl oz	–	70	–
	8 fl oz	–	150	–
	8.45 fl oz	–	160	–
(Minute Maid) grape juice blend	8.45 fl oz	–	130	–
(Mott's)				
grape-apple blend	10 fl oz	–	170	–
(Season's Best) grape	8 fl oz	–	160	–
	10 fl oz	–	190	–
(Seneca)				
purple grape	8 fl oz	–	160	–
white grape	8 fl oz	–	160	–
(Welch's)				
Concord grape cocktail/Juicemakers unfrozen concentrate/prepared	8 fl oz	–	130	–
grape	10 fl oz	–	210	–
	11.5 fl oz	–	240	–
grape-apple	8 fl oz	–	150	–
purple grape	5.5 fl oz	–	120	–
	8 fl oz	–	170	–
Juicemakers	8 fl oz	–	170	–
red grape	8 fl oz	–	170	–
	8.45 fl oz	–	170	–
USDA grape	8 fl oz	–	170	–
white grape				
cranberry	8 fl oz	–	160	–
peach	8 fl oz	–	160	–
raspberry	8 fl oz	–	150	–
regular	5.5 fl oz	–	110	–
	8 fl oz	–	160	–
	8.45 fl oz	–	160	–
WIC	8 fl oz	–	170	–
frozen				
generic/grape/concentrate				
prepared	8 fl oz	–	130	–
undiluted	6 oz	–	395	–
(Seneca) prepared				
blush grape	8 fl oz	–	160	–
purple grape	8 fl oz	–	160	–
white grape	8 fl oz	–	140	–
(Sunkist)	6 fl oz	–	70	–
(Welch's) prepared				
100% grape	8 fl oz	–	160	–
purple grape				
regular	8 fl oz	–	170	–
sweetened	8 fl oz	–	130	–
red grape	8 fl oz	–	170	–
white grape				
regular	8 fl oz	–	170	–
sweetened	8 fl oz	–	140	–
white grape-cranberry	8 fl oz	–	150	–

Food and Description	Amount	Fat Grams	Total Calories	% Fat Calories
white grape-peach	8 fl oz	–	150	–
white grape-raspberry	8 fl oz	–	150	–
GRAPE JUICE DRINK (*See also* FRUIT PUNCH; SOFT DRINK, SOFT DRINK MIX)				
bottled, boxed, or canned				
(Bama)	8.45 fl oz	–	120	–
(Betty Crocker)Squeezit				
grumpy grape	1 bottle	–	110	–
100 Grape	1 bottle	–	90	–
(Capri Sun) pouch	6.75 fl oz	–	100	–
(Chiquita) grape-apple-raspberry liquid concentrate	1.6 fl oz	–	130	–
(Dole)	10 fl oz	–	150	–
(Fruitopia) The Grape Beyond	8 fl oz	–	127	–
(Hi-C)				
box	8.45 fl oz	–	130	–
can	7.7 fl oz	–	110	–
(Juicy Juice)	6 fl oz	–	90	–
	8.45 fl oz	–	130	–
(Minute Maid) grape juice beverage	8 fl oz	–	120	–
(Mott's) drink	10 fl oz	–	170	–
(Powerade)	8 fl oz	–	73	–
(Snapple) Grapeade	8 fl oz	–	120	–
(TreeTop) Juice Rivers grape punch	1 box	–	130	–
(Welch's)				
concord grape juice cocktail	8 fl oz	–	130	–
grape juice cocktail	8 fl oz	–	150	–
	10 fl oz	–	170	–
grape juice drink	8 fl oz	–	130	–
	8.45 fl oz	–	150	–
	10 fl oz	–	170	–
	11.5 fl oz	–	200	–
grape-apple juice cocktail	8 fl oz	–	150	–
grape-apple juice drink	8.45 fl oz	–	150	–
	10 fl oz	–	160	–
	11.5 fl oz	–	210	–
grape-peach juice cocktail	8 fl oz	–	130	–
	10 fl oz	–	160	–
	11.5 fl oz	–	180	–
sparkling red grape juice drink	8 fl oz	–	160	–
sparkling white grape juice drink	8 fl oz	–	160	–
Welchade	8 fl oz	–	130	–
white grape				
juice cocktail	8.45 fl oz	–	160	–
peach				
cocktail	8 fl oz	–	130	–
drink	10 fl oz	–	160	–
raspberry				
cocktail	8 fl oz	–	130	–
drink	10 fl oz	–	160	–
frozen/prepared				
(Mott's) fruit basket cocktail	8 fl oz	–	130	–

Food and Description	Amount	Fat Grams	Total Calories	% Fat Calories
(Seneca) cocktail	10 fl oz	–	130	–
(Welch's)				
juice cocktail/light	8 fl oz	–	50	–
orchard grape apple	8 fl oz	–	150	–
passion blended juice	8 fl oz	–	140	–
Welchade	8 fl oz	–	130	–
white grape				
juice cocktail	8 fl oz	–	140	–
peach juice blend	8 fl oz	–	150	–
raspberry juice blend	8 fl oz	–	150	–
GRAPE LEAVES				
(Alma)				
California	2 leaves	–	10	–
imported	2 leaves	–	10	–
(Fancifoods)	2 leaves	–	5	–
(Krinos)	1 leaf	–	10	–
GRAPE SODA (See SOFT DRINK)				
GRAPEFRUIT				
canned/sections				
generic				
in juice	½ cup	–	46	–
in light syrup	½ cup	–	76	–
in water	½ cup	–	44	–
(Nutradiet)	½ cup	–	40	–
(SW)				
in light syrup	½ cup	–	80	–
natural	⅔ cup	–	50	–
fresh/whole	½ medium	–	38	–
(Chiquita) ruby	½ medium	–	40	–
(Dole)	½ medium	–	50	–
(Ocean Spray)				
pink	½ medium	–	50	–
white	½ medium	–	45	–
GRAPEFRUIT JUICE/JUICE BLEND				
bottled, boxed, or canned				
(Dole) juice blend				
sunripe grapefruit/100%	8 fl oz	–	130	–
	10 fl oz	–	160	–
(Minute Maid)				
grapefruit	8 fl oz	–	100	–
pink grapefruit blend	8 fl oz	–	125	–
100% grapefruit	8 fl oz	–	100	–
(Mott's)	10 fl oz	–	120	–
(Ocean Spray)				
100%				
pink grapefruit	8 fl oz	–	110	–
white grapefruit juice	8 fl oz	–	100	–
ruby red				
& mango	8 fl oz	–	130	–
& tangerine grapefruit	8 fl oz	–	130	–

Food and Description	Amount	Fat Grams	Total Calories	% Fat Calories
(Season's Best)	8 fl oz	–	90	–
	10 fl oz	–	110	–
	11.5 fl oz	–	120	–
(Seneca)	8 fl oz	–	90	–
(S&W)	6 fl oz	–	80	–
	8 fl oz	–	100	–
(TreeTop)	8 fl oz	–	100	–
	10 fl oz	–	130	–
	11.5 fl oz	–	140	–
(Tropicana)				
pure premium				
golden	6 fl oz	–	80	–
	8 fl oz	–	90	–
ruby red	6 fl oz	–	70	–
	8 fl oz	–	100	–
	10 fl oz	–	120	–
ruby red-orange	8 fl oz	–	120	–
Twister				
pink grapefruit	8 fl oz	–	120	–
	10 fl oz	–	140	–
	11.5 fl oz	–	160	–
ruby red-cranberry	8 fl oz	–	120	–
	10 fl oz	–	150	–
(Welch's)	10 fl oz	–	130	–
	11.5 fl oz	–	150	–

GRAPEFRUIT JUICE DRINK (*See also* FRUIT PUNCH)
bottled, boxed, or canned

Food and Description	Amount	Fat Grams	Total Calories	% Fat Calories
(Dole) Pacific pink grapefruit	8 fl oz	–	140	
juice drink	16 fl oz	–	280	
(Ocean Spray) ruby red grapefruit				
juice drink	8 fl oz	–	130	
(Snapple Farms) pink grapefruit				
cocktail	12 fl oz	–	190	
(TreeTop) Desert Ice pink grapefruit				
juice cocktail	8 fl oz	–	120	

frozen/prepared

Food and Description	Amount	Fat Grams	Total Calories	% Fat Calories
(Dole) Pacific pink grapefruit				
juice drink	8 fl oz	–	140	
(Tropicana) Twister/light pink grapefruit				
juice drink	10 fl oz	–	40	

GRAPEFRUIT PEEL /candied — 1 oz | – | 90 | –

GRAVY (*See also* SAUCE; SEASONINGS)
■ **CANNED OR JARRED**

Food and Description	Amount	Fat Grams	Total Calories	% Fat Calories
(Franco-American)				
au jus	¼ cup	0.5	10	45%
beef				
fat-free	¼ cup	–	20	–
slow-roasted	¼ cup	–	20	–
regular	¼ cup	2.0	30	60%
slow-roasted	¼ cup	0.5	25	18%

Food and Description	Amount	Fat Grams	Total Calories	% Fat Calories
brown w/ onions	¼ cup	1.0	25	36%
chicken				
fat-free/slow-roasted	¼ cup	–	20	–
giblet	¼ cup	3.0	40	68%
regular	¼ cup	4.0	40	90%
slow-roasted	¼ cup	1.0	25	36%
mushroom	¼ cup	1.0	20	45%
pork	¼ cup	4.0	45	80%
turkey				
fat-free				
regular	¼ cup	–	20	–
slow-roasted	¼ cup	–	30	–
regular	¼ cup	1.0	25	36%
slow-roasted	¼ cup	1.0	30	30%
generic				
au jus	1 cup	0.5	38	12%
beef	1 cup	5.5	125	40%
brown	1 cup	4.0	100	36%
chicken	1 cup	14.0	190	66%
mushroom	1 cup	6.5	120	49%
turkey	1 cup	5.0	122	37%
(Heinz)				
au jus/bistro style	¼ cup	–	10	–
beef/homestyle				
regular	¼ cup	1.0	25	36%
w/onions	¼ cup	1.0	25	36%
brown/savory	¼ cup	1.0	25	36%
chicken				
classic	¼ cup	1.0	20	45%
fat-free	¼ cup	–	15	–
homestyle				
regular	¼ cup	2.0	35	51%
w/mushrooms & onions	¼ cup	2.0	35	51%
country				
blue ribbon	¼ cup	1.0	25	36%
homestyle	¼ cup	1.0	25	36%
mushroom				
homestyle				
regular	¼ cup	1.0	25	36%
rich	¼ cup	0.5	20	23%
original/rich	¼ cup	0.5	20	23%
pork/homestyle	¼ cup	1.0	25	36%
turkey				
fat-free	¼ cup	–	15	–
homestyle	¼ cup	1.0	25	36%
(Libby's)				
chicken	¼ cup	4.0	60	60%
sausage/country	¼ cup	6.0	80	68%
(Pepperidge Farm) 98% fat-free				
beef	¼ cup	1.0	25	3^%

Food and Description	Amount	Fat Grams	Total Calories	% Fat Calories
chicken				
cream of	¼ cup	1.0	30	30%
golden	¼ cup	1.0	25	36%
rotisserie flavor	¼ cup	1.0	25	36%
seasoned	¼ cup	1.0	30	30%
mushroom/country	¼ cup	0.5	30	15%
turkey	¼ cup	1.0	30	30%

■ **MIX** (Note: Unless stated otherwise, 1 serving of mix = the amount in ¼ cup prepared)

Food and Description	Amount	Fat Grams	Total Calories	% Fat Calories
(Durkee) mix/prepared				
au jus	1 serving	–	5	–
brown				
herb	1 serving	1.0	15	60%
mushroom	1 serving	–	15	–
onion	1 serving	–	10	–
original	1 serving	1.0	10	90%
chicken	1 serving	1.0	20	45%
country	1 serving	2.0	35	51%
homestyle	1 serving	1.0	10	90%
mushroom	1 serving	–	15	–
onion	1 serving	–	10	–
pork	1 serving	–	10	–
sausage	1 serving	2.0	35	51%
Swiss steak	1 serving	–	15	–
turkey	1 serving	–	20	–
(French's) mix/prepared				
au jus	1 serving	–	5	–
brown				
herb	1 serving	1.0	15	60%
original	1 serving	1.0	10	90%
chicken	1 serving	1.0	20	45%
country	1 serving	2.0	35	51%
homestyle	1 serving	1.0	10	90%
mushroom	1 serving	1.0	10	90%
onion	1 serving	1.0	15	60%
pork	1 serving	–	10	–
sausage	1 serving	2.0	35	51%
Swiss steak	1 serving	–	15	–
turkey	1 serving	–	20	–
generic/prepared				
au jus	1 cup	1.0	32	28%
brown	1 cup	2.0	80	23%
chicken	1 cup	2.0	85	21%
mushroom	1 cup	1.0	70	13%
pork	1 cup	2.0	75	24%
turkey	1 cup	2.0	90	20%
(Jimmy Dean) country/mix only	1 Tbs	2.0	40	45%
(Knorr) mix only				
au jus	⅕ pkg	–	15	–

Food and Description	Amount	Fat Grams	Total Calories	% Fat Calories
brown/classic	⅙ pkg	0.5	20	23%
brown & onion lyonnaise	⅕ pkg	0.5	20	23%
chicken	⅕ pkg	1.0	30	30%
hunter mushroom	⅕ pkg	1.0	25	36%
turkey	⅕ pkg	0.5	25	18%
(Lawry's) prepared				
beef	1 cup	1.5	80	17%
brown	1 cup	1.5	95	14%
chicken	1 cup	3.0	100	27%
turkey	1 cup	4.0	100	36%
(Loma Linda) Quik/mix only				
brown	1 Tbs	–	20	–
chicken	1 Tbs	–	20	–
country	1 Tbs	0.5	25	18%
mushroom	1 Tbs	–	15	–
onion	1 Tbs	–	20	–
(McCormick/Schilling) mix only				
au jus	½ tsp	–	5	–
brown				
herb	2 tsp	0.5	20	23%
regular	1 Tbs	0.5	20	23%
chicken	2 tsp	–	20	–
country				
regular	1⅓ Tbs	2.0	45	40%
sausage	4 tsp	1.5	40	34%
homestyle	1 Tbs	1.0	25	36%
mushroom	1 Tbs	0.5	20	23%
onion	2 tsp	0.5	20	23%
pork	1 Tbs	–	25	–
turkey	2 tsp	–	20	–
(Pillsbury) mix only				
brown	2 tsp	–	15	–
chicken	2 tsp	–	15	–
homestyle	2 tsp	–	15	–
GREAT NORTHERN BEAN				
canned				
(Bush's Best)	½ cup	–	70	–
(Eden)	½ cup	<1.0	110	4%
generic	½ cup	0.5	150	3%
(Green Giant)	½ cup	0.5	100	5%
(Joan of Arc)	½ cup	0.5	100	5%
(Luck's)				
mixed w/pinto beans	½ cup	0.5	130	3%
seasoned w/pork	½ cup	3.0	140	19%
(Seneca)	½ cup	0.5	150	3%
dry				
(Bean Cuisine)	½ cup	1.0	115	8%
generic/cooked	½ cup	0.5	105	4%

GREEK SOUP (*See* SOUP)

Food and Description	Amount	Fat Grams	Total Calories	% Fat Calories
GREEN BEAN/SNAP BEAN				
canned				
(Bush's Best)				
Blue Lake	½ cup	–	20	–
cut	½ cup	–	20	–
French style	½ cup	–	20	–
whole	½ cup	–	20	–
w/shelly beans	½ cup	–	35	–
(Del Monte)				
cut				
no salt added	½ cup	–	20	–
regular	½ cup	–	20	–
French style				
no salt added	½ cup	–	20	–
regular	½ cup	–	20	–
seasoned	½ cup	–	20	–
Italian cut	½ cup	–	30	–
whole	½ cup	–	20	–
(Festal)				
cut	½ cup	–	20	–
French style	½ cup	–	20	–
(Freshlike)				
cut	½ cup	–	20	–
French style				
in water/no salt	½ cup	–	20	–
no salt added	½ cup	–	20	–
no salt or sugar added	½ cup	–	20	–
regular	½ cup	–	20	–
generic	½ cup	–	22	–
(Green Giant)				
cut				
50% less sodium	½ cup	–	20	–
regular	½ cup	–	20	–
French style	½ cup	–	20	–
kitchen sliced				
50% less sodium	½ cup	–	20	–
regular	½ cup	–	20	–
(Joan of Arc)				
cut				
50% less sodium	½ cup	–	20	–
regular	½ cup	–	20	–
French style	½ cup	–	20	–
(Libby)				
cut	½ cup	–	20	–
French style	½ cup	–	20	–
whole	½ cup	–	20	–
(S&W)				
cut	½ cup	–	20	–
cut green & wax	½ cup	–	20	–

Food and Description	Amount	Fat Grams	Total Calories	% Fat Calories
dilled	½ cup	–	20	–
French style	½ cup	–	20	–
vertical pack	½ cup	–	20	–
whole	½ cup	–	20	–
(Seneca) all styles	½ cup	–	30	–
(Stokely)				
cut	½ cup	–	20	–
cut/no salt or sugar	½ cup	–	20	–
shellie	½ cup	–	45	–
(Veg-All)				
cut	½ cup	–	20	–
French	½ cup	–	20	–
fresh/raw	½ cup	–	20	–
frozen				
(Birds Eye)				
cut	½ cup	–	25	–
French cut	½ cup	–	25	–
Italian	½ cup	–	30	–
whole				
deluxe	½ cup	–	45	–
farm fresh	¾ cup	–	30	–
(C&W)				
French Cut				
microwave	3 oz	–	25	–
regular	⅔ cup	–	30	–
haricots verts/tiny whole	¾ cup	–	25	–
Italian cut/microwave or regular	¾ cup	–	25	–
petite whole	¾ cup	–	25	–
(Freshlike)				
French style	3 oz	–	25	–
Italian style	3 oz	–	30	–
whole	3 oz	–	25	–
generic	½ cup	–	25	–
(Green Giant)				
cut	¾ cup	–	25	–
Harvest Fresh/cut	⅔ cup	–	25	–
(Seneca) all styles	¾ cup	–	30	–
(Veg-All)				
French	3 oz	–	30	–
Italian	3 oz	–	30	–
whole	3 oz	–	25	–
GREEN ONION (See SCALLION)				
GRENADINE (See COCKTAIL MIXER)				
GRITS (See CORN GRITS)				
GROUND CHERRY				
raw	½ cup	0.5	37	12%
GROUPER				
cooked-dry heat	3 oz	1.0	100	9%
raw	3 oz	0.9	78	10%
GUACAMOLE (See DIP; SEASONINGS)				

Food and Description	Amount	Fat Grams	Total Calories	% Fat Calories
GUAVA/fresh	1 medium	0.5	45	10%
GUAVA, STRAWBERRY				
raw	1 medium	<1.0	4	8%
	1 cup	1.5	169	8%
GUAVA BUTTER	1 Tbs	–	39	–
GUAVA JUICE/JUICE BLEND (See also FRUIT JUICE/JUICE DRINK, MIXED)				
(Kern's) nectar	6 fl oz	–	110	–
(Knudsen) guava-strawberry	8 fl oz	–	110	–
(Libby's) nectar	6 fl oz	–	110	–
(Welch's) frozen, prepared	8 fl oz	–	140	–
GUAVA JUICE DRINK (See also FRUIT JUICE/JUICE DRINK, MIXED; FRUIT PUNCH; SOFT DRINK MIX)				
(Ocean Spray) Mauna Lai Hawaiian Guava Passion	8 fl oz	–	130	–
GUAVA SAUCE/cooked	½ cup	–	43	–
GUINEA HEN/raw				
meat & skin	1 lb	23.0	568	36%
meat only	3.5 oz	2.5	110	20%
GUINEA PIG/raw	3 oz	1.7	82	19%
GUM				
(Bazooka)				
bubble	1 piece	–	15	–
soft				
regular	1 piece	–	30	–
sugarless	1 piece	–	20	–
(Beech-Nut)				
peppermint	1 piece	–	10	–
spearmint	1 piece	–	10	–
(Bubble Yum) bubble gum				
mega	1 piece	–	25	–
sugar-free	1 piece	–	15	–
variety	1 piece	–	25	–
(Bubblicious) assorted	1 piece	–	25	–
(Carefree) sugarless				
bubble gum	1 piece	–	10	–
cinnamon	1 piece	–	5	–
peppermint	1 piece	–	5	–
spearmint	1 piece	–	5	–
variety	1 piece	–	10	–
wintergreen	1 piece	–	10	–
(Chiclets) peppermint	1 piece	–	5	–
(Clorets)	1 piece	–	5	–
(Dentyne)				
Cinnaburst	1 piece	–	10	–
cinnamon	1 piece	–	10	–
regular	1 piece	–	10	–
sugar free	1 piece	–	5	–
(Dubble Bubble) bubble gum	1 piece	–	20	–

Food and Description	Amount	Fat Grams	Total Calories	% Fat Calories
(Eclipse)				
spearmint	2 pieces	–	5	–
winterfresh	2 pieces	–	5	–
(Extra) sugar-free				
bubble gum				
classic	1 piece	–	5	–
original	1 piece	–	5	–
cinnamon	1 piece	–	5	–
peppermint	1 piece	–	5	–
spearmint	1 piece	–	5	–
winter fresh	1 piece	–	5	–
(Freedent)				
peppermint	1 stick	–	10	–
spearmint	1 stick	–	10	–
winterfresh	1 stick	–	10	–
(Fruit Stripe)				
assorted	1 piece	–	10	–
bubble	1 piece	–	10	–
(Hubba Bubba)				
blueberry	1 piece	–	20	–
cola	1 piece	–	20	–
grape				
regular	1 piece	–	20	–
sugar-free	1 piece	–	10	–
original				
regular	1 piece	–	20	–
sugar-free	1 piece	–	15	–
raspberry	1 piece	–	20	–
strawberry	1 piece	–	20	–
generic/candy-coated pieces	12 pieces	–	60	–
(Trident)				
assorted	1 piece	–	5	–
cinnamon	1 piece	–	5	–
fresh mint	1 piece	–	5	–
original	1 piece	–	5	–
spearmint	1 piece	–	5	–
(Wrigley's)				
Big Red	1 stick	–	10	–
Doublemint	1 stick	–	10	–
Juicy Fruit	1 stick	–	10	–
spearmint	1 stick	–	10	–
winter fresh	1 stick	–	10	–

GUMBO (See SOUP; SEASONINGS)

Food and Description	Amount	Fat Grams	Total Calories	% Fat Calories
HADDOCK (*See also* SEAFOOD DINNER/ENTRÉE)				
breaded & fried	3 oz	9.7	194	45%
cooked-dry heat	3 oz	0.8	95	8%
raw	3 oz	0.6	74	7%
smoked	3 oz	0.8	99	7%
HAKE (*See* WHITING)				
HALIBUT (*See also* SEAFOOD DINNER/ENTRÉE)				
Atlantic & Pacific				
batter-fried	3 oz	6.0	153	35%
broiled w/butter	3 oz	6.0	140	39%
cooked-dry heat	3 oz	2.5	119	19%
raw	3 oz	2.0	93	19%
smoked	3 oz	12.7	190	60%
Greenland				
raw	3 oz	12.0	160	68%
HAM (*See also* LUNCHEON MEAT; PORK; TURKEY)				
(Alpine Lace) cooked	2 oz	2.0	60	30%
(DAK) Danish/sliced	2 oz	1.0	40	23%
(Dubuque) canned patties	1 patty	11.0	140	71%
(Eckrich)				
Lean Supreme				
honey-smoked	1 slice	1.0	30	30%
Virginia baked	1 slice	0.5	30	15%
zip pack				
honey & clove	1 slice	1.0	30	30%
Virginia	1 slice	1.0	30	30%
(Fletcher's) Black Forest				
4% fat/fully cooked	3 oz	3.0	100	27%
generic				
cured				
boneless				
extra lean & regular				
cold	1 oz	2.0	45	40%
cold/chopped or diced	1 cup	10.5	230	41%
roasted	3 oz	6.5	140	42%
roasted/chopped or diced	1 cup	10.5	230	41%
extra lean/5% fat				
cold	1 oz	1.0	35	26%
cold/chopped or diced	1 cup	6.0	185	29%
roasted	3 oz	4.0	125	32%
roasted/chopped or diced	1 cup	7.0	200	32%

Food and Description	Amount	Fat Grams	Total Calories	% Fat Calories
regular/11% fat				
cold	1 oz	3.0	50	54%
cold/chopped or diced	1 cup	13.5	255	48%
roasted	3 oz	7.5	150	45%
roasted/chopped or diced	1 cup	12.5	250	45%
whole				
lean				
cold	1 oz	1.5	40	34%
cold/chopped or diced	1 cup	7.0	210	30%
roasted	3 oz	4.0	135	27%
roasted/chopped or diced	1 cup	7.0	220	29%
lean & fat				
cold	1 oz	5.0	70	64%
cold/chopped or diced	1 cup	24.0	345	63%
roasted	3 oz	13.5	210	58%
roasted/chopped or diced	1 cup	22.0	340	58%
canned				
4% fat				
cold	1 oz	1.0	35	26%
cold/chopped or diced	1 cup	6.0	170	32%
roasted	3 oz	4.0	115	31%
roasted/chopped or diced	1 cup	6.5	190	31%
13% fat				
cold	1 oz	3.5	55	57%
cold/chopped or diced	1 cup	16.5	265	56%
roasted	3 oz	12.0	195	55%
roasted/chopped or diced	1 cup	19.5	320	55%
extra lean & regular				
cold	1 oz	2.0	40	45%
cold/chopped or diced	1 cup	9.5	200	43%
roasted	3 oz	6.5	145	40%
roasted/chopped or diced	1 cup	11.0	235	47%
country style center slice/lean &	1 oz	3.5	60	53%
fat/cold	4 oz	13.5	230	53%
patties, grilled	1 patty	17.5	205	77%
steak/extra lean/cold	2 oz	2.0	70	26%
(Healthy Choice) deli meats				
cooked	2 oz	1.5	60	23%
honey	2 oz	1.5	60	23%
smoked	2 oz	1.5	60	23%
Virginia	2 oz	1.5	60	23%
(Hillshire Farm)				
ham/10-oz pkg				
cooked	1 oz	1.0	30	30%
lower salt	1 oz	1.0	30	30%
honey	1 oz	1.0	35	26%
(Hormel)				
chunk ham	2 oz	6.0	90	60%
ham				
Black Label				
canned	3 oz	4.5	100	41%

Food and Description	Amount	Fat Grams	Total Calories	% Fat Calories
chopped				
regular	2 oz	11.0	140	71%
sweet	2 oz	11.0	140	71%
Cure 8½ ham	3 oz	4.5	100	41%
Curemaster	3 oz	3.0	80	34%
deli cooked	2 oz	2.5	60	38%
Light & Lean	2 oz	2.0	50	36%
Primissimo/proscuitti ham	2 oz	7.0	120	53%
Spiral Cure 81 half ham	3 oz	9.0	150	54%
Supreme Cut/canned				
1.5-lb ham	2 oz	3.0	60	45%
3-lb ham	2 oz	3.0	60	45%
patties				
ham	1 patty	16.0	180	80%
ham & cheese	1 patty	17.0	180	85%
(Jone's Dairy Farm)				
Country Carved	3 oz	4.0	100	36%
Ham steak	3 oz	4.0	100	36%
(Kahn's) 97% fat free	1 oz	1.0	30	30%
(Louis Rich) baked cooked dinner slices	1 slice	1.5	80	17%
(Oscar Mayer)				
dinner slices	3 oz	3.0	80	34%
dinner steaks	1 steak	2.0	60	30%
Sweet Morsel smoked boneless	3 oz	15.0	180	75%
(Owens) Ham steak				
1 steak	4 oz	4.0	120	30%
2 slices	1.64 oz	1.5	50	27%
(Russer)				
baked	2 oz	3.0	70	39%
Canadian brand maple	2 oz	2.0	70	26%
honey cured	2 oz	3.0	60	45%
honey & maple cured	2 oz	2.0	70	26%
light smoked	2 oz	2.0	60	39%
smoked Virginia	2 oz	3.0	70	39%
(Schwan's) Haugin's Farm/frozen	2 oz	2.0	60	30%
HAM & CHEESE SPREAD	1 Tbs	2.8	37	68%
HAM SALAD (*See also* LUNCHEON MEAT)				
generic	1 Tbs	2.0	32	56%
	1 oz	4.0	61	59%

HAM SPREAD (*See* LUNCHEON MEAT SPREAD)
HAMBURGER (*See also* BEEF; BEEF DISH/ENTRÉE; BUFFALO; FROZEN ENTRÉE/DINNER; TURKEY; VEGETARIAN FOODS; individual FAST FOOD listings)

frozen or refrigerated				
(Hormel) Quick Meal				
bacon w/cheese	1 burger	22.0	420	47%
cheese	1 burger	20.0	400	45%
plain	1 burger	20.0	350	51%
(Jimmy Dean)				
burger	1 burger	21.0	220	86%
flamed-broiled cheeseburger	1 burger	34.0	540	57%

Food and Description	Amount	Fat Grams	Total Calories	% Fat Calories
mini beef w/cheese	2 burgers	14.0	270	47%
(Simplot) Micro Magic				
cheeseburger	1 burger	21.0	410	46%
plain	1 burger	15.0	340	40%
(White Castle)				
cheeseburger	2 burgers	17.0	310	49%
plain	2 burgers	14.0	270	47%
HASH (See BEEF DISH/ENTRÉE; SAUSAGE DISH; TURKEY ENTRÉE/DINNER)				
HAZELNUT (See also FILBERT)				
(Diamond of California)				
chopped	¼ cup	18.0	200	81%
shelled 1 oz	~22 nuts	18.0	200	81%
HAZELNUT BUTTER/SPREAD				
(Ferrero) Nutella chocolate	1 Tbs	5.0	85	53%
(Roaster Fresh) hazelnut butter	2 Tbs	19.0	200	85%
HERBS (See SEASONINGS; individual listings)				
HERRING (See also HERRING ROE)				
Atlantic				
breaded & fried	3 oz	18.0	279	58%
canned/in tomato sauce	2 oz	6.0	100	54%
cooked-dry heat	3 oz	9.9	172	52%
dried	1 oz	5.0	72	63%
kippered	~1.5 oz	5.0	87	51%
pickled	~½ oz	2.7	39	62%
	3 oz	15.0	220	61%
raw	3 oz	7.7	134	52%
(Lascco) chilled				
sour cream fillet	2 oz	7.0	120	53%
spice cut	2 oz	6.0	110	49%
wine snacks	2 oz	5.0	100	45%
(Nathan's) snacks in wine sauce	¼ cup	4.0	90	40%
Pacific				
cooked-dry heat	3 oz	15.0	215	63%
raw	3 oz	11.8	166	64%
HERRING ROE/raw	3 oz	1.7	111	14%
HICKORY NUT				
dried/shelled	1 oz	18.0	187	87%
HOKI/raw	3.5 oz	0.8	74	10%
HOLLANDAISE SAUCE (See SAUCE)				
HOMINY (See also CORN GRITS)				
canned				
(Allen's)				
golden	½ cup	<1.0	120	4%
Mexican	½ cup	1.0	120	8%
white	½ cup	<1.0	100	5%
(Goya)				
golden	½ cup	–	120	–
white	½ cup	0.5	100	5%
(Sun Vista)				
golden	½ cup	–	70	–

Food and Description	Amount	Fat Grams	Total Calories	% Fat Calories
white	½ cup	0.5	65	7%
(Van Camp's)				
golden	½ cup	1.0	80	11%
white	½ cup	1.0	80	11%
HOMINY GRITS (See CORN GRITS)				
HONEY				
(Bee Maid)				
cinnamon	1 Tbs	–	70	–
natural/creamed	1 Tbs	–	60	–
regular	1 Tbs	–	60	–
(Burleson's)				
clover	1 Tbs	–	60	–
creamed	1 Tbs	–	60	–
natural	1 Tbs	–	60	–
raw	1 Tbs	–	60	–
Rocky Mountain Clover	1 Tbs	–	60	–
generic	1 Tbs	–	64	–
	½ cup	–	512	–
(Golden Blossom)	1 tsp	–	20	–
	1 Tbs	–	60	–
(Knott's Berry Farm)	1 Tbs	–	60	–
	1 oz	–	90	–
(Sioux)	1 Tbs	–	60	–
(Tree of Life)				
alfalfa	1 Tbs	–	60	–
buckwheat	1 Tbs	–	60	–
clover	1 Tbs	–	60	–
honeybear wildflower	1 Tbs	–	60	–
orange	1 Tbs	–	60	–
tupelo	1 Tbs	–	60	–
wildflower	1 Tbs	–	60	–
HONEY BUTTER				
(Downey's)				
cinnamon	1 Tbs	1.0	50	18%
original	1 Tbs	1.0	50	18%
HONEYDEW MELON /fresh				
cut up	1 cup	<1.0	50	9%
(Chiquita) cubed	1 cup	–	70	–
whole	¹⁄₁₀ melon	<1.0	47	10%
(Dole)	¹⁄₁₀ melon	–	50	–
HORSE /meat only				
roasted	4 oz	7.0	200	32%
roasted/chopped	1 cup	3.0	245	11%
HORSERADISH (See also SAUCE)				
fresh/raw	1 oz	–	18	–
jarred				
(Gold's) hot	1 tsp	–	4	–
(Hebrew National)				
red	1 Tbs	–	7	–
	½ cup	–	25	–

Food and Description	Amount	Fat Grams	Total Calories	% Fat Calories
white	1 Tbs	–	7	–
	½ cup	–	25	–
(Kraft)				
cream style	1 tsp	–	–	–
mustard	1 tsp	–	–	–
prepared	1 tsp	–	–	–
sauce	1 tsp	1.5	20	7%
(Rosoff's)				
red	1 Tbs	–	8	–
white	1 Tbs	–	7	–

HOT CROSS BUN (*See* PASTRY)
HOT DOG (*See* FRANKFURTER; individual FAST FOOD listings)
HUMMUS (*See also* DIP)

homemade/USDA Standard Home Recipe	1 cup	21.0	420	45%
mix				
(Casbah) prepared	¼ cup	5.0	120	38%

HUNTER'S SOUP (*See* SOUP)
HUSHPUPPY (*See* BREAD)
HYACINTH BEAN

mature				
boiled	½ cup	0.6	114	4%
raw	½ cup	2.0	350	5%
immature	½ cup	–	20	–

I

Food and Description	Amount	Fat Grams	Total Calories	% Fat Calories

ICE CREAM & ICE CREAM-LIKE FROZEN DESSERTS (*See also* FRUIT ICES, BARS, & POPS; ICE CREAM BARS, SANDWICHES, & FROZEN NOVELTIES; RICE FROZEN DESSERT; SHERBET; TOFU FROZEN DESSERT; YOGURT, FROZEN)

■ **(Baskin-Robbins)**

Blasts				
non-fat				
cappuccino	8 oz	–	90	–
chocolate	8 oz	–	170	–
mocha cappuccino	8 oz	–	120	–
regular				
cappuccino w/whipped cream	8 oz	7.0	160	39%
chocolate w/whipped cream	8 oz	7.0	250	26%
mocha cappy w/whipped cream	8 oz	6.0	180	30%

Food and Description	Amount	Fat Grams	Total Calories	% Fat Calories
Deluxe				
banana strawberry	½ cup	7.0	130	48%
Baseball Nut	½ cup	9.0	160	51%
black walnut	½ cup	11.0	160	62%
blueberry cheesecake	⅓ cup	8.0	150	48%
cherries jubilee	½ cup	7.0	140	45%
chocolate	½ cup	8.0	150	48%
chocolate almond	½ cup	11.0	180	55%
chocolate chip	½ cup	10.0	150	60%
chocolate chip cookie dough	½ cup	9.0	170	48%
chocolate fudge	½ cup	9.0	160	45%
chocolate mousse royale	½ cup	10.0	170	53%
chocolate raspberry truffle	½ cup	9.0	180	45%
chocolate ribbon	½ cup	7.0	140	45%
Chunky Heath Bar	½ cup	10.0	170	53%
cookies 'n cream	½ cup	10.0	160	56%
eggnog	½ cup	8.0	150	48%
English toffee	½ cup	9.0	160	51%
French vanilla	½ cup	10.0	160	56%
fudge brownie	½ cup	11.0	170	58%
German chocolate cake	½ cup	10.0	180	50%
Gold Medal Ribbon	½ cup	8.0	150	48%
Here Comes the Fudge	½ cup	7.0	150	42%
Jamoca	½ cup	9.0	140	58%
Jamoca almond fudge	½ cup	9.0	160	51%
lemon custard	½ cup	8.0	150	48%
mint chocolate chip	½ cup	10.0	150	60%
Oregon blackberry	½ cup	8.0	140	51%
pistachio-almond	½ cup	12.0	170	64%
pralines 'n cream	½ cup	9.0	160	51%
pumpkin pie	½ cup	7.0	130	48%
Quarterback Crunch	½ cup	10.0	160	56%
Reese's peanut butter	½ cup	11.0	180	55%
rocky road	½ cup	10.0	170	53%
rum raisin	½ cup	7.0	140	45%
strawberry shortcake	½ cup	9.0	160	51%
triple chocolate passion	½ cup	11.0	180	55%
vanilla	½ cup	8.0	140	51%
very berry strawberry	½ cup	7.0	130	48%
winter white chocolate	½ cup	9.0	150	54%
world class chocolate	½ cup	9.0	160	51%
Fat-free				
berry innocent cheese	½ cup	–	110	–
check it out cherry	½ cup	–	100	–
chocolate vanilla twist	½ cup	–	100	–
Jamoca swirl	½ cup	–	110	–
FroZone Kids Flavors				
Dirt'n worms	½ cup	8.0	160	45%
Errie I scream	½ cup	8.0	150	48%
Neon sour apple ice	½ cup	–	110	–

Food and Description	Amount	Fat Grams	Total Calories	% Fat Calories
Pear paws	½ cup	10.0	160	56%
Pink bubblegum	½ cup	8.0	150	48%
Skullicious	½ cup	10.0	170	53%
Watermelon ice	½ cup	–	110	–
Low-fat				
espresso 'n cream	½ cup	2.5	100	23%
No sugar added				
call Me Nuts	½ cup	2.0	110	16%
cherry cordial	½ cup	2.0	100	18%
mad about chocolate	½ cup	2.0	100	18%
pineapple coconut	½ cup	1.5	90	15%
thin mint	½ cup	2.5	100	23%
■ (Ben & Jerry's)				
Low-fat				
Blondies are a Swirls Best Friend	½ cup	2.0	200	9%
coconut cream pie	½ cup	2.5	160	14%
Mocha Latte	½ cup	2.0	150	12%
S'mores	½ cup	2.0	190	9%
Original				
Bavinity Divinity	½ cup	18.0	290	56%
Cherry Garcia	½ cup	16.0	260	55%
chocolate chip cookie dough	½ cup	16.0	300	48%
chocolate fudge brownie	½ cup	15.0	280	48%
Chubby Hubby	½ cup	21.0	350	54%
Chunky Monkey	½ cup	19.0	310	55%
Coffee Heath Bar Crunch	½ cup	18.0	310	52%
Dilbert's World Totally Nuts	½ cup	21.0	310	61%
mint w/chocolate cookie	½ cup	17.0	280	55%
New York super fudge chunk	½ cup	21.0	320	59%
Nutty Waffle Cone	½ cup	19.0	310	55%
orange & cream	½ cup	14.0	230	55%
peanut butter cup	½ cup	25.0	380	59%
Phish Food	½ cup	14.0	300	42%
Pistachio Pistachio	½ cup	15.0	240	56%
Southern Pecan Pie	½ cup	19.0	290	59%
Triple Caramel Chunk	½ cup	17.0	290	53%
Vanilla caramel fudge	½ cup	17.0	300	51%
Vanilla Heath Bar Crunch	½ cup	19.0	310	55%
Wavy Gravy	½ cup	20.0	340	53%
World's Best Vanilla	½ cup	16.0	250	58%
Special Batch				
Coffee Hazelnut Swirl	½ cup	19.0	280	61%
2-Twisted ice cream				
Entangled Mints	½ cup	17.0	290	53%
Everything But the O	½ cup	19.0	320	53%
From Russia w/Buzz	½ cup	18.0	280	58%
Half Baked	½ cup	15.0	290	47%
Jerry's Jubilee	½ cup	14.0	260	49%
Monkey Wrench	½ cup	20.0	310	58%
Pulp Addiction	½ cup	13.0	240	49%

Food and Description	Amount	Fat Grams	Total Calories	% Fat Calories
Urban jumble	½ cup	21.0	310	61%
■ **(Borden's)**				
Fat-free				
black cherry	½ cup	–	90	–
chocolate	½ cup	–	100	–
peach	½ cup	–	90	–
strawberry	½ cup	–	90	–
vanilla	½ cup	–	90	–
Olde Fashioned				
Dutch chocolate	½ cup	6.0	130	42%
strawberries'n cream	½ cup	5.0	130	35%
vanilla	½ cup	7.0	130	37%
Regular				
buttered pecan	½ cup	12.0	180	60%
chocolate swirl	½ cup	6.0	130	42%
strawberry	½ cup	6.0	130	42%
Sundae Cone	1 cone	12.0	210	51%
■ **(Breyers)**				
All Natural				
butter almond	½ cup	11.0	160	62%
butter pecan	½ cup	12.0	170	64%
calcium rich natural vanilla	½ cup	7.0	130	48%
caramel praline crunch	½ cup	9.0	170	48%
cherry vanilla	½ cup	7.0	140	45%
chocolate	½ cup	9.0	160	51%
chocolate chip	½ cup	10.0	170	53%
chocolate chip cookie dough	½ cup	10.0	180	50%
chocolate chocolate chip	½ cup	10.0	180	50%
coffee	½ cup	9.0	140	58%
cookies in cream	½ cup	9.0	170	48%
Dulce de Leche	½ cup	7.0	160	39%
French vanilla	½ cup	10.0	160	56%
mint chocolate chip	½ cup	10.0	170	53%
natural cherry vanilla	½ cup	8.0	140	51%
natural peach	½ cup	6.0	130	42%
natural strawberry	½ cup	7.0	130	48%
natural vanilla	½ cup	9.0	150	54%
rocky road	½ cup	9.0	180	45%
vanilla/chocolate/strawberry	½ cup	8.0	140	51%
vanilla fudge twirl	½ cup	8.0	150	48%
All Natural Light				
French chocolate	½ cup	5.0	150	30%
French vanilla	½ cup	4.0	120	30%
mint chocolate chip	½ cup	5.0	140	32%
natural vanilla	½ cup	3.0	120	23%
pralines & caramel	½ cup	3.5	140	23%
rocky road	½ cup	4.5	140	29%
strawberry	½ cup	2.5	110	20%
vanilla-chocolate-strawberry	½ cup	3.0	120	23%

Food and Description	Amount	Fat Grams	Total Calories	% Fat Calories
Breyer's Rainbow				
chocolate rainbow	½ cup	7.0	140	45%
fruit rainbow	½ cup	8.0	140	51%
Fat-free				
vanilla	½ cup	–	90	–
Homemade				
butter pecan	½ cup	11.0	170	58%
double chocolate fudge	½ cup	8.0	170	42%
fudge brownie	½ cup	9.0	180	45%
neapolitan	½ cup	8.0	150	48%
vanilla	½ cup	8.0	140	51%
Ice Cream Parlor				
apple pie w/cinnamon	½ cup	8.0	160	51%
banana split	½ cup	9.0	180	45%
black forest	½ cup	6.0	150	36%
candy bar sundae	½ cup	8.0	170	42%
Chips Ahoy! Chocolate chip cookie	½ cup	8.0	160	45%
coffee & cream	½ cup	8.0	150	48%
double chocolate malt	½ cup	7.0	160	39%
English toffee	½ cup	8.0	180	40%
Hershey's chocolate w/almonds	½ cup	8.0	170	42%
ice cream sandwich	½ cup	7.0	160	39%
marble mint chip	½ cup	8.0	170	42%
Mississippi Mud	½ cup	9.0	180	45%
Oreo cookies & cream	½ cup	8.0	160	45%
raspberry cobbler	½ cup	7.0	150	42%
Reese's peanut butter cups	½ cup	9.0	180	45%
Strawberry shortcake	½ cup	6.0	160	34%
Light Ice Cream				
vanilla	½ cup	4.5	130	31%
No sugar added				
vanilla	½ cup	4.5	90	45%
vanilla fudge twirl	½ cup	4.5	100	41%
vanilla/chocolate/strawberry	½ cup	5.0	90	45%
Viennetta				
chocolate	1 slice	12.0	190	57%
mint	1 slice	11.0	190	52%
vanilla	1 slice	11.0	190	52%
■ (Cascadian Farm) Organic Premium Ice Cream Pints				
banana chocolate nut	½ cup	17.0	230	67%
brownies and cream	½ cup	12.0	200	54%
butter pecan	½ cup	17.0	230	67%
cappuccino	½ cup	11.0	175	57%
double chocolate	½ cup	11.0	195	51%
lava nut crunch	½ cup	13.0	200	59%
vanilla	½ cup	12.0	180	60%
vanilla caramel almond	½ cup	12.0	210	51%
■ (Dreamery)				
Banana Boogie	½ cup	17.0	290	53%
black raspberry avalanche	½ cup	14.0	250	50%

Food and Description	Amount	Fat Grams	Total Calories	% Fat Calories
Blue Ribbon Berry Pie	½ cup	13.0	260	45%
Caramel toffee bar heaven	½ cup	14.0	270	47%
Cashew Praline Parfait	½ cup	13.0	260	45%
chocolate peanut butter chunk	½ cup	18.0	310	52%
chocolate truffle explosion	½ cup	15.0	280	48%
cool mint	½ cup	14.0	280	45%
creme caramel	½ cup	12.0	260	42%
Cuppa Joe	½ cup	13.0	230	51%
Galactic Chocolate Swirl	½ cup	12.0	280	39%
Grandma's Cookie Jar	½ cup	14.0	270	47%
harvest peach	½ cup	11.0	220	45%
Hot Chilly Chili	½ cup	14.0	260	48%
New York strawberry cheesecake	½ cup	13.0	250	47%
Nuts About Malt	½ cup	15.0	280	48%
sticky bun	½ cup	14.0	270	47%
vanilla	½ cup	15.0	260	52%
■ (Dreyer's)				
fat-free				
blueberry cobbler/no sugar added	½ cup	–	100	–
caramel praline crunch	½ cup	–	110	–
chocolate fudge				
no sugar added	½ cup	–	100	–
regular	½ cup	–	120	–
chocolate peanut butter chunk	½ cup	–	120	–
coffee fudge/no sugar added	½ cup	–	100	–
cookie chunk	½ cup	–	110	–
raspberry marble chunk	½ cup	–	110	–
raspberry vanilla swirl/no sugar added	½ cup	–	90	–
vanilla				
no sugar added	½ cup	–	90	–
regular	½ cup	–	100	–
vanilla chocolate swirl/no sugar added	½ cup	–	100	–
vanilla 'n caramel/no sugar added	½ cup	–	100	–
Grand				
light				
butter pecan	½ cup	5.0	120	38%
chocolate fudge mousse	½ cup	4.0	120	30%
Chocolate Raspberry Escape	½ cup	4.0	120	30%
coffee mousse crunch	½ cup	4.0	120	30%
cookie dough	½ cup	4.0	120	30%
cookies 'n cream	½ cup	4.0	120	30%
crazy for caramel	½ cup	4.0	120	30%
espresso fudge chip	½ cup	4.0	120	30%
French silk	½ cup	4.0	120	30%
mint chocolate chips	½ cup	4.0	120	30%
peanut butter cups	½ cup	5.0	130	35%
rocky road	½ cup	4.0	120	30%
S'Mores & More	½ cup	4.0	130	28%
vanilla	½ cup	3.0	100	27%

Food and Description	Amount	Fat Grams	Total Calories	% Fat Calories
low-fat				
chocolate fudge chunk	½ cup	2.0	110	16%
cookies 'n cream	½ cup	2.0	110	16%
espresso chip	½ cup	2.0	100	18%
Heath toffee & caramel	½ cup	2.0	120	15%
rocky road	½ cup	2.0	110	16%
vanilla	½ cup	2.0	100	18%
no sugar added (also see Fat-Free section)				
All About PB	½ cup	6.0	130	42%
butter pecan	½ cup	5.0	110	41%
chips'N swirls	½ cup	3.0	100	27%
double fudge brownie	½ cup	3.0	100	27%
strawberry	½ cup	3.0	90	30%
triple chocolate	½ cup	3.0	100	27%
vanilla	½ cup	3.0	90	30%
regular				
almond praline	½ cup	8.0	170	42%
black cherry vanilla	½ cup	7.0	160	39%
butter pecan	½ cup	10.0	160	56%
chocolate	½ cup	8.0	150	48%
Chocolate Chips!	½ cup	9.0	170	48%
coffee	½ cup	8.0	140	51%
cookie dough	½ cup	9.0	170	48%
cookies 'n cream	½ cup	8.0	150	45%
double fudge brownie	½ cup	7.0	150	42%
Dulce de Leche	½ cup	9.0	160	51%
French vanilla	½ cup	10.0	160	56%
ice cream sandwich	½ cup	4.0	120	30%
Mint Chocolate Chips!	½ cup	9.0	170	48%
mocha almond fudge	½ cup	9.0	170	48%
Neapolitan	½ cup	7.0	140	45%
real strawberry	½ cup	6.0	130	42%
rocky road	½ cup	10.0	170	53%
toasted almond	½ cup	9.0	150	54%
triple chocolate thunder	½ cup	9.0	160	51%
vanilla	½ cup	10.0	150	56%
vanilla bean	½ cup	8.0	140	51%
Homemade Ice Cream				
all natural vanilla	½ cup	7.0	130	48%
apple pie a la mode	½ cup	6.0	140	39%
brownies a la mode	½ cup	7.0	150	42%
caramel peanut brittle	½ cup	7.0	160	39%
chocolate chip cookie jar	½ cup	9.0	170	48%
chocolate cream pie	½ cup	9.0	170	48%
double chocolate chunk	½ cup	9.0	170	48%
eggnog & cream	½ cup	7.0	140	45%
old fashioned butter pecan	½ cup	10.0	160	56%
strawberries & cream	½ cup	6.0	120	45%
vanilla custard	½ cup	8.0	140	51%

Food and Description	Amount	Fat Grams	Total Calories	% Fat Calories
Limited Edition				
baseball sundae	½ cup	8.0	170	42%
blackberry pie Grand light	½ cup	4.0	110	33%
checkered flag sundae	½ cup	9.0	160	51%
Chunky Top Funilla	½ cup	9.0	170	48%
50/50 Bar Grand light	½ cup	2.5	100	23%
Gingerbread Man Grand Light	½ cup	4.0	120	30%
Girl Scouts				
Samoas Cookie	½ cup	8.0	170	42%
Tagalongs Cookie	½ cup	5.0	130	35%
Thin Mint Cookie	½ cup	10.0	170	53%
Halloween Bash	½ cup	8.0	160	45%
Infinity Divinity Grand Light	½ cup	4.0	120	30%
NFL peanut butter blitz	½ cup	10.0	170	53%
peppermint	½ cup	8.0	150	48%
peppermint Grand Light	½ cup	4.0	120	30%
pumpkin	½ cup	7.0	140	45%
■ **(Edy's)**				
fat-free				
blueberry cobbler/no sugar added	½ cup	–	100	–
caramel praline crunch	½ cup	–	110	–
chocolate fudge				
no sugar added	½ cup	–	100	–
regular	½ cup	–	110	–
chocolate peanut butter chunk	½ cup	–	120	–
coffee fudge/no sugar added	½ cup	–	100	–
cookie chunk	½ cup	–	110	–
raspberry marble chunk	½ cup	–	110	–
raspberry vanilla swirl/no sugar added	½ cup	–	90	–
vanilla				
no sugar added	½ cup	–	90	–
regular	½ cup	–	100	–
vanilla chocolate swirl/no sugar added	½ cup	–	100	–
vanilla 'n caramel/no sugar added	½ cup	–	100	–
Grand				
light				
butter pecan	½ cup	5.0	120	38%
chocolate fudge mousse	½ cup	4.0	120	30%
Chocolate Raspberry Escape	½ cup	4.0	120	30%
coffee mousse crunch	½ cup	4.0	120	30%
cookie dough	½ cup	4.0	120	30%
cookies 'n cream	½ cup	4.0	120	30%
crazy for caramel	½ cup	4.0	120	30%
espresso fudge chip	½ cup	4.0	120	30%
French silk	½ cup	4.0	120	30%
Mint chocolate chips!	½ cup	4.0	120	30%
Peanut butter cups!	½ cup	5.0	130	35%
rocky road	½ cup	4.0	120	30%
S'Mores & More	½ cup	4.0	130	28%
vanilla	½ cup	3.0	100	27%

Food and Description	Amount	Fat Grams	Total Calories	% Fat Calories
no sugar added (also see Fat-Free section)				
All About PB	½ cup	6.0	130	42%
butter pecan	½ cup	5.0	110	41%
chips'N swirls	½ cup	3.0	100	27%
double fudge brownie	½ cup	3.0	100	27%
strawberry	½ cup	3.0	90	30%
triple chocolate	½ cup	3.0	100	27%
vanilla	½ cup	3.0	90	30%
regular				
black cherry vanilla	½ cup	7.0	140	45%
butter pecan	½ cup	10.0	160	56%
chocolate	½ cup	8.0	150	48%
Chocolate Chips!	½ cup	9.0	170	48%
chocolate fudge mousse	½ cup	8.0	160	45%
chocolate fudge sundae	½ cup	9.0	170	48%
coffee	½ cup	8.0	140	51%
cookie dough	½ cup	9.0	170	48%
cookies 'n cream	½ cup	8.0	160	45%
double fudge brownie	½ cup	7.0	170	37%
Dulce de Leche	½ cup	7.0	150	42%
Espresso chip	½ cup	8.0	150	48%
French vanilla	½ cup	10.0	160	56%
ice cream sandwich	½ cup	8.0	160	45%
Mint Chocolate Chips!	½ cup	9.0	170	48%
real strawberry	½ cup	6.0	130	42%
rocky road	½ cup	10.0	170	53%
triple chocolate thunder	½ cup	9.0	160	51%
vanilla	½ cup	8.0	140	51%
vanilla bean	½ cup	8.0	140	51%
vanilla chocolate	½ cup	8.0	150	48%
vanilla chocolate strawberry	½ cup	7.0	140	45%
Homemade Ice Cream				
all natural vanilla	½ cup	7.0	130	48%
apple pie a la mode	½ cup	6.0	140	39%
brownies a la mode	½ cup	7.0	150	42%
caramel peanut brittle	½ cup	7.0	160	39%
chocolate chip cookie jar	½ cup	9.0	170	48%
chocolate cream pie	½ cup	9.0	170	48%
double chocolate chunk	½ cup	9.0	170	48%
eggnog & cream	½ cup	7.0	140	45%
old fashioned butter pecan	½ cup	10.0	160	56%
strawberries & cream	½ cup	6.0	120	45%
vanilla custard	½ cup	8.0	140	51%
Limited Edition				
baseball sundae	½ cup	8.0	170	42%
blackberry pie Grand light	½ cup	4.0	110	33%
checkered flag sundae	½ cup	9.0	160	51%
Chunky Top Funilla	½ cup	9.0	170	48%
50/50 Bar Grand light	½ cup	2.5	100	23%
Gingerbread Man Grand Light	½ cup	4.0	120	30%

Food and Description	Amount	Fat Grams	Total Calories	% Fat Calories
Girl Scouts				
Samoas Cookie	½ cup	8.0	170	42%
Tagalongs Cookie	½ cup	5.0	130	35%
Thin Mint Cookie	½ cup	10.0	170	53%
Halloween Bash	½ cup	8.0	160	45%
Infinity Divinity Grand Light	½ cup	4.0	120	30%
NFL peanut butter blitz	½ cup	10.0	170	53%
peppermint	½ cup	8.0	150	48%
peppermint Grand Light	½ cup	4.0	120	30%
pumpkin	½ cup	7.0	140	45%
■ (Eskimo Pie) reduced-fat				
butter pecan	½ cup	7.0	140	45%
chocolate marshmallow	½ cup	4.0	130	28%
fudge ripple	½ cup	4.0	120	30%
neapolitan	½ cup	4.0	110	33%
vanilla				
plain	½ cup	4.0	110	33%
w/cookie wafers	½ cup	4.0	160	23%
■ (Haagen-Dazs)				
Ice Cream Shops/low-fat				
coffee fudge	½ cup	2.5	170	13%
cookies & fudge	½ cup	2.5	180	13%
Ice Cream Shops/regular				
Baileys Irish Cream	½ cup	17.0	270	57%
Belgian chocolate chocolate	½ cup	21.0	330	57%
Brownies a la Mode	½ cup	16.0	280	51%
butter pecan	½ cup	22.0	300	66%
Cappuccino Commotion	½ cup	21.0	310	61%
chocolate	½ cup	17.0	260	59%
chocolate chocolate chip	½ cup	19.0	300	57%
chocolate chocolate mint	½ cup	20.0	300	60%
chocolate Swiss almond	½ cup	20.0	300	60%
coffee	½ cup	17.0	250	61%
coffee mocha chip	½ cup	18.0	270	60%
cookies & cream	½ cup	17.0	270	57%
Cookie dough Dynamo	½ cup	20.0	310	58%
deep chocolate peanut butter	½ cup	24.0	350	62%
Dulce de leche caramel	½ cup	16.0	270	53%
macadamia brittle	½ cup	19.0	280	61%
macadamia nut	½ cup	24.0	320	68%
mint chip	½ cup	18.0	280	58%
pineapple coconut	½ cup	13.0	230	51%
pistachio	½ cup	19.0	280	61%
pralines & cream	½ cup	17.0	280	55%
rum raisin	½ cup	17.0	260	59%
strawberry	½ cup	16.0	250	58%
vanilla	½ cup	17.0	250	61%
vanilla chocolate chip	½ cup	19.0	290	59%
vanilla Swiss almond	½ cup	20.0	290	62%

Food and Description	Amount	Fat Grams	Total Calories	% Fat Calories
Retail Market				
low-fat				
chocolate	½ cup	2.5	170	13%
coffee fudge	½ cup	2.5	170	13%
strawberry	½ cup	2.0	150	12%
vanilla	½ cup	2.5	170	13%
regular				
butter pecan	½ cup	23.0	310	67%
cherry vanilla	½ cup	15.0	240	56%
chocolate	½ cup	18.0	270	60%
chocolate, chocolate chip	½ cup	20.0	300	60%
chocolate, chocolate fudge	½ cup	18.0	290	56%
coffee	½ cup	18.0	270	60%
coffee mocha chip	½ cup	19.0	290	59%
cookies & cream	½ cup	17.0	270	57%
cookie dough chip	½ cup	20.0	310	58%
creme caramel pecan	½ cup	20.0	320	56%
Dulce de leche caramel	½ cup	17.0	290	53%
macadamia brittle	½ cup	20.0	300	60%
mango	½ cup	14.0	250	50%
mint chip	½ cup	19.0	300	57%
pineapple coconut	½ cup	13.0	230	51%
pistachio	½ cup	20.0	290	62%
rum raisin	½ cup	17.0	270	57%
strawberry	½ cup	16.0	250	58%
vanilla	½ cup	18.0	270	60%
vanilla chocolate chip	½ cup	20.0	310	58%
vanilla fudge	½ cup	18.0	290	56%
vanilla Swiss almond	½ cup	20.0	300	60%
sorbet & cream				
orange	½ cup	9.0	200	41%
raspberry	½ cup	9.0	190	43%
■ **(Healthy Choice)**				
butter pecan crunch	½ cup	2.0	120	15%
cappuccino chocolate chunk	½ cup	2.0	120	15%
cappuccino mocha crunch	½ cup	2.0	120	15%
cherry chocolate chunk	½ cup	2.0	110	16%
chocolate chocolate chunk	½ cup	2.0	120	15%
coconut cream pie	½ cup	2.0	120	15%
cookie creme de mint	½ cup	2.0	130	14%
cookies 'n cream	½ cup	2.0	120	15%
fudge brownie	½ cup	2.0	120	15%
mint chocolate chip	½ cup	2.0	120	15%
old fashioned blueberry hill	½ cup	2.0	120	15%
old fashioned butterscotch blonde	½ cup	2.0	140	13%
old fashioned cherry vanilla	½ cup	2.0	120	15%
old fashioned strawberry	½ cup	2.0	110	16%
peanut butter cup	½ cup	2.0	110	16%
praline caramel cluster	½ cup	2.0	130	14%

Food and Description	Amount	Fat Grams	Total Calories	% Fat Calories
rocky road	½ cup	2.0	140	13%
turtle fudge cake	½ cup	2.0	130	14%
vanilla	½ cup	2.0	100	18%
vanilla bean	½ cup	2.0	110	16%
wild raspberry truffle	½ cup	2.0	120	15%
■ (Hood's)				
Fat-free				
chocolate passion	½ cup	–	100	–
classic harlequin	½ cup	–	100	–
double brownie sundae	½ cup	–	120	–
heavenly hash	½ cup	–	120	–
Mississippi mud pie	½ cup	–	130	–
praline pecan delight	½ cup	–	120	–
raspberry blush	½ cup	–	120	–
super strawberry swirl	½ cup	–	100	–
vanilla fudge twist	½ cup	–	120	–
very vanilla	½ cup	–	100	–
Light				
almond praline delight	½ cup	5.0	110	41%
brownie nut sundae	½ cup	5.0	140	32%
Caribbean coffee royale	½ cup	4.0	110	33%
chocolate almond chip	½ cup	5.0	150	32%
chocolate, chocolate chip cookie dough	½ cup	5.0	140	32%
cookies 'n cream	½ cup	4.0	130	28%
Heath Toffee chunk swirl	½ cup	5.0	140	32%
heavenly hash	½ cup	4.0	130	28%
maple sugar shack	½ cup	4.0	130	28%
Massachusetts mud pie	½ cup	5.0	140	32%
raspberry swirl	½ cup	3.0	120	23%
strawberry supreme	½ cup	3.0	110	25%
triple nut cluster sundae	½ cup	5.0	140	32%
vanilla	½ cup	4.0	110	33%
vanilla, chocolate, strawberry	½ cup	4.0	110	33%
Low-fat/No sugar added				
caramel swirl	½ cup	3.0	120	23%
chocolate supreme	½ cup	3.0	120	23%
mocha fudge	½ cup	3.0	110	25%
raspberry swirl	½ cup	3.0	110	25%
vanilla	½ cup	3.0	100	27%
Traditional				
caramel butterscotch blast	½ cup	8.0	160	45%
chocolate	½ cup	7.0	140	37%
chocolate chip	½ cup	9.0	160	51%
coffee	½ cup	7.0	140	37%
cookie dough delight	½ cup	8.0	160	45%
cookies 'n cream	½ cup	8.0	160	45%
egg nog	½ cup	6.0	130	42%
grasshopper pie	½ cup	7.0	160	39%
heavenly hash	½ cup	6.0	140	39%
maple walnut	½ cup	9.0	160	51%

Food and Description	Amount	Fat Grams	Total Calories	% Fat Calories
spumoni	½ cup	9.0	140	58%
strawberry	½ cup	7.0	130	48%
vanilla	½ cup	7.0	140	37%
vanilla chocolate patchwork	½ cup	7.0	140	37%
vanilla chocolate strawberry	½ cup	7.0	140	37%
vanilla fudge	½ cup	6.0	140	39%
■ (Kemp's)				
Fat-free				
caramel praline	½ cup	–	120	–
French silk chocolate	½ cup	–	100	–
fudge marble	½ cup	–	110	–
turtle fudge brownie	½ cup	–	120	–
vanilla	½ cup	–	90	–
Light				
Vanilla				
1 gal tub	½ cup	3.0	100	27%
5 gal tub	½ cup	3.5	120	26%
half gallon carton	½ cup	3.0	100	27%
Premium				
almond praline	½ cup	8.0	160	45%
Bear Tracks	½ cup	9.0	170	48%
butter pecan	½ cup	11.0	170	58%
cookies 'n cream	½ cup	9.0	170	48%
chocolate chip	½ cup	10.0	170	53%
Chocolate Monster	½ cup	8.0	170	42%
Mocha Madness	½ cup	8.0	160	45%
natural vanilla	½ cup	8.0	150	48%
northern exposure	½ cup	11.0	190	52%
old fashioned vanilla	½ cup	8.0	150	48%
vanilla	½ cup	7.0	130	48%
premium fat-free				
caramel nutty crunch	½ cup	0.5	120	4%
fudge marble	½ cup	–	110	–
heavenly hash	½ cup	–	120	–
mint fudge brownie	½ cup	–	110	–
vanilla	½ cup	–	100	–
■ (Lactaid)				
cappuccino swirl	½ cup	8.0	180	40%
classic vanilla	½ cup	9.0	160	51%
creamy butter pecan	½ cup	12.0	190	57%
double chocolate chip	½ cup	10.0	180	50%
mint chocolate chip	½ cup	10.0	170	53%
■ (Mocha Mix)				
Berry Berry Berry	½ cup	6.0	140	39%
Dutch chocolate	½ cup	8.0	140	51%
mocha almond fudge	½ cup	8.0	150	48%
neapolitan	½ cup	7.0	140	45%
strawberry swirl	½ cup	6.0	140	39%
vanilla	½ cup	7.0	140	45%

Food and Description	Amount	Fat Grams	Total Calories	% Fat Calories
■ **(Schwan's)**				
Fat-free/no sugar added ice cream				
strawberry	½ cup	–	70	–
vanilla	½ cup	–	70	–
Low-fat ice cream				
butter crunch	½ cup	3.0	110	25%
praline almondine sundae	½ cup	2.5	120	19%
vanilla	½ cup	2.0	100	18%
Premium ice cream				
banana fudge ripple	½ cup	6.0	140	39%
blackjack cherry	½ cup	8.0	160	45%
butter crunch	½ cup	8.0	150	48%
butter pecan	½ cup	9.0	150	54%
cherry nut	½ cup	7.0	140	45%
cherry vanilla	½ cup	7.0	140	45%
chip & mint	½ cup	8.0	150	48%
chocolate	½ cup	7.0	140	45%
chocolate almond	½ cup	8.0	150	48%
chocolate chip	½ cup	8.0	150	48%
chocolate chip cookie dough	½ cup	8.0	150	48%
chocolate chunk	½ cup	8.0	150	48%
chocolate double fudge brownie	½ cup	7.0	160	45%
chocolate fudge ripple	½ cup	7.0	140	45%
chocolate malt twist	½ cup	7.0	160	45%
chocolate marshmallow ripple	½ cup	6.0	140	39%
Chunky Chocolate Peanut Butter Binge	½ cup	12.0	190	57%
cookies & cream	½ cup	8.0	160	45%
dark sweet cherry	½ cup	6.0	140	39%
honey caramel cashew	½ cup	8.0	170	42%
maple nut	½ cup	9.0	150	54%
mocha almond fudge	½ cup	9.0	170	48%
neapolitan	½ cup	7.0	140	45%
peaches & cream	½ cup	5.0	130	35%
pecan caramel quke (?)	½ cup	9.0	180	45%
pecan praline sundae	½ cup	7.0	150	42%
raspberry rumble	½ cup	8.0	160	45%
rocky road	½ cup	7.0	150	42%
strawberry	½ cup	7.0	140	45%
Summer's Dream	½ cup	5.0	130	35%
vanilla	½ cup	7.0	140	45%
■ **(Starbuck's)**				
Low-fat				
latte	½ cup	3.0	170	16%
mocha mambo	½ cup	3.0	170	16%
Original				
cafe almond fudge	½ cup	13.0	260	45%
cafe biscotti bliss	½ cup	12.0	240	45%
dark roast espresso	½ cup	10.0	220	41%
Italian roast coffee	½ cup	12.0	230	47%
java chip	½ cup	13.0	250	47%

Food and Description	Amount	Fat Grams	Total Calories	% Fat Calories
vanilla mocha chip	½ cup	16.0	270	53%
■ (Sweet 'N Low)				
Fat-free				
chocolate	½ cup	–	70	–
strawberry	½ cup	–	70	–
vanilla	½ cup	–	70	–
■ (Tofutti) Non-dairy				
Low-Fat Supreme				
chocolate fudge	½ cup	2.0	120	15%
coffee marshmallow swirl	½ cup	1.0	100	9%
peach mango	½ cup	1.0	100	9%
strawberry banana	½ cup	1.0	100	9%
vanilla fudge	½ cup	2.0	120	15%
Premium				
better pecan	½ cup	13.0	220	53%
chocolate cookie crunch	½ cup	11.0	210	47%
chocolate supreme	½ cup	11.0	180	55%
vanilla	½ cup	11.0	190	52%
vanilla almond bark	½ cup	13.0	210	56%
vanilla fudge	½ cup	9.0	190	43%
wildberry supreme	½ cup	9.0	190	43%
Three Gallon Bulk Cans				
chocolate supreme	½ cup	11.0	180	55%
vanilla	½ cup	11.0	190	52%
vanilla almond bark	½ cup	13.0	210	56%
wildberry supreme	½ cup	9.0	190	43%
■ (Weight Watchers)				
Cookie Dough Craze	½ cup	3.5	140	23%
Oh! So Very Vanilla	½ cup	2.5	120	19%
Positively Praline Crunch	½ cup	3.0	140	19%
Triple Chocolate Tornado	½ cup	3.5	150	21%

ICE CREAM BARS, SANDWICHES, & FROZEN NOVELTIES (See also FRUIT ICES, BARS, & POPS; RICE FROZEN DESSERT; SHERBET; TOFU FROZEN DESSERT)

Food and Description	Amount	Fat Grams	Total Calories	% Fat Calories
■ (Baskin-Robbins)				
Chillyburger				
chocolate chip	1 piece	11.0	220	45%
mint chocolate chip	1 piece	11.0	220	45%
fountain ice-cream drink				
Cappy Blast w/whipped cream	1 drink	10.0	290	31%
Mocha Cappy Blast w/whipped cream	1 drink	11.0	330	30%
vanilla malt	1 drink	31.0	660	42%
sundae bar				
Jamoca almond fudge	1 bar	17.0	280	55%
peanut butter chocolate	1 bar	27.0	340	71%
pralines 'n cream	1 bar	17.0	280	55%
Tiny Toon bar				
chocolate chip	1 bar	17.0	240	64%
mint chocolate chip	1 bar	17.0	240	64%
vanilla	1 bar	16.0	210	69%

Food and Description	Amount	Fat Grams	Total Calories	% Fat Calories
■ (Ben & Jerry's)				
novelties				
cookie dough	1 pop	24.0	410	53%
Phish Stick	1 pop	18.0	290	56%
S'Mores	1 pop	19.0	330	52%
Totally Nuts	1 pop	29.0	370	71%
vanilla	1 pop	22.0	330	60%
vanilla Heath Bar crunch	1 pop	14.0	330	38%
■ (Breyers)				
Cups				
Cappuccino	½ cup	11.0	190	52%
triple chocolate	½ cup	12.0	180	60%
vanilla	½ cup	11.0	190	52%
vanilla snack size	2.64 oz	15.0	240	56%
Caramel magnum bar	1 bar	22.0	360	55%
Strawberry magnum bar	1 bar	21.0	360	52%
Viennetta				
cappuccino/vanilla	1 piece	11.0	190	52%
triple chocolate	1 piece	12.0	110	98%
vanilla				
2.4 oz	1 piece	11.0	190	52%
2.6 oz	1 piece	15.0	240	56%
■ CARNATION (See (Nestlé) in this section)				
■ (Chiquita)				
fruit & cream bar				
banana	1 bar	2.0	80	23%
blueberry	1 bar	1.0	80	11%
peach	1 bar	1.0	80	11%
raspberry	1 bar	1.0	80	11%
strawberry	1 bar	1.0	80	11%
strawberry-banana	1 bar	2.0	80	23%
■ (Dove)				
bar				
almond				
4 per pkg/3-oz bars	1 bar	19.0	280	61%
individual pkg/3.67-oz bar	1 bar	24.0	350	62%
caramel creme swirl/toffee chips/ 3-oz bar	1 bar	16.0	280	51%
chocolate w/dark chocolate coating				
4 per pkg/3-oz bars	1 bar	17.0	260	59%
individual pkg/3.67-oz bar	1 bar	21.0	330	57%
mocha cashew crunch	1 bar	17.0	260	59%
peppermint w/dark chocolate	1 bar	17.0	290	53%
vanilla				
w/dark chocolate coating				
4 per pkg/3-oz bars	1 bar	17.0	260	43%
individual pkg/3.67-oz bar	1 bar	21.0	330	57%
w/milk chocolate coating				
4 per pkg/3-oz bars	1 bar	17.0	260	43%
individual pkg/3.67-oz bar	1 bar	21.0	330	57%

Food and Description	Amount	Fat Grams	Total Calories	% Fat Calories
w/white coating/3-oz bar	1 bar	17.0	270	57%
bite-size				
cherry royale	5 pieces	21.0	340	56%
double chocolate	5 pieces	23.0	360	58%
eggnog w/dark chocolate	5 pieces	22.0	350	57%
vanilla				
classic	5 pieces	24.0	360	60%
French	5 pieces	23.0	370	56%
seasonal				
green mint & chocolate fudge truffle swirl bar w/dark chocolate coating/3-oz bar	1 bar	17.0	290	53%
Irish creme cordial/bite-size	5 pieces	22.0	340	58%
party peppermint/bite-size	5 pieces	22.0	360	55%
▦ (Eskimo Pie)				
Bars				
chocolate chip w/dark choc coating	1 bar	12.0	180	60%
fudge				
chocolate	1 bar	1.0	60	15%
chocolate vanilla	1 bar	1.0	60	15%
original vanilla				
w/dark chocolate coating	1 bar	11.0	160	62%
w/milk chocolate coating	1 bar	12.0	180	60%
w/dark chocolate coating	1 bar	12.0	180	60%
reduced-fat vanilla				
w/crispy rice	1 bar	8.0	120	60%
w/dark chocolate	1 bar	8.0	120	60%
Ice Cream Cones reduced-fat				
vanilla w/chocolate & peanuts	1 bar	12.0	210	51%
Ice Cream Sandwiches				
Arctic Madness	1 round	16.0	260	55%
Nabisco Snackwell's	1 sandwich	1.5	90	15%
Oreo Big Stuff	1 sandwich	10.0	240	38%
original	1 sandwich	6.0	180	30%
Pudding Bars/variety pack	1 bar	1.5	90	15%
▦ (Good Humor)				
Ice cream bar				
Candy center crunch	1 bar	23.0	300	69%
chocolate eclair bar	3 oz bar	7.0	150	42%
Col. Crunch				
chocolate eclair	1 bar	7.0	150	42%
strawberry	1 bar	8.0	160	45%
cookies'n cream bar	3 oz bar	10.0	190	47%
original	1 bar	13.0	230	51%
premium	1 bar	15.0	240	56%
Reese's peanut butter bar	4 oz bar	19.0	310	55%
	3 oz bar	16.0	250	58%
strawberry shortcake	4 oz bar	10.0	220	41%
	3 oz bar	8.0	160	45%

Food and Description	Amount	Fat Grams	Total Calories	% Fat Calories
toasted almond	4 oz bar	12.0	230	47%
	3 oz bar	10.0	180	50%
Ice cream cone				
American Glory	1 cone	16.0	280	51%
king cone/vanilla	1 cone	14.0	270	47%
Ice cream cups				
Cookies'n cream	1 cup	16.0	300	48%
Ice cream sandwich				
chocolate chip cookie	1 sandwich	15.0	320	42%
giant Neapolitan	1 sandwich	10.0	250	36%
giant vanilla	1 sandwich	9.0	250	32%
Good Humor	1 sandwich	6.0	180	30%
premium cookie	1 sandwich	11.0	290	34%
Specialty				
Number 1 bar	1 bar	11.0	190	52%
Snoopy bar	1 bar	8.0	150	48%
Sprinklers	1 bar	8.0	180	40%
WWF bar	1 bar	10.0	200	45%
Sundae Twist cup/lowfat	1 cup	2.5	160	14%
Variety pack				
dark chocolate	3 oz bar	13.0	180	65%
ice cream cone	4 oz cone	16.0	270	53%
milk chocolate	3 oz bar	12.0	180	60%
sandwich	3 oz sandwich	5.0	160	28%
shortcake bar	2.7 oz	7.0	150	42%
■ (Haagen-Dazs)				
Ice Cream Shops				
Coated				
chocolate & dark chocolate	1 bar	24.0	350	62%
coffee & almond crunch	1 bar	27.0	370	66%
vanilla & almonds	1 bar	28.0	380	64%
vanilla & milk chocolate	1 bar	24.0	340	64%
Uncoated				
chocolate	1 bar	13.0	200	59%
coffee	1 bar	13.0	190	62%
vanilla	1 bar	13.0	190	62%
Retail Stores				
Multipack Bars				
chocolate almond	1 bar	22.0	310	64%
chocolate & dark chocolate	1 bar	20.0	290	62%
chocolate peanut butter swirl	1 bar	23.0	320	65%
coffee & almond crunch	1 bar	22.0	310	64%
cookies & cream crunch	1 bar	22.0	310	64%
Dulce De Leche caramel	1 bar	19.0	300	57%
vanilla & almonds	1 bar	23.0	320	65%
vanilla & dark chocolate	1 bar	20.0	280	64%
vanilla & milk chocolate	1 bar	20.0	280	64%
Single Pack Bars				
chocolate & almonds	1 bar	27.0	380	64%
chocolate & dark chocolate	1 bar	24.0	350	62%

Food and Description	Amount	Fat Grams	Total Calories	% Fat Calories
coffee & almond crunch	1 bar	27.0	370	66%
cookies & cream crunch	1 bar	26.0	370	63%
Dulce de Leche caramel	1 bar	24.0	370	58%
tropical coconut	1 bar	24.0	340	64%
vanilla & almonds	1 bar	28.0	380	66%
vanilla & dark chocolate	1 bar	24.0	350	62%
vanilla & milk chocolate	1 bar	24.0	340	64%
Sorbet & Vanilla Ice Cream				
orange	1 bar	5.0	120	38%
strawberry	1 bar	5.0	110	41%
▩ (Kemps)				
Bar	1 bar	12.0	160	68%
Cookie crunch Jr.				
2.6 oz	1 bar	7.0	100	63%
3 oz	1 bar	8.0	120	60%
Toffee Jr's	1 bar	9.0	120	68%
Ice Cream Cones/vanilla mini	1 cone	10.0	160	56%
Sandwich/vanilla				
mini	1 sandwich	4.0	100	36%
regular	1 sandwich	6.0	170	32%
▩ (Klondike)				
almond bar	1 bar	21.0	310	61%
candy bar swirl	1 bar	21.0	320	59%
Big Bear				
bar				
vanilla	1 bar	17.0	480	32%
cone				
caramel	1 cone	21.0	370	51%
fudge	1 cone	21.0	370	51%
sundae	1 cone	27.0	450	54%
vanilla	1 cone	21.0	350	54%
sandwich				
chocolate chip cookie	7 oz sandwich	21.0	520	36%
neapolitan	4.23 oz sandwich	7.0	200	32%
	7 oz sandwich	11.0	300	33%
vanilla	4.23 oz sandwich	7.0	200	32%
	7 oz sandwich	10.0	290	31%
Heath	1 bar	20.0	300	60%
Ice cream Kone	1 kone	17.0	310	49%
Kombo Kones				
caramel	1 kone	18.0	340	48%
fudge	1 kone	18.0	340	48%
Krunchy bar	1 bar	17.0	270	57%
original ice cream bar	1 bar	20.0	290	62%
sundae cup	1 cup	17.0	280	55%

Food and Description	Amount	Fat Grams	Total Calories	% Fat Calories
Tacos				
Choco Taco	4 oz taco	15.0	200	68%
cookies'n cream	1 taco	15.0	300	45%
■ **(M&M *Mars)**				
Milky Way				
chocolate/milk chocolate/singles				
reduced fat/2-oz bar	1 bar	7.0	140	45%
stick/3-oz bar	1 bar	13.0	220	53%
vanilla/dark chocolate/singles				
reduced fat/2-oz bar	1 bar	7.0	140	45%
stick/3-oz bar	1 bar	13.0	220	53%
Snickers				
bar	1 bar	12.0	190	57%
ice cream cone	1 cone	15.0	290	47%
singles/2-oz bar	1 bar	13.0	200	59%
snack	4 bars	25.0	390	58%
3 Musketeers				
chocolate				
singles/2.75 oz-bar	1 bar	11.0	190	47%
6 per pkg, 2-oz bars	1 bar	9.0	150	54%
vanilla				
singles/2.75 oz bar	1 bar	11.0	190	52%
6 per pkg, 2-oz bars	1 bar	8.0	140	51%
■ **MILKY WAY** (*See* (M&M*Mars) in this section)				
■ **(Nestlé)**				
Bon Bons				
dark chocolate	5 pieces	13.0	190	62%
	8 pieces	21.0	310	61%
	9 pieces	24.0	350	62%
milk chocolate	5 pieces	14.0	200	63%
	8 pieces	23.0	330	63%
	9 pieces	26.0	370	63%
Butterfinger	1 bar	12.0	170	64%
Carnation strawberry sundae cup	6 oz	8.0	200	36%
Cool Creations				
cookies & cream	1 sandwich	11.0	240	41%
Lion King	1 cone	14.0	280	45%
Mickey Mouse bar	2.5 oz	7.0	110	57%
	4 oz	11.0	170	58%
mini sandwich	1 sandwich	5.0	110	41%
Crunch				
bar				
Crunch King	4 oz	19.0	270	63%
ice cream bar				
chocolate	3 oz	14.0	200	63%
vanilla	3 oz	14.0	200	63%
reduced fat	2.5 oz	7.0	130	48%
cone	1 cone	16.0	300	48%
nuggets	8 nuggets	20.0	300	60%

Food and Description	Amount	Fat Grams	Total Calories	% Fat Calories
Drumstick				
chocolate	1 cone	19.0	340	50%
chocolate dipped	1 cone	17.0	340	45%
vanilla	1 cone	20.0	350	51%
vanilla caramel	1 cone	20.0	360	50%
vanilla fudge	1 cone	21.0	370	51%
Flintstones				
cool cream	2.75 oz	2.0	90	20%
push-up				
Pebbles treats	1 pop	6.0	120	45%
sherbet treats	1 pop	2.0	100	18%
Heath Bar	1 bar	12.0	160	68%
■ **(Popsicle)**				
Big Bear				
Sundae cone	1 cone	27.0	450	54%
vanilla bar	1 bar	29.0	480	54%
Creamsicle				
no sugar added				
cherry	1 bar	–	25	–
grape	1 bar	–	25	–
orange	1 bar	–	25	–
Original				
orange	1 bar	3.0	110	25%
raspberry	1 bar	3.0	110	25%
Pop				
orange	1 pop	2.0	80	23%
raspberry	1 pop	2.0	80	23%
Fudge Pop	1 pop	1.0	60	15%
Fudgsicle				
banana bananaza	1 bar	–	60	–
chocolate	1 bar	1.5	120	11%
chocolate vanilla swirl	1 bar	1.5	120	11%
fat-free	1 bar	–	60	–
no sugar added	1 bar	0.5	45	10%
original				
bar	1 bar	1.5	90	15%
pop	1 pop	1.0	60	15%
vanilla	1 bar	2.0	120	15%
Heath bar	1 bar	20.0	300	60%
Kones				
Kombo				
caramel	1 kone	18.0	340	48%
fudge	1 kone	18.0	340	48%
milk chocolate coating	1 cone	17.0	310	49%
Krunch bar	1 bar	17.0	270	57%
Rainbow chocolate pops	1 pop	9.0	130	62%
Sprinklers	1 bar	6.0	130	42%
Sundae cup	1 cup	17.0	280	55%
Tacos				
Choco	1 taco	15.0	300	45%

Food and Description	Amount	Fat Grams	Total Calories	% Fat Calories
cookies'n cream	1 taco	15.0	300	45%
■ (Schwan's)				
Bar				
Caramel Apple Treats	1 bar	1.0	80	11%
chocolate sundae crunch	1 bar	9.0	180	45%
double crunch	1 bar	21.0	260	73%
English toffee	1 bar	14.0	200	57%
fudge stick	1 bar	1.5	110	12%
Gold 'n Nugit	1 bar	16.0	250	58%
Krispie Krunch	1 bar	8.0	120	60%
peanut stick	1 bar	14.0	200	62%
Premium	1 bar	15.0	210	64%
rainbow stick	1 bar	1.0	90	10%
raspberry cordial	1 bar	13.0	210	56%
root beer float	1 bar	2.0	80	21%
Silver Mint	1 bar	10.0	160	56%
strawberry crunch	1 bar	9.0	180	45%
Trim Creations chocolate fudge stick	1 bar	–	50	–
Cone				
chip & min sundae	1 cone	11.0	260	38%
pecan praline sundae	1 cone	12.0	270	40%
rocky road sundae	1 cone	12.0	260	42%
vanilla	1 cone	10.0	210	47%
vanilla fudge chocolate sundae	1 cone	11.0	260	38%
Healthy Creations/Fat-free				
raspberry and orange	1 bar	–	70	–
strawberry kiwi and tropical	1 bar	–	60	–
Ice cream cup				
lemon freeze	½ cup	–	130	–
root beer	1 cup	7.0	270	37%
sundae				
chocolate	1 cup	5.0	120	38%
confetti	1 cup	7.0	140	45%
strawberry	1 cup	5.0	120	38%
vanilla	1 cup	6.0	110	49%
Push-Ems				
Bubble gum	1	1.0	100	9%
candy core	1	1.0	110	8%
chocolate malt	1	2.5	90	25%
orange sherbet	1	1.0	90	10%
strawberry shake	1	2.5	90	25%
Sandwich				
cherry cheesecake	1 sandwich	7.0	190	33%
chocolate chip cookie	1 sandwich	12.0	260	42%
Mississippi mud	1 sandwich	8.0	200	36%
vanilla	1 sandwich	7.0	170	34%

■ SNICKERS (*See* (M&M * Mars) in this section)
■ 3 MUSKETEERS (*See* (M&M * Mars) in this section)

Food and Description	Amount	Fat Grams	Total Calories	% Fat Calories
■ (Weight Watchers)				
Bars				
chocolate mousse	1 bar	1.0	40	23%
chocolate treat	1 bar	1.5	100	14%
English toffee crunch	1 bar	6.0	110	49%
mocha java	1 bar	1.5	80	17%
orange vanilla treat	1 bar	0.5	40	11%
Sandwich/vanilla ice cream	1 sandwich	3.0	150	18%
Sundae				
chocolate chip cookie dough	1 sundae	4.5	190	21%
ICE CREAM CONES & CUPS				
(Baskin-Robbins) cones				
sugar	1 cone	1.0	60	15%
waffle				
fresh-baked	1 cone	2.0	140	13%
large	1 cone	1.5	120	11%
(Colosso)				
bowl	1 bowl	1.0	73	12%
cone	1 cone	1.5	98	14%
(Comet)				
cones				
Oreo chocolate	1 cone	1.0	50	18%
sugar	1 cone	–	40	–
Teddy Grahams cinnamon	1 cone	1.0	50	18%
waffle	1 cone	1.0	70	13%
cups	1 cup	–	40	–
(Delicious Brand)				
Cone/sugar	1 cone	–	45	–
Cups				
Cake				
jumbo	1 cup	–	25	–
rainbow	1 cup	–	20	–
regular	1 cup	–	20	–
(Dutch Mill) chocolate covered	1 cone	5.0	80	56%
(Frookie)				
chocolate	1 cone	0.5	50	9%
honey crunch	1 cone	0.5	45	10%
(Joy)				
cones				
classic	1 cone	1.0	70	13%
sugar	1 cone	–	50	–
cups				
cake				
jumbo	1 cup	–	25	–
regular	1 cup	–	15	–
flavored color	1 cup	–	15	–
(Keebler)				
fudge-dipped cup	1 cup	1.5	35	39%
ice cream cup/vanilla	1 cup	–	15	–
sugar cone	1 cone	0.5	50	9%

Food and Description	Amount	Fat Grams	Total Calories	% Fat Calories
waffle				
bowl	1 bowl	1.0	50	18%
cone	1 cone	1.0	50	18%
(Little Debbie) ice cream cups	1 cup	–	15	–
ICE CREAM SANDWICH (*See* ICE CREAM BARS, SANDWICHES, & FROZEN NOVELTIES)				
ICE CREAM TOPPING (*See also* CREAM; CUSTARD; DIP; WHIPPED TOPPING)				
bottled, canned, or jarred				
(Baskin-Robbins)				
chocolate syrup	2 Tbs	–	90	–
freeze coat/chocolate	1 oz	14.0	180	70%
hot fudge				
fat-free	1 oz	–	90	–
no sugar added	1 oz	–	90	–
regular	1 oz	3.0	100	27%
praline caramel	1 oz	–	90	–
strawberry	1 oz	–	60	–
whipped cream	2 Tbs	2.5	30	75%
(Estee) chocolate syrup	2 Tbs	–	50	–
(Fisher) nut topping/peanut	1 oz	17.0	190	81%
(Hershey)				
Chocolate Shoppe toppings				
banana split fudge	1 Tbs	2.5	70	32%
caramel	2 Tbs	–	100	–
chocolate almond fudge	1 Tbs	2.0	70	26%
chocolate caramel fudge	1 Tbs	0.5	60	8%
chocolate marshmallow fudge	1 Tbs	2.0	70	26%
chocolate mint fudge	1 Tbs	2.0	80	23%
double chocolate fudge	1 Tbs	–	50	–
hot fudge				
fat-free	1 Tbs	–	100	–
regular	1 Tbs	2.5	70	32%
Chocolate Shoppe candy bar sprinkles				
candy coated milk chocolate	1 Tbs	3.0	70	39%
milk chocolate w/almonds	1 Tbs	4.0	80	45%
peanut butter/Reese's	1 Tbs	3.5	70	45%
peppermint patty	1 Tbs	4.0	80	45%
sundae syrup				
chocolate mint	2 Tbs	–	110	–
double chocolate	2 Tbs	–	110	–
syrup				
chocolate				
lite	2 Tbs	–	50	–
malt	2 Tbs	–	100	–
original	2 Tbs	–	100	–
strawberry	2 Tbs	–	100	–
topping/canned				
chocolate fudge	1 Tbs	3.0	70	39%
(Kraft)				
butterscotch	2 Tbs	1.5	130	10%
caramel	2 Tbs	–	120	

Food and Description	Amount	Fat Grams	Total Calories	% Fat Calories
chocolate-flavored	2 Tbs	–	110	–
hot fudge	2 Tbs	4.5	140	29%
pineapple	2 Tbs	–	110	–
strawberry	2 Tbs	–	110	–
(Mrs. Richardson's) hot fudge/fat-free	2 Tbs	–	110	–
(Planter's) nut topping	2 Tbs	9.0	100	81%
(Smucker's)				
butterscotch & caramel syrup				
regular	2 Tbs	–	130	–
sundae	2 Tbs	–	110	–
butterscotch & caramel topping				
regular	2 Tbs	–	130	–
special recipe	2 Tbs	1.0	130	7%
caramel				
fat-free microwaveable	2 Tbs	–	110	–
sundae syrup	2 Tbs	–	110	–
chocolate fudge				
microwaveable	2 Tbs	1.5	130	10%
topping	2 Tbs	1.5	130	10%
chocolate-flavored sundae syrup	2 Tbs	–	110	–
Dove Toppings				
dark chocolate	2 Tbs	5.0	140	32%
milk chocolate	2 Tbs	4.0	130	28%
hot caramel	2 Tbs	3.0	120	23%
hot fudge				
light/fat-free	2 Tbs	–	90	–
microwaveable				
fat-free	2 Tbs	–	110	–
original	2 Tbs	2.5	130	17%
original	2 Tbs	4.0	140	26%
special recipe	2 Tbs	4.0	140	26%
magic shell toppings				
caramel	2 Tbs	18.0	220	74%
chocolate	2 Tbs	18.0	220	74%
chocolate fudge	2 Tbs	18.0	220	74%
cookie dough crunch nut	2 Tbs	18.0	220	74%
peanut butter	2 Tbs	18.0	220	74%
marshmallow topping	2 Tbs	–	120	–
peanut butter caramel	2 Tbs	4.5	150	27%
pecans in syrup	2 Tbs	10.0	170	53%
pineapple topping	2 Tbs	–	110	–
strawberry				
sundae syrup	2 Tbs	–	110	–
topping	2 Tbs	–	100	–
walnuts in syrup	2 Tbs	9.0	170	48%
homemade/USDA Standard Home Recipe				
chocolate sauce	1 Tbs	2.0	55	33%
hard sauce	1.2 oz	6.0	95	57%
lemon sauce	2 Tbs	1.5	60	8%

ICE MILK (*See* ICE CREAM & ICE CREAM-LIKE FROZEN DESSERTS)

Food and Description	Amount	Fat Grams	Total Calories	% Fat Calories

ICE MILK BAR (*See* ICE CREAM BARS, SANDWICHES, & FROZEN NOVELTIES)
ICED TEA (*See* TEA)
ICES (*See* FRUIT ICES, BARS, & POPS)
ICING (*See* CAKE FROSTING/ICING)
INDIAN PUDDING (*See* PUDDING & MOUSSE)
INFANT FORMULA (*See* BABY/INFANT FORMULA)
ITALIAN SAUSAGE (*See* SAUSAGE)

J

Food and Description	Amount	Fat Grams	Total Calories	% Fat Calories
JACKFRUIT /raw	1 medium	–	107	–
JALAPEÑO (*See* MEXICAN FOOD; PEPPER)				
JAM/JELLY/PRESERVES				
(Bama)				
jam/red plum	2 tsp	–	30	–
jelly				
apple	2 tsp	–	30	–
grape	2 tsp	–	30	–
preserves				
peach	2 tsp	–	30	–
strawberry	2 tsp	–	30	–
(Cascadian Farm) organic				
conserves				
fruit-sweetened				
red raspberry	1 Tbs	–	40	–
strawberry	1 Tbs	–	40	–
honey-sweetened				
raspberry	1 Tbs	–	40	–
strawberry	1 Tbs	–	40	–
fancy fruit spreads				
apricot	1 Tbs	–	40	–
blackberry	1 Tbs	–	40	–
blueberry	1 Tbs	–	40	–
concord grape	1 Tbs	–	40	–
dark cherry	1 Tbs	–	40	–
harvest berry	1 Tbs	–	40	–
peach	1 Tbs	–	40	–
plum	1 Tbs	–	40	–
raspberry	1 Tbs	–	40	–

Food and Description	Amount	Fat Grams	Total Calories	% Fat Calories
strawberry	1 Tbs	–	40	–
sweet orange marmalade	1 Tbs	–	40	–
(Country Pure)				
jam				
apricot	2 tsp	–	35	–
blackberry	2 tsp	–	35	–
red cherry	2 tsp	–	35	–
red raspberry	2 tsp	–	35	–
strawberry	2 tsp	–	35	–
(Crosse & Blackwell)				
guava jelly	1 Tbs	–	60	–
mint flavored apple	1 Tbs	–	60	–
orange marmalade	1 Tbs	–	60	–
red currant jelly	1 Tbs	–	60	–
(Empress)				
jam/all flavors	2 tsp	–	35	–
jelly/all flavors	2 tsp	–	35	–
marmalade/California orange	2 tsp	–	35	–
preserves/all flavors	2 tsp	–	35	–
(Estee)				
spreads				
apple spice	1 Tbs	–	10	–
apricot	1 Tbs	–	5	–
blackberry	1 Tbs	–	5	–
cherry	1 Tbs	–	5	–
grape	1 Tbs	–	10	–
orange	1 Tbs	–	10	–
peach	1 Tbs	–	5	–
red raspberry	1 Tbs	–	5	–
strawberry	1 Tbs	–	10	–
(Featherweight) fruit spreads/all flavors	1 Tbs	–	15	–
(Knott's Berry Farm)				
jelly				
jalapeño	1 tsp	–	18	–
jelly/light				
apricot-pineapple	1 tsp	–	8	–
blackberry	1 tsp	–	8	–
raspberry	1 tsp	–	8	–
strawberry	1 tsp	–	8	–
preserves				
apricot	1 tsp	–	18	–
apricot-pineapple	1 tsp	–	18	–
bing cherry	1 tsp	–	18	–
blackberry/seedless	1 tsp	–	18	–
blueberry	1 tsp	–	18	–
boysenberry	1 tsp	–	18	–
Kadota fig	1 tsp	–	18	–
red cherry	1 tsp	–	18	–
red raspberry/seedless	1 tsp	–	18	–
strawberry	1 tsp	–	18	–

Food and Description	Amount	Fat Grams	Total Calories	% Fat Calories
(Mary Ellen)				
jam				
apricot	1 Tbs	–	50	–
blackberry/seedless	1 Tbs	–	50	–
grape	1 Tbs	–	50	–
red raspberry	1 Tbs	–	50	–
strawberry	1 Tbs	–	50	–
jelly				
grape	1 Tbs	–	50	–
strawberry	1 Tbs	–	50	–
(Poiret)				
100% pure fruit spreads				
apple	2 tsp	–	35	–
pear, apricot, apple	2 tsp	–	35	–
pear, black cherry	2 tsp	–	35	–
pear, strawberry	2 tsp	–	35	–
pear, strawberry, apple	2 tsp	–	35	–
(Polaner)				
jam				
grape	1 Tbs	–	40	–
jelly				
apple		–	40	–
currant	1 Tbs	–	40	–
grape	1 Tbs	–	40	–
mint	1 Tbs	–	40	–
raspberry	1 Tbs	–	40	–
strawberry	1 Tbs	–	40	–
preserves				
apricot	1 Tbs	–	40	–
black cherry	1 Tbs	–	40	–
blackberry	1 Tbs	–	40	–
blueberry	1 Tbs	–	40	–
peach	1 Tbs	–	40	–
red raspberry	1 Tbs	–	40	–
strawberry	1 Tbs	–	40	–
(R W Knudsen) all-fruit spread				
organic				
blackberry	1 Tbs	–	50	–
blueberry	1 Tbs	–	50	–
red raspberry	1 Tbs	–	50	–
strawberry	1 Tbs	–	50	–
regular				
apricot	1 Tbs	–	50	–
black cherry	1 Tbs	–	50	–
blackberry	1 Tbs	–	50	–
blueberry	1 Tbs	–	50	–
boysenberry	1 Tbs	–	50	–
Concord grape	1 Tbs	–	50	–
orange	1 Tbs	–	50	–
peach	1 Tbs	–	50	–

Food and Description	Amount	Fat Grams	Total Calories	% Fat Calories
red raspberry	1 Tbs	–	50	–
strawberry	1 Tbs	–	50	–
(Smucker's) fruit spreads				
homestyle/all flavors	1 Tbs	–	45	–
jam/all flavors	1 Tbs	–	50	–
jelly/all flavors	1 Tbs	–	50	–
light fruit preserves/ all flavors	1 Tbs	–	10	–
low-sugar/all flavors	1 Tbs	–	25	–
marmalade/orange	1 Tbs	–	50	–
preserves/all flavors	1 Tbs	–	50	–
Simply Fruit spread/all flavors	1 Tbs	–	40	–
(Welch's)				
jam/all flavors	1 Tbs	–	50	–
jelly/all flavors	1 Tbs	–	50	–
preserves/all flavors	1 Tbs	–	50	–
spread/strawberry	1 Tbs	–	50	–
Totally Fruit				
apricot	1 Tbs	–	35	–
blackberry	1 Tbs	–	35	–
blueberry	1 Tbs	–	35	–
grape	1 Tbs	–	40	–
red raspberry	1 Tbs	–	35	–
strawberry	1 Tbs	–	35	–
JAPANESE FOOD (See ASIAN FOOD)				
JELL-O (See GELATIN)				
JELLY (See JAM/JELLY/PRESERVES)				
JERKY STICKS & STRIPS				
(Bridgford)				
jerky				
hot'n spicy	1.25 oz	2.0	100	18%
original	1.25 oz	2.0	110	16%
teriyaki	1.25 oz	1.0	90	10%
sticks				
bacon & beef	1 oz	12.0	140	77%
beef	1 oz	12.0	140	77%
beef & cheese	1.5 oz	14.0	170	74%
(Frito Lay) Rustlers Roundup				
beef jerky	9 pieces	2.5	40	56%
flamin' hot meat stick	1 serving	3.0	40	68%
smoky steak strip	1 serving	2.0	60	30%
spicy stick	1 serving	8.0	100	72%
(Lance)				
beef				
jerky	1 piece	1.0	25	36%
snack				
.25 oz pkg	1 piece	3.0	35	77%
.40 oz pkg	1 piece	4.5	60	68%
.90 oz pkg	1 piece	10.0	130	69%
beef & cheese stick	1.5 oz pkg	11.0	150	66%

Food and Description	Amount	Fat Grams	Total Calories	% Fat Calories
hot sausage stick				
1.2 oz pkg	1 piece	4.5	60	68%
1.7 oz pkg	1 piece	8.0	120	40%
kippered beef steak				
original	1 pkg	2.5	60	38%
peppered	1 pkg	2.0	60	30%
teriyaki	1 pkg	2.0	60	30%
premium beef jerky/4 oz pkg				
original	¼ pkg	0.5	70	9%
peppered	¼ pkg	0.5	80	6%
teriyaki	¼ pkg	0.5	70	9%
(Pacific Gold) natural				
hot & spicy	1 oz	1.0	90	10%
original	1 oz	1.0	80	11%
teriyaki	1 oz	1.0	80	11%
(Pemmican)				
natural				
hot red pepper	.5 oz bag	–	40	–
	1 oz serving	0.5	80	6%
	1.25 oz bag	1.0	100	9%
	2 oz	1.5	160	8%
original	1.1 oz bag	1.0	80	11%
	1.25 oz bag	1.0	90	10%
	2 oz bag	2.0	150	12%
spicy teriyaki	1 oz serving	1.0	70	13%
	1.25 oz bag	1.0	90	10%
	2 oz bag	2.0	150	12%
sweet mesquite	1 oz serving	1.0	70	13%
	1.25 oz bag	1.0	90	10%
	2 oz bag	2.5	150	15%
tender jerky				
hickory smoked and peppered	1 oz bag	2.0	80	23%
hot red pepper	1 oz bag	2.0	80	23%
teriyaki	1 oz bag	3.0	90	30%
tendered kippered beef steak				
original	1 piece	5.0	110	41%
peppered	1 piece	5.0	110	41%
teriyaki	1 piece	5.0	110	41%
(Shelton's)				
turkey jerky				
hot	½ oz	0.5	50	9%
regular	½ oz	0.5	50	9%
	1 oz	1.0	100	9%
turkey sticks	½ oz	0.5	50	9%
(Slim Jim)				
beef				
steak strips	1 piece	3.0	70	39%
Super Jerk/.31 oz bag	1 piece	2.0	35	51%
Big Jerk	1 piece	1.5	25	54%
Big Slim dry sausage	1 piece	6.0	70	77%

Food and Description	Amount	Fat Grams	Total Calories	% Fat Calories
Giant Jerk/chopped & formed	1 piece	4.0	70	51%
nacho Super Slim dry sausage	1 piece	8.0	100	72%
spicy dry sausage stick				
.89 oz pkg	1 piece	4.0	45	80%
Giant Slim/1 oz bag	1 piece	14.0	150	84%
Super Slim.				
64 oz bag	1 piece	9.0	100	81%
twin pack	1.28 oz pkg	17.0	190	81%
Tabasco	1 piece	8.0	100	72%
JERUSALEM ARTICHOKE				
raw/sliced	½ cup	–	57	–
JEW'S EAR				
dried	½ cup	–	35	–
raw/sliced	½ cup	–	15	–
JICAMA/YAM BEAN-TUBER				
cooked	½ cup	<1.0	46	10%
raw/sliced	1 cup	<1.0	50	9%
JUICE (See FRUIT JUICE/JUICE DRINK, MIXED; individual listings)				
JUJUBE				
dried	3 oz	0.9	246	3%
raw	3 oz	–	68	–

K

Food and Description	Amount	Fat Grams	Total Calories	% Fat Calories
KALE				
fresh/cooked	½ cup	–	21	–
frozen/cooked	½ cup	–	20	–
raw	½ cup	–	17	–
KANPYO/DRIED GOURD STRIP	3 strips	–	49	–
KASHA (See BUCKWHEAT GROATS)				
KELP (See SEAWEED)				
KETCHUP (See CATSUP)				
KIDNEY BEAN				
canned				
(Bush's Best)				
dark red	½ cup	–	70	–
light red	½ cup	–	70	–
(Eden) Organic				
red/no salt added	½ cup	–	100	–

Food and Description	Amount	Fat Grams	Total Calories	% Fat Calories
generic				
dark red	½ cup	<1.0	104	4%
red	½ cup	<1.0	108	4%
(Goya) habichuelas coloradas/red	½ cup	1.0	90	10%
(Green Giant)				
dark red	½ cup	–	110	–
light red	½ cup	–	110	–
(Hain) dark red	½ cup	1.0	95	9%
(Hunt's)	½ cup	0.5	95	5%
(Joan of Arc)				
dark red	½ cup	–	110	–
light red	½ cup	–	110	–
(Libby)	½ cup	–	120	
(Progresso)				
cannellini/white	½ cup	1.0	110	8%
red	½ cup	1.0	110	8%
(S&W) all types	½ cup	1.0	120	8%
(Seneca)	½ cup	0.5	120	4%
(Stokely)				
dark red	½ cup	0.5	120	4%
light red	½ cup	0.5	120	4%
(Trappey's)				
dark red	½ cup	1.0	130	7%
jalapeño	½ cup	1.0	110	8%
light red	½ cup	1.0	120	8%
New Orleans style w/bacon	½ cup	1.0	110	8%
W/chili gravy	½ cup	1.0	110	8%
(Van Camp's)				
dark red	½ cup	–	90	–
light red	½ cup	–	90	–
dry/generic				
boiled				
dark red	½ cup	–	112	–
red	½ cup	–	112	–
raw				
dark red	½ cup	1.0	300	3%
red	½ cup	1.0	310	3%
sprouted/raw				
mature seeds	1 oz	<1.0	8	15%
	½ cup	0.5	30	15%
KIELBASA (See SAUSAGE)				
KINGFISH				
cooked-dry heat	3 oz	11.0	219	4 5%
raw	3 oz	2.6	90	26%
KIWI JUICE/JUICE BLEND (See also FRUIT JUICE/JUICE DRINK, MIXED; FRUIT PUNCH; SOFT DRINK MIX; individual listings)				
(Snapple) kiwi-strawberry				
can	11.5 oz	–	160	
diet	8 fl oz	–	20	–
regular	8 fl oz	–	110	–

Food and Description	Amount	Fat Grams	Total Calories	% Fat Calories
KIWIFRUIT				
fresh/raw	1 medium	<1.0	46	10%
	1 large	<1.0	55	8%
(Dole)	2 medium	1.0	90	10%
KNOCKWURST (*See* FRANKFURTER; SAUSAGE)				
KOHLRABI				
fresh/sliced				
cooked-drained	½ cup	–	24	–
raw	½ cup	–	19	–
KOOL-AID (*See* SOFT DRINK MIX)				
KRAUT (*See* SAUERKRAUT)				
KRAUT JUICE (*See* SAUERKRAUT JUICE)				
KUMQUAT				
fresh/raw	1 medium	–	12	–

L

Food and Description	Amount	Fat Grams	Total Calories	% Fat Calories
LAMB				

(NOTE: All serving sizes are cooked portions, unless otherwise stated. "Lean" means lamb trimmed of all separable fat before cooking. "Lean & fat" means untrimmed and cooked or eaten as purchased. In most cases, 4 ounces of raw meat yields 3 ounces cooked.)

Food and Description	Amount	Fat Grams	Total Calories	% Fat Calories
domestic				
composite cuts/leg & shoulder				
lean				
braised/cubed	3 oz	7.5	190	36%
broiled				
cubed	3 oz	6.0	160	23%
ground	3 oz	17.0	240	64%
stewed/cubed	4 oz	10.0	255	35%
leg/foreshank				
lean				
braised	3 oz	5.0	160	28%
braised/diced	1 cup	8.5	260	29%
broiled/ground	3 oz	17.0	240	64%
stewed/diced	1 cup	8.5	265	29%
lean & fat				
braised	3 oz	11.5	210	49%
braised/diced	1 cup	19.0	340	50%

Food and Description	Amount	Fat Grams	Total Calories	% Fat Calories
stewed	3 oz	11.5	210	49%
leg/shank				
lean				
roasted	3 oz	5.7	155	33%
roasted/diced	1 cup	9.0	250	32%
lean & fat				
roasted	3 oz	10.5	190	50%
roasted/diced	1 cup	17.5	315	50%
leg/sirloin				
lean				
roasted	3 oz	8.0	175	41%
roasted/diced	1 cup	13.0	290	40%
lean & fat				
roasted	3 oz	17.5	250	63%
roasted/diced	1 cup	29.0	410	64%
leg/whole				
lean				
roasted	3 oz	6.5	165	35%
roasted/diced	1 cup	11.0	270	37%
lean & fat				
roasted	3 oz	14.0	220	57%
roasted/diced	1 cup	23.0	360	57%
loin				
lean				
broiled	3 oz	8.5	190	40%
roasted	3 oz	8.5	175	44%
lean & fat				
broiled	3 oz	19.5	270	65%
roasted	3 oz	20.0	265	68%
organs				
brain				
braised	3 oz	8.5	125	61%
pan-fried	3 oz	19.0	235	73%
heart				
braised	3 oz	7.0	160	39%
simmered	3 oz	7.0	160	39%
kidney				
braised	3 oz	3.0	120	23%
liver				
braised	3 oz	7.5	190	36%
pan-fried	3 oz	11.0	205	48%
lung/braised	3 oz	2.5	95	24%
pancreas/braised	3 oz	13.0	200	59%
spleen/braised	3 oz	4.0	135	27%
tongue/braised	3 oz	17.0	235	65%
rib				
lean				
broiled	3 oz	11.0	200	50%
roasted	3 oz	11.0	200	50%
lean & fat				
broiled	3 oz	25.0	305	74%

Food and Description	Amount	Fat Grams	Total Calories	% Fat Calories
roasted	3 oz	25.5	305	75%
shoulder/arm				
lean				
braised	3 oz	12.0	235	46%
broiled	3 oz	7.5	170	40%
roasted	3 oz	8.0	165	44%
shoulder/blade				
lean				
braised	3 oz	14.0	245	51%
broiled	3 oz	9.5	180	48%
roasted	3 oz	10.0	180	50%
lean & fat				
braised	3 oz	21.0	295	64%
broiled	3 oz	17.0	235	65%
roasted	3 oz	17.5	240	66%
shoulder/whole				
lean				
braised	3 oz	7.5	240	28%
braised/diced	1 cup	22.0	400	50%
broiled	3 oz	9.0	180	45%
roasted	3 oz	9.0	175	46%
roasted/diced	1 cup	10.0	320	28%
stewed	3 oz	7.5	240	28%
stewed/diced	1 cup	22.0	400	50%
lean & fat				
braised/diced	1 cup	34.0	485	63%
broiled	3 oz	22.0	315	63%
broiled/diced	1 cup	27.0	390	62%
roasted	3 oz	17.0	235	65%
roasted/diced	1 cup	28.0	385	65%
stewed	3 oz	21.0	295	64%
stewed/diced	1 cup	34.5	485	64%
New Zealand/frozen				
composite cuts				
lean/cooked	3 oz	7.5	175	39%
leg/foreshank				
lean				
braised	3 oz	5.0	160	28%
braised/diced	1 cup	8.5	260	29%
stewed	3 oz	5.0	160	28%
stewed/diced	1 cup	8.5	260	29%
lean & fat				
braised	3 oz	13.5	220	55%
braised/diced	1 cup	22.0	360	55%
stewed	3 oz	13.5	220	55%
stewed/diced	1 cup	22.0	360	55%
leg/whole				
lean				
roasted	3 oz	6.0	155	35%
roasted/diced	1 cup	10.0	255	35%

Food and Description	Amount	Fat Grams	Total Calories	% Fat Calories
lean & fat				
roasted	3 oz	13.0	210	56%
roasted/diced	1 cup	22.0	345	57%
loin				
lean				
broiled	3 oz	7.0	170	37%
roasted	3 oz	7.0	170	37%
lean & fat				
broiled	3 oz	20.5	270	68%
rib				
lean/roasted	3 oz	8.5	165	46%
lean & fat/roasted	3 oz	24.5	290	76%
shoulder/whole				
lean				
braised	3 oz	13.0	245	48%
braised/diced	1 cup	22.0	400	50%
stewed	3 oz	13.0	240	49%
stewed/diced	1 cup	22.0	400	50%
lean & fat				
braised	3 oz	22.0	305	65%
braised/diced	1 cup	35.5	490	65%
stewed	3 oz	21.5	300	65%
stewed/diced	1 cup	35.5	490	65%
LAMB DISH				
homemade/USDA Standard Home Recipe				
curry	1 cup	23.0	460	45%
stew	1 cup	7.0	165	38%
LAMB'S-QUARTERS				
fresh/cooked	1 cup	0.6	29	19%
LARD (*See also* FAT; OIL; PORK)	1 Tbs	12.8	115	100%
	1 cup	205.0	1850	100%
LASAGNA (*See* BEEF DISH/ENTRÉE; FROZEN ENTRÉE/DINNER; PASTA ENTRÉE/DINNER)				
LAVER (*See* SEAWEED)				
LEEK				
freeze-dried	¼ cup	–	3	–
fresh				
cooked	¼ cup	–	8	–
raw	¼ cup	–	16	–
	1 medium	–	17	–
LEMON/fresh	1 medium	–	17	–
	1 large	–	25	–
LEMON JUICE				
bottled				
generic	1 Tbs	–	5	–
	⅓ cup	–	17	–
(Realemon)	1 fl oz	–	6	–
(Seneca)	1 Tbs	–	5	–
fresh	1 Tbs	–	4	–
	⅓ cup	–	20	–

Food and Description	Amount	Fat Grams	Total Calories	% Fat Calories
frozen				
generic	1 Tbs	–	3	–
(Sunkist)	1 oz	–	7	–
LEMON PEEL				
candied				
generic	1 oz	–	90	–
(S&W)	58 pieces	–	80	–
grated	1 Tbs	–	–	–
LEMONADE/LEMONADE-FLAVORED DRINK *(See also* SOFT DRINK; SOFT DRINK MIX; TEA)				
bottled, boxed, or canned				
(Crystal Light)				
pink	8 fl oz	–	5	–
traditional	8 fl oz	–	5	–
(Fruitopia)				
Cranberry Lemonade Vision	8 fl oz	–	120	–
Lemonade Love & Hope	8 fl oz	–	120	–
Pink Lemonade Euphoria	8 fl oz	–	120	–
Raspberry Psychic	8 fl oz	–	120	–
(Knudsen)				
cranberry	8 fl oz	–	120	–
natural	8 fl oz	–	120	–
organic	8 fl oz	–	120	–
(Newman's Own)	8 fl oz	–	110	–
(Snapple)				
pink				
can	11.5 oz	–	160	–
diet	8 fl oz	–	20	–
regular	8 fl oz	–	120	–
regular	8 fl oz	–	120	–
(Tropicana)	8 fl oz	–	120	–
	10 fl oz	–	140	–
	11.5 fl oz	–	160	–
(Welch's)	10 fl oz	–	160	–
	11.5 fl oz	–	190	–
frozen/prepared				
(Minute Maid)				
country style	8 fl oz	–	120	–
cranberry	8 fl oz	–	80	–
pink	8 fl oz	–	120	–
raspberry	8 fl oz	–	110	–
regular	8 fl oz	–	110	–
tropical	8 fl oz	–	120	–
(Mott's)	10 fl oz	–	160	–
(Seneca)	8 fl oz	–	110	–
mix/prepared				
(Country Time)				
Lem'N Berry Sippers sweetened lemonade drink mix				
cranberry-raspberry	8 fl oz	–	90	–
raspberry	8 fl oz	–	90	–

Food and Description	Amount	Fat Grams	Total Calories	% Fat Calories
strawberry	8 fl oz	–	90	–
wildberry	8 fl oz	–	90	–
pink				
sugar-free	8 fl oz	–	5	–
sweetened	8 fl oz	–	70	–
regular				
sugar-free	8 fl oz	–	5	–
sweetened	8 fl oz	–	70	–
(Crystal Light)				
pink	8 fl oz	–	5	–
traditional	8 fl oz	–	5	–
(Kool-Aid) prepared w/sugar and water				
pink	8 fl oz	–	100	–
traditional	8 fl oz	–	100	–
LEMON-LIME DRINK (See SOFT DRINK; SOFT DRINK MIX; SPORTS DRINK)				
LENTIL (See also VEGETARIAN FOODS)				
Canned				
(Eden) w/sweet onion & bay leaf	½ cup	–	90	–
generic				
cooked	½ cup	–	103	–
uncooked	½ cup	–	130	–
(Health Valley) Fast Menu				
hearty lentils garden vegetables	1 container	4.0	150	24%
organic lentils w/tofu weiner	1 container	5.0	170	26%
dry				
(Arrowhead Mills) green or red/raw	¼ cup	–	150	–
generic				
boiled	½ cup	–	115	–
raw	½ cup	1.0	374	2%
split	½ cup	1.0	379	2%
sprouted	½ cup	–	40	–
LENTIL SOUP (See SOUP)				
LETTUCE (See also SALAD GREENS & BLENDS)				
Bibb	med head	–	21	–
butterhead	med head	–	21	–
cos/shredded	½ cup	–	2	–
iceberg	med head	–	70	–
looseleaf or Simpson/shredded	½ cup	–	5	–
romaine/shredded	½ cup	–	4	–
LICHEE NUT/LYCHEE NUT/LITCHI NUT				
dried/shelled	1 oz	<1.0	80	4%
	3 oz	1.0	235	4%
raw	~6 nuts	0.5	40	10%
shelled & seeded	½ cup	0.5	65	7%
LIMA BEAN (See also BUTTER BEAN)				
Canned				
(Aunt Nellie's) Reber butter beans	½ cup	1.0	140	6%
(Bush's Best)				
green	½ cup	–	90	–
green & white	½ cup	–	80	–

Food and Description	Amount	Fat Grams	Total Calories	% Fat Calories
(Del Monte) green	½ cup	–	80	–
(Dennison's) seasoned w/ham & bacon	½ cup	3.5	150	21%
(Freshlike)				
no salt	½ cup	–	80	–
regular	½ cup	–	80	–
(Green Giant) butter	½ cup	–	90	–
(Joan of Arc) butter	½ cup	–	90	–
(Luck's) seasoned w/pork				
giant	½ cup	3.0	150	18%
small	½ cup	2.0	140	13%
(Seneca)	½ cup	–	80	–
(Stokely)	½ cup	–	80	–
Fordhook	½ cup	–	80	–
no salt or sugar added	½ cup	–	80	–
(Trappey's) baby				
green	½ cup	1.0	120	8%
white	½ cup	1.0	120	8%
(Van Camp's)	½ cup	–	80	–
(Veg-All)	½ cup	–	80	–
dried				
baby				
boiled	½ cup	–	115	–
uncooked	½ cup	1.0	330	3%
large				
boiled	½ cup	–	108	–
uncooked	½ cup	0.5	300	2%
frozen				
(Birds Eye)				
baby	½ cup	–	130	–
Fordhook	½ cup	–	100	–
(C&W) baby	½ cup	0.5	90	5%
(Green Giant) baby	½ cup	–	80	–
(Seneca)				
Fordhook	⅔ cup	–	90	–
regular	⅔ cup	–	110	–
(Veg-All)	½ cup	1.0	130	7%
LIMA BEAN DISH				
(Green Giant) frozen in butter sauce	½ cup	1.5	110	12%
LIME	1 medium	–	20	–
LIME JUICE				
bottled				
generic	1 Tbs	–	3	–
	⅓ cup	–	17	–
(Realime)	1 fl oz	–	6	–
fresh	⅓ cup	–	22	–
LIME JUICE DRINK (*See also* SOFT DRINK; SOFT DRINK MIX)				
(Knudsen) Key West lime	8 fl oz	–	100	–
LING				
baked or broiled	3 oz	1.0	95	9%
raw	3 oz	0.5	75	6%

Food and Description	Amount	Fat Grams	Total Calories	% Fat Calories
LINGCOD				
baked or boiled	3 oz	1.0	90	10%
raw	3 oz	1.0	75	12%
LINGUINE (See FROZEN ENTRÉE/DINNER; PASTA ENTRÉE/DINNER; VEGETARIAN FOODS)				
LIQUEUR (See also COCKTAIL; LIQUOR, DISTILLED)				
anisette	¾ fl oz	–	74	–
B&B	1 fl oz	–	94	–
Benedictine	¾ fl oz	–	69	–
brandy/fruit-flavored	1.5 fl oz	–	129	–
brandy/coffee	1.5 fl oz	–	132	–
Cherry Hering	1.5 fl oz	–	120	–
coffee	1.5 fl oz	–	174	–
coffee w/cream	1.5 fl oz	7.0	154	41%
creme de almonde	1.5 fl oz	–	151	–
creme de banana	1.5 fl oz	–	144	–
creme de cacao	1.5 fl oz	–	150	–
creme de cassis	1.5 fl oz	–	122	–
creme de menthe	1.5 fl oz	–	186	–
curaçao	¾ fl oz	–	54	–
Drambuie	1.5 fl oz	–	165	–
gin/citrus	1.5 fl oz	–	114	–
kirsch	1.5 fl oz	–	124	–
maraschino	1.5 fl oz	–	112	–
peppermint schnapps	1.5 fl oz	–	124	–
pernod	1.5 fl oz	–	117	–
rock & rye	1.5 fl oz	–	140	–
sloe gin	1.5 fl oz	–	124	–
Southern Comfort	1.5 fl oz	–	180	–
Tia Maria	1.5 fl oz	–	138	–
triple sec	1.5 fl oz	–	121	–
vodka/citrus	1.5 fl oz	–	150	–
LIQUOR, DISTILLED				
(NOTE: In all cases, the higher the proof [the % of alcohol], the higher the calories.)				
80 proof	1 fl oz	–	67	–
84 proof	1 fl oz	–	70	–
86 proof	1 fl oz	–	72	–
86.8 proof	1 fl oz	–	72	–
90 proof	1 fl oz	–	75	–
90.4 proof	1 fl oz	–	75	–
94 proof	1 fl oz	–	78	–
94.6 proof	1 fl oz	–	79	–
97 proof	1 fl oz	–	81	–
100 proof	1 fl oz	–	83	–
LIVER (See BEEF; CHICKEN; GOOSE; LAMB; PÂTÉ; PORK; TURKEY)				
LIVER LOAF (See LUNCHEON MEAT)				
LIVERWURST (See LUNCHEON MEAT)				
LOBSTER (See also SEAFOOD ENTRÉE/DINNER)				

Food and Description	Amount	Fat Grams	Total Calories	% Fat Calories
fresh				
northern				
boiled	3 oz	0.5	83	5%
	1 cup	0.9	142	6%
raw/~5-oz lobster	1 lobster	1.0	140	6%
spiny				
cooked-moist heat	3 oz	1.5	120	11%
raw	3 oz	1.0	95	10%
frozen				
(Langostino's) lobster tails/small/ cooked	3 oz	1.0	105	9%
LOBSTER, IMITATION				
(Louis Kemp)				
chunk style	½ cup	–	80	–
flake style	½ cup	–	80	–
salad style	½ cup	–	80	–
LOBSTER BISQUE (See SOUP)				
LOBSTER PASTE	1 Tbs	2.0	39	46%
LOBSTER SALAD				
homemade/USDA Standard Home	3 oz	5.5	94	53%
Recipe/made w/mayonnaise, tomato, celery, carrots, onion, & egg				
LOGANBERRY				
canned				
in heavy syrup	½ cup	–	89	–
in water	½ cup	–	40	–
fresh	½ lb	1.5	140	10%
frozen	1 cup	0.5	80	5%
LOGANBERRY JUICE	8 oz	–	100	–
LOQUAT	1 medium	–	5	–
	½ lb	–	65	–
LOTUS ROOT				
cooked	½ cup	–	75	–
raw	10 slices	–	45	–
	1 root	–	60	–
LOTUS SEED				
dried	1 oz	0.5	94	5%
	1 cup	0.6	106	5%
raw	1 oz	–	25	–
LOX (See SALMON)				
LUNCHEON LOAF (See LUNCHEON MEAT)				
LUNCHEON MEAT (See also BEEF; CHICKEN; HAM; LUNCHEON MEAT SPREAD; TURKEY; VEGETARIAN FOODS)				
■ (Alpine Lace)				
Deli Meats				
Fat-free turkey breast	2 oz	–	45	–
97% fat-free ham				
honey	2 oz	2.0	60	30%
regular	2 oz	1.5	60	23%
smoked Virginia Brand	2 oz	1.5	60	23%
97% fat-free roast beef	2 oz	1.5	70	19%

Food and Description	Amount	Fat Grams	Total Calories	% Fat Calories
■ **(Armour)**				
Beef				
dried/95% fat-free	1 oz	1.5	60	27%
Treet luncheon loaf				
Lite	2 oz	8.0	110	65%
original	2 oz	11.0	130	76%
Vienna sausage				
barbecue	2.17 oz	13.0	150	78%
chicken	1.89 oz	9.0	110	74%
hot'n spicy	2.17 oz	13.0	140	78%
jalapeño	1.89 oz	16.0	170	85%
lite	1.89 oz	7.0	90	70%
original	1.89 oz	14.0	150	84%
smoked	1.89 oz	14.0	150	84%
■ **(Bil Mar)**				
beef				
Signature top round				
Cajun beef	2 oz	3.0	70	39%
deli	2 oz	2.0	70	26%
split	2 oz	3.0	70	39%
whole/cap off	2 oz	1.5	50	27%
West Virginia/smoked	6 slices	2.0	60	30%
ham/West Virginia				
honey pork	2 oz	1.5	60	27%
smoked	2 oz	2.0	60	30%
pastrami/West Virginia/smoked	6 slices	1.5	60	27%
turkey/Signature turkey breast				
cozzinni	2 oz	1.0	60	18%
deli	2 oz	0.5	50	9%
honey-smoked/fat-free	2 oz	–	60	–
natural	2 oz	1.5	60	23%
natural/smoked	2 oz	2.0	60	30%
peppered/fat-free	2 oz	–	50	–
reduced sodium	2 oz	–	50	–
skinless	2 oz	0.5	50	9%
smoked	2 oz	–	50	–
whole boneless/foil/raw	4 oz	4.5	140	29%
■ **(Bridgeford)**				
salami/hard	1 oz	12.0	130	83%
■ **(Butterball)**				
Chicken breast				
Chicken Requests/crispy baked	3.5 oz	6.0	180	30%
grilled				
original glazed w/rib meat	3 oz	6.0	130	42%
strips carved	3 oz	3.5	110	29%
Fresh chicken				
breast fillets/boneless				
Italian	4 oz	2.0	120	15%
lemon butter	4 oz	1.0	120	8%
mesquite	4 oz	1.0	120	8%

Food and Description	Amount	Fat Grams	Total Calories	% Fat Calories
teriyaki	4 oz	1.0	120	8%
thin	1 serving	0.5	110	4%
breast tenders/boneless, skinless	8 pieces	<1.0	70	6%
thigh cutlets/boneless, skinless	2.67 oz	6.0	100	54%
whole roasting	5 oz	16.0	220	65%
turkey bologna	1 oz	5.0	60	75%
turkey breast				
skinless				
browned	1 oz	–	25	–
honey-roasted	1 oz	–	30	–
less sodium	1 oz	–	25	–
oven-roasted	1 oz	–	25	–
mesquite	1 oz	0.5	30	15%
smoked	1 oz	–	25	–
skin-on				
honey-roasted	1 oz	1.0	35	26%
less sodium	1 oz	1.0	30	30%
oven-roasted	1 oz	1.0	30	30%
smoked	1 oz	1.0	30	30%
turkey ham				
10% water added	1 oz	1.0	35	26%
25% water added	1 oz	1.5	35	39%
turkey pastrami	1 oz	1.0	35	26%
turkey salami	1 oz	4.0	60	60%
▩ (Carl Buddig)/sliced				
beef				
2.5 oz	1 pkg	5.0	100	45%
4 oz pkg	9 slices	4.0	75	48%
chicken				
lean/sliced				
honey-smoked	2.5 oz	1.0	70	13%
oven-roasted	2.5 oz pkg	1.0	60	15%
regular				
2.5	1 oz pkg	7.0	110	57%
4 oz pkg	9 slices	5.0	85	53%
corned beef				
2.5 oz	1 pkg	5.0	100	45%
4 oz pkg	9 slices	4.0	75	48%
ham				
lean				
brown sugar-baked	2.5 oz pkg	2.0	90	20%
roasted	1 pkg	2.0	90	20%
smoked	1 pkg	2.0	80	23%
honey/4 oz pkg	9 slices	5.0	90	50%
original				
2.5 oz	1 pkg	7.0	120	53%
4 oz pkg	9 slices	5.0	85	53%
smoked	2.5 oz pkg	2.0	80	23%
turkey	2.5 oz	5.0	100	45%
pastrami	2.5 oz pkg	5.0	100	45%

Food and Description	Amount	Fat Grams	Total Calories	% Fat Calories
turkey breast				
lean				
honey-roasted	2.5 oz pkg	1.0	70	13%
oven-roasted				
2.5 oz	1 pkg	1.0	70	13%
4 oz pkg	9 slices	5.0	80	56%
oven-roasted honey	2.5 oz pkg	2.0	90	20%
smoked	2.5 oz pkg	1.0	70	13%
original				
honey-roasted	2.5 oz pkg	6.0	110	49%
regular				
2.5 oz	1 pkg	7.0	110	57%
4 oz pkg	9 slices	5.0	80	56%
oven-roasted, cured				
2.5 oz	1 pkg	7.0	110	57%
4 oz pkg	9 slices	5.0	85	53%
smoked				
2.5 oz	1 pkg	7.0	110	57%
4 oz pkg	9 slices	5.0	80	56%
■ (Deli Perfect)				
beef				
cooked	2 oz	1.0	50	18%
Italian-style	2 oz	1.0	50	18%
chicken breast				
browned	2 oz	1.0	60	15%
plain	2 oz	1.0	60	15%
corned beef	2 oz	1.0	50	18%
ham/Hygrade pixie	2 oz	1.0	45	20%
pastrami/beef	2 oz	1.0	50	18%
turkey breast/natural shape				
browned	2 oz	2.5	60	38%
regular	2 oz	2.5	60	38%
smoked	2 oz	1.5	60	23%
turkey ham	2 oz	2.5	60	38%
turkey roll/white	2 oz	5.0	80	56%
■ (Eckrich)				
bologna				
German	1 oz	7.0	80	90%
regular	1 oz	9.0	100	90%
chicken breast/Lean Supreme				
oven-roasted oil-browned	1 slice	0.5	30	15%
ham/Lean Supreme				
honey & clove	1 slice	1.0	30	30%
honey-smoked	1 slice	1.0	30	30%
Virginia baked	1 slice	1.0	30	30%
turkey breast/Lean Supreme				
oven-roasted oil-browned	1 slice	1.0	30	30%
smoked	1 slice	1.0	30	30%
■ (Galileo)				
salami/Italian dry				
light	5 slices	4.0	60	60%

Food and Description	Amount	Fat Grams	Total Calories	% Fat Calories
thin sliced	5 slices	8.0	110	65%
whole	1 oz	10.0	120	75%
■ GENERIC				
barbecue loaf/beef & pork	1 oz	3.0	49	55%
bologna				
beef	1 oz	8.0	89	81%
beef & pork	1 oz	8.0	89	81%
Lebanon/beef	1 oz	4.0	64	56%
pork	1 oz	5.6	70	72%
Braunschweiger/pork	1 oz	9.0	102	79%
corned beef loaf	1 oz	2.0	43	42%
Dutch loaf	1 oz	5.0	68	66%
headcheese/pork	1 oz	4.0	60	60%
liver cheese/pork	1 oz	7.0	86	73%
liverwurst/pork	1 oz	8.0	93	77%
luxury loaf	1 oz	1.0	40	23%
mother's loaf	1 oz	6.0	80	68%
olive loaf/pork	1 oz	4.7	67	63%
pastrami				
beef	1 oz	8.0	99	73%
turkey	2 oz	3.5	80	39%
peppered loaf/beef, pork	1 oz	1.8	42	39%
pickle & pimiento loaf/pork	1 oz	6.0	74	73%
picnic loaf/pork, beef	1 oz	4.7	66	64%
salami				
cooked				
beef	1 oz	5.9	74	72%
beef & pork	1 oz	5.7	71	72%
turkey	2 oz	7.8	111	63%
dry or hard/pork	1 oz	7.0	85	74%
salt pork/raw	1 oz	22.8	212	97%
souse loaf	1 oz	3.8	51	67%
turkey breast	~1.5 oz	0.7	47	13%
turkey ham	2 oz	2.9	73	36%
turkey roll				
light & dark meat	1 oz	2.0	42	42%
light meat	1 oz	2.0	42	43%
■ (Healthy Choice)				
Boneless honey ham	2 oz	1.5	70	19%
Cold Cuts				
bologna				
beef	1 oz slice	1.0	35	26%
turkey, pork, & beef	1 oz slice	1.0	30	30%
chicken breast				
oven roasted	1 oz slice	–	25	–
smoked	1 oz slice	1.0	35	26%
ham				
baked cooked	1 oz slice	1.0	30	30%
cooked	1 oz slice	1.0	30	30%
honey	1 oz slice	1.0	30	30%

Food and Description	Amount	Fat Grams	Total Calories	% Fat Calories
smoked	1 oz slice	1.0	30	30%
turkey breast				
honey roasted & smoked	1 oz slice	1.0	35	26%
oven roasted	1 oz slice	1.0	30	30%
smoked	1 oz slice	1.0	30	30%
turkey ham				
cured turkey thigh	1 oz slice	1.0	35	26%
Deli				
ham				
cooked	2 oz	1.5	60	23%
honey	2 oz	1.5	60	23%
honey maple	2 oz	1.5	60	23%
honey Virginia	2 oz	1.5	60	23%
smoked	2 oz	1.5	60	23%
poultry				
chicken breast				
browned	2 oz	1.0	60	15%
cooked	2 oz	–	45	–
mesquite	2 oz	0.5	60	8%
turkey breast				
browned	2 ox	1.0	60	15%
honey roasted & smoked	2 oz	–	60	–
oven roasted	2 oz	–	45	–
salsa	2 oz	1.0	60	15%
smoked	2 oz	–	50	–
southwest grill	2 oz	1.0	60	15%
Deli Pre-Sliced				
beef				
corned beef	2 slices	2.0	70	26%
roast	2 slices	1.0	50	18%
ham				
honey cured	2 slices	1.5	60	23%
Virginia Brand	2 slices	1.5	60	23%
turkey breast				
honey roasted & smoked	2 slices	–	50	–
oven roasted	2 slices	–	50	–
Deli Thin Sliced				
beef				
cajun style	2 oz	1.0	60	15%
corned beef	2 oz	1.5	60	23%
medium-cooked	2 oz	1:0	60	15%
pastrami	2 oz	1.5	60	23%
roast beef	2 oz	1.5	60	23%
Italian	2 oz	1.0	60	15%
structured	2 oz	1.0	50	18%
bologna				
w/turkey, pork, & beef	4 slices	1.5	60	23%
chicken breast				
oven roasted	6 slices	–	50	–
smoked	6 slices	1.5	60	23%

Food and Description	Amount	Fat Grams	Total Calories	% Fat Calories
corned beef/chopped & formed	6 slices	1.5	60	23%
ham				
baked cooked	6 slices	1.5	60	23%
cooked	6 slices	1.5	60	23%
honey	6 slices	1.5	60	23%
smoked	6 slices	1.5	60	23%
roast beef/chopped & formed	6 slices	1.5	60	23%
turkey breast				
honey roasted & smoke	6 slices	1.5	60	23%
oven	6 slices	1.5	60	23%
peppered	6 slices	1.5	60	23%
turkey	6 slices	1.5	60	23%
turkey ham cured turkey thigh	6 slices	1.5	60	23%
Fresh				
chicken				
oven roasted	1 oz slice	1.0	30	30%
ham				
cooked	1 oz slice	1.0	30	30%
honey	1 oz slice	1.0	30	30%
roast beef/chopped & formed	1 oz slice	1.0	30	30%
turkey breast				
honey roasted and smoked	1 oz slice	1.0	35	26%
oven roasted	1 oz slice	1.0	30	30%
Hearty Deli Flavor				
chicken breast				
rotisserie season	2 slices	0.5	50	9%
corned beef/zesty	3 slices	1.5	60	23%
ham				
brown sugar/cured	2 slices	1.5	60	23%
honey/baked	2 slices	1.5	60	23%
turkey breast				
roasted	2 slices	0.5	50	9%
■ **(Hebrew National)**				
bologna				
beef				
lite/reduced fat	1 oz	12.0	130	83%
regular/chub	2 oz	15.0	160	84%
sliced	4 slices	16.0	180	80%
lean				
chub	2 oz	5.0	90	50%
sliced	4 slices	5.0	90	50%
chicken/Deli Thin/oven-roasted	1.8 oz	0.5	45	10%
corned beef				
brisket/1st cut	2 oz	3.0	80	34%
Deli Express	2 oz	3.0	90	30%
knockwurst				
beef	1 link	24.0	260	83%
hot jalapeño beef	1 link	24.0	260	83%
pastrami/				
deli slices	2 oz	4.0	90	40%

Food and Description	Amount	Fat Grams	Total Calories	% Fat Calories
1st cut	2 oz	3.0	80	34%
salami/beef				
lean	2 oz	5.0	90	50%
regular/chub	2 oz	14.0	170	74%
sliced	3 slices	13.0	150	78%
turkey breast				
oven-roasted	2 oz	0.5	50	9%
smoked	2 oz	0.5	50	9%
▣ (Hickory Farms)				
salami				
dry or hard	1 oz	10.0	120	75%
Genoa	1 oz	10.0	110	82%
▣ (Hillshire Farm)				
beef/Deli Select				
oven-roasted/cured	2 oz	1.0	60	15%
roast	2 oz	1.0	60	15%
smoked/97% fat-free	2 oz	1.0	60	15%
bologna/Deli Select/light	2 oz	2.0	70	26%
chicken breast/Deli Select				
oven-roasted	2 oz	–	60	–
smoked	2 oz	–	60	–
corned beef/Deli Select	2 oz	1.0	50	18%
ham				
Baked/97% fat free	2 oz	1.5	60	23%
brown sugar baked	2 oz	2.0	70	26%
brown sugar cured, bone in	3 oz	6.0	120	45%
Cajun-style/97% fat free	2 oz	1.5	60	23%
regular	2 oz	2.0	60	30%
honey cured				
spiral sliced	3 oz	6.0	120	45%
spiral sliced brown sugar cured half	3 oz	6.0	120	45%
pastrami				
Deli Select	2 oz	1.0	60	15%
regular	2 oz	1.0	70	13%
pepperoni	18 pieces	14.0	150	84%
salami/hard	~1 oz	9.0	100	90%
summer sausage				
beef				
Old World	2 oz	15.0	180	75%
regular	2 oz	17.0	190	81%
32 oz stick	2 oz	16.0	210	69%
Yard-O-Beef	2 oz	17.0	190	81%
turkey breast				
Deli Select				
honey-roasted	2 oz	–	50	–
mesquite smoked	2 oz	–	50	–
oven-roasted	2 oz	–	50	–
regular				
honey-cured	1 oz	2.0	35	51%
honey-roasted	1 oz	2.0	35	51%

Food and Description	Amount	Fat Grams	Total Calories	% Fat Calories
oven-roasted	1 oz	2.0	35	51%
smoked	1 oz	2.0	35	51%
turkey ham/Deli Select	2 oz	1.0	60	15%
■ (Hormel)				
Beef				
chuck roast	2 oz	2.0	60	30%
dried/Pillow Pack	10 slices	1.0	45	20%
top round roast	2 oz	1.0	50	18%
Chicken/chunk meat				
chicken	2 oz	3.0	70	39%
chicken breast				
no salt	2 oz	1.5	60	23%
regular	2 oz	1.5	60	23%
Corned beef	2 oz	7.0	120	53%
Ham				
chunk meat	2 oz	6.0	90	60%
Black Label				
canned	3 oz	5.0	84	54%
chopped	1 oz	11.0	140	71%
Cure 8½	3 oz	5.0	100	45%
Curemaster	3 oz	3.0	80	34%
deli cooked	2 oz	2.5	60	38%
Light & Lean 97				
half ham	3 oz	2.5	90	25%
sliced	1 slice	1.0	25	36%
patties				
plain	1 patty	17.0	180	85%
w/cheese	1 patty	17.0	190	80%
Pepperoni				
chunk	1 oz slice	13.0	140	84%
sliced	1 oz slice	13.0	140	84%
turkey/Pillow Pack	17 slices	4.0	80	45%
twin	1 oz slice	13.0	140	84%
Salami				
Genoa				
Di Lusso	2 oz	18.0	210	77%
Pillow Pack	2 oz	18.0	210	77%
San Remo	1 oz	9.0	120	68%
hard				
Homeland	1 oz	10.0	110	82%
Pillow Pack	4 slices	10.0	120	75%
Spam				
less salt	2 oz	16.0	170	85%
lite	2 oz	8.0	110	65%
original	2 oz	16.0	170	85%
smoked	2 oz	16.0	170	85%
spread	4 Tbs	11.0	140	77%
Turkey				
chunk meat				
turkey	2 oz	3.0	70	39%

Food and Description	Amount	Fat Grams	Total Calories	% Fat Calories
white turkey	2 oz	1.0	60	15%
deli meat				
Light & Lean 97				
mesquite-smoked	1 slice	0.5	30	15%
sliced	1 slice	0.5	30	15%
Turkey ham/chunk meat	2 oz	4.0	70	51%
Vienna sausage				
chicken	2 oz	9.0	110	74%
original	2 oz	14.0	150	84%
▨ (Johnsonville)				
bologna/country style				
beef ring	2 oz	15.0	170	79%
ring	2 oz	15.0	170	79%
summer sausage				
beef	2 oz	15.0	180	75%
original	2 oz	15.0	180	75%
summer				
garlic	2 oz	15.0	180	75%
Old World	2 oz	16.0	190	76%
▨ (Jones Dairy Farm)				
braunschweiger liverwurst				
light	2 oz	6.0	100	54%
light w/bacon added	1.6 oz	13.0	150	78%
regular	2 oz	16.0	180	80%
spread	2 oz	12.0	150	72%
▨ (Kahn's)				
bologna				
beef				
family pack	1 oz slice	6.0	70	77%
fat-free	1 oz slice	–	30	–
pounder	1 oz slice	8.0	90	80%
regular sliced	1 oz slice	8.0	90	80%
beef n' cheddar/8-oz pkg	1 oz slice	8.0	90	80%
ham/97% fat-free	1 oz slice	1.0	30	30%
pickle loaf	1 oz slice	6.0	70	77%
salami				
beef				
8-oz pkg	1 oz slice	6.0	70	77%
family pack	1 oz slice	5.0	60	75%
cooked/8-oz pkg	1 oz slice	4.0	60	60%
cotto salami/regular sliced	1 oz slice	4.5	60	68%
souse loaf/8-oz pkg	1 oz slice	7.0	90	70%
spice loaf				
beef/family pack	1 oz slice	5.0	60	75%
regular				
8-oz pkg	1 oz slice	7.0	80	79%
family pack	1 oz slice	6.0	70	77%
▨ (Louis Rich)				
Chicken				
breast, oven roasted deluxe	1 slice	0.5	30	15%

Food and Description	Amount	Fat Grams	Total Calories	% Fat Calories
breast & white chicken, oven roasted	1 slice	1.5	35	9%
Carving Board				
classic baked	2 slices	0.5	45	10%
grilled	2 slices	0.5	45	10%
Deli-Thin				
breast, oven roasted	4 slices	1.0	50	18%
white meat, oven roasted	1 slice	1.5	35	9%
Ham/Carving Board				
baked	2 slices	1.5	50	27%
honey-glazed				
thin-carved	6 slices	1.5	70	19%
traditional	2 slices	1.5	50	27%
smoked	2 slices	1.5	45	30%
Turkey				
breast/fully cooked/skinless				
fat-free				
hickory-smoked	2 oz	–	50	–
honey-roasted	2 oz	–	60	–
oven-roasted	2 oz	–	50	–
rotisserie flavor	2 oz	–	50	–
breast/sliced				
Carving Board				
hickory-smoked	2 slices	0.5	40	11%
oven-roasted				
thin-carved	6 slices	0.5	60	8%
traditional carved	2 slices	0.5	40	11%
rotisserie flavor	2 slices	0.5	40	11%
Chunk Specialties				
breast & white turkey, oven-roasted	2 oz	1.0	60	15%
ham	2 oz	3.0	70	39%
pastrami	2 oz	2.0	70	26%
salami/cooked	2 oz	8.0	100	72%
Cold Cuts				
Fat-free				
hickory smoked	1 slice	–	25	–
oven roasted	1 slice	–	25	–
regular				
bologna	1 slice	3.5	50	63%
ham				
chopped	1 slice	2.5	45	50%
honey-cured	1 slice	1.0	30	30%
regular	1 slice	1.0	30	30%
pastrami	1 slice	1.0	30	30%
salami				
cooked	1 slice	2.5	40	56%
cotto	1 slice	2.5	40	56%
white/smoked	1 slice	1.0	30	30%
Deli-Thin breast & white meat				
hickory smoked	4 slices	1.5	50	27%
oven roasted	4 slices	1.0	50	18%

Food and Description	Amount	Fat Grams	Total Calories	% Fat Calories
oven roasted/fat-free	4 slices	–	45	–
regular				
hickory-smoked	1 slice	–	50	–
honey-roasted	1 slice	–	60	
oven-roasted	1 slice	–	50	–
rotisserie flavor	1 slice	–	50	–
■ (Oscar Mayer)				
Authentic Cold Cuts				
braunschweiger, liver sausage	1 slice	9.0	100	81%
ham & cheese loaf	1 slice	5.0	70	64%
ham, chopped	1 slice	3.0	50	54%
head cheese	1 slice	4.0	50	72%
liver cheese, pork fat wrapped	1 slice	10.0	120	75%
luncheon loaf, spiced	1 slice	5.0	70	64%
New England Brand sausage	2 slices	2.5	60	38%
old fashioned loaf	1 slice	4.5	70	58%
olive loaf	1 slice	6.0	70	77%
pepperoni	15 slices	13.0	140	84%
pickle & pimiento loaf	1 slice	6.0	80	68%
salami				
cotto				
beef	1 slice	4.5	60	68%
pork chicken, & beef	1 slice	5.0	70	64%
for beer	3 slices	9.0	110	74%
Genoa	3 slices	9.0	100	81%
hard	3 slices	9.0	100	81%
Machiaeh/beef	2 slices	10.0	120	75%
Summer sausage/Thuringer Cervelat)				
beef	2 slices	12.0	140	77%
meat	2 slices	13.0	140	84%
Cold Cuts/Bologna				
Free/fat-free	1 slice	–	20	–
light				
beef	1 slice	4.0	60	60%
pork chicken, & beef	1 slice	4.0	60	60%
regular				
beef	1 slice	8.0	90	80%
garlic	1 slice	12.0	130	83%
pork, chicken, & beef	1 slice	8.0	90	80%
Wisconsin-made ring	2 oz	16.0	180	80%
FREE brand/fat-free				
bologna	1 slice	–	20	–
chicken breast/oven roasted	4 slices	–	45	–
ham				
baked cooked	3 slices	–	35	–
honey	3 slices	–	35	–
smoked	3 slices	–	35	–
turkey breast				
oven roasted	4 slices	–	40	–
smoked	4 slices	–	40	–

Food and Description	Amount	Fat Grams	Total Calories	% Fat Calories
Lean Meats				
ham				
baked cooked	3 slices	2.5	70	32%
boiled	3 slices	2.5	60	38%
honey	3 slices	2.5	70	32%
lower sodium	3 slices	2.5	70	32%
smoked cooked	3 slices	2.0	60	30%
turkey, white				
oven roasted	1 slice	1.0	30	30%
smoked	1 slice	1.0	30	30%
■ **(The Turkey Store)**				
Oven-Roasted chicken breast	2 oz	1.5	50	27%
Oven Roasted turkey breasts				
browned	2 oz	0.5	50	9%
single lobe browned	2 oz	0.5	60	8%
oven roasted	2 oz	0.5	50	9%
Premium turkey hams				
Black Forest	2 oz	3.0	70	39%
regular	2 oz	3.0	70	39%
Premium seasoned turkey breasts				
cracked pepper	2 oz	–	50	–
Cajun	2 oz	–	50	–
garlic pesto	2 oz	–	50	–
homestyle	2 oz	0.5	50	9%
honey dijon	2 oz	–	50	–
lemon pepper	2 oz	–	50	–
sun dried tomato	2 oz	–	50	–
Rotisserie-Ready turkey breasts				
mini	4 oz	3.0	140	19%
regular size	4 oz	3.0	140	19%
Smoked turkey breasts/natural smoked				
hickory	2 oz	1.0	60	15%
hickory honey cured	2 oz	1.0	60	15%
mesquite	2 oz	1.0	60	15%
Turkey pastrami/95% fat-free	2 oz	3.0	70	39%
■ **(Tyson)** Fat-free Luncheon Meat				
Chicken Breast				
hickory smoked	2 slices	–	35	–
honey-flavored	2 slices	–	35	–
mesquite-flavored	2 slices	–	35	–
oven-roasted	2 slices	–	35	–
peppered	2 slices	–	35	–
■ **SPAM** (See also (Hormel) in this section)				
LUNCHEON MEAT SPREAD (See also PÂTÉ)				
(Armour)				
deviled ham	3 oz	18.0	210	77%
potted meat/all flavors	2.2 oz	5.0	80	56%
	3 oz	9.0	130	62%
generic				
beef	1 Tbs	2.5	34	67%
	1 oz	5.0	67	67%

Food and Description	Amount	Fat Grams	Total Calories	% Fat Calories
chicken	1 oz	3.0	55	49%
deviled ham	¼ cup	18.0	198	82%
ham & cheese	1 Tbs	2.8	37	68%
ham salad	1 oz	4.0	61	59%
pork	1 Tbs	2.5	34	67%
	1 oz	5.0	67	67%
turkey	~2 oz	6.0	100	54%
(Hormel)				
Cure 81 deviled ham	4 Tbs	12.0	150	72%
Hormel				
liverwurst	4 Tbs	10.0	130	69%
potted meat	4 Tbs	8.0	100	72%
(Libby's) Spreadables				
deviled meats	¼ cup	8.0	120	60%
potted meats	3 oz	13.0	160	73%
(Oscar Mayer)				
Braunschweiger liver sausage	2 oz	17.0	190	80%
sandwich spread	2 oz	10.0	130	69%
(Swanson)				
chicken/chunky	¼ cup	8.0	120	60%
(Underwood)				
chicken	2 oz	10.0	140	64%
ham				
deviled	¼ cup	24.0	250	86%
honey	2 oz	10.0	130	69%
regular	2 oz	11.0	140	71%
liverwurst	2 oz	14.0	170	74%
roast beef	2 oz	9.0	130	62%
LUPIN				
boiled	½ cup	2.0	98	18%
raw	½ cup	8.0	330	22%

M

Food and Description	Amount	Fat Grams	Total Calories	% Fat Calories
MACADAMIA NUT				
(Diamond Of California) chopped	¼ cup	24.0	240	90%
(Fisher) Snack'N Serve Nut Bowl				
chocolate covered	1 oz	15.0	200	68%
dry roasted	1 oz	21.0	200	95%

Food and Description	Amount	Fat Grams	Total Calories	% Fat Calories
Generic				
dried	1 oz	21.0	200	95%
dry-roasted	1 oz	21.0	193	98%
oil-roasted	1 oz	21.7	204	96%
(MacFarms of Hawaii)				
chocolate covered	¼ cup	16.0	210	69%
dry roasted/salted	¼ cup	23.0	220	94%
Kona coffee dark chocolate covered	¼ cup	16.0	210	69%
(Mauna Loa)				
brittle	1 oz	8.0	150	48%
chocolate-covered	1 oz	13.0	170	69%
honey-roasted	1 oz	17.0	200	77%
roasted/salted/shelled	1 oz	21.0	210	90%
MACARONI (See PASTA)				
MACARONI & CHEESE (See FROZEN ENTRÉE/DINNER; PASTA ENTRÉE/DINNER; VEGETARIAN FOODS)				
MACAROON (See COOKIE)				
MACE /ground	1 tsp	0.6	8	68%
MACKEREL (See also SEAFOOD ENTRÉE/DINNER)				
Atlantic				
cooked-dry heat	3 oz	15.0	223	61%
raw	3 oz	11.8	174	61%
jack/canned/drained				
(Empress)	4 oz	8.0	140	51%
generic	1 cup	12.0	296	36%
king				
cooked-dry heat	3 oz	5.5	135	37%
raw	3 oz	1.7	89	17%
Pacific/mixed species				
cooked-dry heat	3 oz	8.5	170	45%
raw	3 oz	6.5	135	43%
Spanish				
cooked-dry heat	3 oz	5.0	134	34%
raw	3 oz	5.0	118	38%
MAHI MAHI				
cooked-dry heat	3 oz	1.0	95	9%
Hawaiian-style/frozen/skinless-boneless	4 oz	1.0	100	9%
raw	3 oz	0.6	72	8%
MALT (See BARLEY MALT; MILK MIX)				
MALT LIQUOR (See BEER, ALE, & MALT LIQUOR)				
MAMEY APPLE/MAMMEY APPLE/MAMMEE APPLE				
raw				
peeled/no seeds	3 oz	<1.0	42	6%
whole	1 medium	4.4	445	9%
MANDARIN ORANGE (See also TANGERINE)				
canned				
(Del Monte) in heavy syrup	½ cup	–	80	–
(Dole) in light syrup	½ cup	–	70	–
(Empress)	½ cup	–	80	–

Food and Description	Amount	Fat Grams	Total Calories	% Fat Calories
generic				
in juice	1 cup	–	90	–
in light syrup	1 cup	0.5	125	4%
(S&W)				
natural style	½ cup	–	60	–
sections in heavy syrup	½ cup	–	80	
fresh/raw				
sections	½ cup	–	45	–
whole	1 medium	–	35	–
MANGO				
fresh				
diced or sliced	1 cup	0.5	110	4%
whole	1 medium	0.5	135	3%
frozen				
(C&W) chunks	1 cup	–	90	–
MANGO JUICE/JUICE BLEND/JUICE DRINK (See also FRUIT PUNCH)				
bottled				
(Kern's) nectar	6 fl oz	–	100	–
	11.5 fl oz	–	210	–
(Knudsen)				
Mango Montage	8 fl oz	–	110	–
mango-peach	8 fl oz	–	120	–
(Libby's) nectar	6 fl oz	–	100	–
(Snapple) cocktail				
Mango Mad				
regular	8 fl oz	–	110	–
diet	8 fl oz	–	15	–
(TreeTop) More Mango	8 fl oz	–	120	–
mix/prepared				
(Tang) drink mix/mango flavored	8 fl oz	–	100	–
MANICOTTI (See FROZEN ENTRÉE/DINNER; PASTA ENTRÉE/DINNER)				
MAPLE SYRUP (See also PANCAKE & WAFFLE SYRUP)				
Generic	1 Tbs	–	50	–
MARGARINE, MARGARINE SPREAD, & SPRAY				
(Autumn) spread	1 Tbs	8.0	80	100%
(Blue Bonnet)				
lower fat				
stick	1 Tbs	6.0	50	100%
tub	1 Tbs	4.5	45	100%
regular/soft or stick	1 Tbs	11.0	100	100%
spread				
Better Blend				
stick	1 Tbs	11.0	90	100%
tub	1 Tbs	11.0	90	100%
whipped				
soft	1 Tbs	7.0	70	100%
stick	1 Tbs	7.0	70	100%
(Brummel & Brown) w/yogurt				
tub	1 Tbs	5.0	50	100%
stick	1 Tbs	10.0	90	100%

Food and Description	Amount	Fat Grams	Total Calories	% Fat Calories
(Canola Harvest)				
soft	1 Tbs	11.0	100	100%
stick	1 Tbs	11.0	100	100%
tub	1 Tbs	7.0	60	100%
(Chiffon)				
soft stick	1 Tbs	11.0	100	100%
soft tub	1 Tbs	11.0	100	100%
whipped	1 Tbs	7.0	70	100%
(Fleischmann's)				
corn oil spread				
extra light	1 Tbs	6.0	50	100%
fat-free/squeeze	1 Tbs	–	5	–
light				
soft or stick	1 Tbs	8.0	80	100%
squeeze	1 Tbs	10.0	90	100%
diet	1 Tbs	6.0	50	100%
soft or stick	1 Tbs	11.0	100	100%
whipped	1 Tbs	7.0	70	100%
generic				
hard	1 pat	4.0	35	100%
	1 Tbs	11.0	100	100%
	4 oz	91.0	810	100%
soft	1 Tbs	11.0	100	100%
	4 oz	92.0	813	100%
spread				
40% fat/soft	1 Tbs	5.7	50	100%
	4 oz	44.0	393	100%
60% fat				
hard	1 pat	3.0	25	100%
	1 Tbs	9.0	75	100%
	4 oz	69.0	610	100%
soft	1 Tbs	9.0	75	100%
	4 oz	69.0	613	100%
squeeze	1 tsp	4.0	35	100%
whipped/hard or soft	1 Tbs	7.0	70	100%
(Gold-N-Sweet) canola	1 Tbs	11.0	100	100%
(Gregg's) Gold-n-Soft-Lite spread	1 Tbs	7.0	70	100%
(Hain) safflower				
regular	1 Tbs	11.0	100	100%
unsalted	1 Tbs	11.0	100	100%
(Heartlight) canola	1 Tbs	11.0	100	100%
(Hollywood) safflower				
regular	1 Tbs	11.0	100	100%
unsalted sweet	1 Tbs	11.0	100	100%
(I Can't Believe It's Not Butter)				
light spread				
stick	1 Tbs	6.0	50	100%
tub	1 Tbs	5.0	50	100%
regular	1 Tbs	10.0	90	100%

Food and Description	Amount	Fat Grams	Total Calories	% Fat Calories
soft	1 Tbs	10.0	90	100%
spray	5 sprays	–	–	–
squeeze	1 Tbs	8.0	80	100%
unsalted	1 Tbs	10.0	90	100%
(Imperial)				
A La Mode	1 Tbs	7.5	70	100%
A La Mode stick	1 Tbs	11.0	100	100%
light	1 Tbs	6.0	60	100%
quarters	1 Tbs	11.0	100	100%
Savory Squeeze				
buttery	1 Tbs	10.0	90	100%
garlic & herb	1 Tbs	10.0	90	100%
soft	1 Tbs	11.0	100	100%
soft diet	1 Tbs	6.0	50	100%
whipped	1 Tbs	6.0	50	100%
(Kraft) Touch of Butter				
47% fat/tub	1 Tbs	7.0	60	100%
70% fat/stick	1 Tbs	7.0	60	100%
(Land O'Lakes)				
Country Morning Blend				
stick	1 Tbs	11.0	100	100%
light	1 Tbs	6.0	50	100%
unsalted	1 Tbs	11.0	100	100%
tub				
light	1 Tbs	6.0	50	100%
regular	1 Tbs	11.0	100	100%
premium corn oil				
stick	1 Tbs	11.0	100	100%
tub	1 Tbs	11.0	100	100%
soy oil				
stick	1 Tbs	11.0	100	100%
tub	1 Tbs	11.0	100	100%
spread w/sweet cream				
stick				
salted	1 Tbs	10.0	90	100%
unsalted	1 Tbs	10.0	90	100%
tub	1 Tbs	8.0	80	100%
(Lipton) Take Control				
light	1 Tbs	4.5	40	100%
regular	1 Tbs	6.0	50	100%
(Mazola)				
reduced calorie				
extra light	1 Tbs	6.0	50	100%
light corn oil	1 Tbs	6.0	50	100%
regular	1 Tbs	11.0	100	100%
unsalted	1 Tbs	11.0	100	100%
(Miracle Brand) whipped				
soft	1 Tbs	7.0	60	100%
stick	1 Tbs	7.0	70	100%
(Mrs. Filberts)				
corn oil family spread	1 Tbs	7.0	60	100%

Food and Description	Amount	Fat Grams	Total Calories	% Fat Calories
golden quarters	1 Tbs	11.0	100	100%
soft corn	1 Tbs	11.0	100	100%
soft gold	1 Tbs	11.0	100	100%
vegetable oil	1 Tbs	7.0	65	100%
(Nabisco) Move Over Butter				
stick	1 Tbs	10.0	90	100%
tub	1 Tbs	10.0	90	100%
whipped	1 Tbs	7.0	60	100%
(Nucanola)	1 Tbs	10.0	90	100%
(Nucoa)				
Heart Beat/corn oil	1 Tbs	3.0	25	100%
Smartbeat				
light/unsalted	1 Tbs	3.0	25	100%
squeeze/rat-free	1 Tbs	–	5	–
super light/trans fat-free	1 Tbs	2.0	20	100%
tub/salted and unsalted	1 Tbs	3.0	25	100%
soft	1 Tbs	10.0	90	100%
stick	1 Tbs	11.0	100	100%
(Parkay)				
diet	1 Tbs	6.0	50	100%
liquid				
regular	1 Tbs	9.0	80	100%
spread	1 Tbs	9.0	80	100%
soft or stick	1 Tbs	11.0	100	100%
vegetable oil spread				
40%/light	1 Tbs	7.0	60	100%
50%	1 Tbs	7.0	60	100%
53%	1 Tbs	7.0	70	100%
70%	1 Tbs	10.0	90	100%
whipped/soft or stick	1 Tbs	7.0	70	100%
(Promise)				
extra light	1 Tbs	6.0	50	100%
fat-free	1 Tbs	–	5	–
regular	1 Tbs	10.0	90	100%
sunflower oil	1 Tbs	10.0	90	100%
ultra/tub	1 Tbs	4.0	35	100%
(Saffola)	1 Tbs	11.0	100	100%
(Shedd's Spread)				
churn style tub	1 Tbs	7.0	60	100%
classic 64% spread/stick	1 Tbs	7.0	60	100%
corn oil spread	1 Tbs	7.0	60	100%
Country Crock	1 Tbs	7.0	70	100%
original	1 Tbs	9.0	80	100%
quarters spread	1 Tbs	9.0	80	100%
squeeze	1 Tbs	9.0	80	100%
whipped honey spread	1 Tbs	9.0	90	90%
(Weight Watchers)				
Country Cottage spread/tub	1 Tbs	4.0	45	100%
light spread/tub				
regular	1 Tbs	4.0	45	100%

Food and Description	Amount	Fat Grams	Total Calories	% Fat Calories
sodium-free	1 Tbs	4.0	45	100%
(Willow Run Print) sticks	1 Tbs	11.0	100	100%
MARINADE (*See also* SEASONINGS)				
Bottled or jarred				
(Andre Prost) hot adobo	1 Tbs	–	10	–
(Cardini)				
citrus lime dill	1 Tbs	–	20	–
fajita mesquite	1 Tbs	–	10	–
honey dijon	1 Tbs	–	20	–
red wine	1 Tbs	–	10	–
roasted garlic	1 Tbs	–	10	–
spicy Cajun	1 Tbs	–	10	–
tangy teriyaki	1 Tbs	–	20	–
zesty lemon pepper	1 Tbs	–	15	–
(Girard's) lemon dill	2 Tbs	14.0	130	97%
(Golden Dipt)				
Cajun style	1 Tbs	4.5	60	68%
ginger teriyaki	1 Tbs	3.0	60	45%
honey mustard/fat-free	1 Tbs	–	25	–
honey soy/fat-free	1 Tbs	–	30	–
lemon herb	1 Tbs	9.0	80	100%
white wine Dijon/fat-free	1 Tbs	–	10	–
(House of Tsang) Mandarin marinade	1 Tbs	–	25	–
(KC Masterpiece)				
garlic & herb	1 Tbs	1.5	30	45%
honey teriyaki	1 Tbs	0.5	35	13%
original BBQ	1 Tbs	1.5	40	34%
(Lawry's)				
citrus grill	1 Tbs	–	15	–
Hawaiian	1 Tbs	–	20	–
herb garlic	1 Tbs	–	10	–
lemon pepper	1 Tbs	0.5	10	45%
mesquite	1 Tbs	–	5	–
red wine	1 Tbs	–	5	–
teriyaki	1 Tbs	–	35	–
(Mr. Marinade)				
Cajun	1 Tbs	–	10	–
honey mustard	1 Tbs	–	20	–
Italian	1 Tbs	–	10	–
red wine	1 Tbs	–	15	–
teriyaki	1 Tbs	–	10	–
white wine	1 Tbs	0.5	15	30%
(S&W)				
mesquite	1 Tbs	–	10	–
teriyaki				
lite	1 Tbs	–	25	–
regular	1 Tbs	–	25	–
(T. Marzetti Co.)(See (Cardini) in this section				
Mix/mix only				
(Durkee) beef	⅒ pkg	–	–	–
(French's) meat	⅒ pkg	–	–	–

Food and Description	Amount	Fat Grams	Total Calories	% Fat Calories
(Kikkoman)	1 oz	–	60	–
(Lawry's)				
chicken sauté				
country Dijon	2 Tbs	1.0	40	23%
garlic Italian	2 Tbs	2.0	30	60%
seasoned	1 Tbs	–	10	–
teriyaki	1 Tbs	–	25	–
(Marinade-Magic)				
fajitas	½ tsp	–	5	–
grilled chicken	¾ tsp	–	10	–
lemon beef	½ tsp	–	10	–
(McCormick/Schilling)				
chicken				
Italian	2 tsp	–	20	–
mesquite	2 tsp	–	20	–
fajita	¼ tsp	–	1	–
Grill Mates				
mesquite	2 tsp	–	15	–
Oriental	2 tsp	–	15	–
Southwest	2 tsp	–	15	–
zesty herb	2 tsp	–	10	–
meat/original	1 tsp	–	15	–
(Watkins)				
beef	¼ Tbs	–	5	–
fish & seafood	¼ Tbs	–	10	–
MARINARA SAUCE (*See* SAUCE)				
MARIONBERRY				
(Schwan's) frozen/no sugar	3.5 oz	–	60	–
MARJORAM /dried	1 tsp	–	2	–
MARMALADE (*See* JAM/JELLY/PRESERVES)				
MARSHMALLOW				
(Campfire)				
large	2 pieces	–	40	–
miniature	10 pieces	–	17	–
	24 pieces	–	40	–
generic/large or small	1 oz	–	95	–
(Kraft)				
Funmallows				
large	4 pieces	–	110	–
miniature	10 pieces	–	18	–
	½ cup	–	100	–
Jet Puffed	5 pieces	–	110	–
Miniatures	½ cup	–	100	–
MARSHMALLOW CREME				
(Kraft)	2 Tbs	–	40	–
MATZO (*See* CRACKER; MATZO MEAL & MIX)				
MATZO MEAL & MIX (*See also* SOUP)				
Meal				
(Goodman's)				
matzo ball mix				
50% less salt	2 Tbs	–	50	–

Food and Description	Amount	Fat Grams	Total Calories	% Fat Calories
regular	2 Tbs	–	50	–
Passover	1 cup	1.0	514	2%
(Manischewitz)	1 cup	1.0	510	2%
Mix				
(Manischewitz) matzo ball/mix only	2 Tbs	–	50	–
MAYONNAISE/MAYONNAISE-TYPE DRESSING (*See also* SALAD DRESSING)				
(Bama) regular	1 Tbs	11.0	100	100%
(Bennett's) real	1 Tbs	12.0	110	98%
(Best Foods)				
Dijonnaise blend	1 tsp	1.0	10	90%
light	1 Tbs	5.0	50	90%
real	1 Tbs	11.0	100	99%
reduced fat	1 Tbs	3.0	40	68%
(Estee)	1 Tbs	5.0	50	90%
(Featherweight) soyamaise mayo dressing	1 Tbs	11.0	100	99%
(Hain)				
canola				
light/reduced calorie	1 Tbs	5.0	60	75%
regular	1 Tbs	11.0	100	100%
cold-processed	1 Tbs	12.0	110	98%
eggless	1 Tbs	12.0	110	98%
light	1 Tbs	6.0	60	90%
real	1 Tbs	12.0	110	98%
safflower	1 Tbs	12.0	110	98%
(Hellman's)				
Dijonnaise blend	1 tsp	1.0	10	90%
light	1 Tbs	5.0	50	90%
real	1 Tbs	11.0	100	100%
reduced fat	1 Tbs	3.0	40	68%
(Hollywood)				
canola	1 Tbs	11.0	100	100%
safflower	1 Tbs	11.0	100	98%
(Kraft)				
mayonnaise				
Kraft Free/nonfat	1 Tbs	–	10	–
light	1 Tbs	5.0	50	90%
real	1 Tbs	11.0	100	99%
Miracle Whip				
Free	1 Tbs	–	15	–
light	1 Tbs	3.0	35	77%
original	1 Tbs	7.0	70	90%
(Life All Natural) egg-free	1 Tbs	8.0	70	100%
(Nasoya) tofu Nayonaise	1 Tbs	4.0	40	90%
(Nucoa) Heart Beat corn oil	1 Tbs	4.0	40	90%
(Smart Beat)				
canola oil	1 Tbs	4.0	40	90%
corn oil	1 Tbs	4.0	40	90%
fat-free	1 Tbs	–	10	–
(Spectrum) canola				
eggless lite	1 Tbs	3.0	30	90%

Food and Description	Amount	Fat Grams	Total Calories	% Fat Calories
real	1 Tbs	12.0	100	100%
(Spin Blend)				
cholesterol-free	1 Tbs	4.0	40	90%
dressing	1 Tbs	5.0	60	75%
(Weight Watchers)				
fat free	1 Tbs	–	10	–
light				
low-sodium	1 Tbs	2.0	25	72%
regular	1 Tbs	2.0	25	72%
whipped	1 Tbs	–	15	–
(Westbrae) canola	1 Tbs	11.0	100	99%

MEAL REPLACEMENT (*See* NUTRITIONAL SUPPLEMENT)
MEAT LOAF (*See* FROZEN ENTRÉE/DINNER)
MEAT SEASONING (*See* MARINADE; SEASONINGS)
MEAT SPREAD (*See* LUNCHEON MEAT SPREAD)
MEAT SUBSTITUTE (*See* VEGETARIAN FOODS; individual listings)
MEAT TENDERIZER (*See also* MARINADE; SEASONINGS)

Food and Description	Amount	Fat Grams	Total Calories	% Fat Calories
generic/seasoned	1 tsp	–	2	–
(Tone's)				
seasoned	1 tsp	–	7	–
unseasoned	1 tsp	–	7	–

MEATBALL (*See* BEEF; BEEF DISH/ENTRÉE; FROZEN ENTRÉE/DINNER; PASTA ENTRÉE/DINNER)
MELBA TOAST (*See* CRACKER)
MELON (*See also* individual listings)

Food and Description	Amount	Fat Grams	Total Calories	% Fat Calories
balls/frozen				
(C&W) mixed/no sugar added	⅔ cup	–	40	–
generic				
cantaloupe & honeydew	1 lb	1.0	145	6%
sweetened	1 cup	0.5	245	2%
unsweetened	½ cup	0.5	60	8%

MEXICAN FOOD (*See also* BEEF DISH/ENTRÉE; BREAKFAST SANDWICH; DIP; FROZEN ENTRÉE/DINNER; PASTA ENTRÉE/DINNER; RICE DISH; SAUCE; SEASONINGS; TOMATO; TOMATO SAUCE; TORTILLA CHIPS; VEGETARIAN FOODS)
■ **BEANS** (*See* Chili Beans; Refried Beans in this section)
■ **BURRITO**

Food and Description	Amount	Fat Grams	Total Calories	% Fat Calories
frozen				
(BR Brand)				
bean & choose	5 oz	6.0	290	19%
beef & bean	5 oz	15.0	400	34%
green chili	5 oz	9.0	340	24%
red chili	5 oz	5.0	290	16%
(Don Miguel)				
breakfast				
bacon & egg	1 burrito	27.0	520	47%
sausage	1 burrito	27.0	510	48%
smoked ham	1 burrito	17.0	420	36%
Lean Olé!				
bean & cheese	1 burrito	4.0	380	9%
chicken, beans, & rice	1 burrito	5.0	380	12%

Food and Description	Amount	Fat Grams	Total Calories	% Fat Calories
steak, beans, & hoe	1 burrito	4.0	380	9%
regular				
beef steak & bean w/jalapeño peppers	1 burrito	8.0	350	21%
chicken & cheese	1 burrito	14.0	410	31%
shredded beef & cheese	1 burrito	11.0	390	25%
shredded beef, cheddar cheese sauce, & green chilies				
hot & spicy	1 burrito	7.0	270	23%
regular	1 burrito	6.0	230	23%
skinless chicken	4.5 oz	5.0	240	19%
	7 oz	8.0	360	20%
steak strips/beef steak & bean	1 burrito	8.0	370	19%
3 cheeses/bean & cheese	4.5 oz	8.0	280	26%
	7 oz	13.0	420	28%
(El Charrito)				
bean & cheese				
grande	6 oz	8.0	380	19%
regular	5 oz	8.0	320	23%
beef & bean				
grande	6 oz	16.0	430	33%
regular	5 oz	12.0	350	31%
grande	6 oz	14.0	410	31%
green chili beef & bean	5 oz	16.0	370	39%
green chili grande	6 oz	15.0	410	33%
jalapeño grande	6 oz	15.0	410	33%
red chili beef & bean	5 oz	18.0	380	43%
red chili grande	6 oz	15.0	410	45%
red hot beef	5 oz	17.0	340	45%
red hot beef & bean	5 oz	18.0	540	30%
(El Monterey) reduced fat				
bean & cheese	1 burrito	4.0	220	16%
beef & bean	1 burrito	6.0	240	23%
(Hormel) Quick Meal				
beef & bean	1 burrito	13.0	300	39%
cheese	1 burrito	6.0	250	22%
red chili	1 burrito	11.0	280	35%
(Jimmy Dean) burrito breakfast				
bacon	1 burrito	8.0	260	28%
sausage	1 burrito	8.0	250	29%
(Old El Paso)				
bean & cheese	1 burrito	9.0	290	28%
beef & bean				
hot	1 burrito	10.0	320	28%
medium	1 burrito	10.0	320	28%
mild	1 burrito	9.0	330	25%
(Ruiz)				
beefsteak	1 burrito	6.0	270	20%
chicken	1 burrito	7.0	290	22%

Food and Description	Amount	Fat Grams	Total Calories	% Fat Calories
Monterey shredded beef & cheese (Senor Felix's)	1 burrito	10.0	310	29%
burritos				
black bean	1 burrito	18.0	540	30%
black bean soy	1 burrito	7.0	240	26%
chicken	1 burrito	20.0	520	35%
hot potato	1 burrito	24.0	560	39%
Sonora style/includes sauce	1 burrito	8.0	280	40%
Yucatan style/includes sauce	1 burrito	9.0	310	26%
Mixes and dinner kits				
(Chi-Chi's)				
shells & seasonings	2 shells	7.0	300	21%
(Del Monte) burrito filling mix	½ cup	1.0	110	8%
(Old El Paso)				
kit				
mix & 1 tortilla	1 piece	3.5	190	16%
prepared	1 piece	7.0	280	23%
seasoning/mix only	2 tsp	–	20	–
(Taco Bell) Ultimate bean burrito	1 burrito	5.0	200	23%
■ CHILI (See also BEEF DISH/ENTRÉE; SEASONINGS)				
Canned				
(Armour Star) beef & chicken				
w/beans				
original	7.5 oz	14.0	320	39%
Western style	7.5 oz	14.0	300	42%
w/o beans	7.5 oz	21.0	320	59%
(Chili Man)				
no bean	7.5 oz	27.0	380	64%
w/beans	7.5 oz	17.0	330	46%
white bean	7.5 oz	3.0	150	18%
(Dennison's)				
chicken w/black & pink beans	7.5 oz	6.0	360	15%
con carne				
chunky w/beans	8.88 oz	14.0	330	38%
w/o beans	7.5 oz	18.0	330	49%
hot				
& chunky w/beans	7.5 oz	13.0	320	37%
w/beans	7.5 oz	18.0	370	44%
w/o beans	7.5 oz	18.0	330	49%
mild green chilies	7.5 oz	17.0	370	41%
99% fat-free				
beef w/beans	7.5 oz	2.0	220	8%
turkey w/beans	7.5 oz	3.0	210	13%
vegetarian w/beans	7.5 oz	1.0	180	5%
original	7.5 oz	15.0	350	39%
(Don Miguel) XLNT chili con came w/o beans	⅓ cup	20.0	250	72%

Food and Description	Amount	Fat Grams	Total Calories	% Fat Calories
(Fantastic Foods)				
Chile Ole! Cups				
black bean w/ corn	2.5 oz	2.0	250	7%
nacho chili w/tortillas	2.5 oz	3.0	270	10%
spicy white bean	2.3 oz	2.5	260	9%
vegetarian	¼ cup	6.0	100	54%
(Gebhardt) beef w/beans	1 cup	15.0	320	42%
(Hain) Spicy				
tempeh	7.5 oz	4.0	160	23%
vegetarian				
reduced sodium	7.5 oz	1.0	170	5%
regular	7.5 oz	1.0	160	6%
w/chicken	7.5 oz	2.0	130	14%
(Health Valley) fat-free				
burrito flavor	½ cup	–	80	–
enchilada flavor	½ cup	–	80	–
fajita flavor	½ cup	–	80	–
mild w/black beans	½ cup	–	80	–
mild w/3 beans	½ cup	–	80	–
spicy w/black beans	½ cup	–	80	–
(Hormel)				
w/beans				
chunky	1 cup	7.0	270	23%
hot	1 cup	7.0	270	23%
regular	1 cup	7.0	270	23%
w/o beans				
hot	1 cup	9.0	210	39%
regular	1 cup	9.0	210	39%
turkey				
w/beans	1 cup	3.0	210	9%
w/o beans	1 cup	3.0	190	14%
vegetarian	1 cup	1.0	200	5%
(Libby's) beef				
w/beans	7.5 oz	18.0	330	49%
w/o beans	7.5 oz	15.0	350	39%
(Nile Spice) vegetarian/chili 'n beans				
mild	7 oz	1.0	160	6%
spicy	7 oz	2.0	170	11%
(Old El Paso) beef w/beans	1 cup	7.0	200	32%
(Pritikin) vegetarian chili				
black bean				
mild	1 cup	1.0	230	4%
spicy	1 cup	1.0	230	4%
three bean/mild	1 cup	1.0	230	4%
(ShariAnn's) Organic				
veggie chili				
original	1 cup	1.0	230	4%
spicy	1 cup	1.0	230	4%
(Stagg)				
beef				
classic w/beans	1 cup	17.0	330	46%

Food and Description	Amount	Fat Grams	Total Calories	% Fat Calories
country w/beans	1 cup	16.0	320	45%
double barrell	1 cup	22.0	340	58%
dynamite hot w/beans	1 cup	16.0	330	44%
Laredo w/beans	1 cup	15.0	320	42%
ranchero"I"	1 cup	3.0	240	11%
silver	1 cup	3.0	230	12%
steakhouse straight	1 cup	21.0	330	57%
chicken				
green chili	1 cup	12.0	250	43%
ranch house w/beans	1 cup	9.0	290	28%
vegetable	1 cup	1.0	200	5%
(Worthington) vegetarian	1 cup	15.0	290	47%
Homemade/USDA Standard Home Recipe				
beef	1 cup	15.0	400	34%
Kit/mix/seasoning				
(Bush Brothers) Chili Magic				
chili starter				
Louisiana recipe	4.4 oz	1.5	110	12%
Texas	4.4 oz	2.0	120	15%
Traditional	4.4 oz	1.0	110	8%
(Durkee)				
mild/mix only	1 cup	0.5	30	15%
pot-o-chili/mix only	1 cup	–	30	–
regular/mix only	1 cup	–	30	–
Texas red/mix only	1 cup	1.0	45	20%
(Fantastic Foods) vegetarian				
mix only	⅛ cup	–	50	–
prepared	½ cup	–	50	–
(French's) Chili-O/mix only				
mild	1 cup	0.5	30	15%
onion	1 cup	–	40	–
original	1 cup	–	30	–
Texas style	1 cup	1.0	45	20%
(Hain)				
hot	¼ pkg	1.0	30	30%
medium	¼ pkg	1.0	30	30%
mild	¼ pkg	1.0	30	30%
(Knorr) 4 bean chili/mix only	1 serving	1.5	230	6%
(McCormick/Schilling) mix only				
Cincinnati	⅛ pkg	1.0	80	11%
Texas	⅕ pkg	1.5	50	27%
(Old El Paso) mix only	1 Tbs	0.5	25	18%
(Tabasco) 7 spice chili recipe	½ cup	0.5	50	9%
Microwave container				
(Hormel) micro cup meal				
hot w/beans	1 cup	6.0	220	25%
w/beans	1 cup	6.0	220	25%
w/o beans	1 cup	8.0	190	38%
■ CHILI BEANS (See also individual bean listings)				
(Bush's Best) hot	½ cup	–	70	–

Food and Description	Amount	Fat Grams	Total Calories	% Fat Calories
(Dennison's) in chili gravy	½ cup	–	110	–
(Gebhardt)	½ cup	1.0	115	8%
(Green Giant) spicy	½ cup	1.0	110	8%
(Joan of Arc) spicy	½ cup	1.0	110	8%
(Luck's) pintos in chili gravy	½ cup	1.0	120	8%
(S&W)	½ cup	1.0	130	7%
(Sun Vista)	½ cup	1.0	110	8%
(Van Camp's) Mexican	1 cup	2.5	210	11%

■ **CHILI MAC** (*See* PASTA ENTRÉE/DINNER)
■ **CHILIES** (*See* Peppers in this section)
■ **CHIMICHANGA**
frozen

(Chi-Chi's)				
beef	1 pkg	24.0	630	34%
chicken	1 pkg	19.0	580	29%
(Don Miguel)				
beefsteak & bean				
hot	1 piece	12.0	380	28%
mucho bistec	1 piece	12.0	400	27%
chicken	1 piece	12.0	390	28%
(Old El Paso)				
beef	1 piece	20.0	370	49%
chicken	1 piece	16.0	350	41%
(Posada) sliced beef	1 piece	17.0	380	40%
homemade w/beef & cheese	4 oz	15.6	282	50%

■ **CHURRO**
frozen

(Tio Pepe's) cinnamon/6-oz pkg	1 piece	5.0	110	41%

■ **DIP** (*See* DIP)
■ **DIP**

(Senor Felix's)				
empanadas				
chicken	1	15.0	340	40%
corn & rice	1	13.0	280	42%
pumpkin & mushroom	1	11.0	260	38%
spinach & ricotta	1	12.0	260	42%

■ **ENCHILADA**
frozen

(Chi-Chi's)				
baja	1 pkg	20.0	590	31%
chix suprema	1 pkg	20.0	600	30%
(El Charrito)				
beef				
grande/4 per pkg	16.5 oz	47.0	890	48%
6 per pkg	16.25 oz	49.0	880	50%
3 per pkg	11 oz	31.0	560	50%
beef & cheese/6 per pkg	16.25 oz	42.0	880	43%
cheese				
6 per pkg	16.25 oz	30.0	780	35%
3 per pkg	11 oz	20.0	470	38%

Food and Description	Amount	Fat Grams	Total Calories	% Fat Calories
chicken(3)	11 oz	13.0	440	27%
(Senor Felix's)				
red pepper	1	19.0	420	41%
soy verda	1	24.0	430	50%
supreme soy cheese	1	23.0	460	45%
verde	1	23.0	420	49%
■ **FLAUTA**				
frozen				
(Schwan's) apple	1 flauta	4.5	150	27%
■ **GAZPACHO** (*See* SOUP)				
■ **GUACAMOLE** (*See* DIP)				
■ **MENUDO**				
(Juanita's) hot & spicy	1 cup	7.0	170	37%
(La Costena) beef tripe & hominy stew	1 cup	8.0	180	40%
(Pico Pica)	1 cup	9.0	200	41%
■ **NACHOS**				
Frozen/microwaveable				
(Real Fresh) muy fresco	3.5 oz	9.0	140	51%
(Totino's) Stuffed nachos				
beef & cheese	6 nachos	9.0	220	37%
grande	6 nachos	9.0	210	39%
nacho cheese	6 nachos	10.0	220	41%
taco	6 nachos	10.0	220	41%
Kit				
(Taco Bell) Home Originals				
Ultimate Nachos/prepared	about 12 nachos	11.0	240	41%
■ **PEPPERS**				
(Chi-Chi's)				
diced tomatoes & green chilies	¼ cup	–	20	–
green chili				
diced	2 Tbs	–	10	–
whole	¾ pepper	–	10	–
jalapeño				
wheels	19 pieces	–	10	–
whole	2½ medium	–	10	–
(Del Monte)				
chipotle/in spice sauce	2 Tbs	–	20	–
hot yellow chili	4 peppers	–	10	–
jalapeño				
nachos	2 Tbs	–	5	–
pickled				
sliced	2 Tbs	–	5	–
whole	2 Tbs	–	5	–
whole	2 Tbs	–	5	–
(La Victoria) jalapeño				
marinated	1 Tbs	–	4	–
nacho	1 Tbs	–	2	–
(Old El Paso)				
green chili				
chopped	2 Tbs	–	5	–

Food and Description	Amount	Fat Grams	Total Calories	% Fat Calories
whole	1 medium	–	10	–
jalapeño				
sliced	2 Tbs	–	15	–
whole				
peeled	3 medium	–	10	–
pickled	2 medium	–	5	–
(Ortega)				
green chili				
diced	1 oz	–	10	–
sliced	1 oz	–	10	–
strips	1 oz	–	10	–
whole	1 oz	–	10	–
hot chili				
diced	1 oz	–	10	–
whole	1 oz	–	10	–
(Pancho Villa)				
green chili/diced	2 Tbs	–	5	–
(Rosarita)				
green chili				
diced	2 Tbs	–	5	–
whole	2 Tbs	–	5	–
jalapeño				
diced	2 Tbs	–	5	–
nacho sliced	2 Tbs	–	5	–
whole	2 Tbs	–	10	–
(Trappey)				
jalapeño				
hot sliced	21 slices	–	4	–
whole	2 peppers	–	11	–
serano	7 peppers	–	7	–
(Vlasic)				
jalapeño/Mexican hot	1 oz	–	8	–
Mexican tiny hot	1 oz	–	6	–
■ REFRIED BEANS				
(Chi-Chi's)				
fat-free	½ cup	–	120	–
original	½ cup	3.0	150	18%
(Del Monte) plain	½ cup	2.0	130	14%
(Fantastic Foods)				
Mix only				
Instant refried beans	¼ cup	1.5	130	10%
Rice & Bean Cups				
Tex Mex w/pinto beans/prepared	2.3 oz	2.5	240	9%
(Gebhardt)				
jalapeño	½ cup	2.0	115	16%
traditional	½ cup	2.0	100	18%
(Hain) vegetarian/black bean	½ cup	0.5	110	4%
(Old El Paso)				
beans & cheese	½ cup	3.5	130	17%
beans & green chillies	½ cup	0.5	110	4%

Food and Description	Amount	Fat Grams	Total Calories	% Fat Calories
beans & sausage	½ cup	13.0	200	59%
black beans	½ cup	2.0	120	15%
fat-free	½ cup	–	110	–
regular	½ cup	2.0	110	16%
spicy	½ cup	3.0	140	19%
vegetarian	½ cup	1.0	100	9%
(Rosarita)				
bacon	½ cup	3.0	116	23%
green chile	½ cup	3.0	110	25%
green chiles & lime/no-fat	½ cup	–	100	–
homestyle	½ cup	8.0	140	51%
low-fat black beans	½ cup	<1.0	105	4%
nacho cheese	½ cup	3.0	137	20%
onion	½ cup	3.0	114	23%
original	½ cup	2.5	130	17%
spicy	½ cup	2.5	120	19%
traditional				
99% fat-free	½ cup	2.0	110	16%
no-fat	½ cup	–	100	–
regular	½ cup	3.0	125	22%
vegetarian	½ cup	2.0	120	18%
zesty salsa/no-fat	½ cup	–	120	–
(ShariAnns) Organic				
Refried				
black beans	½ cup	–	110	–
pinto beans w/green chile & lime	½ cup	–	110	–
w/roasted garlic	½ cup	–	110	–
(Taco Bell) Home Originals				
fat-free				
plain	½ cup	–	110	–
w/mild chilies	½ cup	–	110	–
original	½ cup	3.0	140	19%
▣ SALSA (See SAUCE)				
▣ SAUCE				
(Chi-Chi's)				
enchilada	¼ cup	1.5	30	45%
picante				
hot	2 Tbs	–	10	–
medium	2 Tbs	–	10	–
mild	2 Tbs	–	10	–
salsa				
con queso	2 Tbs	7.0	90	70%
hot	2 Tbs	–	10	–
medium	2 Tbs	–	10	–
mild	2 Tbs	–	10	–
taco/thick & chunky	1 Tbs	–	15	–
(Del Monte)				
picante				
hot	2 Tbs	–	10	–
medium	2 Tbs	–	10	–

Food and Description	Amount	Fat Grams	Total Calories	% Fat Calories
salsa				
fire roasted/medium	2 Tbs	–	10	–
garlic	2 Tbs	–	10	–
Mexicana	2 Tbs	–	5	–
taquera	2 Tbs	–	5	–
thick & chunky				
hot	2 Tbs	–	10	–
medium	2 Tbs	–	10	–
mild	2 Tbs	–	10	–
verde	2 Tbs	–	10	–
(Doritos) salsa				
medium	2 Tbs	–	15	–
mild	2 Tbs	–	15	–
(Enrico's)				
picante sauce				
hot	2 Tbs	–	10	–
mild	2 Tbs	–	10	–
salsa				
chipotle	2 Tbs	–	10	–
hot	2 Tbs	–	15	–
medium	2 Tbs	–	10	–
mild	2 Tbs	–	15	–
organic				
hot	2 Tbs	–	15	–
mild	2 Tbs	–	15	–
roasted garlic	2 Tbs	–	10	–
(Fritos) Tostitos Kits				
salsa	1 pkg	15.0	320	42%
salsa con queso	1 pkg	27.0	460	53%
(Guiltless Gourmet) salsa				
Roasted Red Pepper	2 Tbs	–	10	–
Southwestern grill	2 Tbs	–	10	–
(Hain) salsa/green chili				
hot	¼ cup	–	20	–
mild	¼ cup	–	20	–
(Heluva Good Cheese) salsa				
cheese	2 Tbs	6.0	80	68%
thick & chunky				
hot	2 Tbs	–	10	–
mild	2 Tbs	–	10	–
(Hunt's)				
picante				
medium	2 Tbs	–	11	–
mild	2 Tbs	–	11	–
salsa				
alfresco				
medium	2 Tbs	–	10	–
mild	2 Tbs	–	10	–
regular				
hot	2 Tbs	–	27	–

Food and Description	Amount	Fat Grams	Total Calories	% Fat Calories
medium	2 Tbs	–	27	–
mild	2 Tbs	–	27	–
(La Victoria)				
Chile sauce				
red	2 oz	0.5	15	30%
Enchilada				
mild	2 oz	1.0	20	45%
mild green chile	2 oz	–	15	–
Picante	2 Tbs	–	10	–
Salsa				
brava	1 Tbs	–	–	–
ranchera/hot	2 Tbs	–	10	–
red jalapeño	2 Tbs	–	10	–
suprema/medium	2 Tbs	–	15	–
Thick 'n Chunky				
hot	2 Tbs	–	15	–
medium	2 Tbs	–	10	–
mild	2 Tbs	–	10	–
verde/thick 'n chunky/medium	2 Tbs	–	15	–
Victoria/hot	2 Tbs	–	15	–
Taco				
green				
medium	1 Tbs	–	–	–
mild	1 Tbs	–	–	–
red				
medium	1 Tbs	–	5	–
mild	1 Tbs	–	5	–
mild/squeeze bottle	1 Tbs	–	5	–
(Louise's) salsa/fat-free				
BBQ black bean	2 Tbs	–	10	–
black bean	2 Tbs	–	10	–
medium	2 Tbs	–	10	–
mild	2 Tbs	–	10	–
nacho queso	2 Tbs	–	15	–
(Muir Glen) Organic Fat-Free				
hot	2 Tbs	–	10	–
medium	2 Tbs	–	10	–
mild	2 Tbs	–	10	–
(Newman's Own) Bandito salsa				
hot	2 Tbs	–	10	–
medium	2 Tbs	–	10	–
mild	2 Tbs	–	10	–
peach	2 Tbs	–	25	–
pineapple	2 Tbs	–	15	–
roasted garlic	2 Tbs	–	10	–
(Old El Paso)				
enchilada				
green chili	¼ cup	1.5	30	45%
hot	¼ cup	1.0	25	36%
mild	¼ cup	1.5	30	45%

Food and Description	Amount	Fat Grams	Total Calories	% Fat Calories
picante				
regular				
hot	2 Tbs	–	10	–
medium	2 Tbs	–	10	–
mild	2 Tbs	–	10	–
thick & chunky				
hot	2 Tbs	–	10	–
medium	2 Tbs	–	10	–
mild	2 Tbs	–	10	–
salsa				
green chili	2 Tbs	–	10	–
homestyle				
medium	2 Tbs	–	5	–
mild	2 Tbs	–	5	–
pico de gallo				
hot	2 Tbs	–	5	–
medium	2 Tbs	–	5	–
salsa verde/medium	2 Tbs	–	10	–
thick & chunky				
hot	2 Tbs	–	10	–
medium	2 Tbs	–	10	–
mild	2 Tbs	–	10	–
taco				
extra chunky				
medium	1 Tbs	–	5	–
mild	1 Tbs	–	5	–
regular				
hot	1 Tbs	–	5	–
medium	1 Tbs	–	5	–
mild	1 Tbs	–	5	–
tomatoes & green chilies	¼ cup	–	10	–
tomatoes & jalapeños	¼ cup	–	15	–
(Ortega) salsa				
garden style				
medium	2 Tbs	–	10	–
mild	2 Tbs	–	10	–
green chili				
hot	2 Tbs	–	10	–
medium	2 Tbs	–	10	–
mild	2 Tbs	–	10	–
thick & chunky				
medium	2 Tbs	–	10	–
mild	2 Tbs	–	10	–
(Pace)				
Picante sauce				
con Queso	2 Tbs	7.0	90	70%
hot	2 Tbs	–	10	–
medium	2 Tbs	–	10	–
mild	2 Tbs	–	10	–
Salsa				
thick & chunky	2 Tbs	–	10	–

Food and Description	Amount	Fat Grams	Total Calories	% Fat Calories
(Rosarita) Chunky				
Picante				
hot	3 Tbs	–	25	–
medium	3 Tbs	–	25	–
mild	3 Tbs	–	25	–
Salsa/taco				
medium	3 Tbs	–	25	–
mild	3 Tbs	–	25	–
(Ro*Tel) salsa/diced tomatoes &				
green chilies				
extra hot	½ cup	–	20	–
regular	½ cup	–	20	–
(S&W) salsa				
mild	¼ cup	–	16	–
ready-cut tomatoes				
medium	¼ cup	–	20	–
mild	¼ cup	–	20	–
w/chipotle	¼ cup	–	20	–
w/cilantro	¼ cup	–	20	–
(Sun Vista)				
picante				
hot	2 Tbs	–	10	–
mild	2 Tbs	–	5	–
salsa				
hot	2 Tbs	–	5	–
mild	2 Tbs	–	5	–
(Taco Bell) Home Originals				
Hot sauce	1 tsp	–	–	–
Smooth'N Zesty				
picante				
medium	2 Tbs	–	15	–
mild	2 Tbs	–	15	–
Thick'N Chunky				
salsa				
hot	2 Tbs	–	15	–
medium	2 Tbs	–	15	–
mild	2 Tbs	–	15	–
taco				
medium	2 Tbs	–	15	–
mild	2 Tbs	–	15	–
seasoning mix	2 tsp	–	20	–
(Tostitos)				
picante				
hot	2 Tbs	–	15	–
medium	2 Tbs	–	15	–
mild	2 Tbs	–	15	–
salsa				
con queso				
low-fat	2 Tbs	3.0	80	34%
regular	2 Tbs	5.0	80	56%

Food and Description	Amount	Fat Grams	Total Calories	% Fat Calories
hot	2 Tbs	–	30	–
medium	2 Tbs	–	30	–
mild	2 Tbs	–	30	–
restaurant style	2 Tbs	–	30	–
roasted garlic	2 Tbs	–	30	–

■ **SPANISH RICE** (*See* RICE DISH)

■ **TACO** (*See also* BREAKFAST SANDWICH; Taco Seasoning in this section; Taco Shell in this section)

Food and Description	Amount	Fat Grams	Total Calories	% Fat Calories
Boxed kit				
(Chi-Chi's) Dinner Kits				
shells & seasoning				
white	2 shells & seasoning	8.0	200	36%
yellow	2 shells & seasoning	9.0	200	36%
soft taco	2 shells & seasoning	7.0	300	54%
(Old El Paso)				
w/taco shell				
mix & 2 shells only	2 pieces	7.0	140	45%
prepared	2 tacos	13.0	270	43%
w/tortilla				
mix & 2 tortillas only	2 pieces	3.5	210	15%
prepared	2 tacos	10.0	380	24%
(Ortega) Dinner kits				
soft taco	2 shells	5.0	240	19%
12 & 18 count traditional tacos	2 shells	5.0	150	30%
(Pancho Villa)				
mix & 2 shells only	2 pieces	8.0	150	48%
prepared	2 tacos	13.0	270	43%
Frozen				
(Owens) Border Breakfasts				
ham	2 tacos	6.0	90	60%
sausage	2 tacos	12.0	190	57%
(Schwan's) taco barquito	~5 oz	18.0	350	46%
Homemade/USDA Standard Home Recipe				
beef	~3 oz	7.0	153	41%
beef w/cheese	~3 oz	9.0	182	45%

■ **TACO SEASONING** (*See also* SEASONINGS)

Food and Description	Amount	Fat Grams	Total Calories	% Fat Calories
(Durkee) mix only				
family	1 serving	–	10	–
mild	1 serving	–	15	–
regular	1 serving	–	15	–
salad	1 serving	–	20	–
(French's) mix only				
mild	1 serving	–	15	–
onion	1 serving	–	20	–
regular	1 serving	–	15	–
(Old El Paso) mix only				
40% less sodium	2 tsp	–	20	–

Food and Description	Amount	Fat Grams	Total Calories	% Fat Calories
regular	2 tsp	–	20	–
(Ortega)				
mix only	2 Tbs	1.0	90	10%
prepared	1 taco	4.0	60	60%
(Taco Bell) mix only	2 Tbs	–	20	–
■ TACO SHELL				
(Azteca) super	1 shell	12.0	200	54%
(Chi-Chi's)				
white	2 shells	8.0	170	40%
yellow	2 shells	8.0	170	40%
(Gebhardt)	3 shells	8.5	155	32%
(Old El Paso)				
mini	7 shells	10.0	160	56%
regular	3 shells	10.0	170	53%
super	2 shells	12.0	190	57%
white corn	3 shells	10.0	170	53%
(Ortega)				
white corn	2 shells	4.0	120	30%
yellow corn	2 shells	5.0	120	38%
(Pancho Villa)	3 shells	11.0	190	52%
(Rosarita)	3 shells	8.5	155	32%
(Taco Bell) Home Originals	3 shells	5.0	150	36%
■ TAMALE				
canned				
(Derby)	2 tamales	7.0	160	39%
(Gebhardt)				
jumbo	2 tamales	30.0	400	68%
original	2 tamales	22.0	290	68%
(Hormel)				
beef				
hot-spicy	2 tamales	7.0	140	45%
jumbo	2 tamales	10.0	210	43%
regular	2 tamales	7.0	140	45%
chicken	2 tamales	7.0	130	48%
(Old El Paso)	3 tamales	19.0	330	52%
(Senor Felix's) tamales/include 4 tsp sauce				
blue corn & soy cheese	2 tamales	10.0	240	38%
chicken	2 tamales	9.0	240	34%
gourmet vegetarian	2 tamales	9.0	240	34%
(Van Camp's)	8 oz	16.0	290	50%
homemade/USDA Standard Home Recipe				
beef	~2.5 oz	9.5	183	48%
■ TOMATILLO				
canned or jarred				
(La Costena)	4 medium	2.5	40	56%
(La Victoria) entero	1 Tbs	–	10	–
■ TORTILLA				
(Azteca)				
corn	1 small	–	45	–
flour				
8" dia	1 tortilla	3.0	130	21%

Food and Description	Amount	Fat Grams	Total Calories	% Fat Calories
salad bake & fill	1 tortilla	12.0	200	54%
small	1 tortilla	2.0	80	23%
taco salad shell	1 tortilla	12.0	200	54%
(El Charito)				
corn	2 tortillas	1.0	95	9%
flour	2 tortillas	4.0	170	21%
(La Suprema)				
corn				
extra crisp for tacos	2 tortillas	1.5	100	14%
for enchiladas, tostada, tacos	2 tortillas	1.5	100	14%
flour				
angel flour extra soft				
burrito size	1 tortilla	5.0	200	23%
taco size	1 tortilla	4.0	150	24%
(Mission)				
corn				
Estilo Casero				
regular size	1 tortilla	1.0	80	11%
super size	1 tortilla	7.0	190	33%
98% fat-free/fajita-size	1 tortilla	0.5	80	6%
regular size	2 tortillas	1.5	100	14%
super size	1 tortilla	1.0	80	11%
white corn	2 tortillas	1.5	120	11%
flour				
burrito-size				
98% fat-free	1 tortilla	1.5	170	8%
regular-size	1 tortilla	6.0	220	25%
tortillas Caseras	1 tortilla	5.0	185	24%
Estilo Casero				
corditas//burrito size	1 tortilla	9.0	260	31%
sabrositas				
burrito size	1 tortilla	7.0	220	29%
regular size	1 tortilla	5.0	140	32%
super-size	1 tortilla	7.0	190	33%
fajita size	1 tortilla	3.0	100	27%
98% fat free wheat	1 tortilla	2.5	140	16%
soft taco size				
fluffy homestyle	1 tortilla	5.0	180	25%
98% fat-free	1 tortilla	1.0	130	7%
regular-size	1 tortilla	4.0	160	23%
wraps				
garden spinach herb	1 tortilla	6.0	240	23%
southwestern chili	1 tortilla	6.0	240	23%
zesty garlic herb	1 tortilla	6.0	240	23%
(Montecito)				
corn/family-size	1 tortilla	1.5	120	11%
flour/regular-size	1 tortilla	4.0	150	24%
(Old El Paso)				
flour	1 tortilla	3.0	150	18%
soft taco	2 tortillas	4.0	180	20%

Food and Description	Amount	Fat Grams	Total Calories	% Fat Calories
(Tyson)				
corn/enchilada style	1 tortilla	<1.0	50	8%
flour				
burrito style	1 tortilla	4.0	170	21%
fajita style	1 tortilla	2.0	90	20%
large/heat-pressed	1 tortilla	4.0	180	20%
small/hand-stretched	1 tortilla	2.0	105	17%
soft taco	1 tortilla	3.0	120	23%
whole wheat	1 tortilla	3.0	120	23%
■ TORTILLA CHIPS (See TORTILLA CHIPS)				
■ TORTILLA MIX				
(Quaker) corn				
harina, preparada para tortillas	⅓ cup	4.0	160	23%
masa harina	¼ cup	1.0	110	8%
■ TOSTADA				
homemade/USDA Standard Home recipe				
beef	~3 oz	7.0	153	41%
beef w/cheese	~3 oz	9.0	182	45%
■ TOSTADA SHELL				
corn				
(Old El Paso)	1 shell	7.0	130	48%
	3 shells	10.0	160	56%
(Ortega)	2 shells	5.0	130	35%
(Pancho Villa)	1 shell	3.0	55	49%
(Rosarita)	1 shell	3.0	60	45%
MEXICAN POTATO (See JICAMA)				
MILK (See also MILK SUBSTITUTE; RICE DRINK; SOYMILK)				
buffalo	1 cup	17.0	236	65%
carob	1 cup	3.0	160	17%
cow/canned				
condensed/sweetened				
(Borden) Eagle Brand/canned				
creamy chocolate	1.4 oz	2.5	120	19%
fat-free	1.4 oz	–	110	–
low-fat	1.4 oz	1.5	120	11%
original	1.4 oz	3.0	130	21%
(Carnation)	2 Tbs	3.0	130	21%
	3.5 fl oz	8.7	321	24%
	⅓ cup	9.0	318	26%
(Dairy Sweet)	⅓ cup	9.0	320	25%
generic	¼ cup	6.6	244	24%
cow/evaporated				
(Carnation)				
low-fat	2 Tbs	0.5	25	18%
skim	2 Tbs	–	25	–
	½ cup	–	100	–
whole	2 Tbs	2.0	40	45%
generic				
low-fat	¼ cup	1.5	55	25%
skim	¼ cup	–	50	–
whole	¼ cup	4.8	84	51%

Food and Description	Amount	Fat Grams	Total Calories	% Fat Calories
(Milnot)				
skim	2 Tbs	–	25	–
	½ cup	–	100	–
whole	2 Tbs	2.0	40	45%
	½ cup	8.0	150	48%
(Pet)				
regular	½ cup	10.0	170	53%
skim	½ cup	–	100	–
cow/fresh				
(A&P)				
buttermilk	1 cup	1.0	90	10%
1% fat/light	1 cup	3.0	100	27%
2% fat/reduced fat	1 cup	5.0	120	38%
(Blue Bunny)				
fat-free	1 cup	–	90	–
2% reduced-fat				
chocolate milk	1 cup	5.0	180	25%
regular milk	1 cup	5.0	120	38%
(Borden)				
buttermilk/Golden Churn 1.5% fat	1 cup	1.0	120	30%
chocolate-flavored/Dutch low-fat	1 cup	5.0	180	25%
hi-protein 20% fat/reduced fat	1 cup	5.0	140	32%
1% fat/light w/L. acidophilus	1 cup	2.0	100	18%
skim/fat-free/protein-fortified	1 cup	1.0	100	9%
whole	1 cup	8.0	150	48%
(Creamland)				
fat-free	1 cup	–	90	–
1% low-fat	1 cup	1.5	110	12%
2% super reduced fat	1 cup	5.0	140	32%
whole	1 cup	8.0	150	48%
(Crowley)				
buttermilk	1 cup	4.0	110	33%
1% fat/light	1 cup	2.0	100	18%
2% fat/reduced fat	1 cup	5.0	120	38%
(Darigold)				
1% fat/light	1 cup	2.0	100	18%
2% fat/reduced fat	1 cup	5.0	120	38%
generic				
buttermilk/cultured	1 cup	2.0	100	18%
	1 quart	9.0	396	20%
chocolate				
1% fat	1 cup	2.5	160	14%
2% fat	1 cup	5.0	180	25%
whole	1 cup	8.5	210	36%
skim/fat-free				
regular	1 cup	0.6	90	6%
w/nonfat milk solids added	1 cup	0.6	90	6%
1 % fat/light/w/nonfat milk solids added	1 cup	2.4	104	21%
2% fat/reduced fat/w/nonfat milk solids added	1 cup	4.7	125	34%

Food and Description	Amount	Fat Grams	Total Calories	% Fat Calories
whole				
vitamin D	1 cup	8.0	150	48%
w/added calcium	1 cup	8.0	150	48%
(Hershey) chocolate				
Premium low-fat	½ pint	2.5	170	13%
shake	7 fl. oz	4.5	230	18%
2% reduced-fat	½ cup	2.5	100	23%
	1 cup	5.0	130	35%
whole milk	1 cup	9.0	210	39%
(Hood) (See also The Organic Cow of Vermont in this section)				
fat-free				
Sil-ou-et	1 cup	–	80	–
Simply Smart	1 cup	–	90	–
lowfat	1 cup	2.5	120	19%
whole/vitamin D	1 cup	8.0	150	48%
(Knudsen)				
buttermilk/2% fat	1 cup	5.0	120	38%
Nice 'n Light/1% fat/light	1 cup	3.0	130	21%
2% fat/reduced fat	1 cup	5.0	140	32%
(Land O'Lakes)				
buttermilk	1 cup	2.0	100	18%
1% fat/light	1 cup	3.0	100	27%
2% fat/reduced fat	1 cup	5.0	120	38%
(Lucerne) chocolate/2% fat	1 cup	5.0	200	23%
(Nestlé USA) Nesquik/chocolate				
whole	1 cup	8.0	230	31%
(Pet)				
chocolate	1 cup	7.0	200	32%
whole/vitamin D	1 cup	8.0	150	48%
(Pevely)				
chocolate-flavored	1 cup	8.0	210	34%
½% fat	1 cup	1.0	90	10%
(The Organic Cow of Vermont)				
chocolate	1 pint	15.0	280	48%
low-fat	1 cup	2.5	110	20%
reduced-fat	1 cup	5.0	130	35%
skim/fat-free	1 cup	–	90	–
whole				
homogenized	1 cup	8.0	150	48%
not homogenized	1 cup	8.0	150	48%
(Viva) w/extra calcium				
2% fat/reduced fat	1 cup	5.0	120	38%
skim	1 cup	1.0	100	9%
(Weight Watchers) skim/fat-free	1 cup	–	90	–
cow/lactose-reduced (See MILK SUBSTITUTE)				
dry/powdered				
(Alba) nonfat, prepared	1 cup	–	80	–
(Carnation) mix only				
Leche w/vitamin D/evaporated	1 oz	2.0	40	45%
skim	⅓ cup	–	80	–

Food and Description	Amount	Fat Grams	Total Calories	% Fat Calories
generic				
nonfat/skim				
mix only	¼ cup	–	100	–
prepared	1 cup	–	80	–
whole				
mix only	¼ cup	8.5	159	48%
prepared	1 cup	8.5	150	48%
(Milkman) low-fat/prepared	1 cup	1.0	90	9%
	1 quart	5.0	300	12%
(Saco)				
buttermilk				
mix only	4 Tbs	<1	80	5%
prepared	1 cup	<1	80	5%
nonfat milk				
mix only	⅓ cup	–	80	–
prepared	1 cup	–	80	–
(Sanalac) nonfat/prepared	1 cup	–	80	–
goat				
canned evaporated				
(Meyenberg)	4 oz	8.0	150	48%
carton				
powder mixed w/water	1 cup	8.0	150	48%
refrigerated	1 cup	8.0	150	48%
fresh	1 cup	10.0	168	54%
human	1 cup	11.0	170	58%
reindeer	8 fl oz	48.6	580	75%
sheep	8 fl oz	17.0	264	58%
MILK MIX (See also BREAKFAST DRINK; COCOA; MILK SHAKE)				
(Alba)				
chocolate marshmallow	1 pkt	–	60	–
milk chocolate	1 pkt	–	60	–
mocha	1 pkt	–	60	–
(Baker's) chocolate	1 oz	2.0	120	15%
(Carnation) mix only				
banana	2 Tbs	–	90	–
chocolate malted	3 heaping Tbs	1.0	80	11%
	3.5 oz	3.5	375	8%
malted/original	3 heaping Tbs	2.0	90	20%
	3.5 oz	8.5	411	19%
milk chocolate				
fat-free	1 envelope	–	25	–
low-calorie	1 envelope	–	70	–
no sugar added	3 Tbs	–	50	–
regular	3 Tbs	1.0	110	8%
rich chocolate				
original	3 Tbs	1.0	110	8%
w/chocolate marshmallows	3 Tbs	1.0	110	8%
w/marshmallows	3 Tbs	1.0	110	8%
(Featherweight) chocolate	1 pouch	1.0	40	23%

Food and Description	Amount	Fat Grams	Total Calories	% Fat Calories
generic				
carob				
mix only	1 Tbs	<1.0	45	10%
prepared w/whole milk	8 fl oz	9.0	195	42%
chocolate malted				
mix only	1 heaping Tbs	1.0	85	11%
prepared w/whole milk	8 fl oz	9.0	235	35%
chocolate syrup				
prepared w/whole milk	8 fl oz	8.5	232	33%
syrup only	2 Tbs	0.5	82	6%
(Ghirardelli) Prepared w/2% milk				
chocolate hazelnut	1 cup	6.0	210	26%
milk double chocolate	1 cup	5.0	210	21%
mocha	1 cup	6.0	210	26%
white mocha	1 cup	5.0	210	21%
(Hershey)				
Hot Cocoa Collection				
chocolate almond	1 envelope	3.0	150	18%
chocolate mint	1 envelope	3.0	150	18%
chocolate raspberry	1 envelope	3.0	150	18%
Dutch chocolate				
fat-free	1 envelope	–	–	–
original	1 envelope	5.0	160	28%
French vanilla				
fat-free	1 envelope	–	50	–
original	1 envelope	2.5	140	16%
Irish cream	1 envelope	3.0	150	18%
syrup/chocolate malted	2 Tbs	–	100	–
(Land O'Lakes)				
Cappaccino Classics				
amaretto	1 pkt	3.5	130	24%
French vanilla	1 pkt	3.5	140	23%
suprema	1 pkt	3.5	130	24%
Swiss mocha	3.5 oz pkt	10.0	410	22%
Cocoa Classics				
amaretto	1 pkt	7.0	160	39%
Belgian chocolate	1 pkt	4.0	140	26%
black cherry	1 pkt	5.0	150	30%
caramel	1 pkt	5.0	150	30%
cinnamon	1 pkt	5.0	150	30%
coconut creme	1 pkt	5.0	150	30%
French vanilla	1 pkt	5.0	150	30%
hazelnut	1 pkt	5.0	150	30%
Irish cream	1 pkt	5.0	150	30%
macadamia nut	1 pkt	5.0	150	30%
mint	1 pkt	5.0	150	30%
mocha	1 pkt	7.0	160	39%
raspberry	1 pkt	5.0	150	30%
supreme	1 pkt	5.0	150	30%

Food and Description	Amount	Fat Grams	Total Calories	% Fat Calories
(Nestlé) mix only				
Milo chocolate-flavored hot or cold				
drink mix	3 Tbs	2.0	80	23%
Quik				
chocolate				
no sugar added	2 Tbs	1.0	40	23%
regular	2 Tbs	0.5	90	5%
strawberry	2 Tbs	–	90	–
(Ovaltine) chocolate malted				
classic/traditional				
mix only	4 Tbs	–	80	–
prepared w/2% milk	8 fl oz	5.0	210	21%
lite				
mix only	2 Tbs	–	50	–
prepared w/skim milk	8 fl oz	0.6	170	3%
original				
mix only	4 Tbs	–	80	–
prepared w/2% milk	8 fl oz	5.0	210	21%
rich chocolate				
mix only	4 Tbs	–	80	–
prepared w/2% milk	8 fl oz	5.0	210	21%
(PDO) malted/prepared w/whole milk	8 fl oz	5.0	180	25%
(Swiss Miss) mix only				
Bavarian chocolate	1 pkt	–	20	–
Chocolate Sensations	1 pkt	4.0	150	24%
cocoa				
diet	1 pkt	–	25	–
fat-free				
regular	1 pkt	–	50	–
French vanilla	1 pkt	2.5	120	19%
lite	1 pkt	<1.0	70	6%
no sugar added				
regular	1 pkt	1.0	60	15%
regular	1 pkt	3.0	140	19%
sugar-free	¼ cup	1.0	70	13%
double rich	1 pkt	1.0	110	8%
marshmallow lovers				
fat-free	1 pkt	–	60	–
regular	1 pkt	3.0	140	19%
milk chocolate				
regular	1.2 oz pkt	3.0	140	19%
	1 oz pkt	2.5	120	19%
sugar-free	1 pkt	–	50	–
w/marshmallows	1 pkt	2.5	120	19%
mini marshmallows				
regular	1 pkt	1.0	110	8%
sugar-free	1 pkt	1.0	50	18%
rich chocolate				
regular	1 pkt	1.0	110	8%
sugar-free	1 pkt	–	50	–

Food and Description	Amount	Fat Grams	Total Calories	% Fat Calories
white chocolate	1 pkt	1.0	110	8%
(Weight Watchers) chocolate & marshmallow/mix only	1 pkt	–	70	–

MILK SHAKE (*See also* individual FAST FOOD listings)

canned

(Frostee)

| chocolate-flavored drink | 1 cup | 8.0 | 200 | 36% |
| strawberry-flavored drink | 1 cup | 7.0 | 180 | 35% |

(Hood) Shake-Up

chocolate	1 cup	6.0	240	23%
strawberry	1 cup	5.0	220	20%
vanilla	1 cup	5.0	220	20%

(Real) Sport Shake

| chocolate | 10 fl oz | 10.0 | 310 | 29% |
| strawberry | 10 fl oz | 10.0 | 270 | 33% |

fountain drink/made w/whole milk

generic

chocolate	10 fl oz	10.0	360	25%
strawberry	10 fl oz	9.0	350	23%
vanilla	10 fl oz	9.0	340	27%

frozen

| (M&M *Mars) low-fat chocolate-malt | 1 cup | 3.0 | 220 | 12% |

(Micro Magic)

chocolate	11.5 fl oz	8.0	340	21%
strawberry	11.5 fl oz	9.0	340	24%
vanilla	11.5 fl oz	13.0	380	31%

mix

(Alba 77) Dairy Shake/mix only

chocolate	1 pkt	–	70	–
double fudge	1 pkt	0.5	70	6%
strawberry	1 pkt	–	70	–
vanilla	1 pkt	–	70	–
(Weight Watchers) chocolate fudge	1 pkt	1.0	80	11%

refrigerated

(Killer) shake

Choco Loco	8 fl oz	6.0	240	23%
Radically Vanilla	8 fl oz	5.0	220	20%
Totally Chocolate	8 fl oz	5.0	230	20%

MILK SUBSTITUTE (*See also* RICE DRINK; SOYMILK; YOGURT DRINK)

(Better Than Milk)

carob	1 cup	5.0	130	35%
chocolate	1 cup	5.0	125	36%
light	1 cup	–	80	–
natural	1 cup	5.0	90	50%

(Dairy Ease) lactose-reduced milk

skim/fat-free	1 cup	–	90	–
1% fat/light	1 cup	2.0	100	18%
2% fat/reduced fat	1 cup	5.0	120	38%

Food and Description	Amount	Fat Grams	Total Calories	% Fat Calories
(Lactaid) 100% lactose reduced				
chocolate/1% fat	1 cup	2.5	150	15%
regular				
70 Milk				
fat-free	1 cup	–	90	–
low-fat	1 cup	2.5	110	20%
100 Milk				
calcium-fortified	1 cup	<1.0	90	5%
skim/fat-free	1 cup	–	90	–
1% fat/low-fat	1 cup	2.5	110	20%
2% fat/reduced fat	1 cup	5.0	90	50%
whole	1 cup	8.0	150	48%
(Meadow Farms)	1 cup	5.0	120	38%
(Nutritious Foods) First Alternative	1 cup	2.0	90	20%
(Vance's) Darifree nondairy beverage	1 cup		90	–
(VitaMite) non-dairy				
2% fat	1 cup	5.0	110	41%
non-fat	1 cup	–	90	–
MILKFISH /raw	3 oz	6.0	125	43%
MILLET (See also CEREAL; FLOUR)				
(Arrowhead Mills)/hulled	¼ cup	1.5	150	9%
generic/pearl				
cooked	4 oz	1.0	135	7%
	1 cup	2.0	287	6%
dry/raw	1 oz	1.0	107	8%
	1 cup	8.0	756	10%
MINCEMEAT (See PIE FILLING & GLAZE)				
MINERAL WATER (See WATER)				
MINESTRONE (See SOUP)				
MISO				
(Eden)				
barley/mugi	1 Tbs	<1.0	25	18%
brown rice/genmai	1 Tbs	1.0	25	72%
rice/shiro	1 Tbs	1.0	35	51%
soybean/hacho	1 Tbs	2.0	35	51%
soybean & rice/kome	1 Tbs	1.0	25	72%
generic	½ cup	8.5	285	27%
w/barley malt/mugi-koji	1 oz	1.0	55	16%
w/rice maft/kome-koji				
dark yellow	1 oz	1.5	53	25%
sweet	1 oz	1.0	62	15%
w/soybean malt/mame-koji	1 oz	4.0	65	55%
(Westbrae) pasteurized				
barley	1 tsp	–	10	–
brown rice	1 tsp	–	10	–
red	1 tsp	–	10	–
soybean	1 tsp	–	12	–
MOLASSES				
(Brer Rabbit)				
dark	1 Tbs	–	60	–
light	1 Tbs	–	60	–

Food and Description	Amount	Fat Grams	Total Calories	% Fat Calories
generic				
Barbados	1 Tbs	–	54	–
	1 oz	–	111	–
	1 cup	–	889	–
light/1st extraction	1 Tbs	–	50	–
	1 oz	–	103	–
	1 cup	–	827	–
medium/2nd extraction	1 Tbs	–	46	–
	1 oz	–	95	–
	1 cup	–	761	–
treacle/black	1 Tbs	–	53	–
(Mott's) Grandma's				
gold label	1 Tbs	–	70	–
green Label	1 Tbs	–	70	–
(Plantation) blackstrap/3rd extraction	1 Tbs	–	43	–
	1 oz	–	87	–
	1 cup	–	699	–
MONKFISH				
cooked-dry heat	3 oz	2.0	85	21%
raw	3 oz	1.0	64	14%
MOOSE /boneless				
raw	3 oz	4.8	152	28%
roasted	3 oz	1.0	115	8%
roasted/diced	1 cup	1.5	190	7%
MORTADELLA (*See* SAUSAGE)				
MOTH BEAN				
boiled	½ cup	0.5	105	4%
raw	½ cup	1.5	335	4%
MOUNTAIN YAM				
Hawaiian/cooked	1 cup	–	119	–
MOUSSE (*See* PUDDING & MOUSSE)				
MUFFIN (*See also* BREAKFAST SANDWICH; PASTRY, TOASTER)				
■ **FROZEN**				
(Health Valley)				
Fat Free				
almond & date oat bran/Fancy Fruit	1 muffin	4.0	180	20%
apple spice	1 muffin	–	140	–
banana	1 muffin	–	130	–
raisin spice	1 muffin	–	140	–
Regular				
oat bran				
Fancy Fruit blueberry	1 muffin	4.0	140	26%
Fancy Fruit raisin	1 muffin	5.0	180	25%
rice bran				
Fancy Fruit raisin	1 muffin	7.0	210	30%
(Pepperidge Farm)				
oatbran w/apple	1 muffin	7.0	190	33%
banana nut	1 muffin	6.0	170	32%
blueberry	1 muffin	7.0	170	37%
cinnamon swirl	1 muffin	6.0	190	28%
corn	1 muffin	7.0	180	35%

Food and Description	Amount	Fat Grams	Total Calories	% Fat Calories
multi-grain muesli	1 muffin	8.0	200	36%
raisin bran	1 muffin	6.0	170	32%
(Sara Lee)				
food service				
almond paradise/4¼ oz muffin	1 muffin	18.0	410	37%
apple cranberry nut				
large muffin/4¼ oz	1 muffin	23.0	440	47%
small muffin/2⅛ oz	1 muffin	12.0	220	49%
banana nut				
individually wrapped	1 muffin	19.0	380	45%
large muffin/4¼ oz	1 muffin	24.0	430	50%
mini-muffin	2 muffins	8.0	180	40%
reduced fat	1 muffin	10.0	280	32%
small muffin/2⅛ oz	1 muffin	9.0	220	37%
blueberry				
individually wrapped	1 muffin	17.0	380	40%
large muffin/4¼ oz	1 muffin	18.0	400	41%
mini-muffin	2 muffins	9.0	190	43%
reduced fat	1 muffin	9.0	310	26%
small muffin/2⅛ oz	1 muffin	10.0	220	41%
blueberries & cheese streusel/ large muffin/4⅝ oz	1 muffin	18.0	430	38%
bran/individually wrapped	1 muffin	20.0	430	42%
carrot nut				
individually wrapped	1 muffin	23.0	450	46%
large muffin/4¼ oz	1 muffin	21.0	470	40%
cheese streusel				
individually wrapped	1 muffin	19.0	410	42%
large muffin/4¼ oz	1 muffin	22.0	440	45%
small muffin/2⅛ oz	1 muffin	11.0	220	45%
chocolate chunk				
individually wrapped	1 muffin	17.0	410	37%
mini-muffin	2 muffins	9.0	200	41%
small muffin/2⅛ oz	1 muffin	11.0	230	43%
corn				
individually wrapped	1 muffin	25.0	480	47%
large muffin/4¼ oz	1 muffin	26.0	490	48%
mini-muffin	2 muffins	11.0	210	47%
small muffin/2⅛ oz	1 muffin	13.0	240	49%
cranberry nut/mini-muffin	2 muffins	9.0	200	41%
double chocolate chunk/ large muffin/4⅝ oz	1 muffin	18.0	440	37%
lemon poppy seed/large muffin/4¼ oz	1 muffin	22.0	460	43%
oat bran raisin/small muffin/ 2⅛ oz	1 muffin	6.0	190	28%
orange streusel/large muffin/ 4¼ oz	1 muffin	19.0	450	39%
peaches & cheese streusel/ large muffin/4¼ oz	1 muffin	13.0	380	31%

Food and Description	Amount	Fat Grams	Total Calories	% Fat Calories
sweet harvest/large muffin/4¼ oz	1 muffin	24.0	460	47%
retail				
blueberry	1 muffin	11.0	220	45%
corn	1 muffin	14.0	260	48%
(Weight Watchers)				
banana	1 muffin	–	170	–
blueberry	1 muffin	–	160	–
chocolate chocolate chip	1 muffin	2.0	290	9%

■ HOMEMADE

USDA Standard Home Recipe (Note: Unless otherwise noted, homemade muffins were prepared with whole milk)

Food and Description	Amount	Fat Grams	Total Calories	% Fat Calories
apple	2 oz	6.0	165	33%
blueberry	2 oz	6.0	165	33%
bran	2 oz	6.5	160	36%
corn				
prepared w/2% milk	2 oz	6.5	180	33%
prepared w/whole milk	2 oz	7.0	185	34%
orange	2 oz	7.0	180	33%
plain	2 oz	5.0	155	28%

■ MIX

(Arrowhead Mills) mix only

Food and Description	Amount	Fat Grams	Total Calories	% Fat Calories
wheat-free oat bran	⅓ cup	2.5	160	14%
whole grain	⅓ cup	1.0	150	6%
(Betty Crocker)				
Original/box				
apple streusel				
mix only	¼ cup	3.0	160	17%
prepared	1 muffin	8.0	210	34%
banana nut				
mix only	3 Tbs	3.0	140	19%
prepared	1 muffin	6.0	170	32%
cranberry orange				
mix only	¼ cup	1.5	120	11%
prepared	1 muffin	5.0	150	30%
double chocolate				
mix only	¼ cup	7.0	190	33%
prepared	1 muffin	8.0	200	36%
lemon poppyseed				
mix only	¼ cup	2.0	140	13%
prepared	1 muffin	7.0	190	33%
twice the blueberry				
mix only	¼ cup	1.5	110	12%
prepared	1 muffin	4.0	140	26%
wild blueberry				
mix only	¼ cup	1.5	130	10%
prepared	1 muffin	5.0	170	26%
Original/pouch				
apple cinnamon				
mix only	¼ cup	3.5	130	24%
prepared	1 muffin	7.0	170	37%

Food and Description	Amount	Fat Grams	Total Calories	% Fat Calories
banana nut				
mix only	¼ cup	4.0	130	28%
prepared	1 muffin	7.0	170	37%
blueberry				
mix only	¼ cup	2.5	120	19%
prepared	1 muffin	6.0	160	34%
chocolate chip				
mix only	3 Tbs	4.5	130	31%
prepared	1 muffin	8.0	170	42%
corn				
mix only	3 Tbs	1.0	110	8%
prepared	1 muffin	5.0	160	28%
lemon poppy seed				
mix only	¼ cup	2.0	120	15%
prepared	1 muffin	8.0	180	40%
Sweet Rewards				
fat-free				
apple cinnamon				
mix only	¼ cup	–	120	–
prepared	1 muffin	–	120	–
wild blueberry				
mix only	3 Tbs	–	120	–
prepared	1 muffin	–	120	–
low-fat				
apple cinnamon				
mix only	¼ cup	–	120	–
prepared	1 muffin	2.0	140	13%
wild blueberry				
mix only	3 Tbs	–	110	–
prepared	1 muffin	2.0	130	14%
(Dromedary) corn/prepared	1 muffin	4.0	120	30%
(Duncan Hines)				
blueberry				
mix only	½₁₂ pkg	4.0	140	26%
prepared	1 muffin	4.5	150	27%
chocolate chip				
mix only	½₁₂ pkg	7.0	190	33%
prepared	1 muffin	7.0	190	33%
cinnamon swirl				
mix only	½₁₂ pkg	6.0	190	28%
prepared	1 muffin	6.0	200	27%
cranberry orange				
mix only	½₁₂ pkg	4.5	150	27%
prepared	1 muffin	5.0	150	30%
(Flako) corn/prepared	1 muffin	4.0	160	23%
generic/corn/prepared	1 muffin	6.0	145	37%
(Gold Medal) prepared				
Low-Fat				
Morning Glory	1 muffin	1.5	140	10%
Variety	1 muffin	1.5	230	6%
corn	1 muffin	3.5	140	23%

Food and Description	Amount	Fat Grams	Total Calories	% Fat Calories
(Golden Dipt)/prepared				
basic	1 muffin	3.0	120	23%
blueberry	1 muffin	3.0	120	23%
corn	1 muffin	2.0	99	18%
(Hain) Prepared				
Oatbran				
apple cinnamon	1 muffin	3.0	140	19%
banana nut	1 muffin	4.0	140	26%
raspberry spice	1 muffin	3.0	140	19%
(Jiffy)/prepared				
apple cinnamon	1 muffin	7.0	190	33%
banana nut	1 muffin	7.0	180	35%
blueberry	1 muffin	7.0	190	33%
bran w/dates	1 muffin	6.0	170	37%
corn	1 muffin	4.0	180	20%
honey date	1 muffin	5.0	170	26%
oatmeal	1 muffin	7.0	180	35%
(Krusteaz)				
Fat-free				
apple cinnamon				
mix & fruit	¼ cup	–	130	–
prepared	1 muffin	–	130	
banana				
mix	⅓ cup	–	140	–
prepared	2 muffin	–	140	–
blueberry				
mix & fruit	¼ cup	–	130	–
prepared	1 muffin	–	130	–
corn/honey cornbread & muffin				
mix only	¼ cup	–	120	–
prepared	1 muffin	–	120	–
cranberry orange				
mix only	¼ cup	–	140	–
prepared	1 muffin	–	140	–
Low-fat				
apple oat bran				
mix only	⅓ cup	2.0	170	11%
prepared	1 muffin	2.0	170	11%
Original				
almond poppy seed				
mix only	⅓ cup	4.5	170	24%
prepared	1 muffin	5.0	180	25%
apple cinnamon				
mix & fruit	⅓ cup	4.0	160	23%
prepared	1 muffin	4.0	160	23%
blueberry				
mix & fruit	⅓ cup	5.0	170	26%
prepared	1 muffin	6.0	180	30%
blueberry bran				
mix & fruit	⅓ cup	6.0	180	30%
prepared	1 muffin	6.0	190	28%

Food and Description	Amount	Fat Grams	Total Calories	% Fat Calories
honey bran				
mix only	¼ cup	4.0	150	24%
prepared	1 muffin	4.5	160	25%
lemon poppy seed				
mix only	⅓ cup	4.5	170	24%
prepared	1 muffin	5.0	180	25%
oat bran				
mix only	⅓ cup	5.0	190	24%
prepared	1 muffin	5.0	190	24%
wild blueberry				
mix only	⅓ cup	5.0	170	26%
prepared	1 muffin	6.0	180	30%
mix only	⅓ cup	7.0	170	37%
prepared	1 muffin	7.0	190	33%
(Pillsbury)				
apple cinnamon				
mix only	⅓ cup	5.0	170	26%
prepared	1 muffin	5.0	180	25%
banana nut				
mix only	¼ cup	6.0	170	32%
prepared	1 muffin	6.0	170	32%
blueberry/low-fat				
mix only	¼ cup	2.0	150	12%
prepared	1 muffin	2.0	150	12%
blueberry/regular				
mix only	⅓ cup	5.0	170	26%
prepared	1 muffin	5.0	180	25%
cinnamon				
mix only	¼ cup	3.5	140	23%
prepared	1 muffin	4.0	160	23%
strawberry				
mix only	⅓ cup	5.0	170	26%
prepared	1 muffin	5.0	180	25%
wildberry				
mix only	⅓ cup	5.0	170	26%
prepared	1 muffin	5.0	180	25%
■ READY TO SERVE				
(Arnold) English				
Bran'nola	1 muffin	1.5	130	10%
extra crisp	1 muffin	1.0	130	7%
raisin	1 muffin	1.0	130	7%
sourdough	1 muffin	1.0	120	8%
(Dunkin' Donuts)				
English	1 muffin	1.0	130	7%
low-fat				
banana	1 muffin	1.5	240	6%
blueberry	1 muffin	1.5	220	6%
cranberry orange	1 muffin	1.5	230	6%
regular				
apple and spice/low-fat	1 muffin	1.5	240	6%
apple cinnamon pecan	1 muffin	21.0	510	37%

Food and Description	Amount	Fat Grams	Total Calories	% Fat Calories
apple n' spice	1 muffin	12.0	350	31%
banana/low-fat	1 muffin	1.5	250	5%
banana nut	1 muffin	15.0	360	38%
blueberry				
4 oz	1 muffin	12.0	320	34%
6 oz	1 muffin	17.0	490	31%
low-fat	1 muffin	1.5	250	5%
reduced-fat	1 muffin	12.0	450	24%
bran				
low-fat	1 muffin	1.0	240	4%
original	1 muffin	12.0	390	28%
cherry				
low-fat	1 muffin	1.5	250	5%
original	1 muffin	12.0	340	32%
chocolate/low-fat	1 muffin	2.5	250	9%
chocolate chip				
4 oz	1 muffin	17.0	400	38%
6 oz	1 muffin	24.0	590	37%
chocolate hazelnut chunk	1 muffin	26.0	610	38%
corn				
4 oz	1 muffin	15.0	390	35%
6 oz	1 muffin	16.0	500	29%
low-fat	1 muffin	2.5	240	9%
reduced-fat	1 muffin	11.0	460	22%
cranberry orange				
low-fat	1 muffin	1.5	240	6%
original	1 muffin	15.0	470	29%
cranberry orange nut	1 muffin	15.0	350	39%
honey raisin bran	1 muffin	16.0	490	29%
lemon poppyseed	1 muffin	13.0	360	33%
oat-bran	1 muffin	13.0	370	32%
(Earth Grains)				
English				
plain	1 muffin	1.0	150	6%
raisin	1 muffin	1.0	150	6%
wheatberry	1 muffin	1.0	150	6%
whole wheat	1 muffin	2.0	170	11%
(Entenmann's) fat-free				
blueberry	1 muffin	–	120	–
generic				
blueberry	1 muffin	4.0	160	23%
English				
cracked wheat	1 muffin	1.0	158	6%
plain	1 muffin	1.0	140	6%
sourdough	1 muffin	1.0	130	7%
w/raisins	1 muffin	1.0	146	6%
whole wheat	1 muffin	1.6	130	11%
oat bran	1 muffin	4.0	155	23%
(Hostess)				
hearty muffin				
banana nut	1 muffin	31.0	620	45%

Food and Description	Amount	Fat Grams	Total Calories	% Fat Calories
blueberry	1 muffin	28.0	590	43%
chocolate chip	1 muffin	29.0	620	42%
cranberry orange	1 muffin	28.0	590	43%
cream cheese	1 muffin	33.0	620	48%
low-fat muffin				
banana bran	1 muffin	3.0	240	11%
blueberry	1 muffin	2.5	230	10%
mini muffin				
apple cinnamon	3 muffins	9.0	160	51%
banana walnut	3 muffins	9.0	160	51%
blueberry	3 muffins	8.0	150	48%
chocolate chip	3 muffins	9.0	160	51%
cinnamon bites	3 muffins	6.0	130	42%
muffin loaf				
apple spice	1 loaf	18.0	430	38%
banana nut	1 loaf	20.0	460	39%
blueberry	1 loaf	19.0	440	39%
chocolate chip	1 loaf	17.0	400	38%
raspberry	1 loaf	19.0	440	39%
regular muffin				
oat bran	1 muffin	8.0	160	45%
(Oroweat) Master's Best English				
blueberry	1 muffin	1.0	170	5%
cinnamon raisin	1 muffin	1.0	170	5%
extra crisp	1 muffin	0.5	130	3%
health nut raisin	1 muffin	3.0	170	16%
oat bran	1 muffin	1.0	150	6%
oat nut raisin	1 muffin	2.0	160	11%
raisins, dates, pecans	1 muffin	3.0	200	14%
sourdough	1 muffin	1.0	140	6%
winter wheat	1 muffin	8.0	220	33%
(Otis Spunkmeyer)				
Low-Fat 4 oz muffins				
apple cinnamon	½ muffin	3.0	190	14%
banana nut	½ muffin	3.0	180	15%
chocolate chocolate chip	½ muffin	3.0	190	14%
wild blueberry	½ muffin	3.0	180	15%
Low-Fat 2.25 oz muffins				
apple cinnamon	1 muffin	3.5	210	15%
banana nut	1 muffin	3.5	200	16%
chocolate chocolate chip	1 muffin	3.5	210	15%
wild blueberry	1 muffin	3.5	200	16%
Mini Muffins				
banana	3 muffins	8.0	180	40%
blueberry	3 muffins	9.0	170	48%
chocolate chocolate chip	3 muffins	9.0	180	45%
Regular 2.25 oz muffins				
apple cinnamon	1 muffin	13.0	240	49%
banana nut	1 muffin	14.0	270	47%
chocolate chocolate chip	1 muffin	13.0	260	45%
harvest bran	1 muffin	10.0	230	39%

Food and Description	Amount	Fat Grams	Total Calories	% Fat Calories
wild blueberry	1 muffin	13.0	230	51%
Regular 4 oz muffins				
almond poppy seed	½ muffin	12.0	210	51%
apple cinnamon	½ muffin	11.0	220	45%
banana nut	½ muffin	12.0	240	45%
cheese streusel	½ muffin	10.0	220	41%
chocolate chocolate chip	½ muffin	12.0	230	47%
cinnamon spice	½ muffin	13.0	230	51%
corn	½ muffin	13.0	230	51%
harvest bran	½ muffin	9.0	200	9%
lemon	½ muffin	13.0	230	51%
orange	½ muffin	13.0	230	51%
pineapple	½ muffin	12.0	210	51%
wild blueberry	½ muffin	11.0	210	47%
(Pepperidge Farm) English				
cinnamon chip	1 muffin	3.0	160	17%
cinnamon raisin	1 muffin	2.0	150	12%
plain	1 muffin	1.0	140	6%
seven-grain	1 muffin	1.0	135	7%
sourdough	1 muffin	1.0	130	7%
(Roman Meal) English	1 muffin	1.0	130	7%
(Sara Lee) English				
blueberry	1 muffin	1.0	140	6%
cinnamon raisin	1 muffin	1.0	140	6%
classic	1 muffin	1.5	130	10%
sourdough	1 muffin	1.0	135	7%
(Thomas') English				
original				
blueberry	1 muffin	1.0	140	6%
cinnamon raisin	1 muffin	1.0	140	6%
cranberry	1 muffin	1.0	140	6%
honey wheat	1 muffin	1.0	110	8%
oat bran	1 muffin	1.0	120	8%
original	1 muffin	1.0	120	8%
raisin	1 muffin	1.0	140	6%
sourdough	1 muffin	1.0	120	8%
sandwich size				
Onion Em's	1 muffin	1.5	180	8%
original	1 muffin	2.0	190	9%
Sourdough Em's	1 muffin	2.0	200	9%
Wheat Em's	1 muffin	1.5	180	8%
(Wolferman's) English/deluxe				
apple orchard	1 muffin	4.0	270	13%
blueberry	1 muffin	1.0	260	3%
cappuccino	1 muffin	3.0	280	10%
cracked wheat	1 muffin	0.5	250	2%
cranberry citrus	1 muffin	1.0	260	3%
herb	1 muffin	0.5	210	2%
honey & oats	1 muffin	2.0	280	6%
onion	1 muffin	0.5	210	2%
original	1 muffin	0.5	240	2%

Food and Description	Amount	Fat Grams	Total Calories	% Fat Calories
pumpkin	1 muffin	1.5	280	5%
sourdough	1 muffin	0.5	240	2%
sugar plum	1 muffin	1.0	270	3%
tomato & herb	1 muffin	1.5	250	5%
MULBERRY/fresh	1 cup	0.6	61	8%
MULLET/striped				
cooked-dry heat	3 oz	4.0	127	28%
raw	3 oz	3.0	99	27%
MUNG BEAN				
Dried/generic				
boiled	6 oz	–	107	–
raw	½ cup	1.0	361	3%
sprouted				
canned	½ cup	–	8	–
cooked	½ cup	–	13	–
raw	½ cup	–	16	–
stir-fried	½ cup	–	31	–
MUNGO BEAN				
boiled	½ cup	–	95	–
raw	½ cup	2.0	365	5%
MUSHROOM				
canned or jarred				
(BinB) broiled in butter				
pieces & stems	1 can	–	30	–
sliced	1 can	–	30	–
sliced w/garlic	1 can	0.5	35	13%
whole	1 can	–	30	–
(Cara Mia)				
marinated	1 oz	1.0	15	60%
seasoned/whole	1 oz		10	–
(Empress)				
button				
pieces & stems	2 oz	–	14	–
sliced	2 oz	–	14	–
whole	2 oz	–	14	–
straw/broken	2 oz	–	10	–
generic				
Oriental straw	2 oz	–	12	–
shiitake	4 oz	–	45	–
white/canned in butter sauce	2 oz	1.0	30	30%
(Green Giant) white				
pieces & stems	½ cup	–	30	–
sliced	½ cup	–	30	–
whole	½ cup	–	30	–
(Libby's)	1 oz	–	70	–
(Seneca)				
shiitake	½ cup	–	25	–
white				
brine pack	½ cup	–	25	–
marinated				
food service	1 oz	0.5	15	30%

Food and Description	Amount	Fat Grams	Total Calories	% Fat Calories
retail	1 oz	9.0	90	90%
pickled	1 oz	–	5	–
teriyaki-sliced	½ cup	–	80	–
water pack	½ cup	–	25	–
dried				
shiitake	1 piece	<1.0	11	3%
	1 oz	<1.0	84	3%
	1 lb	4.5	1343	3%
fresh				
enoki/raw	1 large	–	2	–
oyster/raw	2 oz	–	14	–
shiitake/cooked	4 oz	–	40	
white				
boiled	½ cup	–	21	–
fried or sautéed in butter	10 small	10.0	100	90%
raw				
pieces	½ cup	–	10	–
whole	1 medium	–	5	–
frozen				
(Freshlike)	3.5 oz	–	30	–
(Seneca)	½ cup	–	20	–
(Veg-All)	3.5 oz	–	30	–

MUSHROOM DISH (*See* FROZEN ENTRÉE/DINNER; VEGETABLES, MIXED; individual FAST FOOD listings)
MUSHROOM SOUP (*See* SOUP)
MUSKELLUNGE/NORTH AMERICAN PIKE

raw	3 oz	2.0	93	19%

MUSKMELON (*See* CANTALOUPE)
MUSKRAT

roasted	3 oz	10.0	200	45%
roasted/diced	1 cup	13.0	260	45%

MUSSEL
fresh/blue

cooked-moist heat	3 oz	3.8	147	23%
raw	3 oz	1.9	73	23%
	1 cup	3.0	129	21%

frozen

(Sanford) New Zealand Greenshell on half	3 oz	2.5	100	23%

MUSTARD

dry	1 tsp	<1.0	12	38%
prepared				
(Best Foods) Dijonnaise	1 tsp	1.0	10	90%
(Featherweight)	1 Tbs	–	–	–
(French's)				
bold 'n spicy	1 Tbs	–	5	–
Dijon	1 tsp	0.5	10	45%
(Grey Poupon)				
country Dijon	1 tsp	–	6	–
Dijon	1 tsp	–	6	–

Food and Description	Amount	Fat Grams	Total Calories	% Fat Calories
Parisian	1 tsp	–	6	–
(Gulden's)				
creamy mild	1 Tbs	–	6	–
Diablo	1 Tbs	–	8	–
spicy brown	1 Tbs	–	8	–
(Hain) stone ground				
no salt added	1 Tbs	1.0	14	64%
regular	1 Tbs	1.0	14	64%
(Hebrew National) deli mustard				
original	1 Tbs	–	4	–
w/horseradish	1 Tbs	–	4	–
(Heinz)				
mild yellow	1 Tbs	–	8	–
spicy brown	1 Tbs	1.0	14	64%
(Hellmann's) Dijonnaise	1 tsp	1.0	10	90%
(Jack Daniel's)				
Dijon/stone ground	1 tsp	–	5	–
hickory smoke	1 tsp	–	5	–
honey Dijon	1 tsp	–	10	–
horseradish	1 tsp	–	5	–
Old No. 7	1 tsp	–	5	–
(Kraft)				
horseradish	1 tsp	–	–	–
prepared	1 tsp	–	–	–
(Luizianne) Creole	1 Tbs	–	10	–
(Plochman's)				
Dijon	1 Tbs	1.0	11	82%
spicy brown	1 Tbs	1.0	11	82%
stone ground	1 Tbs	1.0	11	82%
yellow	1 Tbs	1.0	11	82%
(Reckift & Colman)				
classic yellow	1 tsp	<1.0	4	68%
dry	1 Tbs	2.0	29	62%
French				
bold 'n spicy	1 Tbs	–	5	–
Dijon	1 tsp	0.5	10	45%
(Savoir Faire)				
country style	1 tsp	–	5	–
Dijon	1 tsp	–	5	–
(Watkins)				
country mill	1 tsp	1.0	15	60%
Dusseldorf	1 tsp	–	10	–
horseradish	1 tsp	–	10	–
jalapeño	1 tsp	–	10	–
onion	1 tsp	–	10	–
Parisienne	1 tsp	–	10	–
(Westbrae)				
Mt. Fuji	1 tsp	–	–	–
natural stone-ground	1 tsp	–	–	–
yellow	1 tsp	–	–	–

Food and Description	Amount	Fat Grams	Total Calories	% Fat Calories
MUSTARD GREENS				
canned				
(Allen)	½ cup	1.0	30	30%
(Glory Foods)	½ cup	0.5	50	9%
fresh				
boiled	½ cup	–	11	–
raw	½ cup	–	7	–
frozen				
generic				
boiled/drained	½ cup	–	14	–
chopped	½ cup	–	15	–
	10 oz	–	60	–
(Pictsweet)	3.3 oz	–	20	–
MUSTARD SAUCE (See SAUCE)				
MUSTARD SEED				
yellow/whole	1 tsp	1.0	15	60%
MUSTARD SPINACH /fresh				
boiled-drained	½ cup	–	14	–
raw/chopped	½ cup	–	17	–

N

Food and Description	Amount	Fat Grams	Total Calories	% Fat Calories
NACHOS (See MEXICAN FOOD)				
NAPOLEON (See PASTRY)				
NATAL PLUM (See CARISSA)				
NATTO	½ cup	9.7	187	47%
NAVY BEAN				
canned				
(Bush's Best)	½ cup	–	60	–
(Eden Foods) organic	½ cup	0.5	110	4%
(Luck's) seasoned w/pork	½ cup	4.0	140	26%
(Trappey's) seasoned				
w/bacon	½ cup	2.0	110	16%
w/bacon and jalapeño	½ cup	2.0	110	16%
dried				
boiled	½ cup	0.5	130	3%
raw	½ cup	1.5	345	4%
sprouted/raw	½ cup	–	35	–
NAVY BEAN SOUP (See SOUP)				
NECTARINE /fresh				
sliced	1 cup	1.0	70	13%
whole	1 medium	1.0	70	13%

Food and Description	Amount	Fat Grams	Total Calories	% Fat Calories
NEUFCHATEL CHEESE (See CHEESE; CHEESE SPREAD)				
NEWBURG SAUCE (See SAUCE)				
NONDAIRY FROZEN DESSERT (See ICE CREAM & ICE CREAM-LIKE FROZEN DESSERTS; ICE CREAM BARS, SANDWICHES, & FROZEN NOVELTIES; RICE FROZEN DESSERT; SHERBET; TOFU FROZEN DESSERT)				
NOODLE (See ASIAN FOOD; PASTA)				
NOODLE SOUP (See SOUP)				
NORI (See SEAWEED)				
NUTMEG /ground	1 tsp	0.8	11	66%
NUTRITION BAR (See GRANOLA/GRANOLA-TYPE BAR)				
NUTRITIONAL SUPPLEMENT (See also BREAKFAST BAR, BREAKFAST DRINK; GRANOLA/GRANOLA-TYPE BAR)				
(Boost) canned				
High Protein				
chocolate	8 fl oz	6.0	240	23%
strawberry	8 fl oz	6.0	240	23%
vanilla	8 fl oz	6.0	240	23%
Regular				
butter pecan	8 fl oz	6.0	240	23%
chocolate	8 fl oz	6.0	240	23%
chocolate malt	8 fl oz	6.0	240	23%
chocolate mocha	8 fl oz	6.0	240	23%
strawberry	8 fl oz	6.0	· 240	23%
vanilla	8 fl oz	6.0	240	23%
(California Slim) mix only				
chocolate shake	1 serving	<1.0	100	5%
citrus juice	1 serving	<1.0	90	5%
fruit juice	1 serving	<1.0	90	5%
mocha shake	1 serving	<1.0	100	5%
vanilla shake	1 serving	<1.0	100	5%
(Dynatrim)				
Dutch chocolate				
mix only	1 serving	1.0	100	9%
prepared w/1% milk	8 fl oz	4.0	220	16%
strawberry royale				
mix only	1 serving	1.0	100	9%
prepared w/1% milk	8 fl oz	4.0	220	16%
vanilla royale				
mix only	1 serving	1.0	100	9%
prepared w/1% milk	8 fl oz	4.0	220	16%
Ensure (See (Ross) in this section)				
(Nestlé) Sweet Success				
canned				
creamy milk chocolate	10 fl oz	2.5	200	11%
creamy vanilla delight	10 fl oz	3.0	200	14%
dark fudge chocolate	10 fl oz	2.5	200	11%
mocha supreme	10 fl oz	3.0	200	14%
rich chocolate almond	10 fl oz	2.5	200	11%
strawberries 'n' cream	10 fl oz	3.0	200	14%
strawberry creme	10 fl oz	3.0	220	12%

Food and Description	Amount	Fat Grams	Total Calories	% Fat Calories
instant				
creamy milk chocolate				
mix only	1 scoop	1.0	100	9%
prepared w/skim milk	9 fl oz	1.3	180	7%
creamy vanilla delight				
mix only	1 scoop	–	100	–
prepared w/skim milk	9 fl oz	0.5	180	3%
dark chocolate fudge				
mix only	1 scoop	1.0	100	9%
prepared w/skim milk	9 fl oz	1.3	180	7%
(Nutrament) energy food				
chocolate	12 fl oz	10.0	360	25%
vanilla	12 fl oz	10.0	360	25%
(Nutrashake)				
chocolate	4 fl oz	6.0	200	27%
strawberry				
regular	4 fl oz	6.0	200	27%
w/fiber	6 fl oz	2.0	300	6%
vanilla				
regular	4 fl oz	6.0	200	27%
w/fiber	6 fl oz	2.0	300	6%
(Resource) fruit nutritional drink/prepared				
plus/Swiss chocolate	8 fl oz	13.0	360	33%
regular				
French vanilla	8 fl oz	9.0	250	32%
strawberry	8 fl oz	9.0	250	32%
Swiss chocolate	8 fl oz	9.0	250	32%
(Ross) Ensure				
Glucerna OS				
butter pecan	8 fl oz	11.0	220	45%
chocolate	8 fl oz	11.0	220	45%
vanilla	8 fl oz	11.0	220	45%
high-protein				
banana	8 fl oz	6.0	230	23%
chocolate royale	8 fl oz	6.0	230	23%
chocolate supreme	8 fl oz	6.0	230	23%
French vanilla	8 fl oz	6.0	230	23%
vanilla supreme	8 fl oz	6.0	230	23%
wild berry	8 fl oz	6.0	230	23%
light				
strawberry swirl	8 fl oz	3.0	200	14%
plus				
butter pecan	8 fl oz	11.0	360	32%
chocolate	8 fl oz	11.0	360	32%
coffee	8 fl oz	11.0	360	32%
eggnog	8 fl oz	11.0	360	32%
strawberry	8 fl oz	11.0	360	32%
vanilla	8 fl oz	11.0	360	32%
regular				
black walnut	8 fl oz	6.0	250	22%

Food and Description	Amount	Fat Grams	Total Calories	% Fat Calories
butter pecan	8 fl oz	6.0	250	22%
chocolate	8 fl oz	6.0	250	22%
coffee	8 fl oz	6.0	250	22%
eggnog	8 fl oz	6.0	250	22%
strawberry	8 fl oz	6.0	250	22%
vanilla	8 fl oz	6.0	250	22%
w/calcium/vanilla	8 fl oz	6.0	225	24%
w/fiber				
chocolate	8 fl oz	6.0	250	22%
vanilla	8 fl oz	6.0	250	22%
(Ultra Slim*Fast/Slim Fast)				
Powder				
JumpStart mixed w/1 cup fat-free milk				
chocolate	1 cup	2.0	240	8%
vanilla	1 cup	1.5	240	6%
Regular Slim*Fast powder w/1 cup of fat-free milk				
chocolate	1 cup	1.0	190	5%
chocolate malt	1 cup	1.0	190	5%
vanilla	1 cup	1.0	190	5%
strawberry	1 cup	1.0	190	5%
Ultra Slim*Fast powder/mixed w/1 cup fat-free milk				
cafe mocha	1 cup	1.5	200	7%
chocolate fudge	1 cup	2.0	210	9%
chocolate malt	1 cup	1.5	200	7%
chocolate royale	1 cup	1.5	200	7%
French vanilla	1 cup	1.0	200	5%
fruit juice mixable	1 cup	1.0	220	4%
milk chocolate	1 cup	2.0	210	9%
strawberry supreme	1 cup	1.0	200	5%
Ready-to-drink meal				
apple-cranberry-raspberry	11.5 fl oz	1.5	220	6%
cappussino delight	11 fl oz	1.5	220	6%
chocolate fudge	11 fl oz	3.0	220	12%
chocolate royale	11 fl oz	3.0	220	12%
coffee	11 fl oz	3.0	220	12%
French vanilla	11 fl oz	3.0	220	12%
golden apple	11.5 fl oz	1.5	220	6%
milk chocolate	11 fl oz	3.0	220	12%
orange-pineapple	11.5 fl oz	1.5	220	6%
orange-strawberry-banana	11.5 fl oz	1.5	220	6%
strawberries n'cream	11 fl oz	2.5	220	10%
NUTS (*See* NUTS, FORMULATED; NUTS, MIXED; individual listings)				
NUTS, FORMULATED /wheat based				
macadamia-flavored	1 oz	16.0	176	82%
other flavors	1 oz	18.0	184	88%
unflavored	1 oz	16.0	177	81%
NUTS, MIXED (*See also* ICE CREAM TOPPINGS; individual nut listings)				
(Ann's House of Nuts)				
mixed nuts deluxe, no peanuts				
salted				
	1 oz	16.0	170	85%
	¼ cup	20.0	230	78%

Food and Description	Amount	Fat Grams	Total Calories	% Fat Calories
unsalted	1 oz	16.0	170	85%
	¼ cup	20.0	230	78%
(Diamond) In the shell/assorted nuts	15 nuts	19.0	210	81%
(Eagle)				
honey-roasted/cashew & peanut mix	¼ cup	14.0	180	90%
oil-roasted				
deluxe w/o peanuts	¼ cup	17.0	200	77%
lightly salted	¼ cup	17.0	200	77%
original	¼ cup	17.0	200	77%
(Fisher)				
Favorites glazed nut mix & cashews				
praline	1 oz	12.0	170	64%
toffee	1 oz	11.0	160	62%
Nut Topping	1 Tbs	9.0	100	90%
Nuts & Crunches				
golden crisp	1 oz	7.0	140	45%
honey crunch	1 oz	6.0	140	39%
Nuts & Fruits snack mix				
California style	1 oz	8.0	140	51%
trail style	1 oz	11.0	150	66%
Nuts & Seeds				
Cashews	1 oz	13.0	160	73%
mixed nuts	1 oz	15.0	170	79%
peanuts/butter toffee	1 oz	6.0	130	42%
Snack'N serve nut bowl				
fiesta mix	1 oz	7.0	140	45%
mixed deluxe w/no peanuts	1 oz	16.0	180	80%
pecan cashew mix/chocolate covered	1 oz	17.0	230	67%
generic				
dry-roasted/w/peanuts	1 oz	15.0	170	79%
oil-roasted				
w/peanuts	1 oz	16.0	175	82%
w/o peanuts	1 oz	16.0	175	82%
(Guy's)				
tasty mix	1 oz	7.0	130	48%
w/peanuts	1 oz	16.0	180	80%
(Kettle) Roaster Fresh mixed nuts				
camping	1 oz	10.0	140	64%
chocolate lover's				
natural	1 oz	7.0	130	48%
regular	1 oz	7.0	130	48%
deluxe nut				
no salt	1 oz	16.0	170	85%
w/salt	1 oz	16.0	170	85%
honey cranberry	1 oz	6.0	120	45%
honey roast				
harvest	1 oz	6.0	130	42%
nuts & fruit	1 oz	6.0	120	45%
plain	1 oz	13.0	160	73%

Food and Description	Amount	Fat Grams	Total Calories	% Fat Calories
jalapeño lover's	1 oz	11.0	140	71%
Kenai River	1 oz	13.0	160	73%
orchard harvest	1 oz	5.0	110	41%
raw hikers	1 oz	6.0	120	45%
Scandinavian	1 oz	6.0	120	45%
Southwest BBQ	1 oz	10.0	130	69%
sporting	1 oz	11.0	150	66%
Switzerland	1 oz	7.0	130	48%
traffic trail	1 oz	6.0	120	45%
X-Treme Trail	1 oz	12.0	150	72%
(Planters)				
dry-roasted	1 oz	14.0	170	74%
honey-roasted	1 oz	13.0	140	84%
oil-roasted				
deluxe	1 oz	16.0	170	85%
lightly salted	1 oz	15.0	170	79%
mixed	1 oz	15.0	170	79%
no Brazil nuts				
regular	1 oz	15.0	170	79%
unsalted	1 oz	15.0	170	79%
Select				
cashews w/almonds & macadamias	1 oz	16.0	170	85%
cashews w/almonds & pecans	1 oz	15.0	170	79%
sesame nut mix	1 oz	12.0	150	72%
unsalted	1 oz	15.0	170	79%

Food and Description	Amount	Fat Grams	Total Calories	% Fat Calories
OAT BRAN (See BRAN; CEREAL)				
OATS (See also CEREAL)				
(Arrowhead Mills) groats	¼ cup	3.0	160	17%
generic				
rolled flakes	⅓ cup	2.5	130	17%
steel-cut	¼ cup	3.0	170	16%
whole-grain	1 oz	2.0	110	16%
	1 cup	10.8	607	16%
OCEAN PERCH (See also FROZEN ENTRÉE/DINNER; SEAFOOD ENTRÉE/DINNER)				
Atlantic				
breaded & fried	3 oz	11.0	185	54%

Food and Description	Amount	Fat Grams	Total Calories	% Fat Calories
cooked-dry heat	3 oz	1.8	103	16%
raw	3 oz	1.0	80	11%
OCTOBER BEAN /canned				
(Luck's) seasoned w/pork	½ cup	3.0	140	19%
OCTOPUS (See also SQUID; SEAFOOD ENTRÉE/DINNER)				
cooked-moist heat	3 oz	2.0	140	13%
raw	3 oz	0.9	70	11%
OIL (See also ASIAN FOOD/SAUCES & SEASONINGS; COOKING SPRAY)				
Flavored				
(House of Tsang)				
hot chili sesame	1 tsp	5.0	45	100%
Mongolian fired	1 tsp	5.0	45	100%
pure sesame	1 tsp	5.0	45	100%
Singapore curry	1 tsp	5.0	45	100%
wok	1 tsp	5.0	45	100%
Plain				
all vegetable & fish oils	1 tsp	5.0	45	100%
	1 Tbs	14.0	120	100%
	1 cup	218.0	1927	100%

(NOTE: We all need to watch even our use of "healthier" (less saturated) oils in order to keep our total fat intake within acceptable boundaries. Because it is so important to select the least saturated oil that fits your needs, I have listed the most commonly used oils and fats below, showing the percentages of saturated fat, polyunsaturated fat, and monounsaturated fat in each. Those that contain less saturated fat are listed first. Data are based on information from *USDA Nutritive Value of American Foods in Common Units, 1988.* REMEMBER—NO VEGETABLE OIL CONTAINS CHOLESTEROL!)

Vegetable Oils	% Saturated	% Unsaturated	
		% Poly	% Mono
Canola	7%	35%	58%
Almond	8%	19%	73%
Safflower	9%	78%	13%
Sunflower	11%	69%	20%
Corn	13%	62%	25%
Olive	14%	12%	74%
Walnut	14%	67%	19%
Sesame	15%	43%	42%
Soybean	15%	43%	42%
Margarine			
liquid/tub	17%	37%	46%
stick	20%	33%	47%
whipped	20%	30%	50%
Peanut	18%	33%	49%
Soybean/cottonseed blend	19%	50%	31%
Wheat germ	20%	50%	31%
Shortening (vegetable)	27%	26%	47%
Cottonseed	27%	55%	18%

Vegetable Oils	% Saturated	% Unsaturated % Poly	% Mono
Palm	52%	10%	38%
Cocoa butter	62%	3%	35%
Palm kernel	87%	2%	11%
Coconut	92%	2%	6%

Animal Fats	% Saturated	% Unsaturated
Goose	27%	73%
Chicken	30%	70%
Turkey	30%	70%
Duck	34%	66%
Salt pork	36%	64%
Lard	41%	59%
Beef tallow	52%	48%
Butter		
stick	66%	34%
whipped	69%	31%

OKRA (See also VEGETABLES, MIXED)

Canned				
generic	½ cup	–	25	
(Trappey)				
cocktail				
hot	2 pieces	–	8	–
mild	1 piece	–	9	–
Creole gumbo	½ cup	–	35	–
cut	½ cup	–	25	–
fresh				
boiled	½ cup	–	25	–
raw	½ cup	–	19	–
frozen				
(Freshlike)				
cut	½ cup	–	25	–
whole	½ cup	–	30	–
generic/cooked	½ cup	–	34	–
(Pictsweet)				
cut	3.3 oz	–	25	–
microwave	2.5 oz	–	20	–
(Stilwell) breaded	21 pieces	1.0	70	13%
(Veg-All)				
cut	½ cup	–	25	–
whole	½ cup	–	30	–
OLIVE				
(Alma) black/Greek	2 large	3.0	30	90%
(Angonoa)				
green	2 Tbs	2.5	30	75%
sliced ripe	2 Tbs	2.5	30	75%
(Early California) pitted/all sizes	~1 oz	3.0	30	90%

Food and Description	Amount	Fat Grams	Total Calories	% Fat Calories
(Fancifoods)				
green/stuffed or plain	3 olives	2.0	25	72%
queen/plain	2 colossal	2.0	25	72%
generic				
green/pickled	10 small	3.6	33	98%
	10 large	4.9	45	98%
	10 giant	8.0	76	95%
ripe				
Ascolano				
sliced	1 cup	18.6	174	94%
whole	10 extra large	6.5	61	96%
	10 mammoth	7.7	72	96%
	10 giant	9.5	89	96%
	10 jumbo	11.0	105	94%
Manzanillo				
sliced	1 cup	18.6	174	96%
whole	10 small	4.0	38	95%
	10 medium	4.7	44	96%
	10 large	5.5	51	97%
	10 extra large	6.5	61	96%
Mission				
sliced	1 cup	27.0	248	98%
whole	10 small	5.9	54	98%
	10 medium	6.9	63	99%
	10 large	8.0	73	99%
	10 extra large	9.5	87	98%
Sevillano				
sliced	1 cup	12.8	126	91%
whole	10 giant	6.5	64	91%
	10 jumbo	7.8	76	92%
	10 colossal	9.7	95	92%
	10 super colossal	11.6	114	92%
salt-cured/Greek style/whole	10 medium	6.9	65	96%
	10 extra large	9.5	89	96%
(Krinos)				
Greek/black	2 olives	3.0	35	77%
Kalamata	3 olives	4.0	45	80%
(Lindsay) pickled/pitted				
Ascolano	10 jumbo	6.0	70	77%
	10 colossal	8.0	90	80%
	10 super colossal	10.0	120	75%
Manzanilla	10 small	3.5	40	79%
	10 medium	4.0	45	80%
	10 large	5.0	50	90%
	10 extra large	6.0	65	83%
Mission	10 small	3.5	40	79%
	10 medium	4.0	45	80%

Food and Description	Amount	Fat Grams	Total Calories	% Fat Calories
	10 large	5.0	50	90%
	10 extra large	6.0	65	83%
mixed				
chopped	1 oz	3.0	30	90%
sliced	1 oz	3.0	30	90%
	½ cup	6.5	70	84%
Sevillano	10 jumbo	6.0	70	77%
	10 colossal	8.0	90	80%
	10 super colossal	10.0	120	75%
(Progresso) oil-cured	6 olives	6.0	80	68%
(Reese)				
almond stuffed	4 olives	4.0	35	100%
anchovy stuffed	4 olives	2.0	25	72%
(S&W) ripe				
black/pitted	3 extra large	2.5	25	90%
	3 jumbo	2.0	25	72%
	3 super colossal	4.5	45	90%
green				
Manzanilla/stuffed	3 olives	2.0	25	72%
queen	2 olives	2.0	20	90%
stuffed	1 olive	1.0	10	90%
	2 olives	1.5	15	90%
(Santa Barbara Olive Go.)				
Cajun	0.5 oz	1.5	15	90%
California black	0.5 oz	1.5	15	90%
country	0.5 oz	2.0	25	72%
garlic	0.5 oz	1.5	15	90%
pitted	0.5 oz	2.0	25	72%
stuffed	0.5 oz	1.5	15	90%
Italian/pitted	0.5 oz	1.5	15	90%
jalapeño	0.5 oz	1.5	15	90%
pimento-stuffed martini	0.5 oz	1.5	15	90%
OLIVE LOAF (*See* LUNCHEON MEAT)				
OLIVE OIL (*See* OIL)				
OLIVE SALAD				
(Progresso) drained	2 Tbs	2.5	25	90%
OMELET (*See* EGG DISH/MEAL)				
ONION (*See also* SCALLION; VEGETABLES, MIXED)				
canned or jarred				
(Durkee) French-fried	1 oz	15.0	175	77%
(French's) French fried	1 serving	3.5	45	70%
generic/chopped	½ cup	–	20	–
(Green Giant) whole	½ cup	–	35	–
(Heinz) sweet	1 oz	–	40	–
(S&W)				
cocktail	12 pieces	–	5	–
small/whole	½ cup	–	40	–
tiny/whole	½ cup	–	40	–

Food and Description	Amount	Fat Grams	Total Calories	% Fat Calories
(Vlasic) cocktail				
lightly spiced	1 oz	–	4	–
plain	1 oz	–	4	–
dried				
flakes	1 Tbs	–	16	–
	¼ cup	–	45	–
powder/ground	1 tsp	–	7	–
	1 Tbs	–	23	–
fresh/all types/mature				
cooked	1 cup	–	60	–
raw				
chopped	1 Tbs	–	4	–
	½ cup	–	20	–
whole				
(Dole)	1 medium	–	60	–
frozen				
(Birds Eye) small/whole	½ cup	–	30	–
(C&W) petite/whole	⅔ cup	–	30	–
(Freshlike) whole	3.3 oz	–	35	–
generic	10 oz	–	100	–
ONION, GREEN OR SPRING (See SCALLION)				
ONION DISH (See also FROZEN ENTRÉE/DINNER; VEGETABLES, MIXED; VEGETARIAN FOODS)				
frozen				
(Bland Farms) Vidalia O's	6 rings	7.0	180	35%
(Farm Rich) onion rings				
batter dipped	4 oz	13.0	260	45%
Onion O's	5 pieces	9.0	190	43%
generic/onion rings/pan-fried in oven	7 rings	19.0	285	60%
(Mrs. Paul's) Onion rings	7 rings	10.0	200	45%
(Ore-Ida)				
chopped onions	¾ cup	–	25	–
gourmet onion rings	4 pieces	10.0	210	43%
Onion Ringers	6 rings	11.0	210	47%
ONION POWDER	1 tsp	–	7	–
ONION RINGS (See ONION DISH; individual FAST FOOD listings				
ONION SOUP (See SOUP)				
OPOSSUM				
braised or roasted	3 oz	8	190	38%
roasted/diced	1 cup	14.5	310	42%
ORANGE (See also MANDARIN ORANGE)				
fresh				
California				
navel				
peeled sections	1 cup	–	75	–
whole	1 medium	–	65	–
Valencia				
peeled sections	1 cup	0.5	90	5%
whole	1 medium	–	60	–
(Dole)	1 medium	–	50	–

Food and Description	Amount	Fat Grams	Total Calories	% Fat Calories
Florida				
peeled sections	1 cup	0.5	85	5%
whole	1 medium	<1.0	70	4%
ORANGE DRINK/JUICE DRINK BLEND (*See also* SOFT DRINK; SOFT DRINK MIX; TEA)				
bottled, boxed, or canned				
(Betty Crocker) Squeezit Smarty Arty	6.75 fl oz	–	110	–
(Capri Sun)	6.75 fl oz	–	100	–
(Powerade) orange	8 fl oz	–	72	–
(Snapple)				
hydro orange tangerine	8 fl oz	–	100	–
orangeade	8 fl oz	–	120	–
orange tropic	8 fl oz	–	120	–
Snapple Farms orange grove	11.5 fl oz	–	170	–
sun starfruit orange	8 fl oz	–	120	–
Whipper Snapple orange dream	10 fl oz	–	150	–
(Tropicana) Twister				
orange-cranberry				
light	8 fl oz	–	30	–
	10 fl oz	–	35	–
regular	8 fl oz	–	130	–
	10 fl oz	–	160	–
	11.5 fl oz	–	160	–
orange-peach	8 fl oz	–	120	–
	10 fl oz	–	150	–
orange-raspberry				
light	8 fl oz	–	35	–
	10 fl oz	–	45	–
regular	8 fl oz	–	120	–
	10 fl oz	–	150	–
orange-strawberry-banana	8 fl oz	–	120	–
	10 fl oz	–	140	–
	11.5 fl oz	–	160	–
orange-strawberry-guava	8 fl oz	–	120	–
	10 fl oz	–	140	–
(Welch's) orange-pineapple	11.5 fl oz	–	180	–
	8 fl oz	–	140	–
frozen				
(Tropicana) Twister/concentrate/undiluted				
orange-cranberry	2 fl oz	–	130	–
orange-peach	2 fl oz	–	120	–
orange-raspberry	2 fl oz	–	120	–
orange-strawberry-banana	2 fl oz	–	120	–
(Welch's)				
orange-pineapple-apple	8 fl oz	–	140	–
Juicemaker	8 fl oz	–	130	–
Welchade/orange	8 fl oz	–	140	–
mix				
(Tang) breakfast drink/prepared				
orange	8 fl oz	–	90	

Food and Description	Amount	Fat Grams	Total Calories	% Fat Calories
orange-pineapple	8 fl oz	–	100	–
ORANGE JUICE/JUICE BLEND (*See also* FRUIT PUNCH)				
bottled, boxed, or canned				
(Chiquita)				
Citrus Adventure/orange-tangerine	8 fl oz	–	120	–
tropical orange/light	8 fl oz	–	30	–
(Citrus Hill)				
plus calcium	6 fl oz	–	90	–
select	6 fl oz	–	90	–
(Dole)				
orange juice	10 fl oz	–	140	–
orange juice cooler	8.45 fl oz	–	130	–
generic				
sweetened	8 fl oz	–	119	–
unsweetened	8 fl oz	–	104	–
(Knudsen) orange-mango	8 fl oz	–	110	–
(Minute Maid)				
orange juice				
juice box	8.45 fl oz	–	120	–
refrigerated				
calcium rich	8 fl oz	–	120	–
country style	8 fl oz	–	110	–
premium choice	8 fl oz	–	110	–
country style	8 fl oz	–	110	–
pulp-free	8 fl oz	–	110	–
orange juice blend	8 fl oz	–	125	–
(Ocean Spray)				
100% orange juice	8 fl oz	–	120	–
(Seneca)				
orange	8 fl oz	–	120	–
orange-grapefruit	8 fl oz	–	110	–
orange-pineapple	8 fl oz	–	110	–
(Snapple) Snapple Farms orange grove	12 fl oz	–	170	–
(Sunkist)				
fresh-squeezed	6 fl oz	–	80	–
regular	6 fl oz	–	85	–
(TreeTop)	5.5 fl oz	–	80	–
	8 fl oz	–	120	–
	10 fl oz	–	150	–
	11.5 fl oz	–	170	–
(Tropicana)				
orange-pineapple	8 fl oz	–	130	–
	10 fl oz	–	130	–
Pure Premium				
+ calcium	8 fl oz	–	110	–
+ calcium & vitamin c	8 fl oz	–	110	–
+ fiber	8 fl oz	–	120	–
+ vitamins	8 fl oz	–	110	–
regular	8 fl oz	–	110	–
	10 fl oz	–	130	–

Food and Description	Amount	Fat Grams	Total Calories	% Fat Calories
(Welch's)				
juice	10 fl oz	–	130	–
	11.5 fl oz	–	170	–
juice blend	11.5 fl oz	–	170	–
juice cocktail	8 fl oz	–	120	–
frozen				
generic/concentrate/undiluted	6 oz	<1.0	340	1%
(Minute Maid) concentrate/prepared				
calcium-rich	8 fl oz	–	120	–
country style	8 fl oz	–	110	–
original	8 fl oz	–	110	–
pulp free	8 fl oz	–	110	–
reduced acid	8 fl oz	–	110	–
(Seneca) concentrate/undiluted				
Awake	2 oz	–	120	–
orange	2 oz	–	110	–
orange plus	2 oz	–	130	–
Valencia	2 oz	–	110	–
(Tropicana) concentrate/undiluted				
all types	2 oz	–	110	–
ORANGE PEEL				
candied				
generic	1 oz	–	90	–
(S&W)	58 pieces	–	80	–
fresh	1 Tbs	–	–	–
ORANGE ROUGHY (See also SEAFOOD ENTRÉE/DINNER)				
cooked-dry heat	3 oz	1.0	80	11%
raw	3 oz	6.0	110	50%
OREGANO/ground	1 tsp	–	5	–
ORIENTAL FOOD (See ASIAN FOOD; FROZEN ENTRÉE/DINNER; PASTA ENTRÉE/DINNER; RICE DISH; VEGETARIAN FOODS; individual listings)				
OSTRICH	4 oz	4.0	170	21%
OYSTER (See also SEAFOOD ENTRÉE/DINNER)				
canned				
(Bumble Bee) whole	½ cup	4.0	100	36%
(Chicken of the Sea)				
smoked	2.5 oz	8.0	140	51%
	3 oz	11.0	190	52%
whole	2 oz	3.0	70	39%
(Empress) whole	½ cup	4.0	100	36%
(Geisha) whole	⅓ cup	2.5	60	38%
generic				
Eastern	3 oz	2.0	58	31%
	1 cup	6.0	170	32%
Pacific	1 cup	5.0	220	20%
	12 oz	7.5	310	22%
(Reese) smoked	2 oz	1.0	45	50%
(S&W)				
smoked	2 oz	6.0	100	54%
whole	2 oz	3.0	70	39%

Food and Description	Amount	Fat Grams	Total Calories	% Fat Calories
fresh				
eastern				
battered & fried	3 oz	10.0	180	50%
	6 medium	11.0	175	57%
breaded & fried	3 oz	11.0	170	58%
	6 medium	11.0	175	57%
meat only	1 cup	4.0	160	23%
raw	6 medium	2.0	50	30%
steamed	3 oz	4.5	120	34%
	6 medium			
	~1.5 oz	2.0	60	30%
Pacific/western				
raw	3 oz	2.0	70	26%
steamed	1 medium	1.0	40	23%
	3 oz	4.0	140	26%
OYSTER DISH (*See also* FROZEN ENTRÉE/DINNER; SEAFOOD ENTRÉE/DINNER; SOUP				
homemade/USDA Standard Home Recipe				
oyster stew/6 oysters per cup	1 cup	15.5	235	59%
oysters Rockefeller	4 oysters	2.5	85	26%

Food and Description	Amount	Fat Grams	Total Calories	% Fat Calories
PANCAKE				
Frozen				
(Aunt Jemima)				
blueberry	3 pancakes	3.5	210	15%
buttermilk	3 pancakes	3.5	210	15%
low-fat	3 pancakes	1.5	150	9%
original	3 pancakes	3.5	210	15%
(Downyflake)				
blueberry	3 pancakes	9.0	290	28%
buttermilk	3 pancakes	9.0	280	29%
regular	3 pancakes	9.0	280	29%
(Hungry Jack)				
buttermilk	¼ pkg	4.5	270	15%
(Krusteaz)				
blueberry	1 pancake	2.0	100	18%
buttermilk	4" pancake	1.0	70	13%
	4-½" pancake	2.0	90	20%
mini	6 pancakes	2.5	120	19%

Food and Description	Amount	Fat Grams	Total Calories	% Fat Calories
(Pillsbury) Hungry Jack				
blueberry	3 pancakes	3.5	230	14%
buttermilk	3 pancakes	4.0	240	15%
original				
mini	11 pancakes	4.0	230	14%
regular	3 pancakes	4.0	240	15%
(Swanson)				
Budget Breakfast				
eggs & silver dollar pancakes	1 meal	14.0	250	50%
silver dollar pancakes & sausage	1 meal	18.0	340	41%
Kids' Breakfast Blast				
6 mini pancakes w/syrup	1 meal	8.0	320	23%
Great Starts				
pancakes & sausages	1 meal	25.0	490	46%
pancakes w/bacon	1 meal	20.0	400	45%
(Van's) multigrain/nondairy	2 pancakes	1.5	180	8%
Homemade/USDA Standard Home Recipe				
buckwheat/6" dia	3 pancakes	9.0	410	20%
buttermilk/6" dia	3 pancakes	15.0	490	28%
plain				
4" dia	1 pancake	2.0	62	29%
6" dia	1 pancake	5.0	169	27%
Mix (Note: Unless otherwise stated, data are for dry mix only.)				
(Arrowhead Mills)				
blue corn	⅓ cup	2.0	150	12%
buckwheat	⅓ cup	1.5	140	10%
buttermilk	¼ cup	0.5	120	4%
gluten-free	¼ cup	2.0	130	14%
griddle lite	½ cup	3.0	260	10%
kamut	¼ cup	1.0	130	7%
multigrain	¼ cup	0.5	120	4%
oat bran	⅓ cup	1.5	140	10%
whole grain	¼ cup	0.5	120	4%
wild rice	¼ cup	1.0	140	6%
(Aunt Jemima)				
Pancake batter				
blueberry	½ cup	3.5	250	13%
buttermilk	½ cup	3.5	260	12%
original	½ cup	3.5	250	13%
Pancake & Waffle/mix only				
buckwheat	¼ cup	1.0	120	8%
complete				
buttermilk				
reduced calorie	⅓ cup	1.5	140	10%
regular	⅓ cup	2.0	190	9%
original	⅓ cup	0.5	150	3%
whole wheat	¼ cup	0.5	130	3%
(Betty Crocker)				
complete				
buttermilk				
mix only	⅓ cup	2.5	200	11%

Food and Description	Amount	Fat Grams	Total Calories	% Fat Calories
prepared	3 pancakes	2.5	200	11%
original				
mix only	⅓ cup	3.0	200	14%
prepared	3 pancakes	3.0	200	11%
(Bisquick) Shake'N Pour pancake & waffle mix				
prepared				
blueberry	3 pancakes	3.5	210	15%
buttermilk	3 pancakes	3.0	200	14%
original	3 pancakes	4.0	210	17%
(Feam) pancake & waffle/mix only				
buckwheat	½ cup	3.0	235	12%
Rich Earth	½ cup	2.0	190	10%
7-grain buttermilk	½ cup	2.0	200	9%
stone ground whole wheat	½ cup	2.0	220	8%
unbleached wheat & soya	½ cup	2.0	235	8%
generic/prepared/4" dia				
buckwheat	1 pancake	2.0	60	30%
buttermilk	1 pancake	1.0	75	12%
plain	1 pancake	1.0	75	12%
whole wheat	1 pancake	3.0	90	30%
(Krusteaz)				
blueberry				
mix only	½ cup	3.0	210	13%
prepared	3 pancakes	3.0	210	13%
buttermilk				
fat-free				
mix only	½ cup	–	190	–
prepared	½ cup	–	190	–
original				
mix only	½ cup	3.0	200	14%
prepared	3 pancakes	3.0	200	14%
harvest apple spice				
mix only	½ cup	3.0	210	13%
prepared	3 pancakes	3.0	210	13%
oat bran/lite				
mix only	½ cup	1.0	140	6%
prepared	3 pancakes	1.0	140	6%
oat bran/low-fat				
mix only	½ cup	3.0	230	12%
prepared	3 pancakes	3.0	230	12%
old fashioned				
mix only	¼ cup	0.5	120	4%
prepared	3 pancakes	9.0	230	35%
whole wheat & honey				
mix only	½ cup	2.0	230	8%
prepared	3 pancakes	2.0	230	8%
(Mrs. Butterworth's)				
buttermilk complete				
mix only	⅓ cup	2.0	160	11%
prepared	3-4 pancakes	2.0	160	11%

Food and Description	Amount	Fat Grams	Total Calories	% Fat Calories
country breakfast/mix only				
buttermilk complete	⅓ cup	2.0	160	11%
original	⅓ cup	2.0	170	11%
pancake & waffle				
complete	⅓ cup	2.0	160	11%
original	¼ cup	–	120	–
(Robin Hood) buttermilk				
mix only	⅓ cup	3.0	180	15%
prepared	3 pancakes	6.0	230	23%
(Stone-Buhr)				
buckwheat	¼ cup	1.0	130	7%
oat bran	¼ cup	–	130	–
whole wheat	¼ cup	1.0	120	8%

PANCAKE & WAFFLE MIX (*See also* PANCAKE under Mix)
PANCAKE & WAFFLE SYRUP (*See also* MAPLE SYRUP)

Food and Description	Amount	Fat Grams	Total Calories	% Fat Calories
(Aunt Jemima)				
butter lite	¼ cup	–	100	–
butter rich	¼ cup	–	210	–
lite	¼ cup	–	100	–
original	¼ cup	–	210	
(Brer Rabbit)				
dark	2 Tbs	–	120	–
light	2 Tbs	–	120	–
(Cary's)				
pure maple	2 Tbs	–	100	–
sugar-free	¼ cup	–	35	
(Estee)				
blueberry	¼ cup	–	80	–
maple	¼ cup	–	80	–
(Featherweight) lite				
blueberry syrup	¼ cup	–	80	–
maple	¼ cup	–	80	–
(Golden Griddle)	4 Tbs	–	220	–
(Karo) pancake	1 Tbs	–	60	–
	4 Tbs	–	240	–
(Knott's Berry Farm)	2 Tbs	–	110	–
blackberry	2 Tbs	–	120	–
blueberry				
light	2 Tbs	–	50	–
regular	2 Tbs	–	120	–
boysenberry				
light	2 Tbs	–	50	–
regular	2 Tbs	–	120	–
country	2 Tbs	–	110	–
microwaveable				
light	2 Tbs	–	45	–
w/30% real maple syrup	2 Tbs	–	110	–
strawberry	2 Tbs	–	120	–
(Log Cabin)				
Country Kitchen				
butter	¼ cup	–	210	–

Food and Description	Amount	Fat Grams	Total Calories	% Fat Calories
lite	¼ cup	–	100	–
regular	¼ cup	–	210	–
original				
lite	¼ cup	–	100	–
regular	¼ cup	–	200	–
(Mrs. Butterworth's)	–			
original	¼ cup	–	230	–
reduced-calorie	¼ cup	–	100	
(Mrs. Richardson's)				
lite	¼ cup	–	100	–
original recipe	¼ cup	–	210	–
(Nabisco) Vermont Maid	1 Tbs	–	50	–
(Polaner)				
blueberry	¼ cup	–	200	–
raspberry	¼ cup	–	200	–
strawberry	¼ cup	–	200	–
(S&W) reduced calorie				
blueberry	¼ cup	–	60	–
butter flavor	¼ cup	–	60	–
maple	¼ cup	–	60	–
strawberry	¼ cup	–	60	–
(Smucker's) fruit				
light	¼ cup	–	130	–
natural				
apricot	¼ cup	–	210	–
blackberry	¼ cup	–	210	–
blueberry	¼ cup	–	210	–
boysenberry	¼ cup	–	210	–
red raspberry	¼ cup	–	210	–
strawberry	¼ cup	–	210	–
PAPAW /fresh	½ lb	2.0	194	9%
PAPAYA /fresh				
cubed-peeled	1 cup	–	60	–
whole	½ medium	–	80	–
PAPAYA JUICE/NECTAR (See also FRUIT PUNCH)				
bottled, boxed, or canned				
generic	1 cup	–	145	–
(Goya)	6 fl oz	–	110	–
(Kern's)	6 fl oz	–	110	–
(Knudsen)				
papaya juice				
papaya-lime juice	8 fl oz	–	115	–
nectar	11.5 fl oz	–	210	–
Thirst Quencher	8 fl oz	–	130	–
(Libby's)	6 fl oz	–	110	–
	11.5 fl oz	–	210	–
PAPRIKA /ground	1 tsp	–	6	–
PARFAIT (See CANDY; ICE CREAM BARS, SANDWICHES, & FROZEN NOVELTIES; PUDDING & MOUSSE)				
PARSLEY				
dried	1 tsp	–	1	–

Food and Description	Amount	Fat Grams	Total Calories	% Fat Calories
freeze-dried	any amount	–	–	–
fresh	10 sprigs	–	3	–
	½ cup	–	10	–
PARSNIP /fresh				
cooked	½ cup	–	66	–
raw/sliced	½ cup	–	50	
PASSION FRUIT/GRANADILLA				
fresh	1 medium	–	18	–
	½ lb	–	106	
PASSION FRUIT JUICE/JUICE BLEND (*See also* FRUIT PUNCH)				
fresh				
purple	1 cup	–	126	–
yellow	1 cup	–	149	–
frozen				
(Welch's) passion fruit	8 fl oz	–	140	–
PASTA (*See also* COUSCOUS)				
(Adrienne's) Gourmet/wheat-free & gluten-free				
Papadini Hi-Protein pure Lentil Bean Pasta				
cavatappi	2 oz	0.5	200	2%
conchigliette	2 oz	0.5	200	2%
orzo	2 oz	0.5	200	2%
rotini	2 oz	0.5	200	2%
shipper	2 oz	0.5	200	2%
(American Beauty) dry/uncooked				
angel hair	2 oz	1.0	210	4%
capellini	2 oz	1.0	210	4%
curly roni	2 oz	1.0	210	4%
egg noodles				
extra wide	2 oz	3.0	220	12%
fine	2 oz	3.0	220	12%
krinkly	2 oz	3.0	220	12%
wide	2 oz	3.0	220	12%
elbow roni	2 oz	1.0	210	4%
fettuccine	2 oz	3.0	220	12%
lasagna	2 oz	1.0	210	4%
mostaccioli	2 oz	1.0	210	4%
rainbow shells	2 oz	1.0	210	4%
rainbow twirls	2 oz	1.0	210	4%
roni mac	2 oz	1.0	210	4%
rotelle	2 oz	1.0	210	4%
rotini	2 oz	1.0	210	4%
salad mac	2 oz	1.0	210	4%
seashell	2 oz	1.0	210	4%
shell roni				
large	2 oz	1.0	210	4%
regular	2 oz	1.0	210	4%
shells/medium	2 oz	1.0	210	4%
spaghetti				
regular	2 oz	1.0	210	4%
thin	2 oz	1.0	210	4%

Food and Description	Amount	Fat Grams	Total Calories	% Fat Calories
vermicelli	2 oz	1.0	210	4%
(Azumaya) Noodles/cooked				
Chinese	1 cup	1.0	290	3%
Japanese	1 cup	1.0	290	3%
(CEMAC Foods) Orgran pasta/dry				
Stoneground				
barley & spinach	2.2 oz	1.0	196	5%
brown rice/organic	2.2 oz	1.0	210	4%
buckwheat	2.2 oz	1.0	220	4%
corn & vegetable/gourmet	2.2 oz	1.0	217	4%
garlic & parsley	2.2 oz	1.0	215	4%
rice & millet	2.2 oz	1.0	220	4%
split pea & soya soup shells	1.8 oz	1.0	150	6%
tomato & basil	2.2 oz	1.2	215	5%
vegetable rice/gourmet	2.2 oz	1.4	220	6%
(Contadina) Buitoni/fresh				
Cut pasta/refrigerated				
angel's hair	1¼ cups	2.5	230	10%
fettuccine				
spinach	1¼ cup	2.5	250	9%
traditional	1¼ cup	2.5	230	10%
linguine	1¼ cups	2.5	240	9%
Family Size Favorites/refrigerated				
angel hair pasta	1¼ cup	2.5	230	10%
ravioli/4-cheese	1 cup	9.0	290	28%
tortellini/3-cheese	¾ cup	6.0	250	22%
Filled pasta/refrigerated				
ravioli				
chicken & garlic	1¼ cups	11.0	330	30%
classic beef & garlic	1¼ cups	9.0	330	25%
4-cheese				
light	1 cup	4.0	230	16%
regular	1 cup	9.0	290	25%
garden vegetable/lite	1 cup	5.0	250	18%
parmesan	1¼ cup	9.0	310	26%
tortellini				
cheese				
spinach	¾ cup	6.0	260	21%
3-cheese	¾ cup	6.0	250	22%
herb chicken	¾ cup	7.0	260	23%
tortelloni				
chicken & prosciutto	1 cup	13.0	360	33%
chicken & vegetable	¾ cup	10.0	270	33%
mozzarella & herb	1 cup	9.0	320	25%
mushroom & cheese	1 cup	6.0	290	19%
roasted garlic & cheese	1 cup	8.0	270	27%
sun-dried tomato	1 cup	10.0	320	28%
sweet sausage	1 cup	8.0	320	23%

Food and Description	Amount	Fat Grams	Total Calories	% Fat Calories
(Creamette) dry/uncooked				
egg noodles				
enriched/wide	2 oz	3.0	220	12%
no egg yolk	2 oz	2.5	210	11%
stroganoff	2 oz	2.5	210	11%
wide & broad	2 oz	2.5	210	11%
regular				
dumpling	2 oz	2.5	210	11%
extra wide	2 oz	2.5	210	11%
fine	2 oz	2.5	210	11%
kluski	2 oz	3.0	220	12%
enriched pasta				
elbow macaroni	2 oz	1.0	210	4%
fettuccine	2 oz	1.0	210	4%
lasagna	2 oz	1.0	210	4%
linguini	2 oz	1.0	210	4%
manicotti/8-oz pkg	3 pieces	1.0	180	5%
mostaccioli	2 oz	1.0	210	4%
rainbow rotini	2 oz	1.0	210	4%
ribbons/no egg yolk	2 oz	1.0	210	4%
rigatoni	2 oz	1.0	210	4%
rotini	2 oz	1.0	210	4%
shells/jumbo	6 pieces	1.0	210	4%
spaghetti				
regular	2 oz	1.0	210	4%
thin	2 oz	1.0	210	4%
spinach				
egg	2 oz	3.0	220	12%
no egg	2 oz	1.0	210	4%
tri-color	2 oz	1.0	210	4%
vermicelli	2 oz	1.0	210	4%
(De Boles) Organic-dry/uncooked				
angel hair/Jerusalem artichoke				
garlic & parsley	2 oz	1.0	210	4%
plain	2 oz	1.0	210	4%
tomato				
& basil	2 oz	1.0	210	4%
& lemon pepper	2 oz	0.5	200	3%
& pesto	2 oz	0.5	200	3%
whole wheat	2 oz	2.0	210	4%
elbow style				
plain	2 oz	0.5	200	3%
fettuccine				
garlic & parsley	2 oz	0.5	200	3%
spinach	2 oz	0.5	200	3%
tomato				
& basil	2 oz	0.5	200	3%
& lemon pepper	2 oz	0.5	200	3%
& pesto	2 oz	0.5	200	3%
lasagna/organic	2 oz	0.5	200	3%

Food and Description	Amount	Fat Grams	Total Calories	% Fat Calories
linguine/Jerusalem artichoke	2 oz	1.0	210	4%
penne				
garlic & parsley	2 oz	0.5	200	3%
plain	2 oz	1.0	210	4%
tomato & basil	2 oz	0.5	200	3%
whole wheat	2 oz	2.0	210	9%
ribbon				
eggless	2 oz	0.5	200	3%
garlic & parsley	2 oz	1.0	210	4%
whole wheat	2 oz	2.0	210	9%
rigatoni				
garlic & parsley	2 oz	0.5	200	3%
Jerusalem artichoke	2 oz	1.0	210	4%
tomato & basil	2 oz	0.5	200	3%
whole wheat	2oz	2.0	210	9%
rotini				
Jerusalem artichoke/organic	2 oz	1.0	210	4%
Vegetable				
Garlic & parsley	2 oz	1.0	210	4%
primavera	2 oz	1.0	210	4%
tomato & basil	2 oz	1.0	210	4%
shells/organic	2 oz	0.5	200	3%
spaghetti-style				
garlic & parsley	2 oz	0.5	200	3%
Jerusalem artichoke	2 oz	1.0	210	4%
plain	2 oz	1.0	210	4%
tomato & basil	2 oz	0.5	200	3%
w/spinach	2 oz	0.5	200	3%
whole wheat	2 oz	2.0	210	9%
ziti				
Jerusalem artichoke	2 oz	1.0	210	4%
(De Cecco) dry/cooked				
capellini	4 oz	1.0	210	4%
egg noodle	4 oz	3.0	210	13%
fusilli	4 oz	1.0	210	4%
lasagna	4 oz	1.0	210	4%
linguini	4 oz	1.0	210	4%
penne rigati	4 oz	1.0	210	4%
pennete	4 oz	1.0	210	4%
rigatoni	4 oz	1.0	210	4%
rotelle	4 oz	1.0	210	4%
spaghetti	4 oz	1.0	210	4%
spaghettini	4 oz	1.0	210	4%
spinach wheat	4 oz	1.0	210	4%
(Di Giorno) refrigerated				
Low-fat/cholesterol free				
angel's hair	2 oz	1.5	160	8%
fettuccine				
red bell pepper	2.5 oz	1.5	200	7%
regular	2.5 oz	1.5	200	7%

Food and Description	Amount	Fat Grams	Total Calories	% Fat Calories
spinach	2.5 oz	1.5	190	7%
linguine				
herb	2.5 oz	1.5	200	7%
regular	2.5 oz	1.5	200	7%
Filled/prepared				
ravioli				
4-cheese	1 cup	15.0	350	39%
Italian sausage	1 cup	12.0	350	31%
Light cheese w/tomato & cheese	1 cup	7.0	280	23%
tortellini				
beef & roasted garlic	1 cup	11.0	340	29
3-cheese	¾ cup	7.0	250	25%
tortelloni				
chicken & herbs	1 cup	5.0	270	17%
mozzarella-garlic	1 cup	8.0	300	24%
pesto	1 cup	8.0	320	23%
portabella mushroom	1 cup	7.0	310	20%
(Eden)/dry				
elbows/organic				
whole wheat	2 oz	2.0	210	9%
whole wheat vegetable	2 oz	2.0	210	9%
kudzu				
& sweet potato pasta	2 oz	–	190	–
kiri pasta	2 oz	–	190	–
mung bean/Harusame	2 oz	–	190	–
ribbons durum/organic				
wheat	2 oz	1.0	220	4%
wheat curry	2 oz	1.0	220	4%
wheat paella	2 oz	1.0	220	4%
wheat parsley	2 oz	1.0	220	4%
wheat pesto	2 oz	1.0	220	4%
whole wheat spinach	2 oz	2.0	200	9%
rice pasta bifun	2 oz	1.0	200	5%
shells durum wheat vegetable/organic	2 oz	1.0	210	4%
soba				
100% buckwheat	2 oz	–	200	–
lotus root	2 oz	1.0	190	5%
mugwort	2 oz	1.0	190	5%
regular	2 oz	–	200	–
wild yam jinenjo	2 oz	1.0	190	5%
somen	2 oz	2.0	200	9%
spaghetti/organic				
durum wheat	2 oz	1.0	210	4%
kamut	2 oz	2.0	210	9%
parsley garlic	2 oz	1.0	210	4%
whole wheat	2 oz	2.0	210	9%
spirals/organic				
durum wheat vegetable	2 oz	1.0	210	4%
kamut	2 oz	2.0	210	9%
sesame rice	2 oz	2.0	200	9%

Food and Description	Amount	Fat Grams	Total Calories	% Fat Calories
whole wheat vegetable	2 oz	2.0	210	9%
udon				
brown rice	2 oz	2.0	200	9%
regular	2 oz	2.0	200	9%
(Foulds) No Yolks/dry/uncooked				
egg noodle				
broad	2 oz	0.5	210	2%
substitute	2 oz	2.0	210	9%
(Health Valley) dry/uncooked				
elbows				
whole wheat	2 oz	1.0	202	5%
whole wheat w/4 vegetables	2 oz	1.0	202	5%
lasagna/whole wheat				
spinach	2 oz	1.0	170	5%
w/wheat germ	2 oz	1.0	170	5%
spaghetti				
amaranth	2 oz	1.0	170	5%
oat bran	2 oz	1.0	120	7%
whole wheat	2 oz	1.0	170	5%
whole wheat amaranth	2 oz	1.0	200	5%
whole wheat w/spinach	2 oz	1.0	170	5%
(Hodgson Mill) dry/cooked				
bows/semolina veggie	4 oz	1.0	200	4%
egg noodles				
Semolina veggie	4 oz	3.0	220	12%
whole wheat	4 oz	3.0	220	12%
whole wheat-spinach	4 oz	3.0	220	12%
elbows/whole wheat	4 oz	1.0	190	5%
fettuccine/whole wheat	4 oz	1.0	190	5%
lasagna/whole wheat	4 oz	1.0	190	5%
rotini/semolina veggie	4 oz	1.0	200	4%
shells/medium/whole wheat	4 oz	1.0	190	5%
spaghetti				
whole wheat	4 oz	1.0	190	5%
whole wheat-spinach	4 oz	2.0	190	9%
spirals/whole wheat	4 oz	1.0	190	5%
wagon wheels/semolina veggie	4 oz	1.0	200	4%
(Manischewitz) dry/cooked				
egg noodles				
fine	1½ cups	3.0	220	12%
flakes	⅓ cup	3.0	220	12%
medium	1¼ cups	3.0	220	12%
wide	1¾ cups	3.0	220	12%
large egg bows	⅓ cup	3.0	220	12%
matzo farfel	1 cup	1.0	180	5%
wide cut/yolk-free	1¾ cups	1.0	210	4%
(Martha Gooch) dry/cooked				
egg noodles				
dumplings	4 oz	3.0	220	12%
extra wide	4 oz	3.0	220	12%

Food and Description	Amount	Fat Grams	Total Calories	% Fat Calories
wide	4 oz	3.0	220	12%
elbow macaroni/big	4 oz	1.0	210	4%
rotini	4 oz	1.0	210	4%
shell macaroni	4 oz	1.0	210	4%
spaghetti				
long	4 oz	1.0	210	4%
thin	4 oz	1.0	210	4%
(Monterey Pasta Co.) refrigerated				
ravioli/snow crab	3 oz	3.0	205	13%
(Muellers) dry/uncooked				
egg noodles				
golden rich	2 oz	3.0	220	12%
regular	2 oz	3.0	220	12%
elbows	2 oz	1.0	210	4%
lasagna	2 oz	1.0	210	4%
macaroni	2 oz	1.0	210	4%
ready-cut	2 oz	1.0	210	4%
ruffles	2 oz	1.0	210	4%
sea shells	2 oz	1.0	210	4%
spaghetti				
regular	2 oz	1.0	210	4%
thin	2 oz	1.0	210	4%
tri-color twist trio	2 oz	1.0	210	4%
twists	2 oz	1.0	210	4%
vermicelli	2 oz	1.0	210	4%
wide/yolk-free	2 oz	1.0	210	4%
(Nature's Cuisine) dry/uncooked				
long spaghetti				
artichoke	2 oz	2.0	210	9%
sesame	2 oz	2.0	190	9%
spinach	2 oz	2.0	190	9%
wheat & soya	2 oz	1.0	220	4%
(Pasta La Bella) dry/uncooked				
penne rigate	¾ cup	1.0	210	4%
pepi rigate	¾ cup	1.0	210	4%
radiatore	¾ cup	1.0	210	4%
rotelle	1¼ cups	1.0	210	4%
rotini/garden	¾ cup	1.0	210	4%
shells/medium	¾ cup	1.0	210	4%
spaghetti	2 oz	1.0	210	4%
ziti	2 oz	1.0	210	4%
(Pennsylvania Dutch) dry/uncooked				
alphabets/egg	2 oz	2.5	210	11%
bott boi/egg/no yolks	2 oz	2.5	210	11%
bows/egg	2 oz	2.5	210	11%
egg noodles				
broad	2 oz	2.5	210	11%
fine	2 oz	2.5	210	11%
homestyle	2 oz	2.5	210	11%
kluski	2 oz	3.0	220	12%

Food and Description	Amount	Fat Grams	Total Calories	% Fat Calories
medium	2 oz	2.5	210	11%
stroganoff	2 oz	2.5	210	11%
wide & broad	2 oz	2.5	210	11%
(Quinoa) wheat-free				
elbows	2 oz	2.0	180	10%
garden pagodas	2 oz	2.0	180	10%
pasta	2 oz	2.0	180	10%
rotini	2 oz	1.0	210	4%
shells	2 oz	2.0	180	10%
spaghetti	2 oz	1.0	210	4%
(Reames) frozen				
beef noodle soup noodles	3.3 oz/about 6	2.0	140	13%
egg noodles	¾ cup	2.5	200	11%
hearty homestyle				
chicken noodle	3 oz/about 6	2.0	130	14%
homestyle				
flat dumplings	½ cup	2.0	190	9%
Free	½ cup	–	160	–
original egg	½ cup	2.0	170	11%
quick cook egg noodle	1 cup	2.5	230	10%
(Ronzoni) dry/uncooked				
egg noodles				
regular	2 oz	2.0	210	9%
spinach	2 oz	3.0	220	12%
fettuccini	2 oz	1.0	210	4%
fusilli	2 oz	1.0	210	4%
lasagne	2 oz	1.0	210	4%
macaroni				
regular	2 oz	1.0	210	4%
spinach	2 oz	1.0	210	4%
mostaccioli	2 oz	1.0	210	4%
rigatoni	2 oz	1.0	210	4%
rotelle	2 oz	1.0	210	4%
rotini/tri-color	2 oz	1.0	210	4%
shells				
jumbo	2 oz	1.0	210	4%
medium	2 oz	1.0	210	4%
tubettini	2 oz	1.0	210	4%
(San Giorgio) dry				
light & fluffy				
dumplings	1 oz	1.0	210	4%
egg noodles				
extra wide	1 oz	2.5	210	11%
medium	1 oz	2.5	210	11%
spinach	1 oz	2.5	210	11%
wide	1 oz	2.5	210	11%
regular				
acine di pepe	2 oz	1.0	210	4%
alphabets	2 oz	1.0	210	4%
bowties/egg	2 oz	3.0	210	13%

Food and Description	Amount	Fat Grams	Total Calories	% Fat Calories
capellini	2 oz	1.0	210	4%
tusillucut	2 oz	1.0	210	4%
ditalini	2 oz	1.0	210	4%
elbow macaroni	2 oz	1.0	210	4%
flakes	2 oz	1.0	210	4%
kluske	2 oz	3.0	220	12%
lasagne/rippled	2 oz	1.0	210	4%
linguine	2 oz	1.0	210	4%
mafalda	2 oz	1.0	210	4%
manicotti	2 oz	1.0	210	4%
mixed types				
Italian trio	2 oz	1.0	210	4%
mostaccioli rigati	2 oz	1.0	210	4%
shells/rainbow	2 oz	1.0	210	4%
rigatoni	2 oz	1.0	210	4%
rotelle	2 oz	1.0	210	4%
rotini	2 oz	1.0	210	4%
shells				
jumbo	2 oz	1.0	210	4%
large	2 oz	1.0	210	4%
small	2 oz	1.0	210	4%
spaghetti	2 oz	1.0	210	4%
spaghetini	2 oz	1.0	210	4%
twists/rainbow	1 oz	1.0	210	4%
ziti/cut	1 oz	1.0	210	4%
vermicelli	2 oz	1.0	210	4%
(Westbrae Natural) dry/uncooked				
angel hair/corn	2 oz	2.0	210	9%
elbows/com	2 oz	2.0	210	9%
lasagna/whole wheat/no egg				
plain	2 oz	2.0	210	9%
spinach	2 oz	2.0	210	9%
shells/corn	2 oz	2.0	210	9%
spaghetti				
corn	2 oz	2.0	210	9%
whole wheat/no egg				
plain	2 oz	2.0	210	9%
spinach	2 oz	2.0	210	9%

PASTA ENTRÉE/DINNER (See also ASIAN FOOD; FROZEN ENTRÉE/DINNER; VEGETARIAN FOODS; individual listings)

■ CANNED

(Chef Boyardee)				
ABC's & 123's				
plain	1 cup	1.0	180	3%
w/meatballs	1 cup	11.0	260	38%
beef ravioli				
99% fat-free	1 cup	1.0	210	4%
original	1 cup	3.0	190	14%
Beefaroni	1 cup	7.0	220	29%

Food and Description	Amount	Fat Grams	Total Calories	% Fat Calories
Beefogetti w/meatballs	1 cup	7.0	250	25%
cheese ravioli in tomato sauce	1 cup	3.0	200	14%
dinosaurs				
plain	1 cup	1.0	180	3%
w/meatballs	1 cup	9.0	240	34%
elbows in beef sauce	1 cup	7.0	210	30%
lasagna				
in garden vegetable sauce	1 cup	1.0	170	5%
plain	1 cup	9.0	230	35%
macaroni & cheese	1 cup	5.0	180	25%
pasta rings & meatballs	1 cup	8.0	220	33%
rigatoni	1 cup	6.0	210	26%
rings and franks	1 cup	5.0	190	24%
shells				
w/meat sauce	1 cup	6.0	210	26%
w/mushroom sauce	1 cup	1.0	170	5%
spaghetti & meatballs	1 cup	7.0	230	27%
Spider Man				
plain	1 cup	–	190	–
w/meatballs	1 cup	7.0	230	27%
Tic Tac Toes				
plain	1 cup	–	170	–
w/meatballs	1 cup	10.0	250	36%
(Franco American)				
Original				
beef ravioli w/pasta in tomato & cheese	1 cup	3.5	230	14%
Garfield Pasta w/meatballs	1 cup	11.0	260	38%
spaghettios				
w/meatballs	1 cup	11.0	260	38%
w/sliced franks	1 cup	11.0	250	40%
w/tomato and cheese	1 cup	2.0	190	9%
SportyO's				
w/ meatballs	1 cup	11.0	260	38%
w/tomato and cheese	1 cup	2.0	190	9%
TeddyO's				
w/meatballs	1 cup	11.0	260	38%
w/tomato & cheese	1 cup	2.0	190	9%
Superiore				
beef ravioli in meat sauce	1 cup	8.0	280	26%
hearty twists pasta w/meat sauce	1 cup	5.0	250	18%
spaghetti & meatballs in tomato sauce	1 cup	7.0	260	24%
generic/macaroni & cheese	1 cup	9.6	228	38%
(Hormel)				
chili mac	1 can	9.0	200	41%
lasagna	1 can	14.0	260	48%
spaghetti & meatballs	1 can	7.0	220	29%
(Read) Italian pasta salad	½ cup	2.5	90	25%

Food and Description	Amount	Fat Grams	Total Calories	% Fat Calories
■ **FROZEN**				
(Birds Eye)				
Easy Recipe Creations				
basil herb primavera	1 cup	11.0	260	38%
roasted garlic parmesan	1 cup	10.0	240	38%
tortellini parmigiana	1 cup	12.0	240	45%
Pasta Combos				
classic cheddar	5.3 oz	10.0	200	45%
garlic herb	6.4 oz	11.0	260	38%
Pasta Secrets/prepared				
Italian pesto	1 cup	9.0	240	34%
primavera	1 cup	10.0	230	39%
ranch	1 cup	15.0	300	45%
three cheese	1 cup	8.0	230	31%
white cheddar	1 cup	10.0	240	38%
zesty garlic	1 cup	10.0	240	38%
(Chicago Brother's) gourmet				
lasagna w/meat sauce	1 cup	15.0	310	44%
vegetable lasagna	1 cup	8.0	210	34%
(Fazzio's)				
breaded meat ravioli	6 pieces	6.0	250	22%
cannelloni	10 oz	20.0	410	44%
meat ravioli/toasted	6 pieces	16.0	340	42%
pizza rav's/toasted/pepperoni & sausage	6 pieces	19.0	350	49%
(Formagg)				
penne pasta				
alfredo	⅔ cup	2.0	190	9%
primavera	⅔ cup	2.0	190	9%
(Green Giant)				
Create A Meal/prepared				
beefy noodle	1¼ cups	14.0	350	36%
cheesy pasta & vegetable	1¼ cups	21.0	420	45%
chicken Alfredo	1¼ cups	13.0	400	29%
parmesan herb chicken	1¾ cups	11.0	340	29%
skillet lasagna	1¼ cups	13.0	340	34%
Pasta Accents				
Alfredo	2 cups	8.0	210	34%
creamy cheddar	2⅓ cups	8.0	250	29%
garden herb seasoning	2 cups	7.0	230	27%
garlic seasoning	2 cups	10.0	260	35%
Primavera	2¼ cups	9.0	280	29%
three cheese	2 cups	9.0	300	27%
white cheddar sauce	1¾ cups	9.0	270	30%
(Hanover) pasta salad				
Italian	½ cup	–	60	–
Milano	½ cup	–	60	–
Oriental	½ cup	–	80	–
Primavera	½ cup	–	50	–

Food and Description	Amount	Fat Grams	Total Calories	% Fat Calories
(Renaissance) Cafe Pasta				
jumbo stuffed shells	2 pieces	15.0	290	47%
lasagna				
meat	8 oz	18.0	370	44%
vegetable				
plain	8 oz	7.0	260	24%
w/Italian sausage	8 oz	12.0	320	34%
ravioli				
beef	10 pieces	14.0	330	38%
cheese	10 pieces	10.0	280	32%
tortellini				
beef	1 cup	7.0	260	24%
cheese	1 cup	6.0	240	23%
chicken	1 cup	3.0	210	13%
(Rosetto)				
Cavatelli	1 serving	2.5	270	8%
Gnocchi	1 serving	–	220	–
Manicotti/3-cheese	1 serving	10.0	230	39%
Pasta Primavera				
Alfredo sauce only	1 serving	8.0	110	65%
pasta only	1 serving	3.0	160	17%
Ravioli				
beef				
toasted	1 serving	10.0	220	41%
traditional	1 serving	6.0	270	20%
cheese				
large round	1 serving	7.0	250	25%
original	1 serving	6.0	250	22%
small round	1 serving	8.0	260	24%
toasted	1 serving	10.0	230	39%
chicken	1 serving	3.5	230	14%
Italian sausage	1 serving	6.0	250	22%
Quattro formaggi (four cheeses) w/broccoli				
cheese sauce only	1 serving	6.0	110	49%
pasta only	1 serving	2.5	170	13%
Stuffed Shells				
cheese	1 serving	10.0	240	38%
cheese & broccoli	1 serving	7.0	210	30%
Tortellini				
beef & sausage	1 serving	6.0	260	21%
cheese	1 serving	6.0	270	20%
(Swanson)				
homestyle				
lasagne w/ meat sauce	1 meal	15.0	400	34%
macaroni & cheese	1 meal	19.0	390	44%
spaghetti w/Italian style meatballs	1 meal	18.0	490	33%
macaroni & cheese				
7 oz	1 pkg	8.0	200	36%
12.25 oz	1 pkg	15.0	370	36%

Food and Description	Amount	Fat Grams	Total Calories	% Fat Calories
spaghetti & meat balls	1 meal	17.0	390	39%
■ HOMEMADE				
USDA Standard Home Recipe				
lasagna/~2¼" x 4" piece				
w/meat/~7 oz	1 piece	12.0	325	33%
w/o meat/~8 oz	1 piece	9.5	317	27%
macaroni & cheese	1 cup	22.0	430	46%
manicotti				
w/meat sauce	~5 oz	11.0	235	42%
w/tomato sauce	5 oz	10.0	223	45%
ravioli				
cheese				
w/meat sauce	~9 oz	17.0	360	43%
w/tomato sauce	~9 oz	15.0	340	40%
w/o sauce	~8.5 oz	17.0	430	36%
meat				
w/tomato sauce	~9 oz	17.0	385	40%
w/o sauce	~8.5 oz	23.0	550	38%
rigatoni w/meat sauce	1 cup	16.0	347	41%
spaghetti dinner				
w/meatballs & tomato sauce	1 cup	11.7	332	32%
w/red clam sauce	1 cup	7.0	226	28%
w/tomato sauce & cheese	1 cup	8.8	280	28%
w/white clam sauce	1 cup	19.0	345	50%
MICROWAVE CONTAINER				
(Chef Boyardee) Microwave Main Meals				
beans & pasta	1 meal	1.0	200	5%
beef ravioli suprema	1 meal	4.0	290	12%
cheese ravioli suprema	1 meal	4.0	290	12%
fettuccine	1 meal	9.0	290	28%
lasagna	1 meal	8.0	290	25%
peas & pasta	1 meal	2.0	190	9%
spaghetti suprema	1 meal	7.0	200	7%
tortellini w/meat	1 meal	4.0	220	16%
zesty macaroni	1 meal	8.0	290	25%
ziti in sauce	1 meal	–	210	–
(Dinty Moore) American Classics				
beef ravioli	1 bowl	9.0	300	27%
chicken & noodles	1 bowl	8.0	270	27%
spaghetti w/meatballs	1 bowl	7.0	290	22%
(Hormel)				
Kid's Kitchen				
beefy macaroni	1 cup	6.0	190	28%
cheezy mac & beef	1 cup	7.0	260	24%
macaroni & cheese	1 cup	11.0	270	37%
mini ravioli	1 cup	7.0	240	26%
noodle rings & chicken	1 cup	4.0	150	24%
spaghetti & mini meatballs	1 cup	7.0	220	29%
spaghetti rings	1 cup	2.0	190	9%
spaghetti rings & franks	1 cup	9.0	240	34%

Food and Description	Amount	Fat Grams	Total Calories	% Fat Calories
spaghetti rings & meatballs	1 cup	7.0	230	27%
micro cup meals				
chili mac	1 cup	9.0	200	41%
lasagna	1 cup	6.0	210	26%
macaroni & cheese	1 cup	11.0	260	38%
noodles & chicken	1 cup	9.0	200	41%
ravioli w/tomato sauce	1 cup	6.0	220	25%
■ MIX				
(Annie's)				
Alfredo w/garlic & garden basil				
mix only	½ cup	3.5	200	16%
prepared	¾ cup	9.0	250	32%
mild Mexican shells & cheddar				
mix only	½ cup	3.0	200	14%
prepared	¾ cup	9.0	250	32%
petite pasta shells & cheddar				
mix only	½ cup	3.0	200	14%
prepared	¾ cup	9.0	250	32%
whole wheat shells & cheddar				
mix only	½ cup	4.5	200	20%
prepared	¾ cup	10.0	250	36%
(Bean Cuisine)				
country French beans w/gemelli				
mix only	1 serving	1.0	217	4%
prepared	1 cup	10.5	316	30%
Florentine beans w/bow ties				
mix only	1 serving	2.0	162	11%
prepared	1 cup	5.5	216	23%
pasta & beans w/radiatore				
mix only	1 serving	0.5	162	3%
prepared	1 cup	4.5	215	19%
(Betty Crocker)				
Pasta with Seasoning/prepared				
creamy garlic & herb rotini				
reduced-fat recipe recipe	1 cup	10.0	300	30%
regular recipe	1 cup	16.0	360	40%
creamy homestyle chicken pasta				
low-fat recipe	1 cup	2.5	200	11%
regular recipe	1 cup	3.5	210	15%
garlic Alfredo fettuccine				
reduced-fat recipe	1 cup	7.0	290	22%
regular recipe	1 cup	13.0	340	34%
roasted chicken vegetable penne				
reduced-fat recipe	1 cup	3.5	210	15%
regular recipe	1 cup	7.0	240	26%
three cheese gemelli				
reduced-fat recipe	1 cup	8.0	300	24%
regular recipe	1 cup	12.0	330	33%
tomato parmesan pasta				
reduced-fat recipe	1 cup	4.0	210	17%

Food and Description	Amount	Fat Grams	Total Calories	% Fat Calories
regular recipe	1 cup	10.0	260	35%
Suddenly Salad				
Caesar				
mix only	⅔ cup	1.0	150	6%
prepared				
low-fat recipe	¾ cup	3.0	170	16%
regular recipe	¾ cup	9.0	220	37%
classic				
mix only	¾ cup	1.5	190	7%
prepared				
low-fat recipe	¾ cup	3.5	210	15%
regular recipe	¾ cup	8.0	250	20%
garden Italian/98% fat-free				
mix only	½ cup	1.0	140	6%
prepared	¾ cup	1.0	140	6%
ranch & bacon				
mix only	½ cup	1.5	160	8%
prepared				
low-fat recipe	¾ cup	2.0	180	10%
regular recipe	¾ cup	20.0	330	55%
roasted garlic				
mix only	½ cup	1.5	170	8%
prepared				
low-fat recipe	¾ cup	3.0	200	14%
regular recipe	¾ cup	11.0	260	38%
(Casbah) pasta fasul	1 pkg	1.0	150	6%
(Fantastic Foods) Pasta! Cups/mix only				
creamy garlic	2.2 oz	3.5	240	13%
mac & cheese	2.1 oz	4.5	240	17%
spicy thai	1.9 oz	2.0	200	9%
(Formagg) alternative/mix only				
macaroni & cheese sauce	⅔ cup	2.0	190	9%
pasta Primavera	⅔ cup	2.0	130	9%
penne pasta Alfredo	⅔ cup	2.0	190	9%
vegetable pasta & Caesar Italian garden	⅔ cup	2.0	190	9%
(Golden Grain) Pasta Roni/prepared				
angel hair				
w/herbs	1 cup	13.0	320	37%
w/lemon & butter	1 cup	15.0	360	38%
w/Parmesan cheese	1 cup	14.0	320	39%
broccoli				
Au gratin	1 cup	10.0	280	32%
regular	1 cup	15.0	340	40%
chicken				
& garlic/low-fat	1 cup	3.0	210	13%
regular	1 cup	13.0	310	38%
corkscrew pasta				
w/creamy garlic sauce	1 cup	25.0	420	54%
w/four-cheese sauce	1 cup	19.0	410	42%

Food and Description	Amount	Fat Grams	Total Calories	% Fat Calories
fettuccine				
w/Alfredo sauce				
original	1 cup	25.0	460	49%
reduced-fat	1 cup	8.0	310	23%
w/broccoli au gratin	1 cup	10.0	290	31%
w/chicken sauce	1 cup	13.5	320	38%
w/mild cheddar sauce	1 cup	10.5	300	32%
w/Romanoff sauce	1 cup	19.0	410	42%
w/stroganoff sauce	1 cup	14.0	370	34%
garlic alfredo	1 cup	13.0	360	33%
herb w/butter	1 cup	19.0	380	45%
homestyle chicken	1 cup	6.0	230	23%
linguine				
w/chicken & broccoli	1 cup	16.0	370	39%
w/creamy chicken Parmesan	1 cup	18.0	410	40%
mild cheddar	1 cup	10.0	290	31%
parmesano	1 cup	17.0	390	39%
rigatoni w/white cheddar & broccoli sauce	1 cup	19.0	400	43%
romanoff	1 cup	19.0	400	43%
shells w/white cheddar sauce	1 cup	13.0	310	38%
stroganoff	1 cup	14.0	370	34%
vermicelli w/roasted garlic & olive oil	1 cup	16.0	360	40%
(Hain) Pasta & Sauce/mix only				
creamy Parmesan	¼ pkg	3.0	150	18%
creamy Swiss	¼ pkg	4.0	170	21%
fettuccine Alfredo	¼ pkg	4.0	180	20%
Italian herb	¼ pkg	2.0	110	16%
primavera	¼ pkg	4.0	140	26%
tangy cheddar	¼ pkg	6.0	180	30%
(Knorr) spicy couscous/mix only	¼ pkg	1.0	150	6%
(Kraft)				
Macaroni & cheese/prepared				
deluxe				
four cheese blend	1 cup	10.0	320	28%
light	1 cup	4.5	290	14%
original	1 cup	10.0	320	29%
original				
all shapes	1 cup	18.0	410	40%
light	1 cup	6.0	290	19%
regular	1 cup	18.0	410	40%
Premium				
cheesy Alfredo	1 cup	19.0	410	42%
mild white cheddar	1 cup	19.0	410	42%
Thick'N Creamy	1 cup	19.0	420	41%
three-chese	1 cup	18.0	410	40%
Noodle Classics/prepared				
cheddar cheese	1 cup	19.0	400	43%
savory chicken	1 cup	13.0	340	34%

Food and Description	Amount	Fat Grams	Total Calories	% Fat Calories
Pasta Salads/prepared				
classic ranch w/ bacon	¾ cup	22.0	350	57%
creamy Caesar	¾ cup	21.0	340	56%
garden primavera	¾ cup	8.0	240	30%
herb & garlic	¾ cup	14.0	280	45%
Italian/97% fat free	¾ cup	2.0	190	9%
Parmesan peppercorn	¾ cup	23.0	360	58%
Spaghetti Classics/prepared				
mild Italian	1 cup	2.5	240	9%
spaghetti w/meat sauce	1 cup	10.0	330	27%
tangy Italian	1 cup	2.0	240	8%
zesty cheese	1 cup	2.0	240	8%
Velveeta/prepared				
rotini & cheese w/broccoli	1 cup	16.0	400	36%
shells & cheese				
bacon	1 cup	14.0	360	35%
original	1 cup	13.0	360	33%
salsa	1 cup	14.0	380	33%
(Lipton) prepared				
Noodles & Sauce				
Alfredo	⅔ cup	7.0	250	25%
Alfredo broccoli	⅔ cup	7.0	260	24%
Alfredo carbonara	⅔ cup	7.0	260	24%
beef	⅔ cup	3.5	220	14%
butter	⅔ cup	8.0	260	19%
butter & herb	⅔ cup	7.0	250	25%
cheddar broccoli	⅔ cup	3.5	260	12%
cheese	⅔ cup	4.5	250	16%
chicken	⅔ cup	4.5	240	17%
chicken broccoli	⅔ cup	3.5	260	12%
chicken tetrazzini	⅔ cup	5.0	220	20%
creamy chicken	⅔ cup	6.0	235	23%
Parmesan	⅔ cup	8.0	250	29%
Romanoff	⅔ cup	7.0	265	24%
sour cream & chive	⅔ cup	8.0	260	28%
stroganoff	⅔ cup	4.0	210	17%
Pasta & Sauce				
angel hair				
chicken broccoli	1 cup	8.0	260	28%
parmesan	1 cup	11.0	280	35%
bow tie				
chicken primavera	1 cup	10.0	290	31%
Italian cheese	1 cup	12.0	300	36%
butter & herb	1 cup	10.0	270	33%
cheddar broccoli	1 cup	11.0	340	29%
chicken				
herb parmesan	1 cup	9.0	280	29%
stir fry	1 cup	8.0	270	27%
creamy				
garlic	1 cup	13.0	350	33%

Food and Description	Amount	Fat Grams	Total Calories	% Fat Calories
mushroom	1 cup	11.0	320	31%
cheddar cheese	1 cup	10.0	290	31%
roasted garlic				
chicken	1 cup	10.0	290	31%
& olive oil w/tomato	1 cup	9.0	270	27%
rotini				
primavera	1 cup	12.0	320	34%
three-cheese	1 cup	12.0	320	34%
savory herb w/garlic	1 cup	9.0	280	29%
Sizzle & Stir Skillet Supper/mix only				
mild cheddar chicken & shells	⅙ pkg	6.0	190	28%
savory herbed chicken & bow ties	⅛ pkg	4.0	170	21%
3-cheese Alfredo chicken & penne	⅙ pkg	9.0	220	37%
(Near East) prepared				
Couscous				
herbed chicken	1 cup	3.5	220	14%
Mediterranean curry	1 cup	3.5	220	14%
Moroccan pasta	1¼ cups	6.0	260	21%
Parmesan	1 cup	2.5	220	10%
roasted garlic & olive oil	1 cup	4.5	230	18%
toasted pine nut	1 cup	6.0	230	23%
tomato lentil	1 cup	3.5	220	14%
Creative Grains				
chicken & herbs	1 cup	6.0	270	20%
creamy parmesan	1 cup	7.0	280	23%
roasted garlic	1 cup	5.0	220	20%
roasted pecan & garlic	1 cup	9.0	240	34%
Pastas w/Delicate Sauce				
angel hair/spicy tomato	1 cup	6.0	240	23%
fusilli/parmesan & romano	1 cup	7.0	300	21%
gemelli/tomato parmesan	1 cup	10.0	330	27%
radiatore/basil & herb	1 cup	8.0	260	28%
vermicelli/garlic & olive oil	1 cup	8.0	260	28%
(Ramen) noodles (See SOUP)				
(Uncle Ben's) Country Inn pasta & sauce mix/mix only				
angel hair Parmesan	2.2 oz	5.0	245	18%
broccoli & white cheddar	2.2 oz	5.0	240	19%
butter & herb	2 oz	6.0	230	23%
creamy garlic	2.4 oz	5.0	260	17%
fettuccine Alfredo	2.25 oz	6.0	310	17%
herb linguine	2.2 oz	3.5	240	13%
mushroom fettuccine	2.25 oz	6.0	250	22%
vegetable Alfredo	2.2 oz	4.5	240	17%
Velveeta (See (Kraft) in this section)				

PASTA SAUCE (See SAUCE)
PASTRAMI (See LUNCHEON MEAT)
PASTRY (See also CAKE; DONUT; PASTRY, TOASTER; PASTRY DOUGH; PIE CRUST)
■ **FROZEN OR REFRIGERATED**

(Chef Pierre) food service				
apple dumpling w/cinnamon sauce	1 dumpling	23.0	540	38%

Food and Description	Amount	Fat Grams	Total Calories	% Fat Calories
(Dutch) mini cream puffs	2 pieces	10.0	110	82%
(Morton) Honey Buns				
mini	1 honeybun	8.0	160	45%
original	1 honeybun	13.0	270	43%
(Pepperidge Farm)				
Danish/individually wrapped/pocket				
apple	1 Danish	8.0	220	33%
cheese	1 Danish	14.0	240	53%
cinnamon raisin	1 Danish	12.0	250	43%
raspberry	1 Danish	9.0	210	39%
dumpling				
apple	1 dumpling	11.0	290	34%
cherry	1 dumpling	9.0	280	29%
peach	1 dumpling	11.0	300	33%
(Pillsbury)				
Grands! Sweet Rolls				
caramel rolls	1 roll	10.0	320	28%
cinnamon rolls				
w/butter cream icing	1 roll	12.0	340	32%
w/cream cheese icing	1 roll	11.0	330	30%
w/icing				
original	1 roll	10.0	320	28%
reduced-fat	1 roll	7.0	300	21%
sweet roll				
apple cinnamon roll w/icing	1 roll	5.0	150	30%
caramel roll	1 roll	7.0	170	37%
cinnamon raisin roll w/icing	1 roll	6.0	170	32%
cinnamon roll w/icing				
original	1 roll	5.0	150	30%
reduced-fat	1 roll	3.5	140	23%
orange sweet roll w/icing	1 roll	7.0	170	37%
turnover				
apple	1 turnover	8.0	170	42%
cherry	1 turnover	8.0	170	42%
(Rhodes) cinnamon roll/prepared	1 roll	10.0	240	38%
(Rich's) iced chocolate eclair	1 eclair	9.0	190	43%
(Sara Lee)				
cinnamon roll				
plain	1 roll	15.0	370	36%
icing	1 pkt	–	50	–
coffee cakes				
butter streusel	⅛ cake	12.0	220	49%
cheese/reduced-fat	⅛ cake	6.0	180	30%
crumb	⅛ cake	9.0	220	37%
pecan	⅙ cake	12.0	230	47%
raspberry	⅛ cake	8.0	220	33%
eclair	1 eclair	9.0	190	43%
(Schwan's) cinnamon w/icing	1 roll	4.5	240	17%
■ HOMEMADE				
USDA Standard Home Recipe				
apple dumpling	1 average	16.0	275	52%

Food and Description	Amount	Fat Grams	Total Calories	% Fat Calories
baklava	2 oz	18.0	250	65%
eclair	3.5 oz	14.5	260	50%
strudel	~4 oz	8.0	265	27%
■ READY TO SERVE				
(Dolly Madison) snack				
apple sweet roll	1 roll	6.0	230	23%
bear claw	1 pastry	11.0	310	32%
cherry bun	1 bun	7.0	230	27%
cherry sweet roll	1 roll	6.0	210	26%
cinnamon roll	1 roll	7.0	220	29%
cream cheese Danish	1 Danish	15.0	380	39%
English cruller	1 cruller	14.0	260	48%
honey bun				
3-oz bun	1 bun	20.0	360	50%
3.75-oz bun	1 bun	25.0	450	50%
honey wheat cinnamon roll	1 roll	8.0	240	30%
honey wheat cinnamon twirl	1 pastry	14.0	450	28%
lemon sweet roll	1 roll	7.0	230	27%
pecan roller	1 roll	7.0	210	30%
raspberry sweet roll	1 roll	7.0	230	27%
(Dunkin' Donuts) (*See* DONUTS and DUNKIN' DONUTS in FAST FOOD section)				
(Entenmann's)				
fat-free				
apple bun	1 bun	–	150	–
Black Forest pastry	⅑ pastry	–	140	–
blueberry cheese bun	1 bun	–	140	–
cheese filled ring	⅛ danish	–	120	–
cherry cheese pastry	⅑ danish	–	130	–
cinnamon apple twist	⅛ pastry	–	150	–
lemon twist	⅛ pastry	–	130	–
pineapple cheese				
bun	1 bun	–	140	–
pastry	⅑ danish	–	130	–
raspberry cheese				
bun	1 bun	–	160	–
pastry	⅛ pastry	–	140	–
ring	⅛ danish	–	140	–
raspberry twist	⅛ pastry	–	140	–
original				
apple danish bites	1 danish	7.0	170	37%
apricot rugelach	1 serving	5.0	90	50%
raspberry rugelach	1 serving	5.0	90	50%
reduced-fat				
cinnamon bun	1 bun	4.0	190	19%
crumb delight	⅑ cake	6.0	210	26%
generic				
cinnamon bun/~2 oz				
frosted	1 bun	5.0	185	24%
plain	1 bun	5.0	174	26%
cream puff/2" high/3⅓" dia				
shell only	2 oz	10.0	135	66%

Food and Description	Amount	Fat Grams	Total Calories	% Fat Calories
w/custard filling	1 puff	18.0	303	54%
Danish/4½" dia/~2 oz				
plain	1 Danish	12.0	220	49%
w/fruit	1 Danish	13.0	235	50%
eclair w/custard filling & chocolate icing	1 eclair	13.6	239	51%
hot cross bun/2 oz	1 bun	8.0	190	38%
Napoleon	1 medium	15.0	285	47%
(Lance) snack				
cinnamon roll	4 oz roll	7.0	370	17%
honey bun	3 oz bun	13.0	320	37%
pecan twirl	2 pieces	8.0	210	34%
Swiss roll	1 roll	8.0	160	45%
(Little Debbie) snack				
boxed				
honey bun	1 pkg	13.0	210	56%
pecan spinwheel	1 pkg	4.0	110	33%
individual packages				
honey bun				
3-oz bun	1 bun	23.0	380	54%
3.98-oz bun	1 bun	28.0	460	55%
pecan spinwheel	1 pkg	9.0	220	37%
(Otis Spunkmeyer)				
Cinnamon rolls				
giant	½ roll	13.0	250	47%
4 pack	1 roll	8.0	150	48%
8 pack	1 roll	7.0	140	45%
Crumb Cakes				
apple	1 cake	17.0	410	37%
blueberry	1 cake	17.0	400	38%
cheese	1 cake	21.0	450	42%
Danish				
apple danish/12 pack	1 pastry	12.0	320	34%
bear claw	1 pastry	14.0	250	50%
breakfast claw/8 pack	1 pastry	12.0	240	45%
buttercrumb	1 pastry	13.0	250	47%
cheese/12 pack	1 pastry	18.0	330	49%
cherry/12 pack	1 pastry	16.0	310	46%
cinnamon	1 pastry	13.0	250	47%
fruit	1 pastry	12.0	240	45%
raisin	1 pastry	12.0	240	45%
Mini Loaves				
apple spice	3.75 oz loaf	14.0	370	34%
banana walnut	3.75 oz loaf	25.0	450	50%
chocolate fudge pecan	3.75 oz loaf	21.0	420	45%
(TastyKake) snack				
bear claw				
apple	1 roll	7.0	280	23%
cinnamon	1 roll	8.0	300	24%

Food and Description	Amount	Fat Grams	Total Calories	% Fat Calories
Big Texas Bun	1 bun	9.0	300	27%
cinnamon raisin breakfast bun	1 bun	8.0	330	22%
coffee roll				
glazed	1 roll	9.0	300	27%
vanilla	1 roll	9.0	320	25%
Danish				
cheese	1 danish	14.0	290	43%
lemon	1 danish	14.0	290	43%
raspberry	1 danish	14.0	290	43%
honey bun				
glazed	1 bun	17.0	350	44%
iced	1 bun	17.0	350	44%
PASTRY, TOASTER				
(Kellogg's) Pop Tarts				
low-fat/frosted				
brown sugar cinnamon	1 pastry	3.0	190	14%
chocolate fudge	1 pastry	3.0	190	14%
strawberry				
frosted	1 pastry	3.0	190	14%
unfrosted	1 pastry	3.0	190	14%
Pastry Swirls				
apple cinnamon	1 pastry	11.0	260	38%
cheese	1 pastry	11.0	260	38%
strawberry	1 pastry	11.0	260	38%
regular/frosted				
blueberry	1 pastry	5.0	200	23%
brown sugar/cinnamon	1 pastry	7.0	210	30%
cherry	1 pastry	5.0	200	23%
chocolate fudge	1 pastry	5.0	200	23%
grape	1 pastry	5.0	200	23%
raspberry	1 pastry	5.0	210	21%
s'mores	1 pastry	6.0	200	27%
strawberry	1 pastry	5.0	200	23%
Tropical Blast	1 pastry	5.0	210	21%
vanilla cream	1 pastry	5.0	200	23%
wild berry	1 pastry	5.0	210	21%
Wild Magicburst	1 pastry	6.0	200	27%
wild watermelon	1 pastry	5.0	210	21%
regular/unfrosted				
apple cinnamon	1 pastry	6.0	210	26%
blueberry	1 pastry	5.0	200	23%
brown sugar cinnamon	1 pastry	6.0	210	26%
cherry	1 pastry	5.0	200	23%
milk chocolate graham	1 pastry	6.0	210	26%
raspberry	1 pastry	6.0	210	26%
strawberry	1 pastry	5.0	200	23%
Snack-Stix				
frosted				
berry	1 pastry	4.0	190	19%
strawberry	1 pastry	4.0	190	19%

Food and Description	Amount	Fat Grams	Total Calories	% Fat Calories
(Nabisco)				
Toastettes tarts				
frosted				
apple	1 pastry	5.0	190	24%
blueberry	1 pastry	5.0	190	24%
brown sugar cinnamon	1 pastry	5.0	180	25%
cherry burst	1 pastry	5.0	180	25%
screamin' strawberry				
frosted	1 pastry	5.0	180	25%
unfrosted	1 pastry	5.0	180	25%
super fudge blast	1 pastry	5.0	180	25%
(Pillsbury) Toaster Strudel				
apple	1 pastry	8.0	190	38%
blueberry	1 pastry	8.0	190	38%
caramel apple	1 pastry	8.0	190	38%
cherry	1 pastry	8.0	190	38%
cinnamon	1 pastry	8.0	190	38%
cream cheese	1 pastry	11.0	200	50%
cream cheese & blueberry	1 pastry	10.0	200	45%
cream cheese & strawberry	1 pastry	10.0	200	45%
raspberry	1 pastry	8.0	190	38%
strawberry	1 pastry	8.0	190	38%
wildberry	1 pastry	9.0	190	43%
PASTRY DOUGH (See also PIE CRUST)				
(Athens Foods) mini fillo dough shell	2 shells	2.0	45	40%
(Fillo) pastry dough sheet	1⅓ leaves	–	80	–
(Pepperidge Farm)				
patty shell	1 shell	15.0	210	64%
puff pastry dough sheet	¼ sheet	17.0	260	59%
PÂTÉ (See also VEGETARIAN FOODS)				
(Bonavita) Swiss/vegetarian	1 oz	4.0	60	60%
generic/canned				
chicken liver	1 tbs	1.7	26	59%
	1 oz	3.7	57	58%
goose liver/foie gras				
regular	1 tbs	5.7	60	86%
	1 oz	12.0	131	82%
smoked	1 Tbs	5.5	60	82%
	1 oz	12.0	131	82%
(Sell's) liver	¼ cup	14.0	160	79%
PEA (See also BLACK-EYED PEA; PEA DISH; PIGEON PEA; PURPLE HULL PEA; SNOW PEA; VEGETABLES, MIXED)				
canned				
(Del Monte) sweet				
no salt added	½ cup	–	60	–
regular	½ cup	–	60	–
very young small	½ cup	–	60	–
(Freshlike)				
garden sweet	½ cup	–	50	–
small	½ cup	–	50	–

Food and Description	Amount	Fat Grams	Total Calories	% Fat Calories
generic				
Alaska/early or June				
drained	½ cup	–	75	–
undrained	½ cup	–	67	–
green	½ cup	–	59	–
sweet				
drained	½ cup	–	68	–
undrained	½ cup	–	71	–
(Green Giant) sweet				
50% less sodium	½ cup	–	60	–
regular	½ cup	–	60	–
(LeSueur)				
early	½ cup	–	60	–
sweet				
50% less sodium	½ cup	–	60	–
regular	½ cup	–	60	–
(Luck's) seasoned w/pork				
crowder	½ cup	3.0	120	23%
field peas w/snaps	½ cup	3.0	130	21%
(S&W)				
petit pois/early June	½ cup	–	70	–
sweet	½ cup	–	70	–
(Stokely)				
early/June	½ cup	–	60	–
sweet	½ cup	–	60	–
(Trappey)				
field peas				
w/bacon	½ cup	1.0	90	10%
w/snaps & bacon	½ cup	1.0	110	8%
(Val Vista) early June	½ cup	–	80	–
dried				
(Arrowhead Mills) green split	¼ cup	0.5	170	3%
generic				
split	1 cup	<1.0	280	2%
whole	1 cup	<1.0	280	2%
fresh				
green				
cooked	½ cup	–	67	–
raw	½ cup	–	63	–
split/field				
boiled	½ cup	–	115	–
raw	½ cup	1.0	348	3%
sugarsnap				
(Dole)	½ cup	–	30	–
frozen				
(Birds Eye)				
baby sweet	⅔ cup	0.5	70	6%
butter peas	½ cup	0.5	110	4%
crowder	½ cup	0.5	120	4%
field peas w/snaps	⅔ cup	1.0	130	7%

Food and Description	Amount	Fat Grams	Total Calories	% Fat Calories
green	½ cup	–	50	–
purple hull	½ cup	0.5	110	4%
sugar snap deluxe	½ cup	–	45	–
tender deluxe	½ cup	–	60	–
(C&W)				
petite				
microwave box	⅔ cup	0.5	70	6%
no salt added	⅔ cup	0.5	70	6%
regular	⅔ cup	0.5	70	6%
sugarsnap	⅔ cup	–	35	–
(Green Giant)				
sugarsnap				
Harvest Fresh	⅔ cup	–	50	–
regular	¾ cup	–	35	–
	⅔ cup	–	50	–
sweet				
Harvest Fresh	⅔ cup	–	60	–
regular	⅔ cup	0.5	70	6%
(LeSueur)				
baby early/Harvest Fresh	⅔ cup	–	70	–
baby sweet	⅔ cup	0.5	60	8%
early June	⅔ cup	0.5	60	8%
sugar snap	¾ cup	–	35	–
(Seneca)	⅔ cup	–	80	–
PEA, BLACK-EYED (*See* BLACK-EYED PEA)				
PEA, PIGEON (*See* PIGEON PEA)				
PEA, PURPLE HULL (*See* PURPLE HULL PEA)				
PEA, SNOW (*See* SNOW PEA)				
PEA DISH (*See also* PEA; VEGETABLES, MIXED)				
(LeSueur) frozen in butter sauce				
baby early peas	¾ cup	1.5	90	15%
baby sweet peas	¾ cup	1.5	90	15%
PEACH				
can or cup				
(Del Monte)				
chunky cut				
sweet cinnamon in light syrup	½ cup	–	80	–
cling				
halves				
in extra light syrup/lite	½ cup	–	60	–
in heavy syrup	½ cup	–	100	–
melba/in heavy syrup	½ cup	–	100	–
sliced				
in extra light syrup/lite	½ cup	–	60	–
in heavy syrup	½ cup	–	100	–
in light syrup	½ cup	–	80	–
in natural raspberry-flavored light syrup	½ cup	–	60	–
in pear & peach juices/Fruit Naturals	½ cup	–	60	–

Food and Description	Amount	Fat Grams	Total Calories	% Fat Calories
whole/spiced/in heavy syrup	½ cup	–	100	–
freestone				
halves/in heavy syrup	½ cup	–	100	–
sliced				
in extra light syrup/lite	½ cup	–	60	–
in heavy syrup	½ cup	–	100	–
fruit cups/diced				
in extra light syrup/lite	4 oz	–	50	–
in heavy syrup	4 oz	–	80	–
in pear & peach juices/	4 oz	–	50	–
Fruit Naturals				
Fruit Rageous/naturally-flavored sauce				
Peachy pie peaches	4 oz cup	–	80	
generic				
sliced				
in heavy syrup	1 cup	–	190	–
in juice	1 cup	–	109	–
in water	1 cup	–	58	–
spiced/in syrup	1 cup	–	180	–
whole/in heavy syrup	½ cup	–	90	–
(Hunt's)				
halves	½ cup	–	100	–
sliced	½ cup	–	100	–
(Libby's) lite/in juice				
halves	½ cup	–	50	–
sliced	½ cup	–	50	–
(S&W)				
ready-cut				
California Sun	½ cup	–	80	–
clingstone				
halves/in heavy syrup	½ cup	–	100	–
sliced				
in heavy syrup	½ cup	–	100	–
in peach juice/natural style	½ cup	–	90	–
freestone				
halves/in heavy syrup	½ cup	–	100	–
sliced/in heavy syrup	½ cup	–	100	–
Sweet Memory w/cinnamon	½ cup	–	70	–
Tropical Sun	½ cup	–	80	–
whole/spiced/in heavy syrup	1 peach	–	100	–
dried				
(Del Monte) sun-dried	⅓ cup	–	90	–
generic/halves				
cooked				
w/sugar	½ cup	<1.0	165	3%
w/o sugar	½ cup	<1.0	100	5%
uncooked	½ cup	0.6	191	2%
	10 medium	0.9	341	2%
(Mariani)	¼ cup	–	140	–
(Sun Maid)	¼ cup	–	100	–

Food and Description	Amount	Fat Grams	Total Calories	% Fat Calories
(SunSweet)	¼ cup	–	140	–
fresh				
peeled/sliced	½ cup	–	37	–
whole	1 medium	–	37	–
(Dole)	2 medium	–	70	–
frozen				
(Big Valley) freestone	⅔ cup	–	50	–
(C&W) sliced	⅔ cup	–	50	–
generic/sliced				
sweetened	1 cup	<1.0	235	2%
unsweetened	3.5 oz	<1.0	45	10%
	1 cup	<1.0	132	3%
PEACH BUTTER				
(Smucker's)	1 tsp	–	15	–
PEACH JUICE/JUICE BLEND/JUICE DRINK (*See also* FRUIT PUNCH; SOFT DRINK; SOFT DRINK MIX)				
bottled, boxed, or canned				
(Dole) orchard peach 100% juice blend	8 fl oz	–	140	–
	10 fl oz	–	170	–
(Goya) nectar	6 fl oz	–	110	–
(Kern's) nectar	6 fl oz	–	110	–
(Knudsen)				
After the Fall/Georgia peach	8 fl oz	–	100	–
Thirst Quencher/nectar	8 fl oz	–	120	–
(Libby's) nectar	8 fl oz	–	130	–
(Smucker's)	8 fl oz	–	120	–
(TreeTop) Peach Quake	8 fl oz	–	120	–
frozen/prepared				
(Dole) Orchard Peach 100% juice blend	8 fl oz	–	140	–
(Mott's) Fruit Basket				
orchard peach juice cocktail	8 fl oz	–	130	–
PEANUT				
(Ballpark)	1 oz	15.0	180	75%
(Eagle)				
lightly salted	1 oz	15.0	180	75%
oil honey-roasted	1 oz	13.0	170	69%
roasted	1 oz	15.0	180	75%
(Fisher)				
dry/honey-roasted	1 oz	13.0	170	69%
dry/roasted	1 oz	14.0	170	74%
golden roasted	1 oz	14.0	170	74%
honey-roasted	1 oz	13.0	170	68%
oil-roasted	1 oz	15.0	170	79%
party	1 oz	14.0	160	79%
raw/Chef's naturals	1 oz	11.0	160	62%
salted in shell/shelled	1 oz	14.0	170	74%
Spanish/redskin				
5 oz can	1 oz	15.0	170	79%
12 oz can	1 oz	16.0	180	80%

Food and Description	Amount	Fat Grams	Total Calories	% Fat Calories
(Frito Lay)				
hot	1 oz	16.0	190	76%
salted	1 oz	16.0	200	72%
generic				
all types				
boiled	½ cup	7.0	102	62%
dried	1 oz	14.0	161	78%
dry-roasted				
lite	1 oz	9.0	135	60%
regular	1 oz	13.9	164	76%
honey-roasted	1 oz	13.0	170	69%
oil-roasted	1 oz	13.8	163	76%
	½ cup	35.5	418	76%
Spanish				
oil-roasted	1 oz	14.0	160	78%
	½ cup	36.0	425	76%
raw	1 oz	13.7	162	76%
	½ cup	36.0	415	78%
Valencia				
oil-roasted	1 oz	14.0	165	76%
	½ cup	37.0	424	78%
raw	1 oz	13.0	160	73%
	½ cup	35.0	420	75%
Virginia				
oil-roasted	1 oz	13.7	160	77%
	½ cup	35.0	415	76%
raw	1 oz	13.5	160	76%
	½ cup	35.5	410	78%
(Guy's)				
dry-roasted	1 oz	14.0	170	74%
Spanish/salted	1 oz	14.0	170	74%
(Lance)				
BBQ	2⅛ oz pkg	26.0	360	65%
honey-toasted	1 oz	11.0	160	62%
roasted	1¾ oz	14.0	190	66%
salted				
in shell	1.6 oz	15.0	180	75%
long tube	1 oz	14.0	180	70%
regular	1⅛ oz pkg	15.0	200	68%
	⅞ oz	12.0	150	72%
(Laura Scudder's)				
Spanish	1 oz	15.0	180	75%
Virginia	1 oz	15.0	180	75%
(Planters)				
dry-roasted	1 oz	14.0	170	74%
lightly salted	1 oz	14.0	160	79%
	1.75 oz pkg	25.0	290	78%
unsalted	1 oz	14.0	160	79%
honey dry-roasted	1.7 oz	19.0	260	69%

Food and Description	Amount	Fat Grams	Total Calories	% Fat Calories
honey-roasted				
original	1 oz	13.0	160	73%
reduced-fat	1 oz	7.0	130	48%
oil-roasted	2 oz	24.0	340	64%
cocktail	1 oz	14.0	170	74%
lightly salted	1 oz	15.0	170	79%
	1.8 oz	27.0	300	81%
unsalted	1 oz	14.0	170	74%
fun size	2 bags	15.0	170	79%
heat hot spicy	1 oz	14.0	160	79%
	1.7 oz	25.0	290	78%
	2 oz	29.0	330	79%
heat mild spicy	1 oz	14.0	160	79%
Munch 'N Go singles	2.5 oz	36.0	410	79%
salted	1 oz	15.0	170	79%
Spanish				
oil roasted	1 oz	14.0	170	74%
raw	1 oz	13.0	150	78%
sweet n crunchy	1 oz	7.0	140	45%
(Weight Watchers) honey-roasted	0.7 oz	5.0	100	45%
PEANUT BUTTER				
(Arrowhead Mills) 100% Valencia/sodium-free				
creamy	2 Tbs	15.0	200	68%
crunchy	2 Tbs	15.0	200	68%
(Bama)				
creamy	2 Tbs	17.0	200	77%
crunchy	2 Tbs	17.0	200	77%
(Country Pure)				
chunky	2 Tbs	16.0	190	76%
creamy	2 Tbs	16.0	190	76%
(Erewhon)				
chunky				
regular	2 Tbs	14.0	190	66%
unsalted	2 Tbs	14.0	190	66%
creamy				
regular	2 Tbs	14.0	190	66%
unsalted	2 Tbs	14.0	190	66%
(Estee)				
creamy	2 Tbs	15.0	190	71%
crunchy	2 Tbs	15.0	190	71%
(Featherweight)				
chunky	2 Tbs	15.0	190	71%
creamy	2 Tbs	15.0	190	71%
generic				
chunky	2 Tbs	16.0	188	77%
	½ cup	64.0	760	76%
	1 cup	132.0	1,526	78%
creamy	2 Tbs	16.0	188	77%
	½ cup	64.0	760	76%
	1 cup	131.0	1,526	78%

Food and Description	Amount	Fat Grams	Total Calories	% Fat Calories
(Health Valley)				
chunky				
no salt	2 Tbs	14.0	170	74%
regular	2 Tbs	14.0	170	74%
creamy				
no salt	2 Tbs	14.0	170	74%
regular	2 Tbs	14.0	170	74%
(Jif)				
original				
creamy	2 Tbs	16.0	190	76%
extra crunchy	2 Tbs	16.0	190	76%
reduced fat				
creamy	2 Tbs	12.0	190	57%
crunchy	2 Tbs	12.0	190	57%
Simply Jif				
creamy	2 Tbs	16.0	190	76%
crunchy	2 Tbs	16.0	190	76%
(Knott's Berry Farm)				
creamy	2 Tbs	16.0	190	76%
crunchy	2 Tbs	16.0	190	76%
(Laura Scudder's)				
old fashioned				
creamy				
regular	2 Tbs	16.0	200	72%
unsalted	2 Tbs	16.0	200	72%
nutty				
regular	2 Tbs	16.0	200	72%
unsalted	2 Tbs	16.0	200	72%
reduced fat/creamy	2 Tbs	12.0	220	49%
(Nu Made)				
chunky	2 Tbs	16.0	190	76%
creamy	2 Tbs	16.0	190	76%
(Peter Pan)				
creamy				
regular	2 Tbs	16.0	190	75%
very low sodium	2 Tbs	17.0	200	77%
crunchy				
regular	2 Tbs	16.0	190	75%
very low sodium	2 Tbs	17.0	200	77%
Smart Choice spread				
creamy	2 Tbs	11.0	180	55%
crunchy	2 Tbs	12.0	190	57%
whipped				
creamy	2 Tbs	13.0	150	78%
crunchy	2 Tbs	13.0	150	78%
(President's Choice) Too Good to Be True				
creamy	2 Tbs	18.0	210	77%
crunchy	2 Tbs	18.0	210	77%
(Real)				
creamy	2 Tbs	16.0	190	75%

Food and Description	Amount	Fat Grams	Total Calories	% Fat Calories
crunchy	2 Tbs	16.0	190	75%
(Reese's)				
creamy	2 Tbs	16.0	200	72%
crunchy	2 Tbs	16.0	200	72%
(Roaster Fresh) gourmet/unsalted	2 Tbs	14.0	170	74%
(Skippy)				
reduced fat				
creamy	2 Tbs	12.0	190	57%
super chunk	2 Tbs	12.0	180	60%
roasted honey nut/creamy	2 Tbs	17.0	190	81%
super chunk	2 Tbs	17.0	190	81%
	1 cup	138.0	1560	80%
(Smucker's) All Natural				
Goober peanut butter & jelly	3 Tbs	13.0	230	51%
old fashioned natural				
chunky	2 Tbs	16.0	200	72%
creamy	2 Tbs	16.0	200	72%
original				
chunky	2 Tbs	16.0	200	72%
creamy	2 Tbs	16.0	200	72%
(Westbrae) natural				
chunky				
regular	2 Tbs	16.0	190	76%
no salt	2 Tbs	16.0	190	76%
creamy/no salt	2 Tbs	16.0	190	76%

PEANUT BUTTER FLAVORED BAKING CHIPS (*See* BAKING BITS, CHIPS, CHUNKS, & PIECES)
PEANUT FLOUR (*See* FLOUR)
PEAR

Food and Description	Amount	Fat Grams	Total Calories	% Fat Calories
candied	1 oz	–	86	
canned				
(Del Monte)				
halves				
in extra light syrup/lite	½ cup	–	60	–
in heavy syrup	½ cup	–	100	–
in light syrup/cinnamon flavored	½ cup	–	80	–
in pear juice/Fruit Naturals	½ cup	–	60	–
natural ginger flavor	½ cup	–	90	–
sliced				
in extra light syrup/lite	½ cup	–	60	
in heavy syrup	½ cup	–	100	–
generic/solids & liquid				
in extra heavy syrup	1 cup	<1.0	250	1%
in extra light syrup	1 cup	<1.0	115	2%
in heavy syrup	1 cup	<1.0	190	2%
in juice	1 cup	<1.0	125	1%
in light syrup	1 cup	<1.0	140	2%
in water	1 cup	<1.0	70	2%
(Libby's) lite				
halves	½ cup	–	60	–

Food and Description	Amount	Fat Grams	Total Calories	% Fat Calories
sliced	½ cup	–	60	–
(S&W)				
Bartlett halves/in heavy syrup	½ cup	–	90	–
quartered/in heavy syrup	½ cup	–	90	–
sliced/in pear juice	½ cup	–	80	–
dried				
generic				
cooked				
sweetened	½ cup	0.5	200	2%
unsweetened	½ cup	0.5	165	3%
uncooked	½ cup	0.5	240	1%
(Manani) dried	¼ cup	–	150	–
fresh				
Bartlett	1 medium	1.0	100	9%
California Sun/ready-cut	½ cup	–	80	–
D'Anjou				
sliced	1 cup	0.7	97	6%
whole	1 medium	1.0	120	8%
(Dole)	1 medium	1.0	100	9%
PEAR JUICE/NECTAR				
canned				
(Goya) nectar	6 fl oz	–	120	–
(Kern's) nectar	6 fl oz	–	120	–
(Knudsen) Rogue River pear juice	8 fl oz	–	120	–
(Libby's) nectar	6 fl oz	–	110	–
PECAN				
(Azar)				
chips	1 oz	21.0	210	90%
halves	1 oz	21.0	210	90%
pieces	1 oz	21.0	210	90%
(Diamond of California)				
chips	¼ cup	21.0	220	86%
chopped	¼ cup	21.0	220	86%
halves	¼ cup	21.0	220	86%
shelled	¼ cup	21.0	220	86%
(Fisher)				
chopped	1 oz	19.0	190	90%
ground	1 oz	19.0	190	90%
raw	1 oz	19.0	190	90%
generic				
dried	1 oz	19.0	190	90%
halves	1 cup	73.0	721	91%
dry-roasted	1 oz	18.0	187	87%
large	10 extra large	28.7	277	93%
fresh				
in shell	10 large	24.5	236	93%
shelled	2 oz	40.0	390	92%
chopped	1 Tbs	5.0	52	87%
	1 cup	84.0	811	93%

Food and Description	Amount	Fat Grams	Total Calories	% Fat Calories
ground	1 cup	67.6	653	93%
halves	10 large	6.0	62	87%
	10 jumbo	10.0	96	94%
	10 mammoth	12.8	124	93%
	1 cup	76.9	742	93%
oil-roasted	1 oz	20.0	195	92%
(Planters)				
chips	2 oz	40.0	390	92%
halves				
Gold Measure	2 oz	40.0	390	92%
regular	1 oz	20.0	190	95%
honey-roasted	1 oz	16.0	180	80%
pieces	1 oz	20.0	190	95%
PECAN FLOUR (See FLOUR)				
PEPPER (See also MEXICAN FOOD; PEPPER, GROUND; SEASONINGS)				
canned or jarred				
(Hebrew National)				
filet peppers	1 oz	–	9	–
hot cherry	1 oz	–	11	–
red filet peppers	1 oz	–	9	–
(Heinz)				
banana/hot	1 pepper	–	6	–
hot rings/slices	1 pepper	–	4	–
mild sweet	1 pepper	–	8	–
sweet pepper momentos	1 pepper	–	6	–
(Progresso) drained				
cherry	2 Tbs	2.0	30	60%
fried/sweet w/onions	2 Tbs	1.5	20	68%
hot cherry				
sliced	2 Tbs	2.0	25	72%
whole	1 pepper	–	10	–
pepper salad	2 Tbs	1.0	15	60%
roasted	2 peppers	–	10	–
Tuscan	3 peppers	–	10	–
(Rosoffs) sweet	1 oz	–	9	–
(Schorr's) filet	1 oz	–	9	–
(Trappey's)				
banana				
slices	21 slices	–	6	–
whole	3 peppers	–	6	–
cherry				
hot	2 peppers	–	7	–
mild	2 peppers	–	10	–
hot/in vinegar	15 peppers	–	9	–
jalapeño/hot				
sliced	21 slices	–	4	–
whole	1 pepper	–	11	–
Serrano/hot	3 peppers	–	7	–
tempero/Greek peperoncini/mild	1 pepper	–	5	–
torrido/Santa Fe grande/hot	1 pepper	–	10	–

Food and Description	Amount	Fat Grams	Total Calories	% Fat Calories
(Vlasic)				
banana/hot	1 oz	–	4	–
cherry				
hot	1 oz	–	10	–
mild	1 oz	–	8	–
Greek pepperoncini salad				
hot	1 oz	–	10	–
mild	1 oz	–	4	–
Mexican hot	1 oz	–	8	–
Mexican tiny hot	1 oz	–	6	–
dried				
green	1 Tbs	–	1	–
red	1 Tbs	–	1	–
freeze-dried/sweet red or green	1 Tbs	–	1	–
	½ cup	–	10	–
fresh				
green chili/hot				
chopped	½ cup	–	16	–
whole	1 medium	–	15	–
jalapeño				
chopped	½ cup	–	20	–
whole	2 medium	–	14	–
red chili/hot				
chopped	½ cup	–	17	–
whole	1 medium	–	18	–
red or green/sweet				
chopped	½ cup	–	12	–
whole	1 medium	–	18	–
yellow/sweet				
chopped	10 strips	–	14	–
whole	1 medium	–	50	–
frozen				
(Birds Eye) green & red, stir-fry	3 oz	–	25	–
(C&W) green & red/strips	3 oz	–	25	–
(Southland) sweet				
green, diced	2 oz	–	10	–
green & red/cut	2 oz	–	15	–
PEPPER, GROUND (See also PEPPER; SEASONINGS)				
(Durkee)				
black	1 tsp	–	8	–
red/cayenne	1 tsp	–	8	–
white	1 tsp	–	9	–
generic				
black	1 tsp	–	5	–
	1 Tbs	–	15	–
chili	1 tsp	–	9	–
red/cayenne	1 tsp	–	5	–
	1 Tbs	–	15	–

Food and Description	Amount	Fat Grams	Total Calories	% Fat Calories
white	1 tsp	–	7	–
	1 Tbs	–	20	–
(Lawry's) lemon	1 tsp	–	6	–

PEPPER DISH (*See also* FROZEN ENTRÉE/DINNER; VEGETARIAN FOODS)
homemade/USDA Standard Home Recipe
stuffed pepper

w/beef & bread crumbs	1 medium	10.5	325	29%
w/beef & rice	½ medium	13.0	219	53%
w/rice only	~5 oz	11.9	198	54%

PEPPER POT SOUP (*See* SOUP)
PEPPERONI (*See* SAUSAGE)
PERCH (*See* OCEAN PERCH; SEAFOOD ENTRÉE/DINNER; WHITE PERCH)
PERSIMMON
Japanese/kaki

dried	1 medium	<1.0	93	5%
fresh	1 medium	<1.0	118	4%
native/fresh	1 medium	–	32	–

PESTO SAUCE (*See* SAUCE)
PHEASANT /raw

breast meat	~6 oz	5.9	243	22%
giblets	3 oz	4.0	119	30%
leg meat	~4 oz	4.6	143	29%
meat & skin	~1 lb	42.0	825	46%
meat only	~¾ lb	12.8	470	25%

PHYLLO DOUGH (*See* PASTRY DOUGH)
PICANTE SAUCE (*See* MEXICAN FOOD; SAUCE)
PICCALILLI (*See* PICKLE RELISH)
PICKLE (*See also* PICKLE RELISH)
(Arnold's)
dill

German	1 oz	–	–	–
hot	1 oz	–	–	–
kosher	1 oz	–	–	–
kosher/spears	1 oz	–	–	–
regular	1 oz	–	–	–
hamburger slices	1 oz	–	–	–

(Cascadian Farm)

baby dills	1 oz	–	5	–
baby sweets	1 oz	–	30	–
bread & butter chips	1 oz	–	25	–

Kosher dill
low-sodium

regular	1 oz	–	5	–
spicy	1 oz	–	5	–
slicers	1 oz	–	5	–
whole	1 oz	–	5	–

(Claussen)
bread 'n butter

chips	4 slices	–	20	–
sandwich slices	2 slices	0.5	20	23%

Food and Description	Amount	Fat Grams	Total Calories	% Fat Calories
half sours/New York deli style	½ pickle	–	5	–
hamburger dills slices/chips	10 slices	–	5	–
hearty garlic deli style				
sandwich slices	1 oz	–	5	–
wholes	1 oz	–	5	–
kosher dills				
burger slices	4 slices	–	5	–
halves	½ pickle	–	5	–
mini	1 pickle	–	5	–
sandwich slices	2 slices	–	5	–
slices	4 slices	–	5	–
spears	1 spear	–	5	–
whole	½ pickle	–	5	–
(Del Monte)				
dill				
halves	¼ pickle	–	5	–
hamburger chips	5-½ chips	–	5	–
tiny kosher	1½ pickles	–	5	–
whole	1½ pickles	–	5	–
sweet				
dill chips	5 chips	–	40	–
gherkins	2 pickles	–	40	–
midget	3 pickles	–	40	–
whole				
8- or 22-oz jar	2 pickles	–	40	–
12-oz jar	1 pickle	–	40	–
(Featherweight) dill/whole	1 medium	–	5	–
generic				
bread & butter	3 slices	–	16	–
dill				
deli style halves	1 oz	–	4	–
genuine	1 oz	–	2	–
hamburger	1 oz	–	2	–
whole	1 medium	–	15	–
gherkins	1 small	–	22	–
hamburger chips	1 oz	–	2	–
(Hebrew National)				
half-sour	1 oz	–	4	–
kosher				
barrel cured dill				
hot	1 pouch	–	23	–
regular	1 pouch	–	23	–
chips	1 oz	–	4	–
halves	1 oz	–	4	–
large	1 oz	–	4	–
spears	1 oz	–	4	–
whole	1 oz	–	4	–
kraut sour garlic	1 oz	–	3	–
(Heinz)				
hot garlic	1 oz	–	6	–

Food and Description	Amount	Fat Grams	Total Calories	% Fat Calories
kosher				
dill				
baby	1 oz	–	4	–
chips	1 oz	–	4	–
spears	1 oz	–	4	–
whole	1 oz	–	4	–
halves	1 piece	–	9	–
old fashioned				
chips	1 oz	–	4	–
deli halves	1 oz	–	4	–
whole	1 oz	–	4	–
slices	1 oz	–	3	–
whole	1 oz	–	2	–
pickled cucumbers	2 spears	–	13	–
Polish style				
dill	1 oz	–	4	–
dill/spears	1 oz	–	4	–
Polskie ogorki	1 oz	–	6	–
processed dill	1 oz	–	2	–
sour	1 oz	–	3	–
sweet				
gherkins/midget or regular	1 oz	–	35	–
mixed	1 oz	–	40	–
pickles	1 oz	–	35	–
salad cubes	1 oz	–	30	–
slices	1 oz	–	35	–
sweet cucumber				
slices	1 oz	–	20	–
stix	1 oz	–	25	–
(Mrs. Klein's) fancy imported				
pepperoncini	1 oz	–	5	–
Southern hot mix	1 oz	–	–	–
(Mt. Olive)				
bread & butter	1 oz	–	25	–
dill	1 oz	–	–	–
kosher dill	1 oz	–	–	–
baby	1 oz	–	–	–
chips	1 oz	–	–	–
strips	1 oz	–	–	–
sweet	1 oz	–	35	–
cucumber strips	1 oz	–	20	–
midgets	1 oz	–	35	–
(Rosoff's)				
kosher				
halves	1 oz	–	4	–
whole	1 oz	–	4	–
sour				
half spears	1 oz	–	4	–
halves	1 oz	–	4	–
(Schorr's)				
bread & butter	1 oz	–	12	–

Food and Description	Amount	Fat Grams	Total Calories	% Fat Calories
kosher				
deli	1 oz	–	4	–
halves	1 oz	–	4	–
spears	1 oz	–	4	–
whole	1 oz	–	4	–
sour				
garlic whole	1 oz	–	3	–
half spears	1 oz	–	4	–
halves	1 oz	–	4	–
(Steinfeld's)				
garlic dills	1 oz	–	5	–
Greek pepperoncini	1 oz	–	5	–
homestyle dills	1 oz	–	5	–
kosher				
dills	1 oz	–	5	–
spears	1 oz	–	5	–
Polish dills	1 oz	–	5	–
sandwich builders				
bread & butter	1 oz	–	–	–
kosher dill	1 oz	–	5	–
baby	1 oz	–	5	–
tiny	1 oz	–	5	–
Polish dill	1 oz	–	–	–
zesty dill	1 oz	–	–	–
sweet	1 oz	–	30	–
cucumber chips	1 oz	–	30	–
(Vlasic)				
Half-The-Salt				
hamburger dill chips	1 oz	–	2	–
kosher crunchy dills	1 oz	–	4	–
kosher dill spears	1 oz	–	4	–
sweet butter chips	1 oz	–	30	–
kosher				
baby dills	1 oz	–	4	–
crunchy dills	1 oz	–	4	–
dill gherkins	1 oz	–	4	–
dill spears	1 oz	–	4	–
snack chunks	1 oz	–	4	–
no garlic				
crunchy dills	1 oz	–	4	–
dill spears	1 oz	–	4	–
refrigerated				
deli bread & butter	1 oz	–	25	–
deli dill halves	1 oz	–	4	–
regular				
bread & butter chunks	1 oz	–	25	–
original dills				
original dills	1 oz	–	2	–
Polish snack chunks	1 oz	–	4	–
sweet butter chips	1 oz	–	30	–
sweet butter stix	1 oz	–	18	–

Food and Description	Amount	Fat Grams	Total Calories	% Fat Calories
zesty crunchy dills	1 oz	–	4	–
zesty dill snack chunks	1 oz	–	4	–
zesty dill spears	1 oz	–	4	–
PICKLE RELISH				
(Arnold's) sweet	1 Tbs	–	15	–
(Cascadian Farm)				
dill	1 Tbs	–	5	–
sweet	1 Tbs	–	20	–
(Claussen) sweet	1 Tbs	–	15	–
(Del Monte)				
hamburger	1 Tbs	–	20	–
hot dog	1 Tbs	–	15	–
sweet	1 Tbs	–	20	–
(Hebrew National) sweet/green	1 Tbs	–	18	–
(Heinz)				
piccalilli	1 oz	–	30	–
relish				
dill	1 Tbs	–	–	–
hamburger	1 Tbs	–	15	–
hot dog	1 Tbs	–	15	–
sweet	1 Tbs	–	30	–
(Mt. Olive) sweet	1 Tbs	–	20	–
(Vlasic)				
piccalilli				
green tomato	1 oz	–	35	–
hot	1 oz	–	35	–
relish				
dill	1 oz	–	2	–
hamburger	1 oz	–	40	–
hot dog	1 oz	<1.0	40	11%
India	1 oz	–	30	–
sweet	1 oz	–	30	–
PIE & COBBLER (*See also* PIE CRUST; PIE FILLING & GLAZE)				
■ **FROZEN OR REFRIGERATED**				
(Amy's) apple pie	1 pie	8.0	220	33%
(Banquet) pie				
apple	⅕ pie	13.0	300	39%
banana	⅓ pie	21.0	350	54%
cherry	⅕ pie	14.0	290	43%
chocolate	⅓ pie	20.0	360	50%
coconut cream	⅓ pie	20.0	350	51%
lemon	⅓ pie	20.0	360	50%
mincemeat	⅕ pie	13.0	310	38%
peach	⅕ pie	12.0	260	42%
pumpkin	⅙ pie	8.0	250	29%
(Chef Pierre) food service				
creme de la cream pie				
banana	¹⁄₁₀ pie	17.0	300	51%
cappuccino	⅛ pie	29.0	430	61%
chocolate	⅛ pie	28.0	400	63%

Food and Description	Amount	Fat Grams	Total Calories	% Fat Calories
coconut	1/10 pie	20.0	350	51%
cookies & cream	1/9 pie	28.0	410	61%
double chocolate	1/10 pie	19.0	360	48%
lemon	1/9 pie	24.0	360	60%
toffee crunch	1/9 pie	29.0	430	61%
gourmet silk pie				
chocolate peanut butter	1/8 pie	35.0	500	63%
French silk	1/8 pie	35.0	490	64%
meringue pie				
gourmet				
chocolate	1/10 pie	12.0	320	34%
coconut	1/10 pie	14.0	340	37%
lemon	1/10 pie	8.0	290	25%
regular				
chocolate	1/10 pie	12.0	320	34%
coconut	1/8 pie	14.0	340	37%
lemon	1/8 pie	9.0	290	28%
lime	1/8 pie	15.0	440	31%
lattice top				
apple	1/9 pie	12.0	320	34%
blueberry	1/9 pie	12.0	330	32%
cherry	1/9 pie	12.0	310	35%
peach	1/9 pie	12.0	300	36%
specialty pie				
Boston cream	1/10 pie	7.0	220	29%
chocolate chip pecan	1/8 pie	34.0	560	55%
French coconut	1/8 pie	22.0	490	40%
pumpkin	1/9 pie	11.0	330	30%
Southern pecan	1/8 pie	27.0	570	43%
sweet potato	1/8 pie	19.0	410	42%
traditional 10" pie				
blackberry	1/10 pie	16.0	360	40%
blueberry	1/10 pie	16.0	350	41%
boysenberry	1/10 pie	16.0	360	40%
cherry	1/10 pie	15.0	330	41%
coconut custard	1/8 pie	16.0	320	45%
Dutch apple	1/10 pie	14.0	360	35%
egg custard	1/8 pie	9.0	240	34%
lemon krunch	1/9 pie	17.0	430	36%
mince	1/10 pie	18.0	370	44%
raisin	1/10 pie	16.0	350	40%
red raspberry	1/10 pie	18.0	360	45%
strawberry-rhubarb	1/10 pie	18.0	360	45%
(Edward's)				
Family Recipe				
Georgia pecan				
22 oz	1/8 pie	23.0	450	46%
singles	1/2 pie	23.0	450	46%
lemon meringue				
22 oz	1/8 pie	10.0	380	24%

Food and Description	Amount	Fat Grams	Total Calories	% Fat Calories
34 oz	⅛ pie	9.0	360	23%
singles	½ pie	8.0	280	26%
Gourmet				
apple cheesecake	⅒ pie	17.0	350	44%
keylime				
36 oz	⅛ pie	22.0	440	45%
singles	½ pie	20.0	390	46%
Mississippi mud				
37 oz	⅑ pie	21.0	380	50%
singles	½ pie	18.0	320	51%
pecan cheesecake				
36 oz	⅛ pie	30.0	350	77%
singles	½ pie	27.0	480	51%
Sundae Creations				
caramel crunch	⅙ pie	23.0	450	46%
chocolate dream				
25.5 oz	⅙ pie	30.0	470	57%
singles	½ pie	19.0	300	57%
strawberry supreme	⅙ pie	22.0	410	48%
(Marie Callender's) cobbler				
apple	¼ cobbler	20.0	370	49%
berry	¼ cobbler	21.0	370	51%
cherry	¼ cobbler	19.0	380	45%
peach	¼ cobbler	18.0	360	45%
(Mountain Top)				
apple				
crumb	⅙ pie	13.0	320	37%
old fashioned	⅛ pie	16.0	350	41%
traditional	⅙ pie	16.0	340	42%
blackberry	⅙ pie	16.0	330	44%
blueberry	⅙ pie	16.0	330	44%
cherry				
old fashioned	⅛ pie	16.0	380	38%
traditional	⅙ pie	16.0	340	42%
mincemeat	⅙ pie	16.0	350	41%
peach				
old fashioned	⅛ pie	16.0	360	40%
traditional	⅙ pie	16.0	310	46%
pumpkin				
old fashioned	⅛ pie	10.0	260	36%
traditional	⅙ pie	10.0	250	36%
(Mrs. Smith's)				
Cobblers				
apple	1 serving	9.0	240	34%
blackberry	1 serving	9.0	250	32%
cherry	1 serving	9.0	250	32%
peach	1 serving	9.0	240	34%
Pies				
apple				
Dutch apple crumb	⅛ pie	16.0	360	40%

Food and Description	Amount	Fat Grams	Total Calories	% Fat Calories
old fashioned/special recipe/ 9" pie	⅛ pie	17.0	350	44%
reduced-fat	⅙ pie	8.0	210	34%
blueberry/8" pie	⅙ pie	17.0	330	46%
Boston cream/8" pie	⅛ pie	7.0	180	35%
cherry/old fashioned/special recipe/ 9" pie	⅛ pie	17.0	340	45%
chocolate cream/8" pie	¼ pie	17.0	330	46%
coconut custard/8" pie	⅕ pie	12.0	250	43%
cookies & cream				
chocomint	⅛ pie	19.0	390	44%
droxies	⅛ pie	20.0	390	46%
lemonylemon	⅛ pie	20.0	370	49%
s'mores	⅛ pie	20.0	410	44%
strawbanana	⅛ pie	21.0	380	50%
lemon cream/8" pie	¼ pie	15.0	300	45%
lemon meringue/8" pie	⅕ pie	8.0	300	24%
mince/8" pie	⅙ pie	17.0	380	40%
peach/old fashioned/special recipe/ 9" pie	⅛ pie	17.0	320	48%
pecan				
24 oz box	⅙ pie	23.0	520	40%
36 oz box	⅛ pie	23.0	500	41%
pumpkin custard	⅛ pie	9.0	240	34%
red raspberry/8" pie	⅙ pie	17.0	340	45%
strawberry/8" pie	⅕ pie	11.0	290	34%
strawberry rhubarb/8" pie	⅙ pie	11.0	280	35%
Restaurant Classics				
cappuccino	⅕ pie	19.0	360	48%
French silk	⅕ pie	40.0	560	64%
key lime	⅕ pie	19.0	420	41%
peanut butter silk	⅕ pie	41.0	600	62%
Special Recipe Deep Dish Pies				
apple	serving	15.0	330	41%
cherry	serving	14.0	330	38%
cherry-berry	serving	15.0	330	41%
peach	serving	14.0	330	38%
pumpkin	serving	11.0	280	35%
Southern pecan	serving	26.0	550	43%
Sweet potato	serving	15.0	330	41%
(Pet-Ritz)				
cobbler/homestyle				
apple cinnamon	⅙ cobbler	12.0	280	39%
blackberry	⅙ cobbler	12.0	260	42%
cherry	⅙ cobbler	11.0	300	33%
peach	⅙ cobbler	10.0	240	38%
pie/homestyle				
apple	⅙ pie	16.0	320	45%
banana creme	⅓ pie	18.0	350	46%
cherry	⅙ pie	16.0	310	46%

Food and Description	Amount	Fat Grams	Total Calories	% Fat Calories
chocolate cream	⅓ pie	17.0	340	45%
coconut cream	⅓ pie	18.0	350	46%
Dutch apple	⅙ pie	15.0	340	40%
key lime	⅓ pie	18.0	350	46%
lemon cream	⅓ pie	18.0	350	46%
pumpkin	⅙ pie	9.0	230	35%
(Sara Lee's)				
apple/45% reduced-fat	⅙ pie	8.0	290	25%
chocolate silk supreme	⅕ pie	32.0	500	58%
coconut cream	⅕ pie	31.0	480	58%
Homestyle/9" pie				
apple	⅛ pie	16.0	340	42%
blueberry	⅛ pie	15.0	360	38%
cherry	⅛ pie	15.0	330	41%
Dutch apple	⅛ pie	15.0	350	39%
mince	⅛ pie	17.0	390	39%
peach	⅛ pie	14.0	320	39%
pecan	⅛ pie	24.0	520	42%
pumpkin	⅛ pie	11.0	260	38%
raspberry	⅛ pie	19.0	380	45%
southern sweet potato	⅛ pie	10.0	280	50%
lemon meringue	⅙ pie	11.0	350	28%
Signature Selections				
caramel applenut	1/9 pie	18.0	370	43%
cinnamon French apple	⅒ pie	15.0	360	38%
fruits of the forest	1/9 pie	17.0	340	45%
pumpkin/traditional	⅒ pie	9.0	250	32%
(Schwan's) old fashioned				
apple	1/12 pie	13.0	270	43%
peach	⅒ pie	14.0	320	39%
■ HOMEMADE				
USDA Standard Home Recipe (Note: Pie crust was made with enriched flour & vegetable shortening.)				
fried pie				
apple	4.5 oz	20.0	400	45%
blueberry	4.5 oz	20.0	400	45%
cherry	4.5 oz	20.0	400	45%
lemon	4.5 oz	20.0	400	45%
peach	4.5 oz	20.0	400	45%
strawberry	4.5 oz	20.0	400	45%
regular 9" pie				
apple	⅙ pie	18.0	405	40%
banana cream	⅙ pie	13.0	300	39%
banana custard	⅙ pie	14.0	336	38%
blackberry	⅙ pie	17.0	384	40%
blueberry	⅙ pie	17.0	380	40%
butterscotch	⅛ pie	12.5	304	37%
cherry	⅙ pie	18.0	410	40%
chess	⅙ pie	24.0	485	45%
chocolate	⅙ pie	22.0	433	46%

Food and Description	Amount	Fat Grams	Total Calories	% Fat Calories
chocolate meringue	⅙ pie	18.0	383	42%
coconut cream	⅙ pie	23.0	455	45%
coconut custard	⅙ pie	19.0	357	48%
custard	⅙ pie	17.0	330	46%
grasshopper	⅙ pie	23.0	460	45%
key lime	⅙ pie	19.0	460	37%
lemon chiffon	⅙ pie	13.6	338	36%
lemon meringue	⅙ pie	14.0	355	36%
mincemeat	⅙ pie	18.0	428	38%
peach	⅙ pie	17.0	405	38%
pecan	⅙ pie	32.0	575	50%
pineapple	⅙ pie	17.0	400	38%
pineapple chiffon	⅙ pie	13.0	311	38%
pineapple custard	⅙ Pie	13.0	334	35%
pumpkin	⅙ pie	17.0	320	48%
raisin	⅙ pie	17.0	427	36%
rhubarb	⅙ pie	17.0	400	38%
shoo-fly	⅛ pie	13.0	395	30%
squash	⅙ pie	20.0	360	50%
strawberry	⅙ pie	10.0	246	37%
strawberry-rhubarb	⅛ pie	23.0	430	48%
sweet potato	⅙ pie	17.0	324	47%
vanilla cream	⅛ pie	17.0	350	44%
■ **READY TO SERVE**				
(Aunt Fanny's) individual pie				
apple	1 pie	23.0	460	45%
berry	1 pie	22.0	430	46%
cherry	1 pie	22.0	400	50%
peach	1 pie	22.0	430	46%
(Break Cake) snack/fried pie				
apple	1 pie	14.0	255	49%
cherry	1 pie	14.0	250	50%
(Dolly Madison) snack/packaged				
apple	1 pie	23.0	510	41%
blueberry	1 pie	24.0	520	42%
cherry	1 pie	24.0	530	41%
chocolate	1 pie	27.0	570	43%
lemon	1 pie	25.0	530	42%
peach	1 pie	23.0	500	41%
pecan	1 pie	22.0	540	37%
pineapple	1 pie	22.0	490	40%
(Entenmann's) pie				
original				
apple/homestyle	1 serving	7.0	140	45%
coconut custard	1 serving	8.0	140	51%
snack				
apple	1 pie	14.0	266	47%
apple/fried	1 pie	21.0	404	47%
blueberry/fried	1 pie	21.0	404	47%
cherry	1 pie	14.0	266	47%

Food and Description	Amount	Fat Grams	Total Calories	% Fat Calories
cherry/fried	1 pie	21.0	404	47%
lemon	1 pie	14.0	266	47%
lemon/fried	1 pie	21.0	404	47%
peach/fried	1 pie	21.0	404	47%
strawberry/fried	1 pie	21.0	404	47%
(Hostess) snack/packaged				
apple	1 pie	22.0	480	45%
blackberry	1 pie	21.0	520	36%
blueberry	1 pie	21.0	480	39%
cherry	1 pie	22.0	470	42%
French apple	1 pie	22.0	480	41%
lemon	1 pie	24.0	500	43%
peach	1 pie	21.0	480	39%
pineapple	1 pie	21.0	460	41%
strawberry fruit	1 pie	23.0	510	41%
(Lance) snack/packaged				
apple/fried	3 oz	17.0	330	46%
coconut	3 oz	19.0	370	46%
pecan	3 oz	17.0	350	44%
(Tastykake) snack				
apple	1 pie	11.0	270	37%
blueberry	1 pie	11.0	300	33%
cherry	1 pie	11.0	290	34%
coconut creme	1 pie	21.0	370	51%
French apple	1 pie	11.0	310	32%
lemon	1 pie	13.0	300	39%
peach	1 pie	11.0	280	35%
pineapple	1 pie	12.0	290	37%
pineapple cheese	1 pie	12.0	320	34%
pumpkin	1 pie	14.0	340	37%
strawberry	1 pie	12.0	320	34%
Tastyklair	1 pie	20.0	400	45%
PIE CRUST (*See also* PASTRY)				
■ **FROZEN**				
(Chef Pierre) food service/unbaked				
deep dish/9" crust	⅛ crust	8.0	130	55%
regular/10" crust	⅑ crust	7.0	110	57%
vegetable shortening				
9" crust	⅑ crust	8.0	130	55%
10" crust	⅑ crust	8.0	120	60%
generic/9" crust	⅛ crust	4.8	80	53%
	1 crust	38.0	650	53%
(Mrs. Smith's) 9 inch pastry				
deep dish	⅛ crust	7.0	110	57%
regular	⅛ crust	7.0	100	63%
(Oronoque)				
3" crust/tart shell	1 crust	9.0	140	58%
6" crust	¼ crust	7.0	110	57%
9" deep dish crust	⅛ crust	7.0	100	63%
9" regular	⅛ crust	6.0	80	68%

Food and Description	Amount	Fat Grams	Total Calories	% Fat Calories
(Pepperidge Farm) patty shells	1 shell	15.0	210	64%
(Pet-Ritz) Ready-To-Bake				
deep dish				
all vegetable	⅛ crust	5.0	90	50%
9"	⅛ crust	5.0	90	50%
extra large/9-⅝"	⅛ crust	6.0	110	49%
regular				
all vegetable	⅛ crust	4.5	80	51%
9" crust	⅛ crust	4.0	80	45%
■ **HOMEMADE**				
USDA Standard Home Recipe/9" crust				
cookie-type				
chocolate wafer				
baked	⅛ crust	8.0	140	51%
chilled	⅛ crust	8.0	140	51%
graham cracker				
baked	⅛ crust	7.0	150	42%
chilled	⅛ crust	7.0	150	42%
vanilla water				
baked	⅛ crust	7.5	120	56%
chilled	⅛ crust	7.5	120	56%
regular				
baked	⅛ crust	7.0	120	53%
	1 crust	63.0	960	59%
unbaked	⅛ crust	7.0	115	55%
	1 crust	63.0	920	62%
■ **MIX**				
(Betty Crocker) 9" crust/prepared	⅛ crust	8.0	110	65%
(Flako) mix only	¼ cup	8.0	130	55%
(Jiffy) prepared	⅐ crust	10.0	180	50%
(Krusteaz)				
mix only	2 Tbs	5.0	90	50%
9" crust/baked	⅛ crust	5.0	90	50%
(Nabisco)				
Honey Maid/graham				
9" crust/prepared	⅙ crust	7.0	140	45%
Nilla/cookie crumb				
crumbs only	2 Tbs	2.5	70	32%
9" crust/prepared	⅙ crust	7.0	140	45%
Oreo/cookie crumb				
crumbs only	2 Tbs	3.0	80	34%
9" crust/prepared	⅙ crust	7.0	140	45%
(Pillsbury) mix only	2 Tbs	6.0	100	54%
■ **READY TO USE**				
(Keebler) Ready Crust				
chocolate				
9" pie	⅛ crust	5.0	110	41%
single-serve	1 tart	5.0	110	41%
graham cracker				
9" pit	⅛ crust	5.0	100	45%

Food and Description	Amount	Fat Grams	Total Calories	% Fat Calories
single serve	1 tart	5.0	110	41%
(Pillsbury) refrigerated	⅛ crust	7.0	120	53%
(Wonderslim) fat-free				
chocolate	⅛ crust	–	70	–
original	⅛ crust	–	70	–

PIE FILLING & GLAZE (*See also* PUDDING & MOUSSE)

■ **CANNED OR JARRED**

(Borden) None Such mincemeat				
condensed	¼ pkg	2.0	220	8%
ready to use				
original	⅓ cup	1.0	200	5%
w/brandy & rum	⅓ cup	2.0	220	8%
(Comstock)				
apple				
cinnamon n' spice	⅓ cup	–	110	–
French	⅓ cup	–	100	–
more fruit	⅓ cup	–	80	–
original				
country	⅓ cup	–	90	–
sliced apples	⅓ cup	–	30	–
reduced calorie	⅓ cup	–	50	–
banana cream	⅓ cup	1.5	130	10%
blackberry	⅓ cup	–	110	–
blueberry/MoreFruit	⅓ cup	–	80	–
cherry				
dark sweet	⅓ cup	–	100	–
MoreFruit				
light	⅓ cup	–	60	–
regular	⅓ cup	–	90	–
original				
light	⅓ cup	–	60	–
red ruby	⅓ cup	–	90	–
chocolate cream	⅓ cup	5.0	120	38%
coconut cream	⅓ cup	3.0	110	25%
lemon	⅓ cup	1.5	130	10%
mincemeat	⅓ cup	–	170	–
peach/MoreFruit	⅓ cup	–	80	–
pineapple	⅓ cup	–	110	–
pumpkin				
pie mix	⅓ cup	–	90	–
pure pumpkin	½ cup	–	50	–
raisin/California	⅓ cup	–	120	–
raspberry	⅓ cup	–	100	–
strawberry	⅓ cup	–	100	–
(Libby's) pumpkin pie mix	½ cup	–	100	–
(Musselman's)				
apple				
deluxe	⅓ cup	–	120	–
plus	⅓ cup	–	120	–
turnover/diced	⅓ cup	–	120	–

Food and Description	Amount	Fat Grams	Total Calories	% Fat Calories
apricot	⅓ cup	–	150	–
blackberry				
plus	⅓ cup	–	120	–
regular	⅓ cup	–	120	–
blueberry				
plus	⅓ cup	–	145	–
regular	⅓ cup	–	120	–
boysenberry	⅓ cup	–	120	–
cherry				
plus	⅓ cup	–	110	–
regular	⅓ cup	–	120	–
gooseberry	⅓ cup	–	180	–
lemon				
French	⅓ cup	1.0	180	5%
regular	⅓ cup	2.0	200	9%
mincemeat	⅓ cup	1.0	190	5%
peach				
plus	⅓ cup	–	115	–
regular	⅓ cup	–	150	–
pineapple	⅓ cup	–	110	–
pumpkin	⅓ cup	–	170	–
raisin	½ cup	–	130	–
raspberry				
black	⅓ cup	–	190	–
red	⅓ cup	–	190	–
strawberry				
plus	⅓ cup	–	140	–
regular	⅓ cup	–	120	–
strawberry-rhubarb	⅓ cup	–	120	–
(None Such) Mincemeat See (Borden) in this section)				
(S&W) mincemeat	¼ cup	2.5	180	13%
(Thank You)				
apple				
cinnamon n' spice	⅓ cup	–	110	–
French	⅓ cup	–	100	–
more fruit	⅓ cup	–	80	–
original				
country	⅓ cup	–	90	–
sliced apples	⅓ cup	–	30	–
reduced calorie	⅓ cup	–	50	–
banana cream	⅓ cup	1.5	130	10%
blackberry	⅓ cup	–	110	–
blueberry/MoreFruit	⅓ cup	–	80	–
cherry				
dark sweet	⅓ cup	–	100	–
MoreFruit				
light	⅓ cup	–	60	–
regular	⅓ cup	–	90	–
original				
light	⅓ cup	–	60	–

Food and Description	Amount	Fat Grams	Total Calories	% Fat Calories
red ruby	⅓ cup	–	90	–
chocolate cream	⅓ cup	5.0	120	38%
coconut cream	⅓ cup	3.0	110	25%
lemon	⅓ cup	1.5	130	10%
mincemeat	⅓ cup	–	170	–
peach/MoreFruit	⅓ cup	–	80	–
pineapple	⅓ cup	–	110	–
pumpkin				
pie mix	⅓ cup	–	90	–
pure pumpkin	½ cup	–	50	–
raisin/California	⅓ cup	–	120	–
raspberry	⅓ cup	–	100	–
strawberry	⅓ cup	–	100	–
(Wilderness)				
banana cream	⅓ cup	1.5	100	14%
chocolate cream	⅓ cup	1.5	120	11%
coconut cream	⅓ cup	3.0	110	25%
pumpkin	⅓ cup	–	90	–

■ **MIX** (Note: Unless stated otherwise, 1 serving of mix = the amount in ½ cup prepared.)

Food and Description	Amount	Fat Grams	Total Calories	% Fat Calories
(Calhoun Bend Mill)				
apple-cinnamon crisp/mix only	¼ cup	–	140	–
cherry-oatmeal crunch/mix only	¼ cup	0.5	140	3%
chocolate-fudge/mix only	3 Tbs	5.0	140	32%
peach cobbler/mix only	¼ cup	–	150	–
pecan/mix only	⅛ cup	–	110	–
strawberry				
mix only	1 oz	<1.0	110	4%
prepared	1 serving	7.0	256	25%
(Jell-O) pudding & pie filling				
Americana pudding & custard				
Custard/prepared w/2% milk	½ cup	2.5	140	16%
rice pudding/prepared w/skim milk	½ cup	–	140	–
tapioca pudding/prepared w/skim milk	½ cup	–	130	–
cook & serve				
fat-free/prepared w/skim milk				
chocolate	½ cup	–	130	–
vanilla	½ cup	–	130	–
original/prepared w/2% milk				
banana cream	½ cup	2.5	140	16%
butterscotch	½ cup	2.5	160	14%
chocolate	½ cup	2.5	150	15%
chocolate fudge	½ cup	2.5	150	15%
coconut cream	½ cup	5.0	150	30%
flan	½ cup	2.5	140	16%
lemon/prepared as directed	½ cup	2.0	140	13%
milk chocolate	½ cup	3.0	150	18%
vanilla	½ cup	2.5	140	16%

Food and Description	Amount	Fat Grams	Total Calories	% Fat Calories
sugar-free/reduced calorie-prepared w/2% milk				
chocolate	½ cup	2.5	90	25%
vanilla	½ cup	2.5	80	28%
instant				
fat-free/prepared w/skim milk				
chocolate	½ cup	–	140	–
devil's food	½ cup	–	140	–
vanilla	½ cup	–	140	–
white chocolate	½ cup	–	140	–
fat-free/sugar-free/reduced calorie-prepared w/skim milk				
banana	½ cup	–	70	–
butterscotch	½ cup	–	70	–
chocolate	½ cup	–	80	–
chocolate fudge	½ cup	–	80	–
vanilla	½ cup	–	70	–
vanilla chocolate	½ cup	–	70	–
original/prepared w/2% milk				
banana cream	½ cup	2.5	150	15%
butterscotch	½ cup	2.5	150	15%
chocolate	½ cup	2.5	160	14%
chocolate fudge	½ cup	3.0	160	17%
coconut cream	½ cup	5.0	160	28%
French vanilla	½ cup	2.5	150	15%
lemon	½ cup	2.5	150	15%
pistachio	½ cup	3.0	160	17%
vanilla	½ cup	2.5	150	15%
(McCormick/Schilling) pie glaze mix for				
blueberries	2 oz	–	60	–
peaches	2 oz	–	70	–
strawberries	2 oz	–	70	–
(Nabisco) My-T-Fine/mix only				
butterscotch	1 serving	–	90	–
chocolate	1 serving	–	100	–
chocolate almond	1 serving	1.0	100	10%
chocolate fudge	1 serving	–	100	–
lemon	1 serving	–	90	–
vanilla	1 serving	–	90	–
(Royal) mix only				
cook & serve				
banana cream	1 serving	–	80	–
butterscotch	1 serving	–	90	–
chocolate	1 serving	–	90	–
dark 'n sweet chocolate	1 serving	–	90	–
vanilla	1 serving	–	80	–
instant				
regular				
banana cream	1 serving	–	90	–
butterscotch	1 serving	–	90	–
cherry vanilla	1 serving	–	90	–

Food and Description	Amount	Fat Grams	Total Calories	% Fat Calories
chocolate	1 serving	–	100	–
chocolate almond	1 serving	1.0	120	8%
chocolate chocolate chip	1 serving	1.0	110	8%
chocolate peanut butter	1 serving	1.0	110	8%
dark 'n sweet	1 serving	–	110	–
lemon	1 serving	–	90	–
pistachio	1 serving	1.0	90	10%
strawberry	1 serving	–	100	–
toasted coconut	1 serving	2.0	100	18%
vanilla	1 serving	–	90	–
vanilla chocolate chip	1 serving	1.0	90	10%
sugar-free				
chocolate	1 serving	–	45	–
pistachio	1 serving	–	40	–
vanilla	1 serving	–	40	–

PIEROGI/POTATO DUMPLING (*See* FROZEN ENTRÉE/DINNER)
PIGEON (*See* SQUAB/PIGEON)
PIGEON PEA
dried/mature/shelled

boiled	½ cup	–	100	–
raw	½ cup	1.5	350	4%
fresh				
cooked	½ cup	1.0	90	10%
raw	½ cup	1.5	350	4%
shelled				
boiled-drained	½ cup	1.5	120	11%
raw	½ cup	2.0	155	12%
seeds/immature				
boiled-drained	½ cup	1.0	85	11%
raw	20 seeds	<1.0	10	18%

PIGNOLA (*See* PINE NUT)
PIG'S FEET (*See* PORK; PORK DINNER/ENTRÉE)
PIKE (*See also* PIKE ROE)
northern

cooked-dry heat	3 oz	1.0	95	9%
raw	3 oz	1.0	75	12%
walleye				
cooked-dry heat	3 oz	1.0	100	9%
raw	3 oz	1.0	79	11%

PIKE ROE

northern/raw	3 oz	1.7	110	14%

PILAF (*See* RICE DISH; PASTA ENTRÉE/DINNER)
PIMIENTO /canned

(Dromedary)	1 oz	–	10	–
(Dunbar's)	½ oz	–	4	–
generic				
diced or sliced	4 oz	–	30	–
whole	1 medium	–	11	–
(S&W) whole	2¼ oz	–	20	–

PIÑA COLADA (*See* COCKTAIL)

Food and Description	Amount	Fat Grams	Total Calories	% Fat Calories
PINE NUT				
canned				
(Diamond of California)	1 oz	17.0	180	85%
dried				
pignola	1 oz	14.0	146	86%
pinyon	1 oz	17.0	161	95%
jarred				
(Progresso) pignoli nuts	1 oz	13.0	170	69%
PINEAPPLE				
can or cup				
(Del Monte)				
chunks				
in heavy syrup	½ cup	–	90	–
in juice	½ cup	–	70	–
crushed				
in heavy syrup	½ cup	–	90	–
in juice	½ cup	–	70	–
sliced				
in heavy syrup	2 slices	–	90	–
in juice	2 slices	–	60	–
spears or wedges/in juice	½ cup	–	70	–
tidbits/in juice				
canned	½ cup	–	70	–
snack cup	4 oz	–	60	–
wedges in juice	½ cup	–	70	–
(Dole)				
chunks				
in clarified juice	½ cup	–	60	–
in heavy syrup	½ cup	–	90	–
coarse-cut crushed				
in juice	½ cup	–	70	–
crushed				
in extra heavy syrup	½ cup	–	110	–
in heavy syrup	½ cup	–	90	–
in juice	½ cup	–	70	–
cubes				
in extra heavy syrup	½ cup	–	200	–
in light syrup	½ cup	–	80	–
pieces				
in light syrup	½ cup	–	80	–
sliced				
in clarified juice	2 slices	–	60	–
in heavy syrup	2 slices	–	90	–
90 slices/in light syrup	3½ slices	–	60	–
100-110 slices/in heavy syrup	4 slices	–	90	–
66 slices				
in clarified juice	2½ slices	–	60	–
in heavy syrup	2½ slices	–	90	–
tidbits				
in clarified juice	½ cup	–	60	–

Food and Description	Amount	Fat Grams	Total Calories	% Fat Calories
in heavy syrup	½ cup	–	90	–
in light syrup	½ cup	–	80	–
(Empress)				
chunks	½ cup	–	70	–
crushed	½ cup	–	70	–
sliced	½ cup	–	70	–
generic/sliced or chunks				
in heavy syrup	1 slice	–	45	–
in juice	1 slice	<1.0	35	3%
	1 cup	0.5	150	3%
in water	1 slice	<1.0	19	6%
	1 cup	<1.0	79	6%
(S&W) Hawaiian/sliced/in syrup	2 slices	–	90	–
candied				
(S&W) glace				
slices				
green	1 piece	–	180	–
natural	1 piece	–	180	–
red	1 piece	–	180	–
wedges				
natural	5 pieces	–	80	–
tri-color	5 pieces	–	80	–
fresh	1 slice	<1.0	42	8%
	1 cup	0.7	77	8%
(Chiquita)	1 cup	1.0	90	10%
(Del Monte)	½ cup	–	52	–
	2 slices	–	70	–
(Dole)	2 slices	1.0	90	10%
frozen/generic/chunks				
sweetened	½ cup	–	104	–
unsweetened	3.5 oz	<1.0	50	9%

PINEAPPLE JUICE/JUICE BLEND (*See also* FRUIT PUNCH; PINEAPPLE JUICE DRINK)

Food and Description	Amount	Fat Grams	Total Calories	% Fat Calories
bottled, boxed, or canned				
(Del Monte)				
from concentrate	6 fl oz	–	80	–
	8 fl oz	–	130	–
not from concentrate	8 fl oz	–	110	–
(Dole)				
Juice Cooler	8.45 fl oz	–	130	–
100% juice				
bottled				
pineapple-orange	10 fl oz	–	150	–
pineapple-orange-banana	10 fl oz	–	160	–
pineapple-passion-banana	10 fl oz	–	160	–
canned				
pineapple				
from concentrate	8 fl oz	–	120	–
	6 fl oz	–	80	–
not from concentrate	8 fl oz	–	110	–
pineapple-grapefruit	6 fl oz	–	100	–

Food and Description	Amount	Fat Grams	Total Calories	% Fat Calories
pineapple-orange	6 fl oz	–	100	–
pineapple-orange-banana	6 fl oz	–	100	–
refrigerated				
pineapple	8 fl oz	–	130	–
	6 fl oz	–	90	–
pineapple-orange	8 fl oz	–	120	–
pineapple-orange-banana	4 fl oz	–	70	–
	8 fl oz	–	130	–
pineapple-orange-berry	8 fl oz	–	130	–
pineapple-orange-guava	8 fl oz	–	120	–
pineapple-orange-strawberry	8 fl oz	–	130	–
pineapple-passion-banana	8 fl oz	–	120	–
unfrozen juice concentrate				
reconstituted	6 fl oz	–	80	–
	8 fl oz	–	110	–
single strength	6 fl oz	–	80	–
	8 fl oz	–	110	–
generic	8 fl oz	–	140	–
(Kern's) pineapple-orange-passion fruit	11.5 fl oz	–	210	–
(Knudsen) Thirst Quencher/ pineapple-coconut	8 fl oz	–	130	–
(Minute Maid) drink box	8.45 fl oz	–	130	–
(Mott's) pineapple-orange	10 fl oz	–	170	–
(S&W)	6 fl oz	–	90	–
	8 fl oz	–	110	–
individual serving	12 fl oz	–	180	–
(Seneca)	8 fl oz	–	130	–
frozen				
(Dole) prepared				
100% pineapple juice	8 fl oz	–	130	–
pineapple-grapefruit	8 fl oz	–	130	–
pineapple-orange	8 fl oz	–	120	–
pineapple-orange-banana	8 fl oz	–	130	–
pineapple-orange-berry	8 fl oz	–	130	–
pineapple-orange-guava	8 fl oz	–	120	–
pineapple-orange-strawberry	8 fl oz	–	130	–
pineapple-passion-banana	8 fl oz	–	120	–
pineapple-strawberry	8 fl oz	–	130	–
generic/frozen concentrate				
prepared	8 fl oz	<1.0	130	3%
undiluted	6 oz	<1.0	385	1%
(Welch's) pineapple-banana/prepared	8 fl oz	–	130	–
PINK BEAN				
canned				
(Goya)				
habichuelas rosadas/Spanish style	½ cup	0.5	80	9%
original	½ cup	0.5	80	9%
dried				
boiled	½ cup	0.5	125	4%
raw	½ cup	1.0	360	3%

Food and Description	Amount	Fat Grams	Total Calories	% Fat Calories
PIÑON/PINYON (*See* PINE NUT)				
PINTO BEAN				
canned				
(Bush's)	½ cup	–	60	–
(Eden) Organic				
original	½ cup	–	100	–
spicy/w jalapeño & red peppers	½ cup	–	125	–
(Gebhardt)	½ cup	–	100	–
(Goya) Spanish style	½ cup	0.5	110	4%
(Green Giant)	½ cup	0.5	110	4%
(Hain)	½ cup	1.0	110	8%
(Luck's) seasoned w/pork				
regular	7 oz	3.0	200	14%
	½ cup	4.0	140	26%
w/great northern beans	½ cup	2.0	130	14%
w/onions	½ cup	3.0	150	18%
(Progresso)	½ cup	1.0	130	7%
(Trappey's) w/bacon				
jalapinto	½ cup	1.0	120	10%
original	½ cup	1.0	120	10%
dried/raw				
(Arrowhead Mills)	¼ cup	0.5	150	3%
(Bean Cuisine)	½ cup	1.0	115	8%
generic				
cooked	½ cup	0.5	133	3%
raw	½ cup	1.0	325	3%
sprouted/mature seeds				
boiled-drained	½ cup	0.5	25	18%
raw	½ cup	1.0	65	14%
PINYON (*See* PINE NUTS)				
PISTACHIO				
(Alma) extra jumbo				
natural	1 oz	14.0	160	79%
red	1 oz	14.0	160	79%
(Ann's House Of Nuts) natural	1 oz	14.0	160	79%
(Dole) dry-roasted				
shelled	1 oz	14.0	160	79%
unshelled	1 oz	7.0	90	70%
(Fisher) red	1 oz	15.0	170	79%
generic				
dried	1 oz	13.7	164	75%
	1 cup	61.9	739	75%
dry roasted	1 oz	15.0	172	79%
	1 cup	67.6	776	78%
shelled	1 oz	15.0	168	80%
unshelled	1 oz	7.0	84	75%
(Lance)	⅓ cup	9.0	120	68%
	¼ cup	7.0	100	63%
	2 oz pkg	9.0	120	68%

Food and Description	Amount	Fat Grams	Total Calories	% Fat Calories
(Planters) dry-roasted				
shelled				
Munch 'N Go	2 oz	29.0	330	79%
regular	1 oz	14.0	160	79%
unshelled				
red/salted	1 oz	14.0	160	79%
uncolored	½ cup	14.0	160	79%
	1 oz	14.0	160	79%
	2.25 oz	16.0	190	76%
PITA BREAD (See BREAD)				
PITANGA/BRAZILIAN CHERRY/SURINAM CHERRY				
fresh	2 pieces	<1.0	5	11%
	1 cup	0.7	57	11%
	1 lb	1.6	132	11%
PIZZA (See also FROZEN ENTRÉE/DINNER; VEGETARIAN FOODS; individual FAST FOOD listings.)				
■ **(Celeste)**				
Pizza For One				
cheese	1 pizza	20.0	420	43%
4-cheese				
original	1 pizza	26.0	480	49%
zesty	1 pizza	24.0	470	46%
deluxe	1 pizza	25.0	470	48%
pepperoni	1 pizza	27.0	470	52%
sausage	1 pizza	27.0	530	46%
suprema	1 pizza	27.0	500	49%
vegetable	1 pizza	21.0	420	45%
Pizza/Large				
cheese	¼ pizza	16.0	320	45%
deluxe	¼ pizza	18.0	350	46%
pepperoni	¼ pizza	20.0	350	51%
suprema	⅕ pizza	16.0	290	50%
Pizza/Large Premium				
cheese	¼ pizza	18.0	350	46%
deluxe	¼ pizza	21.0	390	48%
pepperoni	¼ pizza	22.0	380	52%
sausage/pepperoni	¼ pizza	22.0	380	52%
Pizza/Rising Crust				
four cheese	⅙ pizza	10.0	340	26%
supreme	⅙ pizza	17.0	380	40%
three meat	⅙ pizza	17.0	390	39%
pepperoni	⅙ pizza	16.0	380	38%
■ **(Di Giorno)**				
Rising Crust				
8 inch				
chicken supreme	⅓ pizza	9.0	270	30%
four-cheese	⅓ pizza	9.0	260	31%
Italian sausage	⅓ pizza	12.0	300	36%
pepperoni	⅓ pizza	13.0	300	39%
spinach	⅓ pizza	8.0	250	29%

Food and Description	Amount	Fat Grams	Total Calories	% Fat Calories
supreme	⅓ pizza	14.0	310	41%
three meat	⅓ pizza	13.0	310	38%
vegetable	⅓ pizza	8.0	250	29%
12 inch				
four-cheese	⅙ pizza	11.0	320	31%
Italian sausage	⅙ pizza	14.0	360	35%
pepperoni	⅙ pizza	16.0	370	39%
supreme	⅙ pizza	17.0	380	40%
three meat	⅙ pizza	16.0	380	38%
vegetable	⅙ pizza	10.0	310	29%
■ **(Freschetta)**				
8 Inch				
BBQ chicken	½ pizza	11.0	380	26%
garlic chicken	⅓ pizza	9.0	260	31%
four cheese	½ pizza	14.0	390	32%
pepperoni	½ pizza	17.0	420	36%
supreme	⅓ pizza	12.0	290	37%
Thai style	⅓ pizza	8.0	260	28%
vegetable primavera	⅓ pizza	9.0	250	32%
12 Inch				
BBQ chicken	⅕ pizza	12.0	340	32%
four-cheese	⅕ pizza	14.0	380	33%
pepperoni	⅙ pizza	15.0	350	39%
sausage	⅙ pizza	15.0	350	39%
sausage & pepperoni	⅙ pizza	15.0	350	39%
special deluxe	⅙ pizza	15.0	350	39%
supreme	⅙ pizza	15.0	350	39%
vegetable primavera	⅕ pizza	11.0	340	29%
Stuffed Crust				
four-cheese	⅕ pizza	10.0	310	29%
pepperoni	⅕ pizza	13.0	340	34%
sausage & pepperoni	⅕ pizza	13.0	340	34%
supreme	⅕ pizza	13.0	350	33%
vegetable medley	⅕ pizza	8.0	280	26%
■ **(Graindance)**				
pizza/cheese w/whole wheat crust	¼ pizza	8.0	190	38%
■ **(Jack's)**				
Great Combinations/9 Inch				
double cheese	½ pizza	21.0	430	44%
pepperoni & sausage	½ pizza	18.0	380	43%
Great Combinations/12 Inch				
bacon cheeseburger	¼ pizza	18.0	360	45%
double cheese	¼ pizza	19.0	380	45%
pepperoni	¼ pizza	19.0	410	42%
pepperoni & mushroom	¼ pizza	16.0	340	42%
sausage	¼ pizza	18.0	390	42%
sausage & mushroom	¼ pizza	15.0	310	44%
sausage & pepperoni	¼ pizza	19.0	350	49%
supreme	¼ pizza	18.0	350	46%

Food and Description	Amount	Fat Grams	Total Calories	% Fat Calories
Naturally Rising Pizza/9 Inch				
cheese	⅓ pizza	10.0	300	30%
combination w/sausage & pepperoni	¼ pizza	14.0	300	42%
pepperoni	⅓ pizza	16.0	360	40%
sausage	⅓ pizza	16.0	360	40%
the works	¼ pizza	12.0	280	39%
Naturally Rising Pizza/12 Inch				
bacon cheeseburger	⅙ pizza	15.0	350	39%
Canadian style bacon	⅙ pizza	9.0	280	29%
cheese	⅙ pizza	10.0	290	31%
combination w/sausage & pepperoni	⅙ pizza	17.0	360	43%
pepperoni	⅙ pizza	16.0	350	41%
pepperoni supreme	⅙ pizza	16.0	340	42%
sausage	⅙ pizza	15.0	340	40%
spicy Italian sausage	⅙ pizza	14.0	330	38%
the works	⅙ pizza	14.0	330	38%
Original Pizza/12 Inch				
Canadian style bacon	¼ pizza	10.0	280	32%
cheese	⅓ pizza	13.0	350	33%
hamburger	¼ pizza	14.0	300	42%
pepperoni	¼ pizza	15.0	330	41%
sausage	¼ pizza	14.0	300	42%
spicy Italian sausage	¼ pizza	13.0	290	40%
Pizza Bursts				
combination sausage & pepperoni	6 pieces	12.0	250	43%
pepperoni	6 pieces	14.0	260	48%
sausage	6 pieces	12.0	250	43%
supercheese	6 pieces	12.0	250	43%
supreme	6 pieces	13.0	250	47%
■ **(Jenos)**				
Crisp 'n Tasty Pizza				
Canadian-style bacon	1 pizza	19.0	440	39%
cheese	1 pizza	19.0	460	37%
combination	1 pizza	28.0	520	48%
hamburger	1 pizza	25.0	500	45%
pepperoni	1 pizza	27.0	510	48%
sausage	1 pizza	28.0	520	48%
supreme	1 pizza	28.0	520	48%
three meat	1 pizza	26.0	500	47%
■ **(Kid's Kitchen) Pizza Wedges**				
3-cheese	1 cup	7.0	270	23%
cheeseburger	1 cup	5.0	250	18%
pepperoni	1 cup	8.0	260	28%
■ **LEAN CUISINE** (*See* FROZEN ENTRÉE/DINNER)				
■ **LUNCHABLES** (*See* Oscar Mayer in this section)				
■ **(Marie Callender's)** (*See* FROZEN ENTRÉE/DINNER)				
■ **(Michelina's)**				
Pizza singles				
cheese	1 pizza	19.0	380	45%

Food and Description	Amount	Fat Grams	Total Calories	% Fat Calories
combination	1 pizza	22.0	400	50%
pepperoni	1 pizza	22.0	410	48%
supreme	1 pizza	22.0	400	50%
Pizza Snack Rolls				
cheese	6 rolls	12.0	230	47%
combination	6 rolls	12.0	230	47%
four meat	6 rolls	12.0	230	47%
hamburger	6 rolls	11.0	220	45%
nacho cheese	6 rolls	10.0	220	41%
pepperoni	6 rolls	13.0	240	49%
That'za Pizza!				
cheese	1 pizza	18.0	370	44%
pepperoni	1 pizza	21.0	400	47%
■ **(Oscar Mayer) Lunchables/Fun Pack**				
extra cheesey	1 pizza	15.0	450	30%
pizza dunks	1 pizza	14.0	510	25%
pizza swirls	1 pizza	18.0	490	33%
■ **(Pepperidge Farm)**				
Croissant Crust Pizza				
cheese	1 pizza	23.0	430	48%
deluxe	1 pizza	23.0	440	47%
pepperoni	1 pizza	22.0	420	47%
■ **(Red Baron)**				
Bake To Rise				
four-cheese	⅙ pizza	13.0	340	34%
meat trio	⅙ pizza	14.0	360	35%
pepperoni	⅙ pizza	14.0	350	36%
sausage	⅙ pizza	14.0	350	36%
special deluxe	⅙ pizza	14.0	340	37%
supreme	⅙ pizza	16.0	360	38%
Deep Dish Breakfast/5 Inch				
bacon scramble	½ pizza	25.0	440	51%
ham scramble	½ pizza	18.0	360	45%
sausage & gravy	½ pizza	20.0	380	47%
sausage scramble	½ pizza	20.0	380	47%
Western scramble	½ pizza	22.0	400	50%
Deep Dish Single-Serve /5 Inch				
4-cheese	1 pizza	27.0	480	51%
cheese	1 pizza	25.0	460	49%
meat trio	1 pizza	28.0	470	54%
pepperoni	1 pizza	30.0	500	54%
sausage	1 pizza	28.0	480	53%
special deluxe	1 pizza	28.0	470	54%
supreme	1 pizza	27.0	460	53%
vegetable supreme	1 pizza	24.0	440	49%
Original/12 Inch				
Canadian bacon	¼ pizza	19.0	380	45%
cheese	¼ pizza	22.0	420	47%
hamburger	⅕ pizza	18.0	330	55%
Mexican style	⅕ pizza	22.0	360	50%

Food and Description	Amount	Fat Grams	Total Calories	% Fat Calories
pepperoni	¼ pizza	26.0	440	51%
pepperoni deluxe	⅕ pizza	18.0	350	46%
sausage	⅕ pizza	19.0	340	50%
sausage & mushroom	⅕ pizza	18.0	350	46%
sausage & pepperoni	⅕ pizza	21.0	360	53%
special deluxe	⅕ pizza	19.0	340	50%
supreme	⅕ pizza	20.0	350	51%
■ **(San Francisco Foods)**				
Calzones				
bacon, egg, & cheese	½ calzone	20.0	370	49%
5-cheese	½ calzone	11.0	280	35%
ham & cheddar	½ calzone	14.0	340	37%
ham & Swiss	½ calzone	13.0	330	35%
pepperoni	½ calzone	13.0	300	39%
sausage, egg, & cheese	½ calzone	17.0	350	44%
spinach & feta	½ calzone	10.0	280	32%
supreme	½ calzone	16.0	310	46%
western omelette	½ calzone	12.0	300	36%
Stuffed Pizza				
5-cheese	¼ pizza	15.0	420	32%
meat combo	¼ pizza	16.0	430	33%
pepperoni	¼ pizza	16.0	410	35%
spinach & feta	¼ pizza	16.0	400	36%
supreme	¼ pizza	17.0	400	38%
western chicken	¼ pizza	12.0	310	35%
■ **(Schwan's)**				
Deep Dish 10-½ Inch				
four cheese	¼ pizza	13.0	320	37%
Meat Trio	¼ pizza	14.0	330	38%
pepperoni	¼ pizza	16.0	350	41%
supreme	¼ pizza	15.0	340	40%
Deep-dish single-serve pizza				
cheese	1 pizza	26.0	500	47%
pepperoni	1 pizza	30.0	540	50%
sausage	1 pizza	29.0	520	50%
supreme	1 pizza	27.0	490	50%
Self-Rising				
cheese	⅕ pizza	16.0	390	37%
pepperoni	⅙ pizza	16.0	360	40%
supreme	⅙ pizza	16.0	370	39%
Special Recipe Pizza				
Canadian bacon	⅓ pizza	23.0	430	48%
pepperoni	⅓ pizza	28.0	470	54%
sausage	¼ pizza	24.0	380	57%
sausage & pepperoni	¼ pizza	22.0	380	52%
supreme	¼ pizza	22.0	370	54%
■ **(Stouffer's)** (*See* FROZEN ENTRÉE/DINNER)				
■ **(Tombstone)**				
double top pizza				
pepperoni w/double cheese	⅙ pizza	20.0	350	51%

Food and Description	Amount	Fat Grams	Total Calories	% Fat Calories
sausage & pepperoni	⅙ pizza	20.0	360	50%
sausage w/double cheese	⅙ pizza	19.0	350	49%
lower fat pizza				
light				
supreme	⅕ pizza	9.0	270	30%
vegetable	⅕ pizza	7.0	240	26%
original				
9 Inch				
deluxe	⅓ pizza	13.0	280	42%
extra cheese	½ pizza	16.0	380	38%
hamburger	⅓ pizza	13.0	280	42%
pepperoni	⅓ pizza	15.0	300	45%
pepperoni & sausage	⅓ pizza	15.0	300	45%
sausage	⅓ pizza	13.0	280	42%
supreme	⅓ pizza	16.0	310	46%
12 Inch				
Canadian style bacon	¼ pizza	14.0	350	36%
deluxe	⅕ pizza	14.0	310	36%
extra cheese	¼ pizza	15.0	350	39%
hamburger	⅕ pizza	15.0	310	44%
pepperoni	¼ pizza	21.0	400	47%
sausage	⅕ pizza	14.0	300	42%
sausage & mushroom	⅕ pizza	14.0	300	42%
sausage & pepperoni	⅕ pizza	16.0	320	45%
supreme	⅕ pizza	16.0	320	45%
Double-Top				
pepperoni	⅙ pizza	19.0	340	50%
sausage	⅙ pizza	17.0	320	48%
sausage & pepperoni	⅙ pizza	19.0	340	50%
supreme	⅕ pizza	19.0	380	45%
two cheese	⅕ pizza	19.0	380	45%
Light				
supreme	⅕ pizza	9.0	270	30%
vegetable	⅕ pizza	7.0	240	26%
Oven-Rising Crust				
Italian sausage	⅙ pizza	13.0	320	37%
pepperoni	⅙ pizza	15.0	340	40%
supreme	⅙ pizza	14.0	320	39%
three cheese	⅙ pizza	13.0	320	37%
three meat	⅙ pizza	15.0	340	40%
Thin-crust				
four meat combo	¼ pizza	23.0	380	54%
Italian sausage	¼ pizza	22.0	370	54%
pepperoni	¼ pizza	25.0	400	56%
supreme	¼ pizza	22.0	380	52%
supreme taco	¼ pizza	23.0	370	56%
three cheese	¼ pizza	21.0	360	53%
Tombstone For One				
Lower-fat/½ less fat				
cheese	1 pizza	10.0	360	25%

Food and Description	Amount	Fat Grams	Total Calories	% Fat Calories
vegetable	1 pizza	9.0	360	23%
regular				
extra cheese	1 pizza	28.0	520	48%
pepperoni	1 pizza	32.0	550	52%
supreme	1 pizza	32.0	550	52%
■ **(Tony's)**				
Mini Pizza For One				
Canadian bacon	1 pizza	28.0	510	49%
cheese	1 pizza	31.0	560	50%
pepperoni	1 pizza	36.0	610	53%
sausage	1 pizza	37.0	620	54%
sausage & pepperoni	1 pizza	41.0	700	53%
supreme	1 pizza	38.0	640	53%
taco	1 pizza	33.0	590	50%
Stuffed Crust				
four-cheese	⅕ pizza	10.0	310	29%
pepperoni	⅕ pizza	13.0	340	34%
sausage & pepperoni	⅕ pizza	13.0	340	34%
supreme	⅕ pizza	13.0	350	33%
vegetable medley	⅕ pizza	8.0	280	26%
Super Rise				
four-cheese	¼ pizza	13.0	340	34%
meat trio	¼ pizza	17.0	380	40%
pepperoni	¼ pizza	18.0	390	42%
sausage	¼ pizza	18.0	390	42%
sausage & pepperoni	⅕ pizza	18.0	380	43%
supreme	⅕ pizza	15.0	310	44%
W/Italian-Style Pastry Crust				
Canadian bacon	⅓ pizza	22.0	390	51%
cheese	⅓ pizza	21.0	400	47%
four-cheese	⅓ pizza	24.0	410	53%
hamburger	⅓ pizza	25.0	420	54%
meat trio	¼ pizza	21.0	340	56%
pepperoni	⅓ pizza	27.0	430	57%
sausage	⅓ pizza	27.0	440	55%
sausage & mushroom	¼ pizza	19.0	340	50%
sausage & pepperoni	⅓ pizza	28.0	460	55%
supreme	¼ pizza	20.0	330	55%
taco	¼ pizza	22.0	340	58%
■ **(Totino's)**				
Family Size				
cheese	⅓ pizza	16.0	370	39%
combination	¼ pizza	17.0	310	49%
pepperoni	⅓ pizza	22.0	410	48%
sausage	¼ pizza	16.0	300	48%
Party Pizza				
bacon	½ pizza	21.0	380	50%
Canadian style bacon	½ pizza	15.0	330	41%
cheese	½ pizza	14.0	320	39%
combination	½ pizza	21.0	390	48%

Food and Description	Amount	Fat Grams	Total Calories	% Fat Calories
hamburger	½ pizza	20.0	380	47%
pepperoni	½ pizza	21.0	380	50%
sausage	½ pizza	20.0	380	47%
sausage & mushroom	½ pizza	19.0	360	48%
sausage & sliced pepperoni	½ pizza	21.0	390	48%
sliced pepperoni	½ pizza	21.0	380	50%
supreme	½ pizza	21.0	390	48%
three-meat	½ pizza	19.0	360	48%
zesty Italiano	½ pizza	21.0	390	48%
Pizza For One/microwave French Bread				
cheese	1 pizza	11.0	240	41%
combination	1 pizza	18.0	310	52%
pepperoni	1 pizza	16.0	290	50%
sausage	1 pizza	17.0	290	53%
supreme	1 pizza	17.0	300	51%
Pizza Rolls				
cheese	6 rolls	8.0	210	34%
combination	6 rolls	12.0	230	47%
pepperoni	6 rolls	12.0	240	45%
pepperoni supreme	6 rolls	10.0	220	41%
sausage	6 rolls	11.0	230	43%
supreme	6 rolls	10.0	220	41%
three-meat	6 rolls	10.0	220	41%
Select Pizza				
sausage & pepperoni	⅓ pizza	19.0	360	48%
supreme	⅓ pizza	18.0	340	48%
three-cheese	⅓ pizza	14.0	300	42%
two-cheese & Canadian style bacon	⅓ pizza	14.0	310	41%
two-cheese & pepperoni	⅓ pizza	20.0	360	50%
two-cheese & sausage	⅓ pizza	19.0	360	48%
■ **(Weight Watchers)** (*See* FROZEN ENTRÉE/DINNER)				
■ **(Wolfgang Puck)**				
artichoke heart	½ pizza	17.0	340	45%
barbecue chicken				
4-servings pizza	¼ pizza	13.0	370	32%
2-servings pizza	½ pizza	11.0	340	29%
cheese	¼ pizza	10.0	300	30%
four cheeses	½ pizza	15.0	360	38%
grilled vegetable/fat-free	½ pizza	–	200	–
mushroom & spinach	½ pizza	8.0	270	27%
pepperoni & mushroom				
4-servings pizza	¼ pizza	15.0	360	38%
2-servings pizza	½ pizza	15.0	390	35%
sausage & herb	½ pizza	18.0	380	43%
spicy chicken				
4-servings pizza	¼ pizza	18.0	380	43%
2-servings pizza	½ pizza	16.0	360	40%
supreme				
4-servings pizza	¼ pizza	17.0	400	38%
2-servings pizza	½ pizza	17.0	400	38%

Food and Description	Amount	Fat Grams	Total Calories	% Fat Calories
turkey sausage	½ pizza	13.0	320	37%
vegetable				
4-servings pizza	¼ pizza	15.0	360	38%
2-servings pizza	½ pizza	13.0	350	33%
zucchini & tomato	½ pizza	11.0	290	34%
PIZZA CRUST				
(Boboli) Italian bread shell/prebaked/ready to use				
12" size/single or family pack	⅛ shell	3.0	170	16%
thin crust	⅕ shell	3.5	160	20%
(Chef Boyardee) Quick & Easy mix	⅓ pkg	1.5	150	9%
(Jiffy) mix/prepared	¼ crust	3.0	180	15%
(Mama Mary's) fresh baked gourmet				
7" dia	⅙ slice	5.0	200	23%
12" dia				
original	1/12 slice	5.0	200	23%
deep dish	1/12 slice	5.0	200	23%
(Martha White) Mix/crust only				
crispy crust	1 slice	1.0	170	5%
deep pan	1 slice	1.0	150	6%
(Pillsbury) refrigerated	¼ crust	2.5	180	13%
(Ragu) Pizza Quick/mix only	⅓ cup	1.0	130	7%
(Robin Hood) mix/prepared	¼ crust	2.0	160	11%
(Totino's)	¼ crust	7.0	180	35%
PIZZA SAUCE (*See also* SAUCE)				
(Borden) traditional	¼ cup	–	20	–
(Contadina)				
4 cheese	¼ cup	0.5	30	17%
original	¼ cup	–	30	–
pepperoni flavored	¼ cup	1.0	35	26%
squeeze	¼ cup	–	30	–
(Progresso)	¼ cup	1.0	35	26%
(Ragu) Pizza Quick				
chunky mushroom	¼ cup	1.5	40	34%
chunky tomato	¼ cup	1.5	50	27%
garlic & basil	¼ cup	1.5	40	34%
100% natural	¼ cup	1.0	30	30%
pepperoni flavored	¼ cup	2.0	60	30%
traditional	¼ cup	1.5	40	34%
PLANTAIN/BAKING BANANA/COOKING BANANA				
cooked/sliced	1 cup	<1.0	180	3%
raw				
sliced	½ cup	<1.0	90	3%
whole	1 medium	1.0	220	4%
PLUM				
canned				
generic/purple				
in extra heavy syrup				
w/liquid	1 cup	–	265	–

Food and Description	Amount	Fat Grams	Total Calories	% Fat Calories
w/o liquid	½ cup	–	135	–
in heavy syrup				
w/liquid	1 cup	–	230	–
w/o liquid	½ cup	–	115	–
in juice				
w/liquid	1 cup	–	145	–
w/o liquid	½ cup	–	75	–
in light syrup				
w/liquid	1 cup	–	160	–
w/o liquid	½ cup	–	80	–
in water				
w/liquid	1 cup	–	105	–
w/o liquid	½ cup	–	50	–
(S&W) whole purple/in heavy syrup	½ cup	–	130	–
(Solo) prune/plum filling	2 Tbs	–	70	–
(Stokely) in light syrup	½ cup	–	100	–
fresh/raw				
sliced	½ cup	–	90	–
whole	1 medium	<1.0	36	13%
POI	½ cup	–	135	–
POKEBERRY /fresh				
cooked	½ cup	–	16	–
raw	½ cup	–	20	–
POLENTA				
chilled				
(Melissa's)	4 oz	–	100	–
mix				
(Fantastic Foods) Polenta/mix only				
Cups				
Mediterranean	1.8 oz	3.0	200	14%
spicy Mexicana	1.8 oz	3.0	210	14%
Santa Fe	1.9 oz	3.0	220	12%
three cheese	1.8 oz	3.0	210	14%
International Dishes	⅜ cup	5.0	260	17%
POLISH SAUSAGE (See SAUSAGE)				
POLLACK/POLLOCK (See also SEAFOOD ENTRÉE/DINNER)				
Alaskan/walleye				
cooked-dry heat	3 oz	1.0	100	9%
raw	3 oz	0.7	70	9%
Atlantic/raw	3 oz	1.0	80	10%
POMEGRANATE /fresh	1 medium	0.5	104	4%
POMPANO /Florida				
breaded & fried	3 oz	17.0	270	57%
cooked-dry heat	3 oz	10.0	180	50%
raw	3 oz	8.0	140	51%
POP (See COCKTAIL MIXER; SOFT DRINK; SPORTS DRINK)				
POP TART (See PASTRY, TOASTER)				
POPCORN (See also POPCORN BARS & CAKES)				
(NOTE: Unless stated otherwise, data are for popped corn.)				

Food and Description	Amount	Fat Grams	Total Calories	% Fat Calories
(ACT I) microwave				
butter	3 cups	8.0	140	51%
extra butter	3 cups	10.0	160	56%
(Arrowhead Mills) unpopped	¼ cup	2.5	180	13%
(Bag OBeans)				
Apache red				
air-popped	1 cup	<1.0	27	17%
oil-popped	1 cup	1.4	33	38%
Hopi				
air-popped	1 cup	<1.0	27	17%
oil-popped	1 cup	1.4	33	38%
Kiowa black				
air-popped	1 cup	<1.0	27	17%
oil-popped	1 cup	1.4	33	38%
Painted Desert				
air-popped	1 cup	<1.0	27	17%
oil-popped	1 cup	1.4	33	38%
Paiute pearl				
air-popped	1 cup	<1.0	27	17%
oil-popped	1 cup	1.4	33	38%
Zuni				
air-popped	1 cup	<1.0	27	17%
oil-popped	1 cup	1.4	33	38%
(Bearitos) microwave				
all natural buttery	1 cup	4.0	60	60%
	1 bag	31.0	420	66%
lite buttery	1 cup	1.0	30	30%
	1 bag	9.0	230	35%
(Betty Crocker) Pop Secret				
jumbo pop/butter	1 cup	2.5	40	56%
Movie Theater/butter	1 cup	2.5	40	56%
regular				
butter				
light	1 cup	1.0	25	36%
	6 cups	5.0	130	35%
original	1 cup	2.5	35	64%
	4 cups	10.0	150	60%
natural				
light	1 cup	1.0	25	36%
	6 cups	5.0	130	35%
original	1 cup	2.5	35	64%
	4 cups	10.0	150	60%
94% Fat-Free				
butter	6 cups	2.0	110	16%
natural	6 cups	2.0	110	16%
(Black Jewel) microwaveable				
hulless	1¼ cups	8.0	150	48%
(Blue Heaven) microwaveable				
blue corn	2 cups	8.0	130	55%
(Borden) ready to eat				
butter-flavored	1 oz	10.0	150	60%

Food and Description	Amount	Fat Grams	Total Calories	% Fat Calories
tender eating				
baby rice popcorn	1 oz	13.0	170	69%
baby white popcorn	1 oz	13.0	170	69%
yellow popcorn	1 oz	13.0	170	69%
(Cape Cod)				
all natural	3½ cups	9.0	160	51%
old-fashioned butter	3 cups	10.0	170	53%
white cheddar	2⅓ cups	12.0	170	64%
(Chester's)				
microwave				
butter	5 cups	12.0	200	54%
natural	5 cups	12.0	200	54%
prepopped				
butter	3 cups	12.0	160	68%
cheddar cheese	3 cups	13.0	190	68%
(Cracker Jack)				
fat-free				
butter toffee	¾ cup	–	110	–
caramel	¾ cup	–	110	–
original	½ cup	2.0	120	15%
(Crunch & Munch) buttery popcorn w/peanuts				
almond supreme	1 oz	5.0	140	32%
caramel	1 oz	7.0	160	39%
toffee				
buttery	1 oz	6.0	150	36%
fat-free	1 oz	–	110	–
(Featherweight) microwaveable				
lite butter	1 bag	6.0	210	26%
lite natural	1 bag	2.0	160	11%
(Fit Foods) ready to eat	1 oz	–	120	–
decadent caramel	1 oz	–	120	–
(Frookie) Nature's Popcorn				
butter flavor	½ oz	3.0	70	39%
original	½ oz	2.0	70	26%
sour cream & chives	½ oz	3.0	70	39%
white cheddar	½ oz	3.0	80	34%
generic				
air-popped/no butter added	1 cup	–	30	–
caramel-coated				
plain	1 oz	3.0	122	22%
w/peanuts	1.5 oz	5.0	180	25%
oil-popped/no butter added	1 cup	3.0	55	49%
regular				
white/no butter added	4 cups	0.6	77	7%
yellow/no butter added	4 cups	0.8	77	9%
syrup-coated	1 cup	1.0	135	7%
(Greenfield) caramel/fat-free	⅔ cup	–	100	–
(Healthy Choice) microwaveable organic natural				
popped	1 serving	7.0	140	45%

Food and Description	Amount	Fat Grams	Total Calories	% Fat Calories
unpopped	3 Tbs	2.5	120	19%
(Jiffy Pop)				
bag				
butter	5 cups	14.0	180	70%
butter-flavored	5 cups	7.0	140	45%
natural/light	5 cups	7.0	140	45%
white cheddar cheese	5 cups	11.0	170	58%
microwaveable				
butter	3 cups	7.0	140	45%
regular	3 cups	7.0	140	45%
(Jolly Time)				
bag				
white/resealable	1 oz	0.5	100	5%
yellow	1 oz	1.0	100	9%
jar/American's Best				
white	1 oz	0.5	100	5%
yellow	1 oz	1.0	100	9%
microwaveable				
butter				
American's best butter/94% fat-free	1 oz	2.0	90	20%
Blast 'O Butter Theatre Style	1.16 oz	11.0	150	66%
Butter-licious	1.16 oz	9.0	140	58%
cheddar cheese	3 cups	10.0	160	56%
Crispy'N White/natural				
light	3 cups	5.0	120	38%
regular	3 cups	10.0	150	60%
Healthy Pop/94% fat-free butter	3 cups	2.0	90	20%
white & buttery	3 cups	9.0	150	54%
(Lance)				
cheese	⅝ oz	5.0	90	45%
plain	½ oz	5.0	80	56%
	1 oz	5.0	130	35%
white cheddar cheese	⅝ oz	8.0	100	72%
	⅞ oz	11.0	150	66%
	1½ oz	18.0	250	65%
(Lapida's Popcorn Co.) ready to eat				
caramel	2 cups	4.5	140	29%
herb corn	2 cups	11.0	170	37%
(Louise's) fat-free				
apple cinnamon	1 oz	–	100	–
buttery toffee	1 oz	–	100	–
caramel	1 oz	–	100	–
(Michael Seasons) Gourmet Sensations/ready-to-eat				
butter toffee w/pecans & almonds	¾ cup	6.0	130	42%
chocolate covered butter toffee	¾ cup	7.0	140	45%
(Newman's Own) Oldstyle Picture Show				
microwave				
butter				
Butter Boom	3½ cups	11.0	170	58%

Food and Description	Amount	Fat Grams	Total Calories	% Fat Calories
light	3½ cups	3.0	110	25%
natural				
light	3½ cups	3.0	110	25%
no salt	3½ cups	11.0	170	
original	3½ cups	11.0	170	58%
popcorn/plain kernels				
unpopped	3 Tbs	2.0	110	16%
(Old Vienna)				
butter	1 oz	10.0	160	56%
cheese	1 oz	10.0	160	56%
(Orville Redenbacher's) unpopped, unless otherwise specified				
butter toffee popcorn clusters/bag	1 oz	2.5	130	17%
hot air				
popped	3½ cups	–	40	–
unpopped	2 Tbs	1.5	90	15%
microwaveable				
butter				
light	2 Tbs	5.0	110	41%
no salt added	2 Tbs	12.0	160	68%
regular	2 Tbs	12.0	170	64%
Smart Pop/94% fat-free	2 Tbs	2.0	110	16%
cheddar cheese	2 Tbs	9.0	145	43%
homestyle	2 Tbs	11.0	170	58%
movie theater				
butter	2 Tbs	12.0	170	64%
light	2 Tbs	5.0	110	41%
plain	2 Tbs	13.0	175	67%
Pour Over Movie Theater/butter	2 Tbs	14.0	180	70%
natural				
light	2 Tbs	5.0	110	41%
no salt added	2 Tbs	12.0	175	62%
regular	2 Tbs	11.0	15	60%
regular popcorn kernels/unpopped				
original	2 Tbs	1.5	90	15%
white	2 Tbs	1.5	90	15%
(Pop Secret) (*See* Betty Crocker in this section)				
(Poppycock) ready to eat				
popcorn, pecans, & almonds	½ cup	10.0	180	50%
(Pops-Rite)				
butter	3 cups	5.0	90	50%
natural	3 cups	5.0	90	50%
(Smartfood)				
Reduced-fat				
golden butter	3½ cups	4.0	130	28%
white cheddar cheese	3 cups	6.0	140	39%
Regular/white cheddar cheese	2 cups	12.0	190	57%
(Vic's) Corn Popper/ready to eat				
butter				
low-fat	3 cups	1.5	120	11%

Food and Description	Amount	Fat Grams	Total Calories	% Fat Calories
· regular	2½ cups	7.0	150	42%
caramel				
fat-free	1 cup	–	110	–
lite	1 cup	2.0	110	16%
regular	¾ cup	4.0	130	28%
cheese				
white				
lite	2½ cups	6.0	130	42%
regular	2 cups	13.0	180	65%
yellow				
lite	2½ cups	7.0	140	45%
regular	1½ cups	14.0	190	66%
white				
lite				
full salt	2¾ cups	3.0	130	21%
½ salt	2¾ cups	3.0	130	21%
low-fat	3½ cups	1.0	110	8%
regular				
full salt	2½ cups	6.0	150	36%
½ salt	2½ cups	6.0	150	36%
white CDR/low-fat	3½ cups	2.5	110	20%
(Weaver's) Mrs Weaver's home-popped	3 cups	8.0	140	51%
(Weight Watchers)				
microwaveable	1 pouch	1.0	100	9%
ready to eat				
butter	0.66 oz	3.0	90	30%
butter-free	0.9 oz	2.5	110	20%
butter toffee	0.9 oz	3.0	110	25%
caramel	0.9 oz	1.0	100	9%
white cheddar	0.66 oz	4.0	90	40%
(Wise) ready to eat				
buttery cheddar	1 oz	11.0	160	62%
hot cheese flavored	1 oz	9.0	150	54%
lite butter	1 oz	5.0	140	32%
original butter	1 oz	10.0	150	60%
white cheddar cheese	1 oz	11.0	160	62%
POPCORN BARS & CAKES (See also RICE CAKES)				
(Hain)				
butter				
mini	7 cakes	–	60	–
regular	1 cake	1.0	45	20%
caramel/mini	5 cakes	–	60	–
lightly salted/mini	7 cakes	–	50	–
mild cheddar/mini	6 cakes	2.0	70	26%
nacho cheese/regular	1 cake	1.0	45	20%
plain/regular	1 cake	–	35	–
white cheddar/regular	1 cake	1.0	45	20%
(Konriko) popcorn cakes				
butter	1 cake	–	40	–
lightly salted	1 cake	–	40	–

Food and Description	Amount	Fat Grams	Total Calories	% Fat Calories
(Lundberg) Organic				
lightly salted	1 cake	1.0	60	15%
rye w/caraway seeds	1 cake	–	60	–
unsalted	1 cake	1.0	60	15%
(Mother's)				
butter-flavored	1 cake	–	35	–
unsalted	1 cake	–	35	–
(Orville Redenbacher's)				
caramel				
mini	6 cakes	1.0	60	15%
regular	1 cake	–	60	–
chocolate peanut crunch				
mini	6 cakes	1.0	60	15%
regular	1 cake	–	60	–
peanut caramel crunch				
mini	6 cakes	1.0	60	15%
regular	1 cake	–	60	–
(Quaker)				
butter				
mini	6 cakes	1.0	50	18%
regular	1 cake	–	35	–
caramel				
mini	5 cakes	1.0	50	18%
regular	1 cake	–	50	–
cheddar cheese/mini	6 cakes	1.0	50	18%
Monterey Jack				
mini	6 cakes	1.0	50	18%
regular	1 cake	–	40	–
strawberry crunch	1 cake	–	50	–
white cheddar				
mini	6 cakes	1.0	50	18%
regular	1 cake	–	40	–
POPCORN OIL (*See* OIL)				
POPPY SEED (*See also* POPPY SEED FILLING)				
	1 tsp	1.0	15	60%
	1 Tbs	4.0	50	72%
POPPY SEED FILLING				
(Solo)	2 Tbs	4.0	140	26%
POPSICLE (*See* FRUIT ICES, BARS, & POPS; ICE CREAM BARS, SANDWICHES, & FROZEN NOVELTIES)				
PORGY				
beaded & fried	3 oz	13.0	246	48%
cooked-dry heat	3 oz	8.7	172	46%

PORK (*See also* BACON; HAM; LUNCHEON MEAT; PORK DINNER/ENTRÉE; SAUSAGE)
(NOTE: The information listed under Today's Leaner Pork was provided by the National Pork, Livestock, and Meat Board. Following this is nutritional information provided by the United States Department of Agriculture. "Lean" means pork trimmed of separable fat before cooking, "Lean & fat" means untrimmed and cooked or eaten as purchased. Prime cuts have the most fat; choice cuts less; and select cuts the least. In most cases, 4 ounces of raw pork yields approximately 3 ounces cooked. Serving amounts do not include bone.)

Food and Description	Amount	Fat Grams	Total Calories	% Fat Calories
■ **TODAY'S LEANER PORK**				
(Note: Unless otherwise stated, meat has been trimmed of all separable fat and roasted.)				
blade steak	3 oz	10.7	193	50%
center loin chop	3 oz	6.9	165	38%
center rib chop	3 oz	8.3	179	43%
loin chop	3 oz	6.6	173	34%
loin roast	3 oz	6.0	165	33%
rib chop	3 oz	8.3	186	41%
rib roast	3 oz	8.6	182	43%
ribs (country style)	3 oz	12.6	210	54%
sirloin chop	3 oz	5.7	164	31%
sirloin roast	3 oz	8.7	184	43%
tenderloin	3 oz	4.0	139	26%
top loin chop	3 oz	6.6	165	36%
■ **PORK CUTS/FRESH**				
backfat/raw	1 oz	24.0	230	94%
	3.5 oz	84.5	812	94%
backribs/lean & fat/roasted	3 oz	23.0	315	66%
	7.7 oz	58.5	815	65%
belly/raw	1 oz	14.0	150	84%
	1 lb	225.5	2,350	86%
center loin/bone in				
chop				
lean				
braised	3 oz	6.5	175	33%
broiled	3 oz	6.0	170	32%
pan-fried	3 oz	8.0	200	36%
lean & fat				
braised	3 oz	11.0	210	47%
broiled	3 oz	10.0	205	44%
pan-fried	3 oz	13.0	235	50%
roast/roasted				
lean	3 oz	7.0	170	36%
lean & fat	3 oz	10.5	200	47%
composite cuts				
loin & shoulder blade				
lean/cooked	3 oz	7.0	180	35%
lean & fat/cooked	3 oz	11.0	215	46%
ground				
cooked	3 oz	16.0	250	58%
	1 lb	59.0	930	57%
raw	4 oz	22.0	300	66%
leg				
rump half				
lean				
roasted	3 oz	6.5	175	33%
roasted/chopped or diced	1 cup	10.0	280	32%
lean & fat				
roasted	3 oz	11.0	215	46%

Food and Description	Amount	Fat Grams	Total Calories	% Fat Calories
roasted/chopped or diced	1 cup	17.5	340	46%
shank half				
lean				
roasted	3 oz	8.0	185	39%
roasted/chopped or diced	1 cup	13.0	290	40%
lean & fat				
roasted	3 oz	15.5	245	57%
roasted/chopped or diced	1 cup	24.5	390	57%
whole				
lean				
roasted	3 oz	7.5	180	37%
roasted/chopped or diced	1 cup	11.5	285	36%
lean & fat				
roasted	3 oz	13.5	230	53%
roasted/chopped or diced	1 cup	21.5	370	52%
loin				
blade/bone-in/chop				
lean				
braised	3 oz	10.0	190	47%
broiled	3 oz	10.5	200	47%
pan-fried	3 oz	11.5	205	50%
roasted	3 oz	11.0	210	47%
lean & fat				
braised	3 oz	19.5	275	64%
broiled	3 oz	19.0	275	62%
pan-fried	3 oz	21.0	290	65%
roasted	3 oz	19.0	275	62%
center rib				
chop/bone-in				
lean				
braised	3 oz	7.5	175	39%
broiled	3 oz	7.0	190	33%
pan-fried	3 oz	9.0	185	44%
lean & fat				
braised	3 oz	12.0	215	50%
broiled	3 oz	12.0	225	48%
pan-fried	3 oz	13.5	225	54%
chop/boneless				
lean				
braised	3 oz	8.0	180	40%
broiled	3 oz	7.5	185	36%
pan-fried	3 oz	9.5	190	45%
lean & fat				
braised	3 oz	12.5	215	52%
broiled	3 oz	12.0	220	49%
pan-fried	3 oz	14.0	235	54%
roast/bone-in				
lean/roasted	3 oz	9.0	190	43%
lean & fat/roasted	3 oz	12.0	220	49%

Food and Description	Amount	Fat Grams	Total Calories	% Fat Calories
roast/boneless				
lean/roasted	3 oz	7.5	185	36%
lean & fat/roasted	3 oz	11.5	215	48%
ribs/country style				
lean				
braised	3 oz	10.0	200	45%
roasted	3 oz	11.0	210	47%
lean & fat				
braised	3 oz	16.5	250	59%
roasted	3 oz	19.0	280	61%
whole				
lean				
braised	3 oz	7.0	175	36%
broiled	3 oz	7.5	180	38%
roasted	3 oz	7.0	180	35%
lean & fat				
braised	3 oz	11.0	210	47%
broiled	3 oz	11.0	210	52%
roasted	3 oz	11.0	210	52%
shoulder				
arm picnic				
lean				
braised	3 oz	9.5	215	40%
braised/chopped or diced	1 cup	22.0	490	40%
roasted	3 oz	10.0	195	45%
roasted/chopped or diced	1 cup	22.0	435	46%
lean & fat				
braised	3 oz	18.0	280	58%
braised/chopped or diced	1 cup	28.5	445	58%
roasted	3 oz	18.5	270	62%
roasted/chopped or diced	1 cup	29.5	430	62%
Boston blade				
roast				
lean				
raw	1 lb	30.5	555	49%
roasted	3 oz	11.0	200	50%
lean & fat				
raw	1 lb	44.5	705	57%
roasted	3 oz	14.5	230	57%
steak				
lean				
braised	3 oz	12.0	235	47%
broiled	3 oz	9.5	195	44%
lean & fat				
braised	3 oz	16.5	270	55%
broiled	3 oz	12.5	220	51%
whole				
lean				
roasted	3 oz	10.5	200	47%

Food and Description	Amount	Fat Grams	Total Calories	% Fat Calories
roasted/chopped or diced	1 cup	16.5	315	47%
lean & fat				
roasted	3 oz	16.5	250	59%
roasted/chopped or diced	1 cup	26.0	395	59%
sirloin				
chop/bone in				
lean				
braised	3 oz	7.0	170	37%
broiled	3 oz	7.5	180	37%
lean & fat				
braised	3 oz	11.5	210	49%
broiled	3 oz	12.0	220	49%
chop/boneless				
lean				
braised	3 oz	5.0	150	30%
broiled	3 oz	5.0	165	27%
lean & fat				
braised	3 oz	6.5	160	37%
broiled	3 oz	6.0	180	30%
roast/bone in				
lean				
raw	1 lb	19.0	450	38%
roasted	3 oz	8.0	185	39%
lean & fat				
raw	1 lb	32.5	600	49%
roasted	3 oz	12.0	225	48%
roast/boneless	3 oz	5.5	165	30%
lean				
raw	1 lb	22.5	610	33%
roasted	3 oz	6.0	170	32%
lean & fat				
raw	1 lb	26.5	650	37%
roasted	3 oz	7.0	180	35%
spareribs/lean & fat				
braised	3 oz	23.5	340	62%
raw	1 lb	48.5	700	62%
tenderloin				
lean				
broiled	3 oz	4.5	160	25%
raw	1 lb	13.5	545	22%
roasted	3 oz	3.5	140	23%
lean & fat				
broiled	3 oz	6.0	170	32%
roasted	3 oz	4.5	150	27%
top loin				
chop/boneless				
lean				
braised	3 oz	6.5	170	34%
broiled	3 oz	6.0	175	31%
pan-fried	3 oz	8.0	190	38%

Food and Description	Amount	Fat Grams	Total Calories	% Fat Calories
lean & fat				
braised	3 oz	10.0	200	45%
broiled	3 oz	8.5	195	41%
pan-fried	3 oz	11.5	220	47%
roast/boneless				
lean/roasted	3 oz	5.5	165	30%
lean & fat				
raw	1 lb	31.0	690	40%
roasted	3 oz	9.0	195	42%
■ PORK CUTS, ORGAN & OTHER/FRESH				
brain/braised	3 oz	4.5	120	33%
	13.5 oz	18.0	530	31%
chitterlings/chitlins/simmered	3 oz	23.0	260	80%
	6 oz	46.0	520	80%
ear/simmered	1 ear	–	185	–
	15 oz	–	700	–
feet/simmered	2.5 oz	8.0	140	51%
	5 oz	16.0	275	52%
heart				
braised	1 heart	5.0	190	24%
braised/chopped or diced	1 cup	5.5	215	23%
jowl/raw	4 oz	75.0	740	91%
kidney				
braised	3 oz	3.0	130	21%
braised/chopped or diced	1 cup	5.0	215	22%
liver/braised	3 oz	2.5	140	16%
lung/braised	3 oz	2.0	85	21%
pancreas/braised	3 oz	–	190	–
salt pork/cured/raw				
(Country Creek)	2 oz	25.0	260	87%
generic	1 oz	22.0	215	92%
	8 oz	174.0	1700	92%
spleen/braised	3 oz	2.0	130	14%
stomach/raw	4 oz	–	180	–
tail				
raw	4 oz	35.0	430	73%
simmered	3 oz	28.0	340	74%
tongue/braised	3 oz	14.5	230	57%
PORK & BEANS (*See* BEANS, BAKED & VARIETY)				
PORK ENTRÉE/DINNER (*See also* ASIAN FOOD; FROZEN ENTRÉE/DINNER)				
(Delores)				
pickled pork rinds	2 oz	3.0	60	30%
pig's feet	2 oz	6.0	90	60%
Generic/pork brains in milk gravy	⅔ cup	5.0	150	30%
(Grandad's) real bacon rinds	½ oz	1.5	60	23%
Homemade/USDA Standard Home Recipe				
ham croquette	~2 oz	9.8	165	54%
pickled pig's feet	1 oz	4.0	60	60%
	1 lb	67.5	925	66%
(Hormel)				
pickled pig's feet	2 oz	6.0	80	68%

Food and Description	Amount	Fat Grams	Total Calories	% Fat Calories
pickled pork hocks	2 oz	8.0	110	65%
pickled pork tidbits	2 oz	8.0	100	72%
(Schwan's) frozen pork products				
BBQ baby back ribs	5 oz	22.0	370	54%
center cut pork loin chops	5.7 oz	16.0	270	53%
pork loin chop/boneless	6 oz	12.0	250	43%
pork roast/oven-roasted	3 oz	3.0	100	27%

PORK FAT (*See* LARD)
PORK RINDS (*See* PORK ENTRÉE DINNER; SNACKS)
PORK SAUSAGE (*See* SAUSAGE)
POT PIE (*See* BEEF DISH/ENTRÉE; CHICKEN ENTRÉE/DINNER; FROZEN ENTRÉE/DINNER; TURKEY ENTRÉE/DINNER; VEGETARIAN FOODS)
POTATO (*See also* POTATO DISH/ENTRÉE; SWEET POTATO; YAM)

Food and Description	Amount	Fat Grams	Total Calories	% Fat Calories
canned				
(Bush's Best)				
diced	½ cup	–	40	–
sliced	½ cup	–	40	–
whole	½ cup	–	40	–
(Del Monte) new				
sliced	⅔ cup	–	60	–
whole w/liquid	~2 medium	–	60	–
generic/ w/o skin	½ cup	–	54	–
(S&W)	½ cup	–	60	–
(Seneca)	⅔ cup	–	80	–
(Veg All)	½ cup	–	60	–
flakes/granules				
(Betty Crocker) Potato Buds				
original				
mix only	⅓ cup	–	80	–
prepared				
reduced fat recipe	⅔ cup	4.0	120	30%
regular recipe	⅔ cup	8.0	160	45%
generic/mix only				
flakes	1 cup	–	164	–
granules	1 cup	1.0	70	1%
(Hungry Jack) prepared				
complete mashed potatoes	½ cup	1.0	120	8%
flakes/mashed/prepared	½ cup	7.0	160	39%
(Idaho) Mashed Potatoes/prepared w/2% milk and margarine				
flakes	½ cup	6.0	150	36%
granules	½ cup	7.0	160	39%
(Idahoan) mix only				
cheddar/spicy	⅙ pkg	1.0	90	10%
real	⅓ cup	1.0	80	11%
fresh				
baked				
in microwave				
w/skin	1 large	–	212	–
w/o skin	1 large	–	156	–

Food and Description	Amount	Fat Grams	Total Calories	% Fat Calories
in oven				
skin only	1 medium	–	115	–
w/skin	~7 oz	–	220	–
w/o skin	~5.5 oz	–	145	–
boiled				
w/skin	½ cup	–	68	–
w/o skin	½ cup	–	67	–
raw				
w/skin	1 medium	–	110	–
w/o skin	1 medium	–	88	–
	~4.75 oz	–	116	–
frozen				
(C&W) whole red	2 large or 3 small	–	60	–
POTATO CHIPS & SNACKS (*See also* SNACKS)				
(Barbara's)				
no salt added	1¼ cups	10.0	150	60%
regular	1¼ cups	10.0	150	60%
ripple	1¼ cup	10.0	150	60%
yogurt & green onion	1¼ cups	9.0	150	54%
(Borden)				
Calypso/sweet & spicy Caribbean	1 oz	10.0	160	56%
Curlie/plain	1 oz	10.0	150	60%
home fries	1 oz	10.0	150	60%
Krunchers				
jalapeño	1 oz	8.0	140	51%
mesquite barbecue	1 oz	8.0	140	51%
original	1 oz	9.0	150	54%
New York Deli				
jalapeño	1 oz	8.0	140	51%
plain	1 oz	10.0	150	60%
original				
BBQ	1 oz	10.0	160	56%
hot	1 oz	10.0	150	60%
lightly salted	1 oz	10.0	150	60%
onion & garlic	1 oz	10.0	150	60%
salt & vinegar	1 oz	10.0	150	60%
Ranch Fries				
no salt added	1 oz	10.0	150	60%
plain	1 oz	10.0	150	60%
Ridgies				
plain	1 oz	10.0	150	60%
super crispy	1 oz	10.0	150	60%
sour cream & onion/ridged	1 oz	10.0	150	60%
Texas BBQ	1 oz	10.0	150	60%
(Cape Cod)				
no salt	1 oz	10.0	150	60%
original	1 oz	8.0	150	48%
sea salt & vinegar	1 oz	8.0	150	48%

Food and Description	Amount	Fat Grams	Total Calories	% Fat Calories
select	1 oz	6.0	130	42%
sour cream & chive	1 oz	9.0	150	54%
(Fit Foods) baked potato chips				
BBQ	1 oz	–	100	–
original	1 oz	–	100	–
sour cream & chives	1 oz	–	100	–
(French's) Potato Sticks				
bar-b-q	1 oz	12.0	180	60%
original	1 oz	10.0	170	53%
	1.5 oz can	16.0	250	58%
(Frito Lay)				
Lay's baked potato crisps				
BBQ	1 oz	3.0	120	23%
original	1 oz	1.5	110	12%
sour cream & onion	1 oz	3.0	120	23%
Lay's original potato chips				
cheddar cheese	1 oz	10.0	150	60%
classic	1 oz	10.0	150	60%
deli style original	1 oz	10.0	150	60%
Flamin' Hot	1 oz	10.0	150	60%
KC Masterpiece BBQ	1 oz	10.0	150	60%
Limon	1 oz	10.0	150	60%
original	1 oz	10.0	150	60%
salt & vinegar	1 oz	10.0	160	56%
sour cream & onion	1 oz	9.0	160	51%
spicy BBQ	1 oz	9.0	150	51%
toasted onion & cheese	1 oz	10.0	160	60%
unsalted	1 oz	10.0	160	56%
wavy original	1 oz	10.0	160	56%
Ruffles baked potato chips				
cheddar & sour cream	1 oz	3.0	130	21%
regular	1 oz	3.0	130	21%
Ruffles original potato chips				
Buffalo style	1 oz	10.0	160	56%
cheddar & sour cream	1 oz	10.0	160	56%
flamin' hot	1 oz	10.0	150	60%
Flavor Rush				
big BBQ & cheddar	1 oz	10.0	160	56%
zesty sour cream & onion	1 oz	10.0	150	60%
French onion	1 oz	10.0	150	60%
KC Masterpiece BBQ	1 oz	10.0	160	60%
original	1 oz	10.0	150	60%
reduced fat	1 oz	7.0	140	45%
sour cream & onion	1 oz	10.0	150	60%
the works	1 oz	11.0	160	62%
Wow! fat-free potato chips				
Lay's				
mesquite BBQ	1 oz	–	75	–
original	1 oz	–	75	–
sour cream & chive	1 oz	–	80	–

Food and Description	Amount	Fat Grams	Total Calories	% Fat Calories
Ruffles'				
cheddar & sour cream	1 oz	–	75	–
original	1 oz	–	75	–
(Health Valley)				
Country Ripple				
no salt added	1 oz	10.0	160	60%
regular	1 oz	10.0	160	60%
Dip chips				
no salt added	1 oz	10.0	160	60%
regular	1 oz	10.0	160	60%
Natural				
no salt added	1 oz	10.0	160	60%
regular	1 oz	10.0	160	60%
(Jay's)				
Big "J"	1 oz	10.0	150	60%
Big "J" ridged	1 oz	10.0	150	60%
old fashioned kettle cooked	1 oz	9.0	150	54%
(Keebler) potato snack chips				
Ripplin's				
barbecue	12 chips	9.0	150	54%
original	12 chips	11.0	160	62%
ranch	12 chips	9.0	150	54%
Tato Skins				
baked potato	18 chips	8.0	150	48%
cheese n' bacon	18 chips	9.0	150	54%
sour cream n' onion	18 chips	10.0	150	60%
(Kettle Chips) Natural Gourmet				
baked				
honey barbeque	1 oz	1.5	110	12%
lightly salted	1 oz	1.5	110	12%
original				
habanero chili w/ginger	1 oz	8.0	140	51%
honey Dijon	1 oz	8.0	150	48%
lightly salted				
krinkle cut	1 oz	9.0	150	54%
regular	1 oz	9.0	150	54%
New York cheddar w/herbs	1 oz	9.0	150	54%
no salt	1 oz	9.0	150	54%
organically grown	1 oz	9.0	150	54%
salsa w/mesquite/krinkle cut	1 oz	8.0	140	51%
salt & fresh ground pepper/krinkle cut	1 oz	8.0	140	51%
sea salt & vinegar	1 oz	8.0	150	48%
yogurt & green onion	1 oz	8.0	150	48%
(Lance)				
BBQ				
big bag	1 oz	10.0	160	56%
value size	1.5 oz	15.0	230	59%
vending pkg	⅞ oz	9.0	140	58%
	1 oz	10.0	160	62%

Food and Description	Amount	Fat Grams	Total Calories	% Fat Calories
hot fries	⅞ oz	10.0	140	64%
plain				
value size	1½ oz	15.0	240	56%
vending pkg	1 oz	10.0	160	56%
ripple				
plain/vending pkg	1 oz	10.0	160	56%
salt & vinegar				
value size	1.5 oz	16.0	240	60%
vending pkg	1 oz	10.0	160	62%
sour cream & onion				
big bag	1 oz	11.0	160	62%
value size	1.5 oz	16.0	240	60%
vending pkg	1 oz	10.0	160	62%
(Laura Scudder)				
Bar-B-Q	1 oz	10.0	150	60%
for dips	1 oz	10.0	150	60%
Hawaiian	1 oz	9.0	150	54%
natural style	1 oz	10.0	150	60%
plain	1 oz	10.0	150	60%
sour cream & onion	1 oz	9.0	150	54%
(Lay's) (See (Frito Lay) in this section)				
(Louise's) potato chips				
Maui onion/fat-free	1 oz	–	110	–
mesquite BBQ				
fat-free	1 oz	–	110	–
"1g"	1 oz	1.0	110	8%
70% less fat	1 oz	3.0	110	25%
no salt/fat-free	1 oz	–	110	–
original				
fat-free	1 oz	–	110	–
"1g"	1 oz	1.0	110	8%
70% less fat	1 oz	3.0	110	25%
(Michael Season's)				
Gourmet Sensations				
chocolate covered	¾ cup	8.0	140	51%
Kettle-Cooked				
Jalapeño & cheese	1 oz	8.0	150	48%
lightly salted	1 oz	8.0	140	51%
mesquite barbecue	1 oz	8.0	140	51%
Reduced-fat				
cheddar & sour cream	1 oz	7.0	140	45%
honey barbeque	1 oz	6.0	140	39%
lightly salted				
regular	1 oz	6.0	130	42%
ripple	1 oz	6.7	140	43%
salt & vinegar	1 oz	6.0	130	42%
unsalted	1 oz	6.0	130	42%
yogurt & green onion	1 oz	6.0	130	42%
(Mike-Sell's)				
Groovy Party Size	1 oz	9.0	150	54%

Food and Description	Amount	Fat Grams	Total Calories	% Fat Calories
old fashioned family size	1 oz	8.0	150	48%
original family size	1 oz	9.0	150	54%
reduced-fat	1 oz	6.7	140	43%
zesty barbecue	1 oz	9.0	150	54%
(Nabisco) Mr. Phipps				
Tater Crisps				
BBQ	1 oz	4.0	130	28%
original	1 oz	7.0	120	53%
sour cream & onion	1 oz	4.0	130	28%
(Old Vienna)				
Missouri dairy sour cream & onion	1 oz	9.0	150	54%
original/Heartland Pride	1 oz	11.0	180	55%
Ozark hickory	1 oz	10.0	170	53%
Riplets				
grilled steak & onion	1 oz	9.0	150	54%
Heartland Pride	1 oz	10.0	150	60%
red hot	1 oz	9.0	150	54%
Wisconsin cheddar & sour cream	1 oz	10.0	150	60%
(Pik-Nik)				
shoestring potatoes	1.75 oz	18.0	280	58%
	1 oz	11.0	180	55%
(Poore Brothers)				
bar-b-que	1 oz	8.0	140	51%
Cajun	1 oz	8.0	140	51%
dill pickle	1 oz	8.0	140	51%
jalapeño	1 oz	8.0	140	51%
original				
regular	1 oz	10.0	150	60%
unsalted	1 oz	8.0	140	51%
Parmesan & garlic	1 oz	8.0	140	51%
salt & vinegar	1 oz	7.0	130	48%
sour cream & onion	1 oz	8.0	140	51%
(Pringle's) potato crisps				
regular				
BBQ				
fat-free	1 oz	–	70	–
regular	1 oz	11.0	150	66%
Right Crisp	1 oz	7.0	140	45%
Cheez-ums/regular	1 oz	10.0	150	60%
original				
fat-free	1 oz	–	70	–
regular	1 oz	11.0	160	62%
Right Crisp	1 oz	7.0	140	45%
Pizza-Licious/regular	1 oz	11.0	160	62%
ranch				
fat-free	1 oz	–	70	–
regular	1 oz	11.0	150	66%
Right Crisp	1 oz	7.0	140	45%
Salt & vinegar	1 oz	11.0	160	62%
sour cream 'n onion				
fat-free	1 oz	–	70	–

Food and Description	Amount	Fat Grams	Total Calories	% Fat Calories
regular	1 oz	10.0	160	56%
right	1 oz	7.0	140	45%
Ridges				
cheddar n' sour cream	1 oz	10.0	150	60%
mesquite BBQ	1 oz	10.0	150	60%
original	1 oz	10.0	150	60%
Ruffles (*See* Frito Lay in this section)				
(Snyder's)				
Regular chips				
BBQ	1 oz	6.0	150	36%
BBQ Rib	1 oz	7.0	140	45%
cheddar bacon	1 oz	8.0	150	48%
grilled steak & onion	1 oz	6.0	140	39%
hot Buffalo wings	1 oz	7.0	150	42%
Kosher dill	1 oz	6.0	140	39%
no salt	1 oz	10.0	150	60%
original	1 oz	6.0	140	39%
salt & vinegar	1 oz	6.0	140	39%
sausage pizza	1 oz	6.0	150	36%
sour cream & onion	1 oz	7.0	150	42%
unsalted	1 oz	6.0	140	39%
Ripple chips/original	1 oz	6.0	140	39%
(Tato Skins (*See* Keebler in this section)				
(Westbrae)				
original				
no salt	1 oz	8.0	150	48%
salted	1 oz	10.0	150	60%
ripple	1 oz	8.0	150	48%
(Terra) chips				
Blues	1 oz	6.0	140	39%
original	1 oz	7.0	140	45%
spiced	1 oz	5.0	130	35%
sweet potato				
jalapeño	1 oz	7.0	140	45%
mesquite BBQ	1 oz	7.0	140	45%
original/no salt	1 oz	7.0	140	45%
salsa	1 oz	7.0	140	45%
spiced	1 oz	7.0	140	45%
Yukon Gold				
barbecue	1 oz	5.0	130	35%
onion & garlic	1 oz	5.0	130	35%
original	1 oz	5.0	130	35%
salt & pepper	1 oz	5.0	130	35%
salt & vinegar	1 oz	5.0	130	35%
yogurt & green onion	1 oz	5.0	130	35%
(Wise)				
all natural				
regular	1 oz	10.0	150	60%
ridged	1 oz	10.0	150	60%

Food and Description	Amount	Fat Grams	Total Calories	% Fat Calories
regular				
BBQ	1 oz	10.0	160	56%
cottage fries				
no salt added	1 oz	10.0	150	60%
original	1 oz	10.0	150	60%
hot	1 oz	11.0	160	62%
lightly salted	1 oz	10.0	150	60%
New York Deli	1 oz	10.0	150	60%
onion-garlic	1 oz	10.0	150	60%
plain	1 oz	10.0	150	60%
salt & vinegar	1 oz	10.0	150	60%
Smoky Mountain BBQ	1 oz	10.0	150	60%
sour cream & onion	1 oz	9.0	150	54%
Ridgies				
BBQ	1 oz	10.0	150	60%
cheddar & sour cream	1 oz	10.0	160	56%
mesquite	1 oz	10.0	150	60%
original	1 oz	10.0	150	60%
plain	1 oz	10.0	150	60%
sour cream & onion	1 oz	10.0	150	60%
rippled	1 oz	10.0	150	60%

POTATO DISH/ENTRÉE (*See also* FROZEN ENTRÉE/DINNER; SEASONINGS; VEGETARIAN FOODS)

■ **CANNED/JARRED/MICROWAVE CONTAINER**

Food and Description	Amount	Fat Grams	Total Calories	% Fat Calories
(Aunt Nellie's) German potato salad	½ cup	2.0	140	13%
generic				
canned potato salad/homestyle	½ cup	11.0	170	58%
(Hormel)				
scalloped potatoes & ham/canned	1 cup	14.0	240	53%
scalloped potatoes & ham/ microcup meal	1 cup	14.0	240	53%
(Read) potato salad				
German style	½ cup	3.0	120	23%
(Reesur's) potato salad	½ cup	15.0	250	54%

■ **FROZEN OR REFRIGERATED**

Food and Description	Amount	Fat Grams	Total Calories	% Fat Calories
(Bob Evans)				
hash browns	1 serving	–	70	–
home fries	1 serving	–	80	–
mashed	1 serving	8.0	160	45%
(Brighton's) baked potatoes				
broccoli & cheese	10.2 oz	12.0	337	32%
cheese sauce/bacon	9.5 oz	13.0	352	33%
cheese sauce/ham	10.2 oz	12.0	347	31%
classic combination	9.6 oz	13.0	326	36%
(Cascadian Farm)				
country style potatoes	¾ cup	–	80	–
hash browns	1 cup	–	70	–
oven French fries	3 oz	8.0	200	36%
spud puppies	3 oz	8.0	150	48%

Food and Description	Amount	Fat Grams	Total Calories	% Fat Calories
generic				
cottage cut potatoes				
cooked in oven	10 pieces	4.0	109	33%
French-fried/heated	10 pieces	4.0	109	33%
fried in vegetable oil	10 pieces	8.0	158	46%
hash browns				
plain	½ cup	9.0	170	48%
w/butter	3.5 oz	9.0	180	43%
potato puffs	1 puff	0.8	16	45%
scalloped potatoes & ham				
plain	½ cup	6.0	123	44%
w/cheese	½ cup	9.6	177	49%
(Golden) potato pancakes	1 pancake	3.0	70	39%
(Inland Valley)				
French fries				
crinkle cut				
original	3 oz	5.0	150	30%
wedges	3 oz	5.0	150	30%
crispy classics				
colossal crinkles	3 oz	7.0	170	37%
crinkle cuts	3 oz	8.0	190	38%
straight cut	3 oz	7.0	180	35%
crisscut				
regular	3 oz	7.0	160	39%
seasoned	3 oz	11.0	190	52%
curley QQQ's	3 oz	8.0	180	40%
fajita fries	3 oz	8.0	170	42%
Long Branch	3 oz	7.0	160	39%
steak fries/thick cut	3 oz	3.0	110	8%
straight cut	3 oz	4.0	130	28%
tasty QQQ's	3 oz	9.0	190	43%
hash browns				
southern style	3 oz	–	70	–
mashed homestyle				
low-fat	5 oz	3.0	110	25%
portionable	2.28 oz	6.0	150	34%
regular	5 oz	6.0	160	34%
roasted garlic	5 oz	5.0	150	30%
munch skin meals	2 topped skins	15.0	250	54%
potato home browns/patties	2.28 oz	7.0	130	48%
potato stix/shredded	3 oz	10.0	170	53%
Simply Shreds				
O'Brien	1 cup	–	60	–
regular	1 cup	–	70	–
Tasty Q's	1 cup	7.0	160	39%
Tater Babies	3 oz	5.0	130	35%
Tater Puffs/seasoned	10 pieces	7.0	160	39%
Tri-patties/shredded and seasoned	2 oz	4.0	100	36%

Food and Description	Amount	Fat Grams	Total Calories	% Fat Calories
(Larry's) stuffed potatoes				
cheddar cheese	1 potato	9.0	160	51%
combination	1 potato	8.0	160	45%
sour cream & chives	1 potato	8.0	150	48%
(Mrs. Ts) pierogies				
potato & cheese	3 pieces	2.5	180	13%
potato & onion	3 pieces	2.0	180	10%
(Micromagic)				
French fries/low-fat	3 oz	3.0	130	21%
(Oh Boy!)				
cheddar cheese	6 oz	4.0	130	28%
bacon 7 cheese	6 oz	3.0	120	23%
sour cream, onion, & chives	6 oz	2.5	140	16%
(Ore Ida)				
baked/topped/broccoli & cheese	10.25 oz	8.0	310	23%
Crispers!				
Texas	3 oz	7.0	150	42%
original	3 oz	8.0	170	42%
Crispy Crowns	3 oz	8.0	170	42%
Crispy Crunchies	3 oz	8.0	160	45%
fast food fries	3 oz	7.0	160	39%
French fries				
country-style	3 oz	4.5	120	34%
golden crinkles	3 oz	3.5	120	26%
golden fries	3 oz	3.5	120	26%
pixie crinkles	3 oz	4.5	130	31%
shoestrings	3 oz	6.0	150	36%
steak				
country-style	3 oz	3.0	110	25%
regular	3 oz	3.0	110	25%
waffle	3 oz	7.0	150	42%
golden patties	1 patty	8.0	150	48%
golden twirls	3 oz	7.0	160	39%
hash browns				
country style shredded	1¼ cups	–	80	–
microwave	1 serving	6.0	110	49%
shredded	1 patty	–	70	–
Southern style	⅔ cup	–	70	–
toaster	3.5 oz	11.0	210	47%
mashed potatoes	⅔ cup	2.5	90	25%
onion rings/gourmet	4 pieces	10.0	210	43%
oven chips	3 oz	8.0	180	40%
potatoes O'Brien	¾ cup	–	60	–
Snackin'				
Fries				
extra zesty	5 oz	21.0	340	56%
regular	3 oz	12.0	280	39%
tots	3.5 oz	11.0	200	50%

Food and Description	Amount	Fat Grams	Total Calories	% Fat Calories
sweet potatoes/candied				
w/sauce packet	5 oz	–	180	–
Tater Tots				
microwave	3.5 oz	9.0	210	43%
mini	3.5 oz	10.0	180	50%
original	9 pieces	8.0	150	48%
w/onion	9 pieces	8.0	150	48%
twice-baked				
butter flavor	5 oz	6.0	160	34%
cheddar cheese	5 oz	7.0	180	35%
garlic parmesan	5 oz	7.0	180	35%
sour cream & chives	5 oz	7.0	170	37%
wedges w/skin on				
country style	3 oz	4.0	120	30%
regular	3 oz	3.0	110	25%
whipped potatoes/cheese	5 oz	8.0	190	38%
Zesties!	3 oz	7.0	160	39%
Zesty twirls	3 oz	7.0	160	39%
(Simply Potatoes)				
au gratin	¼ pkg	8.0	130	55%
hash browns				
plain	½ pkg	–	70	–
onion	½ pkg	–	70	–
Southwestern style	½ pkg	–	70	–
mashed				
country	¼ pkg	5.0	140	32%
regular	¼ pkg	5.0	140	32%
wedges	½ pkg	–	50	–
■ HOMEMADE				
USDA Standard Home Recipe				
hash brown potatoes	½ cup	10.0	165	55%
mashed potatoes				
made w/whole milk	½ cup	0.6	81	7%
made w/whole milk & butter	½ cup	4.0	94	38%
potato pancakes/made w/butter & milk	1 pancake	12.6	495	23%
potato salad				
made w/mayonnaise	½ cup	10.0	179	50%
made w/mustard	½ cup	6.0	120	45%
potatoes au gratin	½ cup	9.0	160	51%
potatoes O'Brien/made w/bread crumbs & butter	½ cup	1.0	79	11%
scalloped potatoes				
made w/butter	½ cup	4.5	105	39%
made w/cheese	½ cup	9.5	175	49%
■ MIX				
(Betty Crocker) prepared by regular recipe				
Mashed potatoes				
butter & herb	½ cup	8.0	160	45%
Potato Buds/original	⅔ cup	8.0	160	45%

Food and Description	Amount	Fat Grams	Total Calories	% Fat Calories
chicken & herb	½ cup	7.0	150	42%
four cheese	½ cup	7.0	150	42%
roasted garlic	½ cup	8.0	150	48%
sour cream & chives	½ cup	7.0	150	42%
Mashed potatoes & gravy				
hearty beef	¾ cup	7.0	170	37%
roasted chicken	¾ cup	7.0	180	35%
Specialty Potatoes				
au gratin	½ cup	6.0	150	36%
broccoli au gratin/homestyle	½ cup	6.0	140	39%
cheddar cheese/homestyle	½ cup	2.5	120	19%
cheddar 'n bacon	½ cup	6.0	150	36%
cheddar & sour cream	½ cup	3.0	130	21%
cheesy scalloped/homestyle	½ cup	6.0	140	39%
chicken & vegetable	⅔ cup	6.0	160	34%
hash brown	½ cup	8.0	190	38%
julienne	½ cup	6.0	150	36%
ranch	½ cup	6.0	160	34%
scalloped				
8.25 oz box	½ cup	6.0	150	36%
5 or 20-oz box	½ cup	6.0	160	34%
sour cream 'n chive	½ cup	7.0	160	39%
three cheese	½ cup	6.0	150	36%
twice-Baked/cheddar & bacon	⅔ cup	11.0	210	47%
(Fantastic) Stuffed Mashed Potato Cups/dry mix only				
broccoli & cheddar	1.7 oz	3.0	190	14%
garlic & herbs	1.7 oz	3.0	180	15%
jalapeño jack cheese	1.8 oz	3.0	200	14%
sour cream & chives	1.7 oz	3.0	190	14%
sweet creamery butter	1.8 oz	3.0	200	14%
white cheddar cheese	1.7 oz	3.0	190	14%
(Good Harvest) dry mix only				
country French	½ cup	1.0	100	9%
southern Italian	½ cup	0.5	110	4%
vegetable & herb	½ cup	0.5	110	4%
(Hungry Jack) prepared by regular recipe				
Casseroles				
Au gratin	1 serving	4.5	150	27%
cheddar & bacon	1 serving	4.5	150	27%
cheesy scalloped	1 serving	5.0	150	30%
creamy scalloped	1 serving	5.0	150	30%
sour cream & chives	1 serving	6.0	160	34%
Mashed potatoes w/gravy				
w/brown gravy	¾ cup	8.0	170	42%
w/chicken gravy	¾ cup	8.0	180	40%
Potato Pancake/prepared	3 pancakes	1.5	90	15%
(Idahoan) prepared				
au gratin	½ cup	5.0	130	35%
hash brown				
quick one-pan	½ cup	7.0	140	45%

Food and Description	Amount	Fat Grams	Total Calories	% Fat Calories
regular	½ cup	7.0	140	45%
mashed/cheddar	½ cup	5.0	140	32%
scalloped				
sour cream & chives	½ cup	5.0	130	35%
traditional	½ cup	7.0	140	45%
(Manischewitz) potato pancake/mix only	3 Tbs	1.0	80	11%
(Panni) mix only				
Bavarian potato dumpling	⅐ pkg	–	80	–
Bavarian potato pancake	¹⁄₁₂ pkg	–	50	–
POTATO PANCAKE (*See* POTATO DISH/ENTRÉE)				
POTATO SNACKS (*See* POTATO CHIPS & SNACKS)				
POTATO SOUP (*See* SOUP)				
POTATO STARCH				
(Manischewitz)	½ cup	–	285	–
POTTED MEAT (*See* LUNCHEON MEAT; LUNCHEON MEAT SPREAD)				
POULTRY SEASONING (*See also* SEASONINGS)				
generic	1 tsp	–	5	–
POUT, OCEAN				
raw	3 oz	1.0	70	13%
PRESERVES (*See* JAM/JELLY/PRESERVES)				
PRETZEL				
(Bakers Best) soft/frozen				
Dutch twists	2.5 oz twist	1.0	180	5%
(Borden)				
fat-free				
thins	6 pieces	–	100	–
ultra thin	8 pieces	–	100	–
low-fat mini				
cheddar	21 pieces	1.5	110	12%
mustard & honey	21 pieces	1.5	110	12%
(Cape Cod) no-fat multigrain	30 pretzels	–	110	–
(Crunch'N Munch) low-fat bag or box				
toffee sweet & crunchy	1 oz	1.0	120	8%
(Good Health) peanut butter–filled	8 pieces	6.0	140	39%
(Gus) soft baked/frozen				
sticks	1 pretzel	1.0	210	4%
twists	1 pretzel	1.0	210	4%
(Keebler)				
butter				
braids	22 pretzels	1.0	100	9%
knots	7 pretzels	1.0	100	9%
mini knots	18 pretzels	1.0	100	9%
traditional				
Bavarian	3 pretzels	2.0	120	15%
knots	7 pretzels	1.0	110	8%
(Lance)	1¼ oz	1.0	140	6%
(Laura Scudder's)				
Bavarian	1 oz	1.0	110	8%
sticks	1 oz	1.0	110	8%
twists	1 oz	1.0	110	8%

Food and Description	Amount	Fat Grams	Total Calories	% Fat Calories
(Louise's) fat-free sourdough	1 oz	–	90	–
(Michael Season's) O.G.'s Organic				
honey mustard nuggets	1 oz	<1.0	120	3%
lightly salted				
mini	1 oz	<1.0	110	3%
sticks	1 oz	<1.0	110	3%
twists	1 oz	<1.0	110	3%
sesame garlic nuggets	1 oz	1.0	120	8%
unsalted				
mini	1 oz	<1.0	110	3%
twists	1 oz	<1.0	110	3%
Mister Salty (See Nabisco in this section)				
(Mike Sell's) Dutch oven-baked	1 oz	2.0	130	14%
pretzel nuggets/fat-free sourdough	1 oz	0.5	110	5%
pretzel thins/fat-free	1 oz	–	110	–
pretzel twists/mini	1 oz	1.5	110	12%
(Mrs. Manischewitz) Bagel Pretzel				
everything onion	4 pretzels	–	110	–
garlic	4 pretzels	–	110	–
onion	4 pretzels	–	110	–
original	4 pretzels	–.	110	–
(Nabisco)				
Mr. Phipps Pretzel Chips				
fat-free	16 pieces	–	100	–
lower sodium	16 pieces	3.0	120	23%
original	16 pieces	3.0	120	23%
Mister Salty				
chips	1 oz	3.0	110	23%
Dutch	1 oz	1.0	120	8%
fat-free				
chips	1 oz	–	100	–
regular	1 oz	–	110	–
sticks or twists	1 oz	–	110	–
mini	1 oz	1.0	110	8%
(Nestlé USA) Pretzel Flipz				
milk chocolate covered	1 oz	6.0	130	42%
peanut butter fudge covered	1 oz	4.0	120	30%
white fudge covered	1 oz	6.0	140	39%
(Newman's Own)				
Bavarian	1 pretzel	–	90	–
rounds				
regular	1 oz	1.0	110	8%
salt & pepper	1 oz	1.0	110	8%
sticks	1 oz	1.0	110	8%
(Planter's) twists	1 oz	0.5	100	5%
	1.5 oz	1.0	160	6%
(Pocket Pretzels) peanut butter-filled	1 oz	4.0	126	29%
(Quinlan)				
beer	1 oz	1.0	110	8%
logs	1 oz	1.5	110	12%

Food and Description	Amount	Fat Grams	Total Calories	% Fat Calories
mini				
fat-free	1 oz	–	100	–
regular	1 oz	1.0	110	8%
nuggets	1 oz	1.0	110	8%
rods	1 oz	1.0	110	8%
sourdough				
fat-free				
no salt added	1 pretzel	–	80	–
regular	1 pretzel	–	80	–
low-fat/hard	1 oz	1.0	90	10%
sourdough/honey mustard & onion	1 oz	8.0	150	48%
sticks	1 oz	1.0	110	8%
thins				
party	1 oz	1.0	110	8%
plain	1 oz	1.0	110	8%
sourdough	1 oz	–	100	–
tiny thins				
cheese	1 oz	1.0	110	8%
party	1 oz	1.0	110	8%
plain	1 oz	1.0	110	8%
ultra thins/fat-free	1 oz	–	110	–
(Rokeach)				
Dutch	1 oz	–	110	–
no salt	1 oz	–	110	–
party canister	1 oz	1.0	110	8%
(Rold Gold)				
fat-free				
thins	1 oz	–	110	–
tiny twists	1 oz	–	100	–
regular				
classic				
cheddar cheese/tiny twists	1 oz	1.0	110	8%
honey mustard/tiny twists	1 oz	1.0	110	8%
sticks	1 oz	–	100	–
thin twists	1 oz	1.0	110	8%
tiny twists	1 oz	1.0	110	8%
hard sourdough	1 oz	0.5	100	5%
rods	1 oz	1.0	110	8%
sourdough nuggets	1 oz	–	100	–
snack mix	¾ cup	8.0	160	45%
(Seyfert's) butter/rods	1 oz	1.0	110	8%
(Snyder's)				
Nibblers				
garlic bread	1 oz	3.0	130	21%
honey mustard & onion	1 oz	3.0	130	21%
oat bran	1 oz	1.0	110	8%
sourdough original/savory	1 oz	3.0	130	21%
old fashioned hard	1 oz	–	110	–
Old Tyme				
regular	1 oz	–	118	–
unsalted	1 oz	–	110	–

Food and Description	Amount	Fat Grams	Total Calories	% Fat Calories
Pieces				
buttermilk ranch	1 oz	5.0	130	35%
cheddar cheese	1 oz	6.0	130	42%
creamy caramel	1 oz	5.0	130	35%
honey BBQ	1 oz	5.0	130	35%
honey mustard & onion	1 oz	7.0	140	45%
jalapeño	1 oz	5.0	140	32%
pepperoni pizza	1 oz	8.0	150	48%
sourdough honey BBQ	1 oz	5.0	130	35%
sourdough specials	1 oz	1.0	120	8%
Pretzel dips				
creamy white fudge mini's	1 oz	6.0	130	42%
real milk chocolate mini's	1 oz	6.0	130	42%
Pretzels				
golden cheese nibbler	1 oz	2.0	130	14%
hard soughdough	1 oz	–	100	
homestyle	1 oz	1.0	120	8%
honey wheat nibbler	1 oz	2.0	100	18%
log	1 oz	1.0	110	8%
mini	1 oz	–	110	–
nibbler	1 oz	–	120	–
oat bran	1 oz	1.0	110	8%
rod	1 oz	1.0	120	8%
snaps	1 oz	1.0	120	
thin	1 oz	–	110	–
unsalted				
hard sourdough	1 oz	–	100	
mini	1 oz	–	110	–
nibbler	1 oz	–	120	–
old tyme	1 oz	1.0	120	8%
Stix				
old fashion dipping	1 oz	–	100	–
olde tyme pretzel	1 oz	1.0	120	8%
very thins	1 oz	–	110	–
(SuperPretzel) soft-baked/frozen				
pretzels				
bites	5 bites	0.5	140	3%
original	2.16 oz	1.0	170	5%
	2.52 oz	1.0	190	5%
Softstix				
cheddar	2 stix	2.5	140	16%
nacho	2 stix	2.0	110	16%
pizza	2 stix	2.0	110	16%
(Weight Watchers) Smart Snackers				
oat bran pretzel nuggets	1.5 oz pkg	3.0	170	16%
PRICKLY PEAR	1 medium	0.5	42	11%
PROSCIUTTO (See SAUSAGE)				
PRUNE				
canned				
generic/in heavy syrup	5 medium	<1.0	90	2%
	1 cup	<1.0	240	2%

Food and Description	Amount	Fat Grams	Total Calories	% Fat Calories
(S&W) in heavy syrup	8 pieces	–	210	–
dried				
(Del Monte) uncooked				
pitted	2 oz	–	140	–
unpitted	2 oz	–	120	–
(Dole) pitted	¼ cup	–	110	–
generic				
cooked				
sweetened	1 cup	<1.0	225	2%
unsweetened	1 cup	<1.0	294	2%
uncooked/pitted	10 medium	<1.0	201	2%
(Mariani)				
large	¼ cup	1.0	140	6%
pitted	¼ cup	1.0	140	6%
(Sun Sweet)				
bite-size breakfast	¼ cup	–	140	–
medium	¼ cup	–	140	–
orange essence/pitted	6 medium	–	100	–
pitted	¼ cup	–	140	–
PRUNE JUICE /bottled or canned				
(Del Monte) unsweetened	8 fl oz	–	170	–
(Mott's)				
country style	6 fl oz	–	130	–
unsweetened	6 fl oz	–	130	–
(S&W) unsweetened	8 fl oz	–	180	–
(Seneca)	8 fl oz	–	180	–
(Sun Sweet)				
regular	8 fl oz	–	180	–
w/prune pulp	8 fl oz	–	170	–
PUDDING & MOUSSE (*See also* CUSTARD; PIE FILLING & GLAZE)				
■ **HOMEMADE**				
(Note: Unless otherwise stated, homemade puddings were prepared with whole milk.)				
USDA Standard Home Recipe				
apple brown Betty	1 cup	7.6	325	21%
blancmange	4.5 oz	5.0	150	30%
bread pudding w/raisins	1 cup	16.0	495	29%
chocolate				
prepared w/2% milk	½ cup	4.0	205	18%
prepared w/whole milk	½ cup	5.0	220	20%
corn	½ cup	5.0	130	35%
Indian pudding/baked	½ cup	4.5	120	34%
mousse/chocolate	½ cup	30.0	447	60%
rice pudding w/raisins	½ cup	4.0	220	16%
tapioca	½ cup	5.0	190	23%
vanilla	½ cup	4.0	130	31%
Yorkshire				
prepared w/skim milk	3.5 oz	4.0	90	40%
prepared w/whole milk	3.5 oz	5.0	105	43%

Food and Description	Amount	Fat Grams	Total Calories	% Fat Calories
■ **MIX** (Note: Unless stated otherwise, 1 serving of mix = the amount in ½ cup prepared.)				
(D-Zerta)				
chocolate				
mix only	1 serving	–	20	–
prepared w/skim milk	½ cup	–	60	–
(Jell-O) pudding & pie filling				
Americana pudding & custard				
Custard/prepared w/2% milk	½ cup	2.5	140	16%
rice pudding/prepared w/skim milk	½ cup	–	140	–
tapioca pudding/prepared w/skim milk	½ cup	–	130	–
cook & serve				
fat-free/prepared w/skim milk				
chocolate	½ cup	–	130	–
vanilla	½ cup	–	130	–
original/prepared w/2% milk				
banana cream	½ cup	2.5	140	16%
butterscotch	½ cup	2.5	160	14%
chocolate	½ cup	2.5	150	15%
chocolate fudge	½ cup	2.5	150	15%
coconut cream	½ cup	5.0	150	30%
flan	½ cup	2.5	140	16%
lemon/prepared as directed	½ cup	2.0	140	13%
milk chocolate	½ cup	3.0	150	18%
vanilla	½ cup	2.5	140	16%
sugar-free/reduced calorie-prepared w/2% milk				
chocolate	½ cup	2.5	90	25%
vanilla	½ cup	2.5	80	28%
instant				
fat-free/prepared w/skim milk				
chocolate	½ cup	–	140	–
devil's food	½ cup	–	140	–
vanilla	½ cup	–	140	–
white chocolate	½ cup	–	140	–
fat-free/sugar-free/reduced calorie-prepared w/skim milk				
banana	½ cup	–	70	–
butterscotch	½ cup	–	70	–
chocolate	½ cup	–	80	–
chocolate fudge	½ cup	–	80	–
vanilla	½ cup	–	70	–
vanilla chocolate	½ cup	–	70	–
original/prepared w/2% milk				
banana cream	½ cup	2.5	150	15%
butterscotch	½ cup	2.5	150	15%
chocolate	½ cup	2.5	160	14%
chocolate fudge	½ cup	3.0	160	17%
coconut cream	½ cup	5.0	160	28%
French vanilla	½ cup	2.5	150	15%

Food and Description	Amount	Fat Grams	Total Calories	% Fat Calories
lemon	½ cup	2.5	150	15%
pistachio	½ cup	3.0	160	17%
vanilla	½ cup	2.5	150	15%
(Knorr) Alsa International Desserts/mix only				
dark chocolate	¼ pkg	4.0	80	45%
milk chocolate	¼ pkg	4.0	80	45%
white chocolate	¼ pkg	3.5	70	45%
(Lundberg) Elegant Rice Pudding/mix only				
cinnamon raisin	½ cup	–	70	–
coconut	½ cup	2.0	70	26%
honey almond	½ cup	0.5	70	6%
(McCormick/Schilling) pie glaze mix for				
blueberries	2 oz	–	60	–
peaches	2 oz	–	70	–
strawberries	2 oz	–	70	–
(Nabisco) My-T-Fine/mix only = amount of mix in 1 serving prepared				
butterscotch	1 serving	–	90	–
chocolate	1 serving	–	100	–
chocolate almond	1 serving	1.0	100	10%
chocolate fudge	1 serving	–	100	–
lemon	1 serving	–	90	–
vanilla	1 serving	–	90	–
vanilla tapioca	1 serving	–	80	–
(Royal) mix only = the amount of mix in 1 serving prepared.)				
cook & serve				
banana cream	1 serving	–	80	–
butterscotch	1 serving	–	90	–
chocolate	1 serving	–	90	–
dark 'n sweet chocolate	1 serving	–	90	–
vanilla	1 serving	–	80	–
regular				
banana cream	1 serving	–	90	–
butterscotch	1 serving	–	90	–
cherry vanilla	1 serving	–	90	–
chocolate	1 serving	–	100	–
chocolate almond	1 serving	1.0	120	8%
chocolate chocolate chip	1 serving	1.0	110	8%
chocolate peanut butter	1 serving	1.0	110	8%
dark 'n sweet	1 serving	–	110	–
lemon	1 serving	–	90	–
pistachio	1 serving	1.0	90	10%
strawberry	1 serving	–	100	–
toasted coconut	1 serving	2.0	100	18%
vanilla	1 serving	–	90	–
vanilla chocolate chip	1 serving	1.0	90	10%
sugar-free				
chocolate	1 serving	–	45	–
pistachio	1 serving	–	40	–
vanilla	1 serving	–	40	–

Food and Description	Amount	Fat Grams	Total Calories	% Fat Calories
■ **READY TO SERVE**				
generic/can or cup				
banana	½ cup	4.0	150	24%
butterscotch	½ cup	4.0	150	24%
chocolate	½ cup	4.0	190	19%
egg custard	½ cup	6.0	140	39%
fudge	½ cup	4.0	190	19%
lemon	½ cup	2.0	170	11%
rice	½ cup	3.0	150	18%
tapioca	½ cup	4.0	140	26%
vanilla	½ cup	4.0	150	24%
(Hunt's)				
Snack Pack				
banana	1 snack	6.0	160	34%
butterscotch	1 snack	6.0	155	35%
chocolate				
fat-free	1 snack	–	96	–
regular	1 snack	6.0	170	32%
chocolate fudge	1 snack	6.0	170	32%
chocolate marshmallow	1 snack	6.0	155	35%
lemon	1 snack	3.0	165	16%
milk chocolate	1 snack	6.0	165	33%
swirl				
chocolate caramel	1 snack	6.0	170	32%
chocolate peanut butter	1 snack	6.0	165	33%
milk chocolate	1 snack	6.0	165	33%
s'mores	1 snack	6.0	155	35%
tapioca				
fat-free	1 snack	–	95	–
regular	1 snack	6.0	150	36%
vanilla				
fat-free	1 snack	–	95	–
regular	1 snack	6.0	165	33%
vanilla-chocolate swirl				
fat-free	1 snack	–	100	–
regular	1 snack	5.0	165	33%
(Imagine) Rice Dream pudding cups				
banana	1 cup	3.0	140	19%
butterscotch	1 cup	3.0	140	19%
chocolate	1 cup	3.0	160	17%
lemon	1 cup	3.0	140	19%
(Jell-O) Pudding Snacks				
Fat-free				
chocolate	1 snack	–	100	–
chocolate/vanilla swirls	1 snack	–	100	–
devil's food	1 snack	–	100	–
rocky road	1 snack	–	100	–
tapioca	1 snack	–	100	–
vanilla	1 snack	–	100	–

Food and Description	Amount	Fat Grams	Total Calories	% Fat Calories
Handi-Snacks				
banana	1 snack	3.5	120	26%
butterscotch	1 snack	3.5	120	26%
chocolate				
fat-free	1 snack	–	90	–
regular	1 snack	3.5	130	24%
tapioca	1 snack	3.5	120	26%
vanilla				
fat-free	1 snack	–	90	–
regular	1 snack	3.5	120	26%
Original				
chocolate	1 snack	5.0	160	28%
chocolate marshmallow	1 snack	5.0	160	28%
chocolate/vanilla swirls	1 snack	5.0	160	28%
tapioca	1 snack	4.0	140	26%
vanilla	1 snack	5.0	160	28%
(Kozy Shack) cups				
banana	4 oz	3.0	130	21%
chocolate				
light	4 oz	1.0	110	8%
regular	4 oz	4.0	140	26%
rice	4 oz	3.0	130	21%
tapioca	4 oz	3.0	140	19%
vanilla				
light	4 oz	1.0	110	8%
regular	4 oz	3.0	130	21%
(Musselman's)				
banana	4 oz	5.0	150	30%
butterscotch	4 oz	7.0	170	37%
chocolate	4 oz	7.0	180	35%
chocolate fudge	4 oz	8.0	180	40%
rice	4 oz	3.0	120	23%
tapioca	4 oz	6.0	140	39%
vanilla	4 oz	7.0	170	37%
(Rice Dream) See (Imagine) in this section				
(Swiss Miss)				
Pudding Snacks				
butterscotch	1 snack	6.0	180	30%
chocolate				
fat-free	1 snack	–	100	–
light	1 snack	1.0	100	9%
regular	1 snack	6.0	180	30%
chocolate fudge				
light	1 snack	1.0	100	9%
regular	1 snack	6.0	220	25%
chocolate sundae	1 snack	7.0	220	29%
chocolate vanilla parfait	1 snack	6.0	165	33%
chocolate vanilla swirl	1 snack	6.0	170	32%
milk chocolate fudge parfait	1 snack	6.0	165	33%

Food and Description	Amount	Fat Grams	Total Calories	% Fat Calories
pie lover's pudding/chocolate cream pie	1 snack	6.0	150	36%
tapioca				
fat-free	1 snack	–	90	
regular	1 snack	5.0	160	28%
vanilla				
light	1 snack	1.0	100	9%
regular	1 snack	7.0	190	33%
vanilla-chocolate parfait				
light	1 snack	1.0	100	9%
regular	1 snack	6.0	180	30%
vanilla sundae	1 snack	7.0	200	32%
PUMMELO/POMELO				
fresh				
sections	1 cup	–	70	–
whole	1 medium	–	230	–
PUMPKIN				
canned				
(Comstock)	½ cup	–	50	–
(Festal)	½ cup	1.0	40	23%
(Libby's) solid pack	½ cup	0.5	60	8%
(Stokely)	½ cup	–	40	–
fresh				
boiled-mashed	1 cup	–	48	–
raw/cubed	1 cup	–	30	–
PUMPKIN BUTTER				
(Smucker's)	1 tsp	–	12	–
PUMPKIN FLOWER				
cooked	½ cup	<1.0	10	45%
raw	½ cup	<1.0	5	90%
PUMPKIN LEAVES/cooked	½ cup	<1.0	7	64%
PUMPKIN PIE SPICE (See also SEASONINGS)				
generic	1 tsp	–	6	–
PUMPKIN SEEDS				
dried/hulled	1 oz	13.0	155	75%
	1 cup	63.0	747	76%
kernels/roasted				
(David)	¼ cup	13.0	160	73%
generic	1 oz	12.0	150	72%
	1 cup	95.6	1185	72%
whole/roasted	1 oz	5.5	127	39%
	1 cup	12.0	285	38%
PUNCH (See FRUIT PUNCH; SOFT DRINK; SOFT DRINK MIX)				
PURPLE HULL PEA				
canned (Allens Fresh)	½ cup	0.5	100	5%
frozen (Frosty Acres)	3.3 oz	–	130	–
PURSLANE				
boiled	½ cup	–	10	–
raw	1 cup	–	7	–

Q

Food and Description	Amount	Fat Grams	Total Calories	% Fat Calories
QUAIL/raw				
breast meat only	~2 oz	1.7	69	22%
meat & skin-raw	~4 oz	13.0	210	56%
meat only	~3 oz	4.0	123	29%
QUICHE (See EGG DISH/MEAL)				
QUINCE/fresh	1 medium	–	53	–
QUINOA (See also FLOUR; PASTA; QUINOA SEED)				
whole grain/dry				
(Eden)	¼ cup	3.5	180	18%
generic	1 oz	1.6	106	14%
	1 cup	10.0	637	14%
QUINOA SEED				
(Arrowhead Mills)	¼ cup	2.0	140	13%

R

Food and Description	Amount	Fat Grams	Total Calories	% Fat Calories
RABBIT				
domesticated/meat only				
roasted	3 oz	5.5	130	38%
roasted/chopped or diced	1 cup	9.0	220	37%
stewed	3 oz	7.0	175	36%
stewed/chopped or diced	1 cup	12.0	290	37%
wild/meat only				
stewed	3 oz	3.0	150	18%
stewed/chopped or diced	1 cup	5.0	245	18%
RACCOON/meat only				
roasted	3 oz	12.5	220	51%
roasted/chopped or diced	1 cup	20.0	355	51%
RADICCHIO/raw/shredded	½ cup	–	5	–
RADISH				

Food and Description	Amount	Fat Grams	Total Calories	% Fat Calories
dried				
Chinese	¼ cup	–	75	–
daikon	¼ cup	–	75	–
fresh				
Black	1 oz	–	5	–
Chinese				
cooked-drained/sliced	½ cup	–	15	–
raw				
sliced	½ cup	–	10	–
whole	1 medium	–	60	–
daikon				
cooked-drained/sliced	½ cup	–	15	–
raw				
sliced	½ cup	–	10	–
whole	1 medium	–	60	–
red/raw	10 pieces	–	7	–
	½ cup	–	13	–
(Dole)	7 medium	–	20	–
white icicle/raw				
sliced	½ cup	–	7	–
whole	1 medium	–	2	–
RADISH LEAVES	1 oz	–	15	–
RADISH SPROUTS	½ cup	0.5	8	56%
RAISIN (See also SNACK MIX)				
(Del Monte)				
golden	¼ cup	–	130	–
natural	¼ cup	–	120	–
	1.5 oz box	–	140	–
	1 oz box	–	90	–
yogurt raisin snack bag				
strawberry	0.9 oz	3.0	110	25%
vanilla yogurt	0.9 oz	3.0	110	25%
(Dole)				
California/seedless	¼ cup	–	130	–
dark/seedless	½ cup	–	250	–
golden	½ cup	–	250	–
generic				
dark				
ground/uncooked				
loose	1 cup	–	578	–
packed	1 cup	<1.0	780	1%
seedless				
loose	1 cup	0.5	435	1%
packed	1 cup	1.0	495	1%
w/seeds				
loose	1 cup	1.0	430	2%
packed	1 cup	1.0	490	2%
golden/seedless				
loose	1 cup	0.5	438	1%
packed	1 cup	1.0	498	1%

Food and Description	Amount	Fat Grams	Total Calories	% Fat Calories
(S&W)				
dark/seedless	¼ cup	–	130	–
golden/seedless	¼ cup	–	130	–
(Sun Maid)				
baking	¼ cup	–	120	–
dark/seedless				
regular	¼ cup	–	130	–
golden w/seeds	½ cup	–	250	–
muscat	½ cup	1.0	270	3%
snack box	1.5 oz	–	130	–
RASPBERRY				
canned/generic				
in heavy syrup	1 cup	<1.0	234	2%
in water	1 cup	2.0	110	16%
fresh				
black	1 cup	2.0	100	18%
red	1 cup	0.7	61	10%
(Dole)	1 cup	–	45	–
frozen				
(Big Valley)	⅔ cup	–	80	–
(Birds Eye) red/in lite syrup	4.5 oz	–	90	–
(C&W) red/sweetened	1 cup	–	50	–
generic				
sweetened	1 cup	<1.0	255	2%
	10 oz	<1.0	290	2%
unsweetened	3.5 oz	<1.0	50	9%
RASPBERRY JUICE/JUICE BLEND (See also FRUIT PUNCH; LEMONADE; SOFT DRINK; SOFT DRINK MIX)				
bottled, boxed, or canned				
(Dole) country raspberry 100% juice blend				
bottled	8 fl oz	–	140	–
	10 fl oz	–	180	–
refrigerated	4 fl oz	–	70	–
	8 fl oz	–	140	–
(Knudsen)				
raspberry float	8 fl oz	–	140	–
raspberry-peach	8 fl oz	–	115	–
(Smucker's)				
juice	8 fl oz	–	120	–
juice sparkler	10 fl oz	–	130	–
fresh/black	4 fl oz	–	50	–
frozen/prepared				
(Dole) country raspberry 100% juice blend	8 fl oz	–	140	–
generic	6 fl oz	–	90	–
RASPBERRY JUICE DRINK (See also FRUIT PUNCH; LEMONADE; SOFT DRINK; SOFT DRINK MIX; TEA)				
bottled, boxed, or canned				
(Betty Crocker) Squeezit/blue raspberry	6.76 fl oz	–	110	–

Food and Description	Amount	Fat Grams	Total Calories	% Fat Calories
(Dole) Raspberry-Lemon Splash	8 fl oz	–	120	–
	16 fl oz	–	250	–
(Snapple) Raspberry-peach drink	8 fl oz	–	120	–
frozen				
(Dole) Raspberry-Lemon Splash				
juice drink	8 fl oz	–	120	–
(Seneca) raspberry-cranapple				
juice cocktail	8 fl oz	–	140	–

RAVIOLI (*See* BEEF DISH/ENTRÉE; FROZEN ENTRÉE/DINNER; PASTA ENTRÉE/DINNER; VEGETARIAN FOODS)

RED BEAN (*See also* BEANS, BAKED & VARIETY; RICE DISH)

canned				
(Bush's Best)	½ cup	–	70	–
generic	½ cup	–	100	–
(Green Giant) dry beans in brine	½ cup	0.5	100	5%
(Hunt's) small	½ cup	0.5	90	5%
(Joan of Arc) dry beans in brine	½ cup	0.5	100	5%
(Van Camp's)	1 cup	1.0	195	5%
dry				
(Bean Cuisine)	½ cup	1.0	115	8%

RED BEAN SOUP (*See* SOUP)

REFRIED BEANS (*See* MEXICAN FOOD)

RELISH (*See* CHUTNEY; CORN DISH; PICKLE RELISH)

RENNIN PRODUCTS	1 tablet	–	1	–
	1 pkg	–	12	–

RHUBARB

fresh				
cooked-sweetened	1 cup	–	280	–
raw/diced	½ cup	–	13	–
frozen				
generic/cooked w/sugar	1 cup	–	278	–

RICE (*See also* ASIAN FOOD; RICE DISH)

(A Taste of Thai) prepared				
brown jasmine	½ cup	–	220	–
coconut ginger	½ cup	1.0	325	3%
garlic basil	½ cup	1.0	270	3%
soft jasmine	½ cup	–	160	–
(Arrowhead Mills) dry				
basmati/long-grain	¼ cup	–	150	–
brown				
long-grain	¼ cup	1.0	150	6%
medium-grain	¼ cup	1.0	160	6%
short-grain	¼ cup	–	170	–
(Colavita) arborio/dry	1 ounce	–	100	–
(Fantastic Foods) Elegant Grains/dry				
arborio	¼ cup	–	160	–
basmati				
brown	¼ cup	1.5	160	8%
white	¼ cup	–	160	–
jasmine				
brown	¼ cup	1.5	160	8%

Food and Description	Amount	Fat Grams	Total Calories	% Fat Calories
white	¼ cup	–	160	–
generic				
brown				
long-grain				
cooked	½ cup	0.9	108	7%
dry	½ cup	2.7	342	7%
medium-grain				
cooked	½ cup	<1.0	109	6%
dry	½ cup	2.5	343	6%
glutinous				
cooked	½ cup	<1.0	117	1%
dry	½ cup	0.5	342	1%
white				
long-grain				
instant				
cooked	½ cup	<1.0	180	3%
dry	½ cup	<1.0	230	2%
parboiled				
cooked	½ cup	<1.0	100	2%
dry	½ cup	0.5	340	1%
regular				
cooked	½ cup	<1.0	131	2%
dry	½ cup	<1.0	338	1%
raw	1 cup	0.7	672	1%
medium-grain				
cooked	½ cup	<1.0	133	1%
dry	½ cup	0.5	350	1%
raw	1 cup	0.8	708	1%
short-grain				
cooked	½ cup	<1.0	133	1%
dry	½ cup	0.5	358	1%
raw	1 cup	0.8	726	1%
wild				
cooked	½ cup	<1.0	83	3%
dry	½ cup	<1.0	285	3%
raw	4 oz	<1.0	400	1%
(Mahatma)				
brown/dry	1 oz	–	110	–
instant				
cooked, w/o butter or margarine	½ cup	–	110	–
dry	1 oz	–	110	–
white /dry	1 oz	–	100	–
(Minute)				
brown/instant whole grain				
dry	½ cup	1.5	170	8%
prepared, w/o butter or margarine	⅔ cup	1.5	170	8%
long-grain and wild/seasoned w/herbs/prepared	1 cup	0.5	230	2%
white				
boil-in-bag				
dry	½ bag	–	190	–

Food and Description	Amount	Fat Grams	Total Calories	% Fat Calories
prepared, w/o butter or margarine	1 cup	–	190	–
original				
dry	½ cup	–	160	–
prepared, w/o butter or margarine	¾ cup	–	160	–
premium long-grain				
dry	½ cup	–	160	–
prepared, w/o butter or margarine	1 cup	–	160	–
(MJB) brown				
quick/cooked	½ cup	1.0	110	8%
(Pacific International)				
brown calrose/medium grain	1.6 oz	2.0	160	11%
calrose enriched/medium grain	1.6 oz	–	155	–
enriched long-grain	1.6 oz	–	155	–
jasmine	1.6 oz	–	155	–
(Riceland)				
brown/natural extra long-grain	1.5 oz	1.0	150	6%
enriched				
extra long-grain	1.67 oz	–	160	–
medium grain plum & tender	1.67 oz	–	170	–
perfected long-grain/parboiled	1.67 oz	–	170	–
(S&W) dry				
brown				
long-grain	¼ cup	1.0	150	6%
quick	½ cup	1.0	150	6%
white/long-grain	¼ cup	–	100	–
wild	½ cup	1.0	110	8%
(Success)				
brown				
boil-in-bag/prepared	½ cup	1.0	150	6%
10-minute/prepared	½ cup	1.0	190	5%
brown & wild/dry	½ cup	1.0	190	5%
white/natural long-grain				
precooked/prepared	½ cup	–	190	–
(Texmati)				
brown	¼ cup	1.0	170	5%
Jasmati	¼ cup	–	150	–
Kasmati	¼ cup	0.5	150	3%
light brown	¼ cup	1.0	170	5%
risotto	¼ cup	–	150	–
Royal Blend	¼ cup	–	160	–
white/long-grain	¼ cup	0.5	150	3%
(Uncle Ben's)				
brown/cooked	1 serving	1.0	160	6%
white				
aromatic/cooked	½ cup	–	100	–
boil-in-bag/dry	⅓ cup	0.5	170	3%
converted/dry	¼ cup	–	170	–
Rice-in-an-Instant	½ cup	0.5	190	2%
wild/combinations/fast-cooking				
brown & wild	1 serving	1.0	120	8%

Food and Description	Amount	Fat Grams	Total Calories	% Fat Calories
(Vita Fiber) rice grain	1 oz	6.0	100	54%
RICE BRAN (See also CEREAL)				
crude	½ cup	8.5	130	59%
RICE BRAN OIL				
generic	1 Tbs	14.0	120	100%
(Hollywood)	1 Tbs	14.0	120	100%
RICE CAKES (See also POPCORN BARS & CAKES)				
(Hain)				
Mini				
apple cinnamon	5 cakes	–	60	–
barbeque	5 cakes	3.0	70	39%
cheese	5 cakes	2.0	60	30%
honey nut	5 cakes	–	60	–
nacho	5 cakes	2.0	70	26%
plain				
original	5 cakes	–	60	–
no salt added	5 cakes	–	60	–
ranch	6 cakes	3.0	70	39%
teriyaki	5 cakes	–	50	–
Regular				
5-grain	1 cake	–	40	–
plain				
no salt added	1 cake	–	40	–
original	1 cake	–	40	–
sesame				
no salt added	1 cake	–	40	–
original	1 cake	–	40	–
(Lundberg)				
Organic				
lightly salted	1 cake	1.0	60	15%
unsalted	1 cake	1.0	60	15%
Premium				
lightly salted	1 cake	1.0	60	15%
unsalted	1 cake	1.0	60	15%
Sesame/lightly salted	1 cake	–	60	–
(Mother's)				
Mini				
apple	5 cakes	–	50	–
caramel	5 cakes	–	50	–
cinnamon	5 cakes	–	50	–
plain/unsalted	7 cakes	–	60	–
Regular				
multigran/lightly salted	1 cake	–	35	–
rye/unsalted	1 cake	–	35	–
wheat/unsalted	1 cake	–	35	–
(Orville Redenacher's) Mini cakes				
butter	8 cakes	1.0	60	15%
caramel	7 cakes	–	50	–
nacho	8 cakes	1.0	60	15%
peanut caramel	7 cakes	1.0	60	15%

Food and Description	Amount	Fat Grams	Total Calories	% Fat Calories
(Pritikin)				
Mini/apple crisp	5 cakes	–	50	–
Regular				
multigrain				
regular	1 cake	–	35	–
unsalted	1 cake	–	35	–
plain				
regular	1 cake	–	35	–
unsalted	1 cake	–	35	–
sesame				
low sodium	1 cake	–	35	–
unsalted	1 cake	–	35	–
(Quaker)				
Mini rice snacks				
apple cinnamon	8 cakes	–	60	–
BBQ	10 cakes	2.0	70	26%
caramel corn	7 cakes	–	60	–
cheddar cheese	9 cakes	2.5	70	32%
chocolae crunch	7 cakes	1.0	60	15%
creamy ranch	10 cakes	2.5	70	32%
nacho	9 cakes	2.5	70	32%
sour cream & onion	10 cakes	2.5	70	32%
Regular				
apple cinnamon	1 cake	–	50	–
banana nut crunch	1 cake	–	50	–
buttered popcorn	1 cake	–	35	–
caramel apple	1 cake	0.5	60	8%
caramel chocolate chip	1 cake	1.0	60	15%
caramel corn	1 cake	–	50	–
chocolate crunch	1 cake	1.0	60	15%
cinnamon streusel	1 cake	1.0	60	15%
peanut butter	1 cake	1.0	60	15%
plain				
salt-free	1 cake	–	35	–
salted	1 cake	–	35	–
strawberry crunch	1 cake	–	50	–
white cheddar corn	1 cake	0.5	45	10%
(Roman Meal) Mini cakes				
apple	8 cakes	–	50	–
caramel	8 cakes	–	50	–
honey nut	8 cakes	–	50	–
(Too Good To Be True) Mini cakes				
(Westbrae Natural)				
double sesame	1 cake	<1.0	30	15%
sesame garlic	1 cake	<1.0	30	15%
teriyaki	1 cake	<1.0	30	15%
RICE DISH (See also ASIAN FOOD; FROZEN ENTRÉE/DINNER; MEXICAN FOOD)				
■ CANNED				
(Old El Paso) Spanish rice	1 cup	1.0	130	7%
(Van Camp's) Spanish rice	1 cup	4.0	160	23%

Food and Description	Amount	Fat Grams	Total Calories	% Fat Calories
■ FROZEN				
(Green Giant) Rice & Vegetable Combinations				
cheesy rice & broccoli	1 pkg	5.0	300	15%
oriental rice	1 pkg	12.0	340	32%
rice medley	1 pkg	4.0	280	13%
rice pilaf	1 pkg	3.5	230	14%
white & wild rice	1 pkg	6.0	280	19%
(Uncle Ben's) Rice bowls				
BBQ beef	1 bowl	4.5	430	9%
chicken bombay	1 bowl	5.0	440	10%
chicken vegetable	1 bowl	5.0	360	13%
honey Dijon chicken	1 bowl	3.5	400	8%
southwestern style black beans & vegetables	1 bowl	4.5	360	11%
spicy Beef & Broccoli	1 bowl	4.5	370	11%
sweet & sour chicken	1 bowl	3.0	380	7%
Szechuan chicken	1 bowl	4.0	360	10%
teriyaki chicken	1 bowl	5.0	430	10%
teriyaki stir fry w/vegetables	1 bowl	3.0	360	8%
■ MIX				
(Betty Crocker) prepared as directed				
Rice w/Seasoning				
cheddar & broccoli	1 cup	10.0	310	29%
chicken herb	1 cup	5.0	270	17%
creamy herb risotto	1 cup	12.0	320	34%
garden vegetable pilaf	1 cup	6.0	240	23%
herb rice & barley medley	⅓ cup	1.0	180	5%
long train & wild rice pilaf	1 cup	5.0	220	20%
Southwestern rice	1 cup	6.0	250	22%
(Casbah) pilaf/prepared				
nutted	1 cup	3.0	220	12%
original	1 cup	1.0	200	5%
Spanish	1 cup	1.0	200	2%
(Fantastic Foods) dry mix only				
Pilaf				
Basmati	¼ cup	–	170	–
4 grain	½ cup	1.0	160	6%
Hacienda Spanish	⅜ cup	1.0	160	6%
organic	¼ cup	0.5	170	3%
vegetable chicken	¼ cup	–	170	–
Rice & beans				
Bombay curry/cup	2.4 oz	1.5	250	5%
Cajun/cup	2.3 oz	3.0	230	12%
Caribbean black beans	1 pkg	1.5	230	6%
Jamaican				
side dish	⅓ cup	1.5	140	10%
spicy w/black beans/cup	2.4 oz	1.5	250	5%
New Orleans	⅓ cup	1.5	130	10%
Tex-Mex/cup	2.3 oz	2.5	240	9%
Risotto				
classico	¼ cup	2.0	140	13%

Food and Description	Amount	Fat Grams	Total Calories	% Fat Calories
Tuscany mushroom (Farm House) mix only	¼ cup	1.0	130	7%
beans & rice				
w/Mexican pinto beans	⅓ cup	1.0	190	5%
w/red beans	⅓ cup	1.0	180	5%
w/Spanish black beans	⅓ cup	1.0	200	5%
broccoli au gratin	⅓ cup	2.0	210	9%
chicken	⅓ cup	1.5	180	8%
herb & butter	⅓ cup	2.0	210	9%
long grain & wild	⅓ cup	2.0	200	9%
Mexican	⅓ cup	1.0	180	5%
rice pilaf	⅓ cup	1.0	200	5%
Spanish rice	⅓ cup	1.5	180	8%
(Golden Grain) prepared according to pkg directions				
Rice-A-Roni				
beef & mushroom	1 cup	7.0	290	22%
beef flavor				
⅓ less salt	1 cup	5.0	280	16%
regular	1 cup	9.0	310	26%
broccoli	1 cup	10.0	280	32%
broccoli au gratin				
⅓ less salt	1 cup	11.0	320	31%
regular	1 cup	17.0	360	43%
chicken & broccoli	1 cup	6.0	230	23%
chicken & garlic	1 cup	9.0	260	31%
chicken & mushroom	1 cup	14.0	360	35%
chicken & vegetables	1 cup	7.0	290	22%
chicken flavor				
low-fat	1 cup	3.0	210	9%
⅓ less salt	1 cup	5.0	280	16%
original	1 cup	9.0	310	26%
fried rice				
⅓ less salt	1 cup	3.5	260	12%
regular	1 cup	11.0	320	31%
herb & butter	1 cup	9.0	320	25%
herb roasted chicken	1 cup	9.0	260	31%
long grain & wild rice	1 cup	6.0	240	23%
long grain & wild pilaf	1 cup	6.0	240	23%
Long Grain & Wild Rice chicken w/almonds	1 cup	8.0	300	24%
Mexican style	1 cup	8.0	260	28%
Oriental stir-fry	1 cup	6.0	290	19%
red beans & rice	1 cup	7.0	290	22%
rice pilaf	1 cup	9.0	310	26%
savory chicken vegetable/low-fat	1 cup	3.0	210	13%
Spanish rice	1 cup	8.0	270	27%
stroganoff	1 cup	15.0	360	38%
white cheddar & herbs	1 cup	13.0	340	34%
(Goodman's) Rice & Vermicelli/prepared for beef	¾ cup	1.0	160	6%

Food and Description	Amount	Fat Grams	Total Calories	% Fat Calories
for chicken	¾ cup	1.0	160	6%
(Kashi) 7 whole grain & sesame pilaf/cooked	½ cup	3.0	170	26%
(Knorr) dry mix only				
Mexican style	1.95 oz	1.0	200	5%
rice & black beans	2.28 oz	1.0	220	4%
rice & pinto beans	2.28 oz	1.0	230	4%
yellow	2.28 oz	0.5	230	2%
(Konriko) wild pecan rice	⅕ box	1.0	160	6%
(Lipton) mix only				
Rice & Sauce				
alfredo broccoli	½ pkg	5.0	240	19%
beef	½ pkg	1.5	220	6%
beef broccoli	½ pkg	1.5	220	6%
Cajun style	½ pkg	1.5	220	6%
Cajun style w/rice and beans	½ pkg	1.5	260	5%
cheddar broccoli	½ cup	3.0	230	12%
chicken				
broccoli	½ pkg	2.5	230	10%
flavored	½ pkg	2.5	230	10%
fried rice	½ pkg	2.0	240	8%
& parmesan risotto	½ pkg	2.5	220	10%
creamy chicken	½ pkg	5.0	240	19%
creamy garlic parmesan risotto	½ pkg	5.0	250	18%
herb & butter	½ pkg	4.5	230	18%
long grain & wild rice				
mushroom & herb	½ pkg	2.0	250	7%
original	½ pkg	1.5	230	6%
medley	½ pkg	2.5	220	10%
pilaf	½ pkg	1.5	210	6%
scampi style	½ pkg	2.5	220	10%
Spanish	½ pkg	1.5	210	6%
teriyaki	½ pkg	2.0	220	8%
Sizzle & Stir				
lemon garlic chicken	⅙ pkg	3.5	180	18%
Spanish chicken	⅙ pkg	4.0	190	19%
Teriyaki stir-fry chicken	⅙ pkg	4.5	200	20%
(Luzianne) dinner kit/mix only				
Ètouffee	¼ box	1.0	200	5%
gumbo	⅕ box	1.0	160	6%
jambalaya	⅕ box	1.0	160	6%
shrimp Creole	⅕ box	0.5	150	3%
(Mahatma) dry mix only				
black bean	2 oz	1.5	200	7%
broccoli & cheese	2 oz	2.0	200	9%
jambalaya	2 oz	1.0	190	5%
long grain & wild rice	2 oz	1.0	190	5%
pilaf	2 oz	–	190	–
Spanish	2 oz	1.0	180	5%
yellow	2 oz	–	190	–

Food and Description	Amount	Fat Grams	Total Calories	% Fat Calories
(Mayacamas) Just Enough				
chicken w/broccoli	1 cup	–	100	–
rice jalapeño	1 cup	–	130	–
(MJB) prepared				
fried rice Oriental	½ cup	1.0	110	8%
herb & butter	½ cup	1.0	100	9%
Mexican style	½ cup	–	120	–
rice pilaf	½ cup	1.0	110	8%
savory beet	½ cup	1.0	100	9%
savory chicken	½ cup	1.0	100	9%
(Near East) rice pilaf/prepared				
brown rice	1 cup	5.0	220	20%
chicken flavor	1 cup	3.5	210	15%
curry	1 cup	4.0	220	16%
garlic & herb	1 cup	3.5	220	14%
lentil	1 cup	3.0	200	14%
long grain & wild rice	1 cup	3.0	210	13%
Mediterranean black bean & rice	1 cup	5.0	270	17%
Mediterranean chicken-w/wild rice	1 cup	3.0	210	13%
red beans & rice	1 cup	3.5	220	14%
rice pilaf	1 cup	3.0	210	13%
Spanish rice	1 cup	6.0	290	19%
toasted almond	1 cup	5.0	220	20%
wheat	1 cup	4.5	220	18%
wild mushroom & herb	1 cup	3.5	220	14%
(Old El Paso)				
Mexican rice				
cheesy				
mix only	½ cup	3.5	420	8%
prepared	4 oz	3.5	420	8%
regular				
mix only	½ cup	2.0	410	4%
prepared	4 oz	2.0	410	4%
Spanish rice				
mix only	½ cup	2.0	410	4%
prepared	4 oz	2.0	410	4%
(Pritikin)				
Mexican	⅓ cup	2.0	200	9%
Oriental	⅓ cup	1.5	190	7%
Rice-A-Roni (*See* (Golden Grain) in this section)				
(Success) prepared				
beef Oriental	½ cup	–	100	–
broccoli & cheese	½ cup	–	120	–
brown & wild	½ cup	–	120	–
chicken	½ cup	–	100	–
pilaf	½ cup	–	120	–
Spanish	½ cup	–	110	–
(Suzi Wan) prepared, w/o butter or margarine				
chicken flavor				
w/broccoli	½ cup	1.0	120	8%

Food and Description	Amount	Fat Grams	Total Calories	% Fat Calories
w/vegetables	½ cup	1.0	120	8%
dinner recipe				
sweet & sour	½ cup	1.0	130	7%
teriyaki	½ cup	1.0	120	8%
(Tony Chachere's) dry mix only				
butter beans & rice/old fashioned	¼ pkg	1.0	170	5%
Creole mix				
gumbo	¾ oz	–	70	–
Jambalaya	1.39 oz	–	140	–
Louisiana dirty rice	⅕ pkg	–	160	–
New Orleans red beans & rice	¼ pkg	–	100	–
Southern white beans & rice	¼ pkg	1.0	170	5%
(Uncle Ben's)				
Country Inn/mix only				
broccoli almondine	1.2 oz	1.5	125	11%
broccoli rice au gratin	1.1 oz	2.0	115	16%
chicken				
homestyle chicken & vegetables	1.2 oz	3.0	140	19%
stock rice	1.1 oz	1.0	125	7%
w/wild rice	1.1 oz	1.0	110	8%
creamy chicken				
& mushroom	1.2 oz	3.0	140	19%
& wild rice	1.3 oz	1.5	135	10%
green bean & almondine casserole	1.2 oz	2.0	130	14%
herbed rice au gratin	1.1 oz	2.0	120	15%
rice Florentine	1.1 oz	1.5	120	11%
vegetable pilaf	1.2 oz	1.0	115	8%
(Vigo) dry mix only				
black beans & rice	⅓ cup	0.5	190	2%
pinto beans & rice	⅙ cup	2.0	200	9%
red beans & rice	⅓ cup	–	190	–
Santa Fe beans & rice	⅓ cup	2.0	200	9%
yellow rice	⅓ cup	1.0	190	5%
(Zatarain's)				
gumbo w/rice				
mix only	3 Tbs	–	150	–
prepared	1 cup	–	150	–
New Orleans jambalaya				
mix	3 Tbs	–	150	–
prepared	1 cup	–	150	–
RICE DRINK				
(Don Jose) Hor Chata nondairy	6 oz	4.0	120	30%
(Grainaissance) Amazake				
almond	8 fl oz	4.0	200	18%
apricot	8 fl oz	–	160	–
cocoa-almond	8 fl oz	3.0	200	14%
mocha java	8 fl oz	2.0	180	10%
sesame	8 fl oz	1.0	200	5%
vanilla pecan	8 fl oz	4.0	200	18%

Food and Description	Amount	Fat Grams	Total Calories	% Fat Calories
(Rice Dream)				
carob	8 fl oz	2.5	150	15%
chocolate	8 fl oz	3.0	170	21%
original	8 fl oz	2.0	130	14%
vanilla				
enriched	8 fl oz	2.0	120	15%
regular	8 fl oz	2.0	130	14%
RICE FLOUR (See FLOUR)				
RICE FROZEN DESSERT				
(Rice Dream)				
Dream Bar				
chocolate/chocolate	1 bar	15.0	270	50%
chocolate nutty	1 bar	18.0	270	60%
strawberry	1 bar	13.0	250	47%
vanilla	1 bar	14.0	270	47%
vanilla nutty	1 bar	18.0	260	62%
Nondairy frozen dessert				
cappuccino	½ cup	6.0	150	36%
carob almond	½ cup	8.0	170	40%
carob chip	½ cup	6.0	150	36%
cherry vanilla	½ cup	6.0	150	36%
chocolate	½ cup	7.0	150	42%
chocolate chip	½ cup	8.0	170	42%
cocoa marble fudge	½ cup	6.0	150	36%
cookies N' Dream	½ cup	7.0	170	37%
mint carob chip	½ cup	8.0	170	42%
mint chocolate chip	½ cup	8.0	170	42%
Neapolitan	½ cup	6.0	150	36%
orange vanilla swirl	½ cup	6.0	150	36%
strawberry	½ cup	5.0	140	32%
vanilla	½ cup	6.0	150	36%
vanilla Swiss almond	½ cup	8.0	180	40%
Rice Dream nondairy Pies				
chocolate	1 pie	17.0	320	48%
mint	1 pie	18.0	320	51%
mocha	1 pie	17.0	320	48%
vanilla	1 pie	17.0	320	48%
Rice Dream Supreme				
cappuccino almond fudge	½ cup	8.0	170	42%
cherry chocolate chunk	½ cup	7.0	170	37%
chocolate almond chunk	½ cup	8.0	170	42%
chocolate fudge brownie	½ cup	7.0	170	37%
double espresso bean	½ cup	7.0	160	39%
mint chocolate cookie	½ cup	8.0	170	42%
peanut butter cup	½ cup	8.0	180	40%
pralines N'Dream	½ cup	9.0	180	45%
RICE NOODLE (See ASIAN FOOD)				
RICE POLISH /stirred & spooned into cup	1 cup	13.0	278	42%
RICE PUDDING (See PUDDING & MOUSSE)				
RICE SYRUP (See also PANCAKE & WAFFLE SYRUP)				

Food and Description	Amount	Fat Grams	Total Calories	% Fat Calories
(Lundberg) Sweet Dreams	1 Tbs	<1.0	40	7%

RIGATONI (*See* PASTA; PASTA ENTRÉE/DINNER)
ROAST BEEF (*See* BEEF, LUNCHEON MEAT)
ROAST BEEF HASH (*See* BEEF; DISH/ENTRÉE)
ROAST BEEF SPREAD (*See* LUNCHEON MEAT SPREAD)
ROASTING BAGS, SEASONED (*See* SEASONINGS)
ROCKFISH
Pacific/mixed species

Food and Description	Amount	Fat Grams	Total Calories	% Fat Calories
cooked	3 oz	2.0	110	16%
raw	3 oz	1.0	80	11%

ROLL (*See also* CROISSANT; PASTRY; SCONE)
■ **BROWN & SERVE**
(Arnold) Francisco

Food and Description	Amount	Fat Grams	Total Calories	% Fat Calories
sourdough	1 roll	1.0	100	10%
(Country Hearth) krusty				
Italian	1 roll	4.0	170	21%
plain	1 roll	4.0	170	21%
generic				
cloverleaf	1 roll	1.9	84	20%
(Pepperidge Farm)				
bakery/French	½ roll	2.0	180	10%
European Bake Shoppe				
club	1 roll	1.0	100	9%
French	½ roll	2.0	180	10%
hearth	1 roll	1.0	50	18%
(Roman Meal)	2 rolls	2.0	140	13%
(Wonder) Rolls				
du Jour				
cracked wheat	1 roll	1.0	100	9%
crusty Italian	1 roll	0.5	90	5%
sourdough	1 roll	0.5	90	5%
w/buttermilk	1 roll	2.0	80	23%
Wonder				
sourdough	1 roll	1.5	70	13%
wheat	1 roll	1.5	80	17%
white	1 roll	0.5	80	6%

■ **FROZEN**
(Cole's)

Food and Description	Amount	Fat Grams	Total Calories	% Fat Calories
garlic	1 roll	5.0	100	45%
generic/dough, baked				
Parker House	1 roll	1.0	75	12%
(Mama Bella) garlic dinner	1 roll	4.0	130	28%
(Pepperidge Farm)				
garlic & cheese	1 roll	5.0	130	35%
(Rhodes) bread dough, baked				
cinnamon roll	1 roll	10.0	240	38%
Texas dinner				
wheat	1 roll	3.0	140	19%
white	1 roll	3.0	150	18%

Food and Description	Amount	Fat Grams	Total Calories	% Fat Calories
white dinner	1 roll	2.0	100	18%
(Sara Lee) food service				
hard				
light rye	1 roll	1.0	80	11%
malt rye	1 roll	1.0	80	11%
sandwich kaiser	¼ roll	4.0	170	21%
white/assorted	1 roll	2.0	80	23%
soft				
butterfly	1 roll	3.0	90	30%
cloverleaf	1 roll	3.0	90	30%
crescent	1 roll	5.0	100	5%
finger	3 rolls	5.0	170	27%
Parker House	3 rolls	5.0	170	27%
sesame seed	1 roll	3.0	70	39%
white	1 roll	2.0	90	20%
■ HEAT & SERVE				
(Pepperidge Farm) Brown'N Serve				
butter crescent	1 roll	6.0	110	49%
golden twist	1 roll	5.0	110	41%
■ HOMEMADE				
USDA Standard Home Recipe				
cloverleaf/2½" dia	1 roll	3.0	120	23%
dinner/soft white	1 roll	3.0	120	23%
popover	1 roll	3.7	90	37%
■ MIX				
generic				
popover/prepared	1 roll	5.0	170	26%
(Pillsbury)				
hot roll				
mix only	¼ cup	1.0	110	17%
prepared	1 roll	3.0	130	21%
■ READY TO SERVE				
(Arnold)				
Arnold				
deli				
Kaiser	1 roll	2.0	170	11%
onion	1 roll	2.0	170	11%
dinner				
country white				
12 per pkg	1 roll	1.0	50	18%
24 per pkg	1 roll	1.5	110	12%
enriched 24 per pkg	1 roll	2.5	120	19%
w/sesame seeds	2 rolls	1.0	50	18%
Dutch egg	1 roll	3.0	130	21%
hamburger				
8 per pkg	1 roll	2.0	130	14%
12 per pkg	1 roll	2.0	120	15%
hot dog				
New England style	1 roll	2.0	110	16%

Food and Description	Amount	Fat Grams	Total Calories	% Fat Calories
regular				
8 per 11-oz pkg	1 roll	2.0	100	18%
8 per 12-oz pkg	1 roll	2.0	110	16%
12 per pkg	1 roll	2.0	110	16%
Italian Savoni/8-inch	1 roll	3.0	210	13%
kaiser sandwich				
w/sesame seeds	1 roll	3.5	140	23%
onion				
premium	1 roll	1.0	180	5%
soft	1 roll	–	140	–
potato				
dinner	1 roll	1.5	110	12%
hot dog	1 roll	2.0	120	15%
Italian	1 roll	3.5	280	11%
plain	1 roll	2.0	140	13%
sandwich/soft				
Dutch sesame/8 per pkg	1 roll	3.0	170	16%
original/12 per pkg	1 roll	3.0	130	21%
plain	1 roll	2.0	150	12%
Bran'nola				
bun w/bran	1 roll	2.0	130	14%
buns	1 roll	1.0	100	9%
dinner/white	1 roll	1.0	70	13%
hot dog	1 roll	1.5	110	12%
Francisco				
French				
6" roll	1 roll	3.0	210	13%
mini	1 roll	2.0	130	14%
kaiser	1 roll	1.0	180	5%
sourdough	1 roll	1.0	100	9%
steak	1 roll	2.0	170	11%
super sub loaf	1-oz slice	0.5	70	6%
3" roll	1 roll	1.0	90	10%
Levy Old Country				
kaiser	1 roll	2.0	170	11%
onion	1 roll	3.0	160	17%
sub	1 roll	2.0	180	10%
(August Brothers)				
dinner				
wheat	1 roll	2.0	100	18%
white				
10 per pkg	1 roll	2.0	90	20%
16-oz pkg	1 roll	1.0	90	10%
hamburger				
wheat	1 roll	2.0	130	14%
white	1 roll	2.5	140	16%
kaiser	1 roll	2.0	160	11%
onion	1 roll	2.0	160	11%
sesame	1 roll	2.5	170	13%

Food and Description	Amount	Fat Grams	Total Calories	% Fat Calories
steak	1 roll	2.5	170	13%
sub	1 roll	2.5	170	13%
(Awrey's)				
dinner	1 roll	1.0	60	15%
Black Forest	1 roll	1.0	50	18%
cracked wheat	1 roll	1.0	50	18%
crusty	1 roll	1.0	70	13%
poppy seed	1 roll	1.0	60	15%
sesame seed	1 roll	1.0	60	15%
sandwich/oat bran	1 roll	2.0	120	15%
(Brownberry)				
Brownberry				
hot dog				
sliced	1 roll	2.0	110	16%
wheat	1 roll	2.0	110	16%
sandwich				
potato	1 roll	2.5	150	15%
wheat	1 roll	2.0	130	14%
white	1 roll	2.5	140	16%
Francisco International				
dinner	1 roll	1.0	120	8%
French/6" roll	1 roll	1.0	170	5%
kaiser	1 roll	1.0	170	5%
Hearth				
assorted	1 roll	1.5	120	11%
kaiser	1 roll	2.5	150	15%
National/white sandwich				
plain	1 roll	2.5	140	16%
w/sesame seeds	1 roll	3.0	140	19%
(Colombo)				
49er				
sour	1 roll	<1.0	90	5%
sweet	1 roll	2.0	95	19%
Luigi/twin pack	1 roll	1.5	145	9%
steak				
sour	1 roll	2.0	200	9%
sweet	1 roll	3.0	200	14%
(Earth Grains)				
French	1 roll	1.0	100	9%
kaiser	1 roll	2.0	190	10%
onion	1 roll	2.0	190	10%
submarine	½ roll	1.0	180	5%
generic				
cloverleaf	1 roll	1.6	83	17%
cracked wheat	1 roll	<1.0	95	8%
dinner/white				
hard	1 roll	1.6	156	9%
soft	1 roll	2.0	85	21%
egg	1 roll	2.0	110	16%

Food and Description	Amount	Fat Grams	Total Calories	% Fat Calories
French	1 roll	1.0	130	7%
hamburger				
multigrain	1 roll	2.0	115	16%
reduced calorie	1 roll	1.0	85	11%
white	1 roll	2.0	125	14%
hard	1 roll	2.0	170	11%
hot cross bun	1 roll	4.0	200	18%
hot dog				
multi-grain	1 roll	2.0	115	16%
reduced calorie	1 roll	1.0	85	11%
regular	1 roll	2.0	125	14%
kaiser	1 roll	2.0	170	11%
oat bran	1 roll	2.0	80	23%
potato roll	1 roll	2.0	130	14%
rye	1 roll	1.0	80	11%
sourdough	1 roll	1.0	130	7%
whole wheat	1 roll	1.0	93	10%
(Hollywood) dark	1 roll	–	40	–
(Holsum) hamburger	1 roll	2.0	120	15%
(Home Pride)				
buns				
potato/1.5 oz	1 bun	1.0	110	8%
wheat				
1.89 oz	1 bun	2.0	140	13%
2.5 oz	1 bun	2.5	180	13%
dinner rolls				
wheat/1.6 oz	2 rolls	3.0	140	19%
white/1.6 oz	1 roll	1.0	130	7%
(Lewis) Italian crispy dinner	1 roll	1.0	100	18%
(King's Hawaiian)				
honey wheat	1 roll	2.0	90	20%
regular	1 roll	2.0	90	20%
(Martin's)				
Big Marty				
poppy	1 roll	2.0	170	11%
sesame	1 roll	2.0	170	11%
hoagie				
plain	1 roll	3.0	240	11%
sesame	1 roll	3.0	240	11%
potato				
dinner	1 roll	1.0	100	9%
long	1 roll	1.0	140	6%
party	1 roll	1.0	50	18%
potato/sliced	1 roll	1.0	90	30%
sandwich	1 roll	1.0	140	6%
whole wheat	1 roll	2.0	160	11%
(Oroweat)				
health nut	1 roll	3.0	160	17%
master's best/winter wheat	1 roll	4.0	160	23%

Food and Description	Amount	Fat Grams	Total Calories	% Fat Calories
(Pepperidge Farm)				
bakery				
dinner				
country style classic	1 roll	1.0	50	18%
hearty potato classic	1 roll	2.5	80	28%
finger				
w/poppy seeds	3 rolls	4.5	150	27%
w/sesame seeds	3 rolls	4.5	150	27%
frankfurter				
Dijon	1 roll	3.0	140	19%
side-sliced	1 roll	2.5	140	16%
top-sliced	1 roll	2.5	140	16%
garlic & cheese	1 roll	5.0	130	35%
hamburger/sliced	1 roll	2.5	130	17%
hoagie				
deli classic soft	1 roll	4.0	200	18%
multigrain	1 roll	4.0	200	18%
Parker House	3 rolls	4.0	150	24%
party	5 rolls	4.0	170	21%
sandwich				
hearty	1 roll	5.0	230	20%
multigrain	1 roll	3.0	150	18%
onion/sliced	1 roll	3.0	150	18%
potato	1 roll	4.0	160	23%
sliced w/sesame seeds	1 roll	3.0	140	19%
sourdough	1 roll	3.5	170	19%
seven grain French	1 roll	2.0	80	23%
sourdough French	1 roll	1.0	100	9%
(Rainbo) hog dog/white	1 roll	1.5	100	14%
(Roman Meal)				
dinner	2 rolls	2.0	140	13%
hamburger	1 roll	2.0	120	15%
hotdog	1 roll	2.0	110	16%
(Vie De France)				
baguette/mini	1 baguette	1.5	240	6%
French	1 roll	0.5	120	4%
(Wonder)				
buns				
enriched white	1.5 oz bun	1.5	110	12%
	2 oz bun	2.0	150	12%
	2.5 oz bun	3.0	190	14%
	3 oz bun	3.0	220	12%
multigrain	1 bun	2.0	140	13%
wheat	1.5 oz bun	2.0	120	15%
	1.89 oz bun	2.0	140	13%
	2.5 oz bun	2.5	180	13%
yellow	1 bun	2.5	160	14%
country grain hot	1 roll	1.0	100	9%
dinner rolls				
honey rich	1 roll	1.5	100	14%

Food and Description	Amount	Fat Grams	Total Calories	% Fat Calories
wheat	2 rolls	3.0	140	19%
white	1 roll	1.0	130	7%
French				
club	1 roll	1.5	120	11%
hoagie	1 roll	2.5	220	10%
grain				
club	1 roll	1.5	120	11%
hoagie	1 roll	3.0	220	12%
hotdog				
bun	1 roll	2.0	110	16%
roll	1 roll	2.0	80	11%
kaiser				
buns	1 bun	3.0	180	15%
hoagie	1 roll	2.5	220	10%
regular	1 roll	1.5	150	9%
potato buns	1 bun	1.0	110	8%
sourdough				
club	1 roll	1.5	120	11%
hoagie	1 roll	2.5	220	10%
steak	1 roll	2.5	190	12%
■ REFRIGERATED				
(Pillsbury)				
crescent				
Grands!	1 roll	15.0	270	50%
original	1 roll	6.0	110	49%
reduced-fat	1 roll	4.5	100	41%
dinner				
wheat	1 roll	2.0	100	18%
white	1 roll	2.0	110	16%
ROOT BEER (See SOFT DRINK)				
ROSE APPLE /fresh	3.5 oz	<1.0	25	11%
ROSELLE /raw	½ cup	–	15	–
ROSEMARY /dried	1 tsp	–	4	–
ROTINI (See PASTA; PASTA ENTRÉE/DINNER)				
ROUGHY (See ORANGE ROUGHY; SEAFOOD ENTRÉE/DINNER)				
RUM (See LIQUOR, DISTILLED)				
RUTABAGA /fresh				
boiled-drained				
cubed	½ cup	–	30	–
mashed	½ cup	–	40	–
raw	½ cup	–	25	–
RYE (See also FLOUR; CEREAL; LIQUOR, DISTILLED)				
(Arrowhead Mills)flakes/rolled	⅓ cup	0.5	110	4%
generic/whole-grain	1 cup	4.0	565	6%

S

Food and Description	Amount	Fat Grams	Total Calories	% Fat Calories
SABLEFISH				
raw	3 oz	13.0	165	71%
smoked	3 oz	17.0	220	70%
SAFFLOWER MARGARINE/SPREAD (*See* MARGARINE, MARGARINE SPREAD, & SPRAY)				
SAFFLOWER MEAL	1 oz	0.7	97	6%
SAFFLOWER OIL (*See* OIL)				
SAFFLOWER SEEDS				
kernels/dried	1 oz	11.0	150	66%
SAFFRON				
dried	1 tsp	–	2	–
SAGE				
ground	1 tsp	–	4	–
SALAD DRESSING (*See also* MAYONNAISE/MAYONNAISE-TYPE DRESSING)				
■ **HOMEMADE**				
USDA Standard Home Recipe				
cooked/made w/margarine	1 Tbs	2.0	25	72%
French	1 Tbs	10.0	90	100%
vinegar & oil	1 Tbs	8.0	70	100%
■ **MIX** (Note: Unless otherwise stated, mixes were prepared as directed on package.)				
(Andre Frost) A Taste of Thai				
spicy peanut	2 Tbs	1.5	40	34%
(Good Seasons) prepared, as directed				
cheese garlic	2 Tbs	15.0	140	96%
garlic & herbs	2 Tbs	15.0	140	96%
gourmet				
Caesar	2 Tbs	16.0	150	96%
Parmesan Italian	2 Tbs	16.0	150	96%
honey				
French				
fat-free	2 Tbs	–	20	–
regular	2 Tbs	15.0	160	84%
mustard				
fat-free	2 Tbs	–	20	–
regular	2 Tbs	15.0	150	90%
Italian				
mild	2 Tbs	15.0	150	90%
reduced-calorie	2 Tbs	1.0	50	18%
regular	2 Tbs	15.0	140	96%
zesty				
reduced-calorie	2 Tbs	1.0	50	18%

Food and Description	Amount	Fat Grams	Total Calories	% Fat Calories
regular	2 Tbs	15.0	140	96%
Mexican spice	2 Tbs	15.0	140	96%
Oriental sesame	2 Tbs	16.0	150	96%
roasted garlic	2 Tbs	15.0	140	96%
zesty herb/fat-free	2 Tbs	–	20	–
(Hain) No Oil/prepared				
bleu cheese	1 Tbs	–	14	–
buttermilk	1 Tbs	–	11	–
Caesar	1 Tbs	–	6	–
French	1 Tbs	–	12	–
garlic & cheese	1 Tbs	–	6	–
herb	1 Tbs	–	2	–
Italian	1 Tbs	–	2	–
thousand island	1 Tbs	–	12	–
(Hidden Valley)				
bacon				
mix only	1/16 pkg	–	10	–
prepared	2 Tbs	12.0	120	90%
blue cheese				
mix only	1/16 pkg	–	100	–
prepared	2 Tbs	12.0	120	90%
honey Dijon				
mix only	1/16 pkg	–	15	–
prepared	2 Tbs	12.0	120	90%
original				
buttermilk				
mix only	1/16 pkg	–	–	–
prepared	2 Tbs	11.0	110	90%
low-fat				
mix only	1/16 pkg	–	10	–
prepared	2 Tbs	1.0	30	30%
milk				
mix only	1/16 pkg	–	5	–
prepared	2 Tbs	12.0	120	90%
reduced calorie				
mix only	1/16 pkg	–	5	–
prepared	2 Tbs	6.0	70	77%
ranch Italian				
mix only	1/16 pkg	–	15	–
prepared	2 Tbs	14.0	140	90%
(Lawry's) mix only				
Caesar	1 pkg	3.0	75	36%
Italian				
regular	1 pkg	<1.0	45	4%
w/cheese	1 pkg	2.0	75	24%
(Macayamas) mix only (Note: 1 serving of mix = the amount in 1 Tbs prepared.)				
Italian supreme	1 serving	<1.0	8	56%
(Weight Watchers) mix only (Note: 1 serving of mix = the amount in 2 Tbs prepared.)				
blue cheese	1 serving	–	10	–
French	1 serving	–	–	–

Food and Description	Amount	Fat Grams	Total Calories	% Fat Calories
Italian				
creamy	1 serving	–	5	–
regular	1 serving	–	–	–
Russian	1 serving	–	–	–
Thousand Island	1 serving	–	–	–
■ READY TO USE				
(Andre Prost) A Taste of Thai				
Mexican chipotle	1½ Tbs	9.0	100	81%
spicy peanut	¼ cup	8.0	120	60%
(Annie's) wild herbal organics				
balsamic	2 Tbs	10.0	100	90%
cilantro & lime	2 Tbs	10.0	100	90%
cowgirl ranch	2 Tbs	8.0	90	80%
gingerly	2 Tbs	10.0	100	90%
shiitake & sesame	2 Tbs	13.0	120	98%
vinaigrette				
ginger & chamomile	2 Tbs	13.0	130	90%
honey & turmeric	2 Tbs	15.0	170	79%
raspberry	2 Tbs	9.0	110	74%
yogurt/no-fat	2 Tbs	–	20	–
(Ayla's) fat-free				
creamy dill	2 Tbs	–	15	–
French	2 Tbs	–	10	–
garlic & onion	2 Tbs	–	10	–
Italian				
creamy	2 Tbs	–	15	–
regular	2 Tbs	–	10	–
Russian	2 Tbs	–	10	–
spicy Indonesian	2 Tbs	2.5	35	64%
(Bernstein's)				
Fat-Free				
creamy herb ranch	2 Tbs	–	30	–
cheese & garlic itlian	2 Tbs	–	10	–
Light Fantastic				
cheese fantastico	2 Tbs	1.5	25	54%
classico Italian	2 Tbs	1.5	25	54%
Italian w/cheese	2 Tbs	2.0	25	72%
Oriental	2 Tbs	1.5	60	23%
Parmesan garlic ranch	2 Tbs	2.5	50	45%
restaurant ranch	2 Tbs	2.0	45	40%
Regular				
balsamic Italian	2 Tbs	11.0	110	90%
Caesar/creamy	2 Tbs	13.0	120	98%
cheese fantastico	2 Tbs	10.0	100	90%
cheese & garlic Italian	2 Tbs	11.0	110	90%
chunky blue cheese	2 Tbs	13.0	120	98%
creamy roasted garlic	2 Tbs	15.0	150	90%
French vinaigrette	2 Tbs	10.0	100	90%
herb & garlic Italian	2 Tbs	13.0	130	90%
herb garden French	2 Tbs	11.0	130	76%

Food and Description	Amount	Fat Grams	Total Calories	% Fat Calories
Parmesan garlic ranch	2 Tbs	14.0	140	90%
red wine & garlic Italian	2 Tbs	11.0	110	91%
restaurant recipe Italian	2 Tbs	12.0	120	90%
Roquefort	2 Tbs	14.0	130	97%
wine country Italian	2 Tbs	11.0	110	91%
(Bertolli) olive oil				
creamy	2 Tbs	12.0	120	90%
original	2 Tbs	16.0	160	90%
zesty	2 Tbs	14.0	140	90%
(Best)				
Citrus Splash				
orange vinaigrette	2 Tbs	7.0	80	79%
Oriental orange	2 Tbs	7.0	90	70%
ruby red ginger	2 Tbs	7.0	90	70%
tangerine	2 Tbs	6.0	80	68%
tangerine balsamic	2 Tbs	7.0	80	79%
Regular				
Caesar				
creamy	2 Tbs	18.0	170	95%
fat-free	2 Tbs	–	30	–
original	2 Tbs	9.0	100	81%
chardonnay vinaigrette	2 Tbs	4.0	50	72%
French				
creamy	2 Tbs	16.0	160	90%
fat-free	2 Tbs	–	45	–
garlic ranch	2 Tbs	15.0	140	96%
honey Dijon				
fat-free	2 Tbs	–	50	–
Italian				
fat-free	2 Tbs	–	15	–
herb ranch	2 Tbs	14.0	130	97%
original	2 Tbs	11.0	110	90%
ranch				
creamy	2 Tbs	15.0	140	96%
Dressing-To-Go	1.5 oz pkg	21.0	200	95%
fat-free	2 Tbs	–	45	–
spring onion	2 Tbs	14.0	130	97%
raspberry vinaigrette/fat-free	2 Tbs	–	35	–
roasted tomato balsamic vinaigrette	2 Tbs	10.0	100	90%
thousand island/creamy	2 Tbs	13.0	130	90%
(Brianna's) homestyle				
blush wine vinaigrette	2 Tbs	6.0	100	54%
poppy seed	2 Tbs	10.0	130	69%
real French vinaigrette	2 Tbs	10.0	130	69%
(Cardini's)				
Dressing & Marinade				
Italian	2 Tbs	13.0	120	98%
lemon herb	2 Tbs	13.0	130	90%
lime dill	2 Tbs	14.0	130	97%
pesto pasta	2 Tbs	14.0	140	90%

Food and Description	Amount	Fat Grams	Total Calories	% Fat Calories
Natural				
Caesar	2 Tbs	17.0	150	100%
Parmesan ranch	2 Tbs	15.0	150	90%
roasted red pepper	2 Tbs	11.0	110	90%
Romano cheese Italian	2 Tbs	13.0	130	90%
spicy French	2 Tbs	11.0	130	76%
Original				
balsamic vinaigrette	2 Tbs	16.0	150	96%
Caesar				
fat-free	2 Tbs	–	40	–
light	2 Tbs	7.0	80	79%
low-fat	2 Tbs	1.5	45	30%
regular	2 Tbs	17.0	160	96%
Parmesan/low-fat	2 Tbs	2.0	45	40%
poppy seed	2 Tbs	1.0	35	26%
red wine & vinegar	2 Tbs	8.0	90	80%
roasted garlic	2 Tbs	14.0	130	97%
summer honey mustard	2 Tbs	14.0	150	84%
The Source herb French dressing	2 Tbs	13.0	130	90%
(Dorothy Lynch) homestyle/ reduced calorie	2 Tbs	–	60	–
(Estee)				
creamy French	2 Tbs	–	10	–
Italian	2 Tbs	–	5	–
(Girard's)				
balsamic vinaigrette/fat-free	2 Tbs	–	25	–
Caesar				
fat-free	2 Tbs	–	40	–
light	2 Tbs	7.0	80	79%
champagne/light	2 Tbs	5.0	60	75%
Oriental	2 Tbs	11.0	120	83%
raspberry/fat-free	2 Tbs	–	50	–
red wine vinaigrette/fat-free	2 Tbs	–	20	–
(Hain)				
buttermilk/old fashioned	1 Tbs	7.0	70	90%
Canola				
garden tomato	1 Tbs	6.0	60	90%
Italian	1 Tbs	5.0	50	90%
spicy French mustard	1 Tbs	5.0	50	90%
tangy citrus	1 Tbs	5.0	50	90%
Caesar				
creamy	1 Tbs	6.0	60	90%
low-salt	1 Tbs	6.0	60	90%
cucumber dill	1 Tbs	7.0	70	90%
French				
creamy	1 Tbs	6.0	60	90%
garlic & sour cream	1 Tbs	7.0	70	90%
honey & sesame	1 Tbs	5.0	60	75%
Italian/creamy				
no salt added	1 Tbs	8.0	80	90%

Food and Description	Amount	Fat Grams	Total Calories	% Fat Calories
regular	1 Tbs	8.0	80	90%
traditional	1 Tbs	8.0	80	90%
traditional/no salt added	1 Tbs	8.0	80	90%
Italian cheese vinaigrette	1 Tbs	6.0	55	98%
savory herb/no salt added	1 bs	10.0	90	100%
Thousand Island	2 Tbs	9.0	110	74%
vinaigrette				
raspberry	2 Tbs	–	12	–
white wine	2 Tbs	–	25	–
(Hellman's)				
Citrus Splash Dressings				
orange vinaigrette	2 Tbs	7.0	80	79%
Oriental orange	2 Tbs	7.0	90	70%
ruby red ginger	2 Tbs	7.0	90	70%
tangerine	2 Tbs	6.0	80	68%
tangerine balsamic	2 Tbs	7.0	80	79%
Regular Dressings				
blue cheese/chunky	2 Tbs	15.0	140	96%
Caesar				
fat-free	2 Tbs	–	30	–
original	2 Tbs	9.0	100	81%
chardonnay vinaigrette	2 Tbs	4.0	50	45%
French				
fat-free	2 Tbs	–	45	–
creamy	2 Tbs	16.0	160	90%
garlic ranch	2 Tbs	15.0	140	96%
honey Dijon/fat-free	2 Tbs	–	50	–
Italian				
fat-free	2 Tbs	–	15	–
creamy	2 Tbs	16.0	150	96%
herb ranch	2 Tbs	14.0	130	97%
original	2 Tbs	11.0	110	90%
ranch				
fat-free	2 Tbs	–	45	–
creamy	2 Tbs	15.0	140	96%
Dressing-To-Go	1.5 oz pkg	21.0	200	95%
raspberry vinaigrette/fat-free	2 Tbs	–	35	–
roasted tomato balsamic vinaigrette	2 Tbs	10.0	110	90%
thousand island	2 Tbs	13.0	130	90%
(Henri's)				
bacon & tomato	2 Tbs	10.0	130	69%
Caesar				
ranch classic	2 Tbs	15.0	140	96%
creamy				
fat-free	2 Tbs	–	50	–
French				
fat-free	2 Tbs	–	40	–
light/low-fat	2 Tbs	2.0	70	26%
original classic	2 Tbs	11.0	100	99%
roasted tomato	2 Tbs	12.0	130	83%

Food and Description	Amount	Fat Grams	Total Calories	% Fat Calories
honey mustard				
classic	2 Tbs	6.0	60	90%
fat-free	2 Tbs	–	50	–
Italian				
creamy garlic/zesty	2 Tbs	9.0	110	74%
fat-free	2 Tbs	–	15	–
traditional classic	2 Tbs	10.0	100	90%
peppercorn ranch/thick & creamy	2 Tbs	17.0	170	90%
ranch				
peppercorn classic	2 Tbs	16.0	150	96%
Southwest classic	2 Tbs	10.0	100	90%
ranch chef's recipe				
classic	2 Tbs	16.0	150	96%
creamy garden classic	2 Tbs	13.0	160	73%
fat-free	2 Tbs	–	45	–
Russian robust	2 Tbs	10.0	120	75%
Tas-tee private blend				
classic	2 Tbs	9.0	110	74%
light/low-fat	2 Tbs	2.0	60	30%
original	2 Tbs	9.0	110	74%
teriyaki ginger classic	2 Tbs	7.0	80	75%
thousand island				
classic	2 Tbs	9.0	100	81%
fat-free	2 Tbs	–	35	–
vinaigrette				
mustard classic	2 Tbs	8.0	90	80%
raspberry/fat-free	2 Tbs	–	35	–
tomato classic	2 Tbs	9.0	90	90%
(Herb Magic)				
creamy cucumber	2 Tbs	–	15	–
Italian	2 Tbs	–	10	–
sweet & sour	2 Tbs	–	35	–
vinaigrette	2 Tbs	–	10	–
zesty tomato	2 Tbs	–	15	–
(Hidden Valley)				
blue cheese/fat-free	2 Tbs	–	20	–
coleslaw/fat-free	2 Tbs	–	35	–
creamy Parmesan/fat-free	2 Tbs	–	30	–
French/low-fat	2 Tbs	1.0	35	26%
honey Dijon/fat-free	2 Tbs	–	35	–
original ranch				
low-fat	2 Tbs	3.0	40	68%
reduced calorie	2 Tbs	7.0	80	95%
Parmesan Italian/fat-free	2 Tbs	–	20	–
ranch Italian /reduced calorie	2 Tbs	5.0	50	90%
Thousand Island/low-fat	2 Tbs	1.0	35	26%
(Hollywood)				
buttermilk/old fashioned	1 Tbs	8.0	75	85%
Caesar	1 Tbs	7.0	70	90%
Dijon vinaigrette	1 Tbs	6.0	60	90%

Food and Description	Amount	Fat Grams	Total Calories	% Fat Calories
French/creamy	1 Tbs	7.0	70	90%
Italian				
cheese	1 Tbs	8.0	80	90%
creamy	1 Tbs	9.0	90	90%
regular	1 Tbs	9.0	90	90%
poppy seed ranchers	1 Tbs	8.0	75	96%
Thousand Island	1 Tbs	6.0	60	90%
(Ken's) Steak House				
fat-free				
honey Dijon	2 Tbs	–	40	–
peppercorn	2 Tbs	–	40	–
raspberry pecan	2 Tbs	–	45	–
sun-dried tomato vinaigrette	2 Tbs	–	60	–
lite				
Caesar w/imported anchovies	2 Tbs	6.0	70	77%
country French	2 Tbs	5.0	90	50%
creamy Parmesan w/cracked peppercorn	2 Tbs	9.0	90	90%
honey mustard	2 Tbs	4.0	70	51%
raspberry walnut vinaigrette	2 Tbs	6.0	80	68%
red wine vinegar & olive oil	2 Tbs	5.0	50	90%
(Kraft)				
bacon & tomato				
regular	2 Tbs	14.0	140	90%
blue cheese				
flavored/fat-free	2 Tbs	–	45	–
Roka	2 Tbs	13.0	130	90%
buttermilk ranch	2 Tbs	16.0	150	96%
Caesar				
classic	2 Tbs	11.0	110	90%
Italian				
fat-free	2 Tbs	–	25	–
original	2 Tbs	10.0	100	90%
ranch	2 Tbs	11.0	110	90%
Catalina				
fat-free	2 Tbs	–	35	–
original	2 Tbs	10.0	120	75%
w/honey	2 Tbs	11.0	130	76%
coleslaw	2 Tbs	11.0	130	76%
creamy garlic	2 Tbs	11.0	110	90%
cucumber ranch				
⅓ less fat/reduced-fat	2 Tbs	7.0	70	90%
original	2 Tbs	15.0	140	96%
French style				
creamy	2 Tbs	15.0	160	84%
fat-free	2 Tbs	–	45	–
regular	2 Tbs	12.0	120	90%
garlic				
creamy	2 Tbs	11.0	110	90%
ranch	2 Tbs	19.0	180	95%

Food and Description	Amount	Fat Grams	Total Calories	% Fat Calories
honey Dijon				
fat-free	2 Tbs	–	45	–
regular	2 Tbs	10.0	110	82%
Italian				
creamy				
⅓ less fat/reduced-fat	2 Tbs	7.0	70	90%
fat-free	2 Tbs	–	50	–
house w/olive oil blend	2 Tbs	12.0	120	90%
regular	2 Tbs	11.0	110	90%
regular				
deliciously right/reduced calorie	2 Tbs	7.0	70	90%
fat-free	2 Tbs	–	20	–
house	2 Tbs	12.0	120	90%
oil-free/fat-free	2 Tbs	–	5	–
presto	2 Tbs	15.0	140	96%
tomato & herb	2 Tbs	9.0	100	90%
zesty	2 Tbs	11.0	110	90%
ranch				
buttermilk	2 Tbs	16.0	150	96%
cucumber	2 Tbs	15.0	150	90%
peppercorn				
fat-free	2 Tbs	–	545	–
regular	2 Tbs	18.0	170	95%
regular				
⅓ less fat/reduced-fat	2 Tbs	11.0	110	90%
fat-free	2 Tbs	–	50	–
regular	2 Tbs	18.0	170	95%
sour cream & onion	2 Tbs	18.0	170	95%
red wine vinegar/fat-free	2 Tbs	–	15	–
Russian	2 Tbs	10.0	130	69%
salsa				
ranch	2 Tbs	13.0	130	90%
zesty garden	2 Tbs	6.0	70	77%
sour cream & onion				
fat-free	2 Tbs	–	50	–
original	2 Tbs	18.0	170	95%
thousand island				
⅓ less fat/reduced-fat	2 Tbs	4.5	70	58%
fat-free	2 Tbs	–	40	–
regular	2 Tbs	10.0	110	82%
w/bacon	2 Tbs	12.0	130	83%
(Lawry's)				
Caesar				
creamy	2 Tbs	14.0	130	97%
regular	2 Tbs	13.0	130	90%
Italian	2 Tbs	14.0	140	90%
red wine vinaigrette	2 Tbs	7.0	90	70%
San Francisco w/Romano cheese	2 Tbs	13.0	120	98%
(Life) all natural				
avocado w/tofu	1 Tbs	7.0	70	90%

Food and Description	Amount	Fat Grams	Total Calories	% Fat Calories
creamy egg salad/egg-free	1 Tbs	4.0	40	90%
garlic w/tofu	1 Tbs	7.0	70	90%
tofu	1 Tbs	7.0	75	84%
(Maple Grove Farms)				
balsamic vinaigrette				
fat-free	2 Tbs	–	10	–
w/maple syrup	2 Tbs	–	50	–
Caesar				
all natural	2 Tbs	12.0	110	98%
lite	2 Tbs	5.0	70	64%
Greek/fat-free	2 Tbs	–	25	–
honey Dijon/fat-free	2 Tbs	–	45	–
honey mustard				
lite	2 Tbs	5.0	80	56%
Vermont	2 Tbs	9.0	120	68%
lemon'n dill/lite	2 Tbs	5.0	80	56%
pesto Parmesan/lite	2 Tbs	5.0	70	64%
poppyseed/fat-free	2 Tbs	–	45	–
raspberry vinaigrette/fat-free	2 Tbs	–	35	–
shitake w/roasted garlic	2 Tbs	16.0	150	96%
sun-dried tomato w/roasted garlic	2 Tbs	1.0	35	26%
Vermont				
Parmesan & cracked pepper	2 Tbs	11.0	120	83%
sweet 'N sour	2 Tbs	7.0	110	57%
(Marie's)				
blue cheese				
chunky	2 Tbs	19.0	180	95%
fat-free	2 Tbs	–	30	–
lite	2 Tbs	7.0	100	63%
original	2 Tbs	18.0	170	95%
Caesar				
creamy	2 Tbs	18.0	180	90%
cole slaw	2 Tbs	13.0	150	78%
feta cheese & herb	2 Tbs	17.0	170	90%
ranch/creamy	2 Tbs	20.0	190	95%
raspberry vinaigrette/fat-free	2 Tbs	–	35	–
Roquefort classic premium recipe	2 Tbs	20.0	190	95%
Marzetti (*See* (T. Marzetti) in this section)				
(Nasoya) vegi dressings				
dill/creamy	2 Tbs	5.0	60	75%
Italian/creamy	2 Tbs	5.0	60	75%
sesame garlic	2 Tbs	5.0	60	75%
thousand island	2 Tbs	4.0	60	60%
(Naturally Fresh)				
fat-free				
balsamic vinaigrette	2 Tbs	–	5	–
honey ranch	2 Tbs	–	25	–
lemon vinaigrette	2 Tbs	–	25	–
ranch	2 Tbs	–	20	–
raspberry vinaigrette	2 Tbs	–	25	–

Food and Description	Amount	Fat Grams	Total Calories	% Fat Calories
thousand island	2 Tbs	–	20	–
lite				
peppercorn ranch	2 Tbs	8.0	80	89%
ranch	2 Tbs	8.0	80	89%
regular/poppyseed	2 Tbs	13.0	150	78%
(Newman's Own)				
balsamic vinaigrette	2 Tbs	9.0	90	90%
Caesar				
Creamy	2 Tbs	18.0	170	95%
original	2 Tbs	16.0	150	96%
Italian				
light	2 Tbs	4.0	45	80%
original	2 Tbs	16.0	150	96%
olive oil & vinegar	2 Tbs	16.0	150	96%
Parisienne Dijon lime	2 Tbs	13.0	120	98%
ranch	2 Tbs	15.0	140	96%
(Oriental Chef)				
honey orange	2 Tbs	6.0	80	68%.
original French	2 Tbs	6.0	80	68%
snappy ginger	2 Tbs	8.0	80	90%
tangy soy	2 Tbs	8.0	70	100%
(Ott's)				
buttermilk ranch	2 Tbs	14.0	140	90%
Italian	2 Tbs	18.0	180	90%
original				
fat-free	2 Tbs	–	35	–
reduced calorie	2 Tbs	1.5	50	27%
regular	2 Tbs	6.0	80	68%
poppy seed				
fat-free	2 Tbs	–	45	–
regular	2 Tbs	7.0	90	70%
(Peggy Jane's)				
fruit salad	2 Tbs	4.0	70	51%
garden herb	2 Tbs	8.0	90	80%
ground peppercorn	2 Tbs	17.0	160	96%
honey mustard	2 Tbs	12.0	120	90%
Oriental chicken salad	2 Tbs	12.0	130	83%
poppy seed	2 Tbs	9.0	120	68%
raspberry low-fat	2 Tbs	2.0	50	36%
roasted garlic Caesar	2 Tbs	15.0	140	96%
sesame	2 Tbs	10.0	120	75%
sun-dried tomato	2 Tbs	9.0	100	81%
(Pfeiffer)				
balsamic vinaigrette	2 Tbs	9.0	100	90%
blue cheese	2 Tbs	18.0	170	95%
buttermilk & herb	2 Tbs	20.0	180	100%
Caesar				
house	2 Tbs	16.0	150	96%
light	2 Tbs	1.0	20	45%
original	2 Tbs	13.0	120	98%

Food and Description	Amount	Fat Grams	Total Calories	% Fat Calories
coleslaw	2 Tbs	16.0	170	85%
French				
California				
fat-free	2 Tbs	–	40	–
regular	2 Tbs	12.0	140	77%
original				
fat-free	2 Tbs	–	20	–
light	2 Tbs	2.0	40	45%
regular	2 Tbs	13.0	150	78%
garlic/roasted vinaigrette	2 Tbs	10.0	130	69%
honey Dijon	2 Tbs	12.0	140	77%
Italian				
creamy	2 Tbs	17.0	160	96%
garlic	2 Tbs	10.0	100	90%
original				
fat-free	2 Tbs	–	20	–
light	2 Tbs	4.0	50	72%
regular	2 Tbs	10.0	100	90%
ranch				
California	2 Tbs	12.0	140	77%
Dijon	2 Tbs	18.0	170	95%
garden	2 Tbs	17.0	160	96%
original				
fat-free	2 Tbs	–	25	–
light	2 Tbs	7.0	80	79%
regular	2 Tbs	16.0	150	96%
peppercorn				
fat-free	2 Tbs	–	25	–
original	2 Tbs	19.0	180	95%
red wine vinaigrette	2 Tbs	9.0	90	90%
Russian	2 Tbs	14.0	140	90%
sweet & sour	2 Tbs	13.0	160	73%
Thousand Island				
fat-free	2 Tbs	–	45	–
light	2 Tbs	5.0	70	64%
original	2 Tbs	14.0	140	90%
(Pritikin)				
Dijon balsamic vinaigrette	2 Tbs	–	30	–
French style	2 Tbs	–	30	–
honey Dijon	2 Tbs	–	45	–
honey French	2 Tbs	–	40	–
Italian	2 Tbs	–	20	–
raspberry	2 Tbs	–	35	–
(S&W) Vintage Lites/fat-free				
Italian balsamic	2 Tbs	–	35	–
raspberry blush	2 Tbs	–	40	–
red wine & herb	2 Tbs	–	40	–
white wine & herb	2 Tbs	–	40	–
(Seven Seas)				
blue cheese/chunky	2 Tbs	13.0	130	90%

Food and Description	Amount	Fat Grams	Total Calories	% Fat Calories
Caesar				
classic	2 Tbs	10.0	100	90%
creamy	2 Tbs	15.0	140	96%
Green Goddess	2 Tbs	13.0	130	90%
herb vinaigrette	2 Tbs	15.0	140	96%
herbs & spices	2 Tbs	9.0	90	90%
honey mustard	2 Tbs	10.0	110	82%
Italian				
creamy				
fat-free	2 Tbs	–	50	–
regular	2 Tbs	12.0	120	90%
regular/fat-free	2 Tbs	–	10	–
two cheese	2 Tbs	7.0	70	90%
Viva				
fat-free	2 Tbs	–	10	–
regular	2 Tbs	9.0	90	90%
w/olive oil	2 Tbs	5.0	50	90%
ranch				
fat-free	2 Tbs	–	45	–
reduced calorie	2 Tbs	9.0	100	90%
regular	2 Tbs	17.0	160	96%
raspberry vinaigrette	2 Tbs	–	30	–
red wine vinegar	2 Tbs	–	15	–
red wine vinegar & oil				
reduced calorie	2 Tbs	5.0	60	75%
regular	2 Tbs	9.0	90	90%
Russian/Viva	2 Tbs	16.0	150	96%
(Simply Delicious) Organic				
ginger plum	2 Tbs	10.0	110	82%
herb garlic	2 Tbs	10.0	110	82%
honey mustard	2 Tbs	10.0	110	82%
miso sesame	2 Tbs	11.0	110	90%
tofu poppyseed	2 Tbs	10.0	110	82%
(T. Marzetti)				
balsamic vinaigrette	2 Tbs	9.0	100	90%
blue cheese	2 Tbs	18.0	170	95%
buttermilk & herb	2 Tbs	20.0	180	100%
Caesar				
house	2 Tbs	16.0	150	96%
light	2 Tbs	1.0	20	45%
original	2 Tbs	13.0	120	98%
coleslaw	2 Tbs	16.0	170	85%
French				
original				
fat-free	2 Tbs	–	20	–
light	2 Tbs	2.0	40	45%
regular	2 Tbs	13.0	150	78%
California				
fat-free	2 Tbs	–	40	–
regular	2 Tbs	12.0	140	77%

Food and Description	Amount	Fat Grams	Total Calories	% Fat Calories
garlic/roasted vinaigrette	2 Tbs	10.0	130	69%
honey Dijon	2 Tbs	12.0	140	77%
Italian				
creamy	2 Tbs	17.0	160	96%
garlic	2 Tbs	10.0	100	90%
original				
fat-free	2 Tbs	–	20	–
light	2 Tbs	4.0	50	72%
regular	2 Tbs	10.0	100	90%
ranch				
California	2 Tbs	12.0	140	77%
Dijon	2 Tbs	18.0	170	95%
garden	2 Tbs	17.0	160	96%
original				
fat-free	2 Tbs	–	25	–
light	2 Tbs	7.0	80	79%
regular	2 Tbs	16.0	150	96%
peppercorn				
fat-free	2 Tbs	–	25	–
original	2 Tbs	19.0	180	95%
red wine vinaigrette	2 Tbs	9.0	90	90%
Russian	2 Tbs	14.0	140	90%
sweet & sour	2 Tbs	13.0	160	73%
Thousand Island				
fat-free	2 Tbs	–	45	–
light	2 Tbs	5.0	70	64%
original	2 Tbs	14.0	140	90%
(Walden Farms) fat-free				
bleu cheese	2 Tbs	–	25	–
Caesar	2 Tbs	30		
French	2 Tbs	–	30	–
honey Dijon vinaigrette	2 Tbs	–	25	–
Italian				
creamy w/Parmesan	2 Tbs	–	25	–
regular				
no sugar added	2 Tbs	–	–	–
regular	2 Tbs	–	10	–
sodium-free	2 Tbs	–	10	–
w/sun-dried tomato	2 Tbs	–	15	–
ranch				
regular	2 Tbs	–	25	–
w/sun-dried tomato	2 Tbs	–	25	–
Russian	2 Tbs	–	30	–
Thousand Island	2 Tbs	–	20	–
vinaigrette				
balsamic	2 Tbs	–	15	–
raspberry	2 Tbs	–	20	–
(Weight Watchers) Salad Celebrations/fat-free				
French	2 Tbs	–	40	–
honey Dijon	2 Tbs	–	45	–

Food and Description	Amount	Fat Grams	Total Calories	% Fat Calories
Italian				
creamy	2 Tbs	–	30	–
regular	2 Tbs	–	10	–
ranch	2 Tbs	–	35	–
(Western)				
French				
creamy	2 Tbs	11.0	140	71%
fat-free	2 Tbs	–	45	–
lite	2 Tbs	2.5	70	32%
The Original	2 Tbs	12.0	150	72%
w/bacon flavor	2 Tbs	11.0	140	71%
(Wish Bone)				
balsamic vinaigrette	2 Tbs	5.0	60	75%
berry vinaigrette	2 Tbs	4.5	50	81%
blue cheese				
chunky				
fat-free	2 Tbs	–	35	–
regular	2 Tbs	17.0	170	90%
Just 2 Good	2 Tbs	2.0	45	40%
Regular	2 Tbs	17.0	170	90%
Caesar				
classic	2 Tbs	10.0	110	82%
creamy	2 Tbs	18.0	180	90%
Just 2 Good				
classic	2 Tbs	2.0	40	45%
creamy	2 Tbs	2.0	40	45%
creamy roasted garlic				
fat-free	2 Tbs	–	40	–
regular	2 Tbs	13.0	140	84%
French				
deluxe	2 Tbs	11.0	120	83%
Just 2 Good				
deluxe	2 Tbs	2.0	45	40%
sweet 'n spicy	2 Tbs	2.0	50	36%
sweet 'n spicy				
regular	2 Tbs	12.0	140	77%
honey Dijon/Just 2 Good	2 Tbs	2.0	50	36%
Italian				
classic house	2 Tbs	14.0	140	90%
creamy				
fat-free	2 Tbs	–	10	–
regular	2 Tbs	10.0	110	82%
Just 2 Good				
country	2 Tbs	2.0	30	60%
Parmesan basil	2 Tbs	2.0	40	45%
regular	2 Tbs	2.0	35	51%
original				
fat-free	2 Tbs	–	10	–
regular	2 Tbs	8.0	80	90%
robusto	2 Tbs	8.0	90	80%

Food and Description	Amount	Fat Grams	Total Calories	% Fat Calories
olive oil vinaigrette	2 Tbs	5.0	60	75%
Oriental	2 Tbs	1.0	35	26%
Parmesan & onion	2 Tbs	10.0	110	82%
ranch				
fat-free	2 Tbs	–	40	–
Just 2 Good	2 Tbs	2.0	40	45%
original	2 Tbs	17.0	160	96%
red wine vinaigrette/fat-free	2 Tbs	–	35	–
roasted garlic vinaigrette	2 Tbs	5.0	60	75%
Russian	2 Tbs	6.0	110	49%
sun-dried tomato vinaigrette	2 Tbs	5.0	60	75%
Thousand Island				
Just 2 Good	2 Tbs	2.0	60	30%
regular	2 Tbs	12.0	140	77%
white wine vinaigrette	2 Tbs	4.5	60	68%

SALAD GREENS & BLENDS
(Dole)

Food and Description	Amount	Fat Grams	Total Calories	% Fat Calories
Classic mixes				
classic				
coleslaw	3 oz	–	25	–
greener selection	3 oz	–	15	–
iceberg	3 oz	–	15	–
peeled mini carrots	3 oz	–	40	–
shredded				
carrots	3 oz	–	40	–
red cabbage	3 oz	–	25	–
Complete Salads				
Oriental	3.5 oz	6.0	120	45%
Caesar				
creamy garlic	3.5 oz	15.0	170	79%
family	3.5 oz	15.0	170	79%
regular	3.5 oz	15.0	170	79%
Romano	3.5 oz	13.0	150	18%
sunflower ranch	3.5 oz	16.0	170	85%
Complete Salads w/light dressing				
Caesar				
original	3.5 oz	7.0	100	63%
roasted garlic	3.5 oz	7.0	100	63%
zesty Italian	3.5 oz	6.0	100	54%
Costco & Foodservice				
chopped romaine	3 oz	–	15	–
classic & romaine blend	3 oz	–	15	–
iceberg lettuce	3 oz	–	15	–
Great Restaurant Salads				
all American toss	3.5 oz	1.0	50	18%
classic Greek marinade	3.5 oz	8.0	100	72%
Mediterranean marinade	3.5	8.0	90	80%
tomato & mozzarella medley	3.5 oz	2.0	60	30%
triple cheese toss	3.5	5.0	80	56%

Food and Description	Amount	Fat Grams	Total Calories	% Fat Calories
Lunch For One				
classic ranch	7 oz	29.0	350	75%
Caesar	5.75 oz	23.0	290	71%
Italian/low-fat	7 oz	1.5	130	10%
Special Blends				
American	3 oz	–	15	–
European	3 oz	–	15	–
French	3 oz	–	15	–
Italian	3 oz	–	15	–
Mediterranean	3 oz	–	15	–
romaine	3 oz	–	15	–
Tuscany	3 oz	–	15	–
Verona	3 oz	–	10	–
(Et Tu Caesar) U.S.A. salad kit w/dressing & croutons				
Caesar				
light	1 oz	6.0	90	60%
original	1 oz	12.0	140	77%
Greek/authentic	1 oz	9.0	120	90%.
Italian Balsamic	1 oz	8.0	120	60%
Waldorf	1 oz	8.0	110	65%
(Fresh Express)				
American	3 oz	–	20	–
Caesar	3 oz	11.0	140	71%
European	3 oz	–	20	–
garden	3 oz	–	20	–
Italian	3 oz	–	20	–
Oriental	3 oz	8.0	120	60%
Riviera	3 oz	–	10	–
spinach	3 oz	3.0	130	21%

SALAD TOPPINGS & MIXES (*See also* BACON BITS, CHIPS, & PIECES; CROUTONS; SEASONINGS)

Food and Description	Amount	Fat Grams	Total Calories	% Fat Calories
(Betty Crocker) Suddenly Salad/prepared				
Caesar				
low-fat recipe	¾ cup	3.0	170	16%
regular recipe	¾ cup	9.0	220	8%
classic pasta				
low-fat recipe	¾ cup	3.5	210	15%
regular recipe	¾ cup	8.0	250	29%
garden Italian/98% fat-free	¾ cup	1.0	140	6%
ranch & bacon				
low-fat recipe	¾ cup	2.0	180	10%
regular recipe	¾ cup	20.0	330	55%
roasted garlic Parmesan				
low-fat recipe	¾ cup	3.0	200	9%
regular recipe	¾ cup	11.0	260	38%
(Hidden Valley) Salad Crispins				
bacon & onion	1 Tbs	1.0	35	26%
cheddar & onion	1 Tbs	1.0	35	26%
Italian Parmesan	1 Tbs	1.0	35	26%

Food and Description	Amount	Fat Grams	Total Calories	% Fat Calories
ranch	1 Tbs	1.0	35	26%
sour cream & herb	1 Tbs	1.0	35	26%
(McCormick/Schilling) Salad Toppins				
garden	1⅓ Tbs	1.0	30	30%
Oriental	1⅓ Tbs	2.0	40	45%
original	1⅓ Tbs	1.5	35	39%
SALAMI (*See* LUNCHEON MEAT; SAUSAGE)				
SALMON (*See also* SALMON SPREAD; SEAFOOD ENTRÉE/DINNER)				
canned				
(Bumble Bee)				
Keta	3.5 oz	8.0	160	45%
Pink				
regular	¼ cup	5.0	90	50%
skinless	¼ cup	2.0	70	26%
red	¼ cup	7.0	110	57%
(Chicken Of The Sea)				
pink/skinless-boneless				
in spring water	2 oz	2.0	60	30%
	2.8 oz	2.0	80	23%
traditional	2 oz	5.0	90	50%
red/traditional	2 oz	7.0	110	57%
(Deming's) Alaska				
keta	½ cup	5.0	140	32%
pink	½ cup	6.0	140	39%
red	½ cup	9.0	170	48%
generic				
Atlantic				
drained	3 oz	2.8	173	15%
solids & liquid	8 oz	6.0	268	20%
	15 oz	12.0	500	22%
chum	3 oz	4.7	120	35%
(Libby's)				
pink				
boneless	⅓ cup	2.0	70	26%
w/bones	¼ cup	5.0	90	50%
red/sockeye	¼ cup	7.0	110	57%
(S&W) red/sockeye	¼ cup	7.0	110	57%
	3.75 oz	11.0	190	52%
fresh				
Atlantic				
cooked-dry heat	3 oz	7.0	155	41%
raw	3 oz	5.5	120	41%
chinook/lox				
raw	3 oz	9.0	155	29%
smoked	3 oz	3.7	100	33%
chum/keta/raw	3 oz	3.0	100	27%
coho				
cooked-moist heat	3 oz	6.5	160	36%
raw	3 oz	5.0	125	36%

Food and Description	Amount	Fat Grams	Total Calories	% Fat Calories
pink				
cooked-dry heat	3 oz	4.0	130	27%
raw	3 oz	3.0	100	27%
red/sockeye				
cooked-dry heat	3 oz	9.0	185	44%
raw	3 oz	7.0	143	44%
frozen				
(Healthy Desire) salmon burgers	1 burger	1.2	100	11%
smoked				
chinook	3 oz	3.7	100	33%
generic	3 oz	8.0	150	48%
SALMON SPREAD				
(Vita) smoked	¼ cup	5.0	180	25%
SALSA (See also MEXICAN FOOD/SAUCE)				
(Robert Rothchild Berry Farm)				
basil raspberry	1.1 oz	–	40	–
hot raspberry	1.1 oz	–	40	–
raspberry	1.1 oz	–	40	–
SALSIFY				
fresh/sliced				
cooked-drained	½ cup	–	46	–
raw	½ cup	–	55	–
SALT (See also SEASONINGS)				
(Durkee)				
seasoned				
lite	½ tsp	–	–	–
regular	½ tsp	–	–	–
unseasoned	½ tsp	–	–	–
(Hain) sea salt				
iodized	1 tsp	–	–	–
plain	1 tsp	–	–	–
generic				
iodized	any amount	–	–	–
kosher	any amount	–	–	–
plain	any amount	–	–	–
seasoned	1 tsp	–	2-10	–
(McCormick/Schilling)				
Salt 'n Spice	¼ tsp	–	–	–
SALT PORK (See PORK)				
SALT SUBSTITUTE (See also SEASONINGS)				
(Durkee) seasoned	½ tsp	–	–	–
(Estee) Salt It	⅛ tsp	–	–	–
(Featherweight)				
plain	¼ tsp	–	–	–
seasoned	¼ tsp	–	–	–
generic				
seasoned	1 tsp	–	2	–
seasoned/no salt	1 tsp	–	4	–
unseasoned	1 tsp	–	–	–

Food and Description	Amount	Fat Grams	Total Calories	% Fat Calories
(Health Valley) Instead of Salt	1 tsp	–	–	–
(Lawry's)				
plain	1 tsp	–	10	–
seasoned	1 tsp	–	3	–
(McCormick/Schilling) Salt-Less				
seasoned	¼ tsp	–	–	–
unseasoned	¼ tsp	–	–	–
(Morton)				
plain	1 tsp	–	<1	–
seasoned	1 tsp	–	4	–
SANDWICH (*See* BREAKFAST SANDWICH; FROZEN ENTRÉE/DINNER; HAMBURGER; VEGETARIAN FOODS; Individual FAST FOOD listings)				
SANDWICH SPREAD (*See also* LUNCHEON MEAT SPREAD)				
(Best Foods)	1 Tbs	5.0	50	90%
(Hellman's)	1 Tbs	5.0	50	90%
Sandwich Spread				
original	1 Tbs	4.0	50	72%
reduced-fat	1 Tbs	2.5	35	64%
SAPODILLO				
tropical American	1 medium	1.9	140	12%
	1 cup	2.0	178	10%
SAPOTE/fresh	1 medium	1.5	300	5%
SARDINE				
(Chicken of the Sea)				
Fancy Brisling				
in water	2.9 oz	10.0	150	60%
w/hot sauce	3.75 oz	16.0	220	65%
w/mustard	3.75 oz	20.0	260	69%
w/oil	2.9 oz	16.0	220	65%
tall sardines in water	2 oz	3.0	80	34%
(Del Monte) in tomato sauce	1 fish	3.0	50	54%
(Empress) Norway/boneless & skinless				
in olive oil	3.8 oz	38.0	420	81%
in soy oil	4.4 oz	45.0	500	81%
generic				
canned				
Atlantic/in soy oil w/bone	2 pieces	2.8	50	50%
	3.2 oz	11.0	192	52%
Pacific/in tomato sauce w/bone	~3 oz	44.0	658	60%
(S&W)				
Norwegian brisling/drained	1.86 oz	13.0	160	73%
skinless-boneless	1.69 oz	6.0	100	54%
(Underwood)				
in mustard sauce	3.73 oz	12.0	180	60%
in soybean oil	2.96 oz	16.0	220	65%
in tomato sauce	3.73 oz	11.0	180	55%
(Viking's Delight) brisling/in olive oil				
drained	3.75 oz	20.0	260	69%
undrained	3.75 oz	42.0	460	82%

Food and Description	Amount	Fat Grams	Total Calories	% Fat Calories
SAUCE (*See also* ASIAN FOOD/SAUCES & SEASONINGS; BARBECUE SAUCE; GRAVY; MARINADE; MEXICAN FOOD; PASTA ENTRÉE/DINNER; SEASONINGS; SOUP, TOMATO; TOMATO SAUCE)				
■ **HOMEMADE**				
USDA Standard Home Recipe				
clam	½ cup	22.0	275	72%
white				
medium	1 cup	31.0	405	69%
thick	1 cup	39.0	495	71%
thin	1 cup	22.0	305	65%
■ **MIX**				
(Andre Prost) A Taste of Thai/mix only				
peanut sauce	¼ envelope	1.5	45	30%
tangy hot sweet & sour sauce	¼ envelope	–	45	–
(Durkee)				
dry mix only				
chicken				
cacciatore	1/10 pkg	–	10	–
Mexican salsa	1/10 pkg	–	10	–
mushroom	⅛ pkg	–	15	–
sweet & sour	1/9 pkg	–	20	–
enchilada	⅛ pkg	–	10	–
fish				
lemon pepper dill	⅙ pkg	0.5	20	23%
tomato basil	1/7 pkg	–	15	–
sloppy joe	⅙ pkg	–	20	–
spaghetti	⅕ pkg	–	15	–
American-style	⅙ pkg	–	15	–
Family-style	1/10 pkg	–	20	–
w/mushrooms	⅕ pkg	–	15	–
zesty	⅕ pkg	–	20	–
white	¼ pkg	0.5	20	23%
prepared according to pkg directions				
A la king	1cup	4.0	60	60%
cheese				
nacho	2 Tbs	2.0	25	72%
original	¼ cup	2.0	25	72%
hollandaise	2 Tbs	–	10	–
white	¼ cup	1.0	20	45%
(French's) mix only				
cheese	¼ pkg	0.5	25	16%
enchilada	1/7 pkg	–	15	–
holandaise	1/10 pkg	–	10	–
sloppy joe	⅙ pkg	–	20	–
spaghetti				
all-American	⅕ pkg	–	20	–
Italian	⅕ pkg	–	15	–
mushroom	⅕ pkg	1.0	20	45%
thick	⅙ pkg	–	10	–

Food and Description	Amount	Fat Grams	Total Calories	% Fat Calories
stroganoff	¼ pkg	2.0	45	40%
zesty pasta	⅕ pkg	–	20	–
generic				
bearnaise/prepared w/milk & butter	1 cup	68.0	700	87%
cheese sauce				
mix only	1.2 oz	9.0	158	51%
prepared w/milk	1 cup	17.0	307	50%
curry sauce				
mix only	1 oz	6.5	121	48%
prepared w/milk	1 cup	14.7	270	49%
hollandaise/prepared				
made w/butter & water	1 cup	19.7	237	75%
made w/vegetable oil, milk, & butter	1 cup	68.0	703	87%
stroganoff				
mix only	1.6 oz	4.0	161	22%
prepared w/milk & water	1 cup	10.7	271	36%
sweet & sour/prepared	1 cup	–	295	–
teriyaki				
mix only	1 pkg	1.0	30	30%
prepared	1 Tbs	<1.0	8	7%
	1 cup	1.0	131	7%
(Knorr) mix only				
Classic Sauce				
bearnaise	⅒ pkg	–	10	–
bourguignonne	⅙ pkg	1.0	40	23%
chicken Dijon	⅙ pkg	1.0	30	30%
curry	⅕ pkg	1.5	30	45%
demi-glace	⅕ pkg	1.0	30	30%
goulash	1⅓ Tbs	1.0	35	26%
hollandaise	⅒ pkg	–	10	–
lemon dill	⅕ pkg	1.0	30	30%
mushroom	⅕ pkg	1.0	20	45%
mustard herb	¼ pkg	1.5	40	34%
Newburg	⅕ pkg	0.5	20	23%
peppercorn	⅕ pkg	1.0	25	36%
sauerbraten	⅙ pkg	1.0	35	26%
white	⅑ pkg	1.0	25	36%
pasta sauce				
Alfredo	⅙ pkg	1.5	35	39%
carbonara	⅙ pkg	2.0	30	60%
creamy cheddar	⅓ pkg	3.0	60	45%
four cheese	⅙ pkg	2.0	30	60%
garlic herb	⅙ pkg	2.0	35	51%
parma rosa	½ oz	2.5	60	38%
pesto				
creamy	⅕ pkg	1.0	25	36%
original	⅓ pkg	0.5	15	30%
sun-dried tomato	¼ pkg	0.5	35	13%

Food and Description	Amount	Fat Grams	Total Calories	% Fat Calories
tomato basil	⅓ pkg	1.0	70	13%
(Lawry's) mix only				
chicken saute/garlic Italian w/roasted garlic & basil	2 Tbs	2.0	30	60%
pasta sauce				
Alfredo	1 pkg	13.0	225	52%
pesto	2 tsp	2.0	20	90%
rich & thick	1 pkg	2.0	145	12%
w/mushrooms	1 pkg	1.5	145	9%
stroganoff	1 pkg	<1.0	125	2%
Weekday Gourmet Sauce				
chicken dijon	⅓ pkg	3.0	80	34%
peppercorn steak w/green peppercorns	⅙ pkg	3.0	40	68%
(Mayacamas) dry mix only				
Gourmet sauce				
demi-glace	1 Tbs	<1.0	6	75%
hollandaise	1 Tbs	<1.0	6	75%
honey mustard	1 Tbs	<1.0	6	75%
Pasta Passions				
chicken fettuccine	¼ pkg	–	20	–
classic alfredo	¼ pkg	1.0	25	36%
peppered lemon	¼ pkg	–	25	–
pesto Genovese	¼ pkg	–	15	–
spicy Testarosa	¼ pkg	–	25	–
Pasta sauce				
Alfredo	1 Tbs	<1.0	8	56%
creamy				
clam	1 Tbs	<1.0	6	75%
pesto	1 Tbs	<1.0	8	56%
pesto	1 Tbs	<1.0	8	56%
Skillet Toss Mix				
black olive pesto	1½ Tbs	<1.0	40	11%
dried tomato	1½ Tbs	<1.0	35	13%
garden skillet	1½ Tbs	<1.0	40	11%
green olive pesto	1½ Tbs	<1.0	40	11%
mushroom	1½ Tbs	<1.0	30	15%
seafood skillet	1½ Tbs	<1.0	40	11%
spicy skillet	1½ Tbs	<1.0	40	11%
Sonoma Grills				
cabernet pepper	¼ pkg	–	20	–
fiesta kabob	¼ pkg	–	25	–
pesto chicken	¼ pkg	–	20	–
southwest 3-pepper	¼ pkg	–	25	–
(McCormick)				
Chicken Sauce Blends/dry mix only				
Dijon	¼ pkg	1.5	40	34%
Italian	⅙ pkg	–	20	–

Food and Description	Amount	Fat Grams	Total Calories	% Fat Calories
mesquite	⅙ pkg	–	20	–
piccata	1⅓ Tbs	–	25	–
stir fry	⅙ pkg	–	20	–
teriyaki	¼ pkg	1.0	40	23%
McCormick Collection/prepared				
country Dijon	¼ cup	2.0	45	40%
hollandaise	2 Tbs	5.0	60	75%
hunter	¼ cup	9.0	110	74%
lemon & dill	¼ cup	2.5	45	50%
pepper medley	¼ cup	1.5	30	45%
white	¼ cup	3.0	60	45%
Pasta Sauce Blend/dry mix only				
Alfredo	⅓ pkg	2.0	60	30%
Sauces/dry mix only				
beef stroganoff	⅛ pkg	–	15	–
hollandaise	⅒ pkg	–	15	–
spaghetti				
w/mushroom	⅕ pkg	–	25	–
(Old Bay) mix only				
crab classic	1 Tbs	1.0	30	30%
dash o' lemon	¼ tsp	–	–	–
salmon classic	5 tsp	1.5	40	34%
seas'n easy				
garlic & herb	1 Tbs	–	25	–
lemon dill	1 Tbs	–	30	–
seafood marinara	1 Tbs	–	25	–
tuna classic	1 Tbs	1.0	30	30%
(Spice Islands) mix only				
Alfredo	½ pkg	2.5	45	50%
garlic & herb	¼ pkg	–	15	–
pesto	¼ pkg	0.5	15	30%
Primavera	⅕ pkg	1.5	30	45%
tomato pesto	¼ pkg	–	15	–
(Weight Watchers) lemon butter/mix only	¼ pkg	–	5	–
■ READY TO USE				
(A.1.) steak sauce				
bold	1 Tbs	–	20	–
original	1 Tbs	–	15	–
thick & hearty	1 Tbs	–	25	–
(Andre Prost) A Taste of Thai				
chili sauce				
green	1 tsp	–	10	–
red	1 tsp	–	10	–
garlic chili pepper	1 tsp	–	–	–
mole fiesta	1 Tbs	1.5	35	39%
peanut (satay)	2 Tbs	3.0	50	54%
seasoning fish	1 Tbs	–	15	–
tomatillo chile	1 tsp	–	2	–
(Armour Star) sloppy joe/meatless	¼ cup	–	30	–

Food and Description	Amount	Fat Grams	Total Calories	% Fat Calories
(Aunt Millie's) spaghetti sauce				
family style				
chunky tomato & Italian spice	½ cup	1.5	90	15%
w/ground beef	½ cup	2.5	100	23%
w/sliced mushrooms	½ cup	1.0	80	11%
marinara	½ cup	2.5	70	32%
meatless/traditional				
meat-flavored	½ cup	3.0	80	34%
mushroom	½ cup	2.0	70	26%
regular	½ cup	0.5	70	6%
sweet pepper & Italian sausage	½ cup	2.0	60	30%
(Barilla) pasta sauce				
green & black olive	½ cup	3.5	80	39%
lasagna	½ cup	3.0	210	13%
marinara	½ cup	3.5	80	39%
mushroom & garlic	½ cup	3.5	80	39%
roasted garlic & onion	½ cup	3.5	80	39%
spicy pepper	½ cup	3.5	80	39%
sweet peppers & garlic	½ cup	3.5	80	39%
tomato & basil	½ cup	3.5	80	39%
(Bennett's)				
cocktail sauce	¼ cup	2.0	80	23%
hot seafood sauce	2 Tbs	–	50	–
(Best Foods) Tartar sauce				
low-fat	2 Tbs	1.5	15	90%
original	2 Tbs	7.0	80	79%
(Chun King)				
hot teriyaki sauce	1 Tbs	–	17	–
soy sauce	1 Tbs	–	10	–
(Classico) pasta sauce				
Alfredo				
Di Roma	¼ cup	10.0	110	82%
roasted garlic	¼ cup	10.0	110	82%
tomato	¼ cup	3.5	60	53%
four cheese	½ cup	4.0	70	51%
Italian sausage & fennel	½ cup	5.0	90	50%
portobello mushroom	½ cup	1.5	70	19%
spicy red pepper	½ cup	2.5	60	38%
spinach & cheese	½ cup	4.5	80	51%
sweet peppers & onions	½ cup	4.0	70	51%
tomato & basil	½ cup	1.0	50	18%
tomato & pesto	½ cup	6.0	90	60%
(Contadina) Buitoni/refrigerated pasta sauce				
Alfredo				
light	¼ cup	5.0	80	56%
mushroom	¼ cup	7.0	100	63%
original	¼ cup	16.0	180	80%
garden vegetable/red	½ cup	–	40	–
marinara sauce/red	½ cup	4.0	80	45%

Food and Description	Amount	Fat Grams	Total Calories	% Fat Calories
mushroom marinara	½ cup	2.5	70	32%
pesto/w/basil				
original	¼ cup	24.0	290	74%
reduced-fat	¼ cup	18.0	230	70%
roasted garlic marinara/red	½ cup	2.0	60	30%
tomato herb parmesan	½ cup	8.0	130	55%
w/sun-dried tomatoes	¼ cup	15.0	190	71%
(Crosse & Blackwell) sauce				
brandied hard	2 Tbs	8.0	180	40%
mint	1 Tbs	–	5	–
seafood cocktail	¼ cup	–	100	–
shrimp	¼ cup	–	110-	
steak	1 Tbs	–	20	–
Worcestershire	1 Tbs	–	5	–
(Del Monte)				
chili sauce	1 Tbs	–	20	–
pasta sauce/d'Italia				
seafood cocktail sauce	¼ cup	–	100	–
sloppy joe sauce				
hickory flavor	¼ cup	–	70	–
original recipe	¼ cup	–	70	–
spaghetti sauce				
four cheese	½ cup	1.5	70	19%
garlic & herb/chunky	½ cup	1.5	60	27%
Italian herb/chunky	½ cup	1.0	60	15%
w/garlic & onion	½ cup	1.0	80	11%
w/green peppers				
& mushrooms	½ cup	1.0	80	11%
w/meat	½ cup	1.0	60	15%
w/mushrooms	½ cup	0.5	60	8%
tomato & basil	½ cup	1.0	70	13%
traditional	½ cup	0.5	60	8%
(Di Giorno) pasta sauce/refrigerated				
Alfredo				
Light	¼ cup	9.0	140	51%
regular	¼ cup	18.0	180	90%
basil pesto	¼ cup	31.0	320	87%
four cheese	¼ cup	15.0	160	84%
garlic pesto	¼ cup	33.0	340	87%
marinara	½ cup	–	70	–
plum tomato cream sacue	½ cup	13.0	160	73%
plum tomato & mushroom	½ cup	–	60	–
roasted red bell pepper cream	¼ cup	10.0	140	64%
traditional meat	½ cup	6.0	120	45%
(Durkee) Famous Sandwich				
& Salad Sauce	1 Tbs	6.0	60	90%
(Eden) organic				
pasta sauce	½ cup	2.5	80	28%

Food and Description	Amount	Fat Grams	Total Calories	% Fat Calories
soy sauce/shoyu				
reduced sodium	½ tsp	–	2	–
regular	½ tsp	–	2	–
(Enrico's)				
Alfredo Sauce				
original	¼ cup	2.5	80	28%
w/olives	¼ cup	2.5	80	28%
Pasta sauces				
All natural sauces				
garlic marinara	½ cup	2.0	65	28%
garlic & sun dried tomato	½ cup	2.0	60	30%
mushrooms	½ cup	<1.0	55	8%
peppers & mushrooms	½ cup	1.5	70	19%
tomato basil	½ cup	2.0	65	28%
traditional				
fat-free				
no salt	½ cup	–	60	–
regular	½ cup	–	70	–
no salt added	½ cup	<1.0	55	8%
original	½ cup	<1.0	55	8%
Modei cuisine sauces				
garlic marinara	½ cup	4.0	75	48%
herbed marinara	½ cup	4.0	75	48%
organic marinara	½ cup	4.0	75	48%
tomato walnut	½ cup	5.0	80	56%
Organic sauces				
bountiful basil	½ cup	–	50	–
garlic lovers	½ cup	–	50	–
mushroom madness	½ cup	–	60	–
traditional	½ cup	–	45	–
Original sauces				
marinara style	½ cup	1.0	60	15%
meat flavor	½ cup	1.0	60	15%
mushrooms	½ cup	1.0	60	15%
sausage flavor	½ cup	1.0	60	15%
traditional	½ cup	1.0	60	15%
Pizza Sauces				
regular	¼ cup	–	30	–
roasted garlic	¼ cup	1.0	40	23%
(Escoffier)				
Diable	1 Tbs	–	20	–
Robert	1 Tbs	–	20	–
(Five Brothers) pasta sauce				
Alfredo				
creamy	¼ cup	9.0	100	90%
tomato	¼ cup	4.0	70	51%
w/mushrooms	¼ cup	7.0	80	79%
4-cheese/quattro formaggio	¼ cup	9.0	90	90%
5-cheese	½ cup	3.0	90	90%

Food and Description	Amount	Fat Grams	Total Calories	% Fat Calories
grilled				
eggplant	½ cup	3.0	100	27%
summer vegetable	½ cup	5.0	80	56%
marinara w/burgundy wine	½ cup	3.0	80	34%
Mediterranean tomato & olive	½ cup	4.0	80	45%
Mushroom & garlic	½ cup	3.0	90	30%
oven roasted garlic & onion	½ cup	1.5	70	19%
pesto, creamy	¼ cup	9.0	100	90%
spicy pepper trio	½ cup	3.0	80	34%
(French's) Worcestershire sauce				
original	1 Tbs	–	10	–
smoky	1 Tbs	–	10	–
generic				
cheese/canned	2 oz	4.0	60	60%
clam				
red	¼ cup	1.5	40	34%
white	¼ cup	4.8	60	72%
cream/white	½ cup	9.0	118	69%
soy sauce				
shoyu	1 Tbs	–	9	–
	¼ cup	–	30	–
tamari	1 Tbs	–	11	–
	¼ cup	–	35	–
tartar sauce	1 Tbs	8.0	75	96%
(Girard's) Seafood Shop				
cocktail	2 Tbs	1.0	90	10%
tartar sauce	2 Tbs	15.0	140	96%
(Great Impressions)				
horseradish	2 Tbs	14.0	140	90%
seafood				
creole	1 Tbs	–	20	–
dipping	1 Tbs	–	17	–
Polynesian	1 Tbs	<1.0	40	11%
(Green Giant) sloppy joe sandwich sauce				
sauce only	¼ cup	–	50	–
w/meat	1 sandwich	11.0	200	50%
(Healthy Choice) pasta sauce				
Alfredo/creamy	¼ cup	3.0	45	60%
flavored w/meat	½ cup	1.0	50	18%
garlic & herbs	½ cup	–	50	–
garlic & onion/extra chunky	½ cup	–	40	–
Italian vegetable/extra chunky	½ cup	–	40	–
mushroom				
extra chunky	½ cup	–	40	
original	½ cup	–	50	–
mushroom & sweet peppers/super chunky	½ cup	–	45	–
super tomato, mushroom, & garlic	½ cup	–	45	–
traditional	½ cup	–	50	–
vegetable primavera/super chunky	½ cup	–	45	–

Food and Description	Amount	Fat Grams	Total Calories	% Fat Calories
(Heinz)				
chili sauce	1 Tbs	–	15	–
Heinz 57 steak sauce				
hickory smoke	1 Tbs	–	10	–
regular	1 Tbs	–	10	–
horseradish	1 Tbs	7.0	75	84%
seafood	¼ cup	–	60	–
Worcestershire	1 tsp	–	–	–
(Hellman's) tartar sauce				
low-fat	2 Tbs	1.5	403	34%
original	2 Tbs	7.0	80	79%
(Hoffman House)				
chili sauce	1 Tbs	–	10	–
shrimp & seafood	1 Tbs	4.5	110	35%
tartar	2 Tbs	12.0	130	83%
(House Of Tsang)(See ASIAN FOOD)				
(Hunt's)				
Chicken Sensations cooking sauce				
BBQ flavor	1 Tbs	3.0	35	77%
Italian garlic	1 Tbs	3.0	30	90%
lemon herb	1 Tbs	3.0	30	90%
Southwestern	1 Tbs	3.0	30	90%
Manwich				
barbecue	¼ cup	1.0	60	15%
bold	¼ cup	1.0	65	14%
original	¼ cup	0.5	35	13%
thick & chunky	¼ cup	–	45	–
spaghetti sauce				
classic Italian				
garlic & onion	½ cup	2.0	50	36%
Italian w/Parmesan	½ cup	2.0	50	36%
tomato & basil	½ cup	2.0	50	36%
chunky				
Italian style vegetables	½ cup	1.0	65	14%
marinara	½ cup	1.5	60	23%
tomato, garlic, & onion	½ cup	1.0	60	15%
homestyle				
flavored w/meat	½ cup	2.5	60	38%
mushroom	½ cup	2.5	60	38%
traditional	½ cup	2.5	60	38%
Italian sausage	½ cup	3.0	80	34%
Italian style cheese & garlic	½ cup	2.5	65	35%
old country				
flavored w/meat	½ cup	2.0	65	28%
garlic & herbs	½ cup	3.0	65	42%
Italian style vegetables	½ cup	3.0	65	42%
mushroom	½ cup	3.0	55	49%
traditional	½ cup	2.0	55	44%
original				
flavored w/meat	½ cup	2.0	65	28%

Food and Description	Amount	Fat Grams	Total Calories	% Fat Calories
mushroom	½ cup	2.0	65	28%
traditional	½ cup	2.0	65	28%
steak sauce	1 Tbs	–	10	–
(Jake's) World Famous				
cocktail	¼ cup	0.5	45	10%
tartar sauce	2 Tbs	15.0	140	96%
(Just Rite) Hot dog	¼ cup	3.0	50	54%
(Kaukauna) nacho cheese	1 oz	6.0	80	68%
(Kikkoman)				
marinade & sauce				
roasted garlic teriyaki	1 Tbs	–	25	–
teriyaki	1 Tbs	–	20	–
teriyaki lite	1 Tbs	–	15	–
soy sauce				
lite	1 Tbs	–	10	–
milder	1 Tbs	–	10	–
regular	1 Tbs	–	10	–
stir-fry	1 Tbs	–	20	–
sweet & sour	1 Tbs	–	35	–
teriyaki baste & glaze				
regular	2 Tbs	–	50	–
w/honey & pineapple	2 Tbs	–	80	–
Tonkatsu sauce	1 Tbs	–	20	–
(Knorr) grilling & broiling sauce				
spicy plum	⅛ bottle	–	60	–
(Kraft)				
Kraft				
sandwich spread & burger sauce				
reduced fat	1 Tbs	0.0	35	64%
regular	1 Tbs	4.0	50	72%
Sauceworks				
cocktail	¼ cup	0.5	60	9%
horseradish	1 tsp	1.5	20	68%
sweet 'n sour	2 Tbs	–	60	–
tartar sauce				
fat-free	2 Tbs	–	25	–
natural lemon & herb flavor	2 Tbs	16.0	150	96%
original	2 Tbs	9.0	90	90%
(La Choy)				
bead molasses	1 Tbs	–	50	–
brown gravy	¼ cup	–	275	–
plum	1 Tbs	–	25	–
soy sauce/lite	1 Tbs	–	15	–
stir-fry				
Mandarin soy sauce	½ cup	–	70	–
sweet & sour	½ cup	–	140	–
Szechwan	½ cup	–	80	–
teriyaki	½ cup	–	95	–

Food and Description	Amount	Fat Grams	Total Calories	% Fat Calories
sweet & sour				
duck sauce	2 Tbs	–	60	–
original	2 Tbs	–	60	–
teriyaki				
lite	1 Tbs	–	18	–
original	1 Tbs	–	16	–
(Lea & Perrins)				
steak				
garlic peppercorn	1 Tbs	–	25	–
private label	1 Tbs	–	15	–
sweet & spicy	1 Tbs	–	25	–
Worcestershire				
original	1 tsp	–	5	–
white wine	1 tsp	–	–	–
(Litehouse)				
barbecue	2 Tbs	–	35	–
salsa	2 Tbs	–	10	–
seafood cocktail	2 Tbs	–	25	–
stir-fry	2 Tbs	–	45	–
tartar sauce	2 Tbs	14.0	130	97%
(Maple Grove Farms) marinade & grilling sauces				
hickory maple	1 Tbs	–	20	–
honey teriyaki/fat-free	2 Tbs	–	15	–
lemon w/cracked peppercorn	1 Tbs	1.0	15	60%
mesquite/fat-free	1 Tbs	–	10	–
original honey mustard	1 Tbs	4.0	60	60%
Vermont sweet 'n sour	2 Tbs	8.0	120	60%
(Manwhich) (See (Hunt's) in this section)				
(Maull's) steak				
mild	1 Tbs	–	20	–
original	1 Tbs	–	20	–
(Millina's Finest) fat-free organic pasta sauce				
garlic garlic	½ cup	–	40	–
hot n spicy	½ cup	–	48	–
sweet pepper & onion	½ cup	–	41	–
tomato & basil	½ cup	–	45	–
zesty basil	½ cup	–	45	–
(Muir Glen) organic low-fat pasta sauce				
balsamic roasted onion	½ cup	0.5	50	9%
cabernet marinara	½ cup	0.5	50	9%
chunky tomato style	½ cup	0.5	50	9%
garden vegetable	½ cup	1.0	50	18%
garlic & onion	½ cup	0.5	55	8%
garlic roasted garlic	½ cup	0.5	50	9%
green olive	½ cup	1.5	60	23%
green pepper & mushroom	½ cup	2.0	70	26%
Italian herb	½ cup	0.5	55	8%
mushroom marinara	½ cup	–	45	–

Food and Description	Amount	Fat Grams	Total Calories	% Fat Calories
portabella mushroom	½ cup	–	50	–
roasted red pepper	½ cup	1.5	60	23%
Romano cheese	½ cup	2.5	90	25%
sun-dried tomato	½ cup	1.0	55	16%
sweet pepper & onion	½ cup	–	40	–
tomato basil	½ cup	1.0	50	18%
(Nestlé) (See (Contadina) in this section)				
(Newman's Own) pasta sauce				
Bombolina tomato & fresh basil	½ cup	5.0	100	45%
5-Cheese	½ cup	3.0	90	30%
FRA Diavolo hot & spicy	½ cup	3.0	70	39%
Marinara	¼ cup	2.0	60	30%
mushroom marinara	½ cup	2.0	60	30%
roasted garlic & peppers	½ cup	2.5	70	32%
Socarooni	½ cup	2.0	60	30%
(Old Bay)				
cocktail	¼ cup	0.5	110	4%
tartar sauce	2 Tbs	12.0	130	83%
(Prego) pasta sauce				
Extra chunky				
fresh mushroom	½ cup	5.0	150	30%
garden combination	½ cup	2.0	100	18%
garlic supreme	½ cup	4.5	140	29%
mushroom & diced tomatoes	½ cup	3.0	110	25%
mushroom & extra spice	½ cup	4.0	120	30%
mushroom & green pepper	½ cup	4.5	129	34%
mushroom supreme	½ cup	4.5	130	31%
roasted garlic Parmesan	½ cup	1.5	120	11%
tomato, onion, & garlic	½ cup	3.5	110	29%
tomato supreme	½ cup	4.0	130	28%
vegetable supreme	½ cup	4.0	120	30%
Regular				
diced onion & garlic	½ cup	4.5	120	34%
flavored w/meat	½ cup	6.0	140	39%
hamburger	½ cup	4.0	120	30%
Italian sausage & garlic	½ cup	5.0	120	38%
made w/mushrooms	½ cup	5.0	150	30%
marinara	½ cup	6.0	110	49%
mushroom & garlic	½ cup	2.0	110	16%
mushroom Parmesan	½ cup	3.5	130	24%
pepperoni	½ cup	4.5	120	34%
roasted garlic & herb	½ cup	3.5	110	29%
roasted red pepper & garlic	½ cup	3.5	110	29%
three cheese	½ cup	2.0	100	18%
tomato & basil	½ cup	3.0	110	25%
tomato Parmesan				
no salt added	½ cup	6.0	110	49%
regular	½ cup	3.5	140	23%
traditional	½ cup	4.5	140	29%
vegetable supreme/extra chunky	½ cup	3.0	90	30%

Food and Description	Amount	Fat Grams	Total Calories	% Fat Calories
(Pritikin) pasta sauce				
tomato basil	½ cup	–	30	–
traditional	½ cup	–	30	–
(Progresso)				
pasta sauce				
Alfredo/authentic	½ cup	15.0	200	68%
creamy clam	½ cup	6.0	110	49%
lobster	½ cup	7.0	100	63%
marinara/authentic	½ cup	4.0	100	36%
pizza	¼ cup	–	20	–
red clam	½ cup	1.0	60	15%
white clam	½ cup	10.0	140	64%
white clam/authentic	½ cup	10.0	150	60%
(Ragu)				
Cheese Creations				
Alfredo				
classic	¼ cup	12.0	120	90%
light	¼ cup	6.0	80	68%
double cheddar	¼ cup	10.0	110	82%
four cheese	¼ cup	11.0	120	83%
roasted garlic Parmesan	¼ cup	11.0	120	83%
Chicken Tonight simmer sauce				
chicken cacciatore	½ cup	1.5	70	19%
country French chicken	½ cup	1.5	120	11%
creamy mushroom	½ cup	6.0	80	68%
honey mustard	½ cup	0.5	60	8%
sweet & sour chicken	½ cup	–	150	–
pasta sauce				
chunky gardenstyle				
garden combination sweet bell	½ cup	3.5	110	29%
mushroom/super	½ cup	3.5	120	26%
mushroom & green pepper	½ cup	3.5	110	29%
mushroom & onion	½ cup	3.5	120	26%
tomato, garlic & onion	½ cup	3.5	120	26%
vegetable primavera	½ cup	3.5	110	29%
hearty				
chopped tomato olive oil & garlic	½ cup	5.0	100	45%
flavored w/saute	½ cup	5.0	100	45%
Parmesan & Romano	½ cup	4.0	90	40%
red wine & herb	½ cup	3.0	80	34%
roasted garlic	½ cup	3.0	100	27%
sauteed onion & garlic	½ cup	4.0	90	40%
sauteed onion & mushroom	½ cup	4.0	80	45%
six cheese	½ cup	4.0	90	40%
sweet Italian sausage & cheese	½ cup	5.0	100	40%
tomato herb	½ cup	3.5	80	39%
light				
mushroom & garlic/chunky	½ cup	–	60	–
roasted garlic & primavera	½ cup	–	70	–

Food and Description	Amount	Fat Grams	Total Calories	% Fat Calories
tomato & basil				
no sugar added	½ cup	–	50	–
regular	½ cup	–	50	–
tomato & herb	½ cup	–	60	–
Robusto!				
chopped tomato, olive oil, & garlic	½ cup	5.0	100	45%
Parmesan & Romano	½ cup	4.0	90	40%
red wine & herbs	½ cup	3.0	120	23%
roasted garlic	½ cup	3.0	120	23%
saut'eed beef, onion & garlic	½ cup	5.0	100	45%
saut'eed onion & garlic	½ cup	4.0	90	40%
saut'eed onion & mushroom	½ cup	4.0	80	45%
7 herb tomato	½ cup	3.5	80	39%
6 cheese	½ cup	4.0	90	40%
spicy red pepper	½ cup	4.0	90	40%
sweet Italian sausage & cheese	½ cup	5.0	100	45%
spaghetti sauce/Old World style				
flavored w/meat	½ cup	5.0	90	50%
marinara	½ cup	4.5	80	51%
mushroom	½ cup	3.0	80	39%
traditional	½ cup	3.5	80	39%
(S&W) cooking sauce				
mesquite steakhouse	1 Tbs	–	10	–
Oriental stir-fry	1 Tbs	20		
seafood cocktail	1 Tbs	20		
Southwestern fajitas	1 Tbs	–	10	–
steakhouse chili	1 Tbs	–	15	–
teriyaki				
lite	1 Tbs	–	25	–
regular	1 Tbs	–	25	–
Sauceworks (See (Kraft) in this section)				
(Snow's)				
Welsh rarebit cheese	½ cup	11.0	170	58%
Newburg w/sherry	⅓ cup	8.0	120	60%
(Tabasco) chili recipe/7 spice	½ cup	0.5	50	9%
(Texas Best)				
grilling sauces				
Mesa habanero mustard	2 bs	–	60	–
Pueblo roasted pepper	2 Tbs	–	50	–
Santa Fe serrano	2 Tbs	–	35	–
Sedona chipotle	2 Tbs	–	50	–
hot sauce	1 tsp	–	–	–
steak sauce	1 Tbs	–	15	–
(Uncle Ben's) marinade & sauce				
Cantonese orange ginger	1 Tbs	–	25	–
Chinese black bean	1 Tbs	0.5	15	30%
French four peppercorn	1 Tbs	0.5	15	30%
Jamaican island	1 Tbs	1.0	15	60%
Japanese roasted garlic	1 Tbs	–	10	–

Food and Description	Amount	Fat Grams	Total Calories	% Fat Calories
Thai peanut satay	1 Tbs	1.0	25	36%
SAUERKRAUT /canned or jarred				
(Bush's Best)				
Bavarian kraut	½ cup	–	60	–
deli style kraut	½ cup	–	20	–
shredded kraut	½ cup	–	20	–
(Claussen)	¼ cup	–	5	–
(Del Monte)				
Baverian style	2 Tbs	–	15	–
original	2 Tbs	–	–	–
(Eden)	½ cup	–	25	–
(Hebrew National)				
gallon kraut	½ cup	–	25	–
regular	2 Tbs	–	50	–
(Libby's)				
Bavarian w/caraway seeds	2 Tbs	–	15	–
crispy	2 Tbs	–	5	–
(Rosoffs)	½ cup	1.0	50	18%
(S&W)	2 Tbs	–	5	–
	½ cup	–	25	–
(Schon's) new kraut	½ cup	1.0	50	18%
(Seneca)				
Bavarian	1 oz	–	10	–
original	1 oz	–	5	–
(Stokely)				
Bavarian	½ cup	–	30	–
shredded & chopped	½ cup	–	20	–
(Vlasic) old fashioned	1 oz	–	4	–
SAUERKRAUT JUICE /canned				
(S&W)	10 fl oz	–	35	–
SAUSAGE (*See also* FRANKFURTER; LUNCHEON MEAT; SAUSAGE DISH; SAUSAGE STICK)				
■ (Aidell's)				
Andouille Cajun/cooked	1 link	17.0	220	70%
Burmese curry/cooked	1 link	15.0	220	61%
chicken				
& apple/fresh	1 link	8.0	110	65%
& apple/smoked	1 link	16.0	220	65%
& turkey/New Mexico smoked	1 link	16.0	220	65%
& turkey/Thai				
fresh	1 link	16.0	200	72%
smoked	1 link	16.0	220	65%
& turkey w/sun-dried tomatoes & basil				
fresh	1 link	15.0	200	68%
smoked	1 link	15.0	200	68%
Creole hot/cooked	1 link	16.0	220	65%
hunters/cooked	1 link	19.0	240	71%
Italian/fresh				
hot	1 link	18.0	230	70%

Food and Description	Amount	Fat Grams	Total Calories	% Fat Calories
mild	1 link	18.0	230	70%
lamb & beef w/rosemary/fresh	1 link	16.0	220	65%
lemon chicken/cooked	1 link	16.0	220	65%
Mexican chorizo beef/fresh	1 link	37.0	400	83%
■ (Amour Swift-Eckrich)				
Brown 'n serve veggie breakfast links/frozen	⅓ pkg	3.0	90	30%
Vienna sausage				
in BBQ sauce	3 sausages	14.0	160	81%
in beef stock	3 sausages	16.0	170	77%
in hot sauce	3 sausages	15.0	170	81%
smoked	3 sausages	16.0	170	85%
25% less fat	3 sausages	11.0	130	78%
■ (Ball Park)				
smoked sausage				
Burner Hot & spicy	3.25 oz	18.0	220	74%
skinless	3.25 oz	18.0	220	74%
■ (Bilinski's)				
chicken				
& spinach w/garlic & fennel	1 link	3.0	100	27%
& vegetable	1 link	2.0	80	23%
chicken/Italian w/peppers & onions	1 link	4.0	120	30%
■ (Bob Evans)				
Brown & Serve				
country lite	3 links	8.0	120	60%
original	3 links	14.0	160	79%
■ (Butterball)				
turkey sausage				
bratwurst	1 link	10.0	170	53%
breakfast				
links	2 links	5.0	90	50%
original	3 links	9.0	120	68%
Italian				
hot	1 link	10.0	170	53%
sweet	1 link	10.0	170	53%
Polish	1 link	10.0	170	53%
salami	1 oz	4.0	60	60%
■ (Galileo)				
pepperoni/pizza-size	9 slices	13.0	140	84%
salami/Italian dry				
light	5 slices	4.0	60	60%
thin sliced	5 slices	8.0	110	65%
whole	1 oz	10.0	120	75%
summer/smoked	2 oz	16.0	190	76%
■ GENERIC				
beerwurst/beer salami				
beef	1 oz	6.8	75	81%
pork	1 oz	4.0	55	66%
Berliner/beef & pork	1 oz	4.9	65	68%

Food and Description	Amount	Fat Grams	Total Calories	% Fat Calories
blood	1 oz	9.8	107	82%
bratwurst/pork, cooked	1 oz	7.0	85	74%
	3-oz link	22.0	256	77%
chorizo	~2-oz link	23.0	273	76%
honey roll/beef	1 oz	3.0	52	52%
Italian/pork/cooked	3 oz	21.0	268	71%
kielbasa				
pork or beef	1 oz	7.7	88	79%
skinless	1 oz	16.0	180	80%
knockwurst/pork & beef	3 oz	16.0	210	69%
mortadella/beef & pork	1 oz	7.0	88	72%
pepperoni/pork & beef	1 oz	12.0	135	80%
	~9 oz	110.0	1248	79%
Polish/pork	1 oz	8.0	92	78%
10" long/1.5" dia	1 sausage	6.5	74	79%
pork				
brown & serve/link/~1 oz	1 link	5.0	50	90%
country style/cooked				
links/0.5 oz each	1 link	8.0	96	75%
patties/1 oz each	1 patty	8.0	100	72%
fresh/cooked				
link	1 oz	11.0	118	84%
patty	1 oz	8.0	100	72%
raw				
links/1 oz each	1 link	11.0	118	84%
patties/2 oz each	1 patty	23.0	238	87%
smoked links				
4" long/1⅛" dia	1 link	22.6	265	73%
2" long/¾" dia	1 link	5.0	62	73%
pork & beef				
fresh, cooked				
links/2" long/¾" dia	1 link	5.0	55	82%
patties/~1 oz each	1 patty	10.0	110	82%
luncheon/pork & beef	~1 oz	4.8	60	72%
salami				
cooked				
beef	1 oz	5.9	74	72%
beef & pork	1 oz	5.7	71	72%
turkey	2 oz	7.8	111	63%
dry or hard/pork	1 oz	7.0	85	74%
salt pork/raw	1 oz	22.8	212	97%
summer				
beef	~1 oz	7.6	86	80%
cervelat	1 oz	8.5	98	78%
Thuringer	1 oz	8.5	98	78%
turkey	1 oz	3.5	52	61%
Vienna/canned				
beef	1 sausage	4.0	45	80%
chicken	7 sausages	28.0	315	80%

Food and Description	Amount	Fat Grams	Total Calories	% Fat Calories
pork	1 sausage	4.0	45	80%
■ (Healthy Choice)				
low-fat/smoked				
links	2 oz	2.0	70	26%
patties	2 oz	2.0	70	26%
Polska kielbasa	2 oz	2.0	70	26%
■ (Hebrew National)				
kishka	2 oz	11.0	160	62%
knocks				
beef	1.75 oz	24.0	260	83%
beef jalapeño	1.75 oz	24.0	260	83%
Polish/beef	1.75 oz	21.0	240	79%
	4 oz	28.0	320	79%
salami/beef				
lean				
chub	2 oz	5.0	90	50%
sliced	2 oz	5.0	90	50%
regular				
midget chub	2 oz	14.0	170	74%
sliced/6 oz pkg	3 slices	13.0	150	78%
■ (Hickory Farms)				
salami				
dry or hard	1 oz	10.0	120	75%
Genoa	1 oz	10.0	110	82%
■ (Hillshire Farm)				
beef & cheddar/Flavorseal	2 oz	15.0	190	71%
bratwurst				
beer	2 oz	17.0	190	81%
fresh	2 oz	17.0	190	81%
fully cooked	2 oz	16.0	170	85%
light	2 oz	11.0	150	66%
plain	2 oz	17.0	190	81%
smoked	2 oz	17.0	190	81%
spicy	2 oz	17.0	180	85%
cheddarwurst				
bun size	2 oz	18.0	200	81%
lite	2.7 oz	15.0	190	71%
original	2 oz	17.0	190	81%
country recipe/Flavorseal	2 oz	16.0	180	80%
hot				
cheddar hots/80% fat free	2 oz	12.0	150	72%
Hot Links				
beef	2 oz	17.0	190	81%
lite	2 oz	15.0	190	71%
Italian				
hot				
light	2 oz	11.0	150	66%
regular	2 oz	17.0	180	85%
mild				
light	2 oz	11.0	150	66%

Food and Description	Amount	Fat Grams	Total Calories	% Fat Calories
regular	2 oz	17.0	190	81%
Italian dry	~1 oz	7.0	90	70%
knockwurst	2 oz	16.0	180	80%
Mexican-style				
lower fat	2 oz	11.0	150	66%
original	2 oz	17.0	190	81%
pepperoni	~1 oz	10.0	110	82%
Polska kielbasa				
bun size	2 oz	16.0	180	80%
80% fat free	2 oz	10.0	130	69%
Flavorseal				
beef	2 oz	17.0	190	81%
lite	2 oz	11.0	130	73%
mild	2 oz	17.0	190	81%
regular	2 oz	17.0	190	81%
turkey	2 oz	5.0	90	50%
lite	2.7 oz	15.0	190	71%
Lit'l Polskas	2 oz	16.0	180	80%
lower fat	2 oz	11.0	150	66%
original	2 oz	17.0	190	81%
salami/hard	~1 oz	9.0	100	90%
smoked				
bun size				
beef	2 oz	16.0	180	80%
regular	2 oz	16.0	180	80%.
80% fat free	2 oz	10.0	130	69%.
Flavorseal				
beef	2 oz	16.0	180	80%
hot	2 oz	16.0	180	80%
Italian	2 oz	18.0	200	81%
lite	2 oz	11.0	130	73%
regular	2 oz	17.0	190	81%
turkey	2 oz	15.0	190	71%
Lit'l Smokies				
beef	2 oz	16.0	180	80%
cheddar	2 oz	16.0	180	80%
light	2 oz	8.0	120	60%
original	2 oz	16.0	180	80%
original	2 oz	18.0	190	85%
summer				
beef	2 oz	17.0	190	81%
light	2 oz	12.0	150	72%
original	2 oz	16.0	180	80%
w/cheese	2 oz	18.0	200	81%
yard-o-beef	2 oz	17.0	190	81%
■ (Hormel)				
breakfast/Little Sizzlers/cooked				
brown 'n serve				
links	3 links	22.0	230	86%

Food and Description	Amount	Fat Grams	Total Calories	% Fat Calories
patties	2 patties	18.0	190	85%
links	3 links	20.0	210	86%
patties/cooked	2 patties	22.0	230	86%
pork/hot & spicy/cooked	3 links	22.0	230	86%
Genoa salami	2 oz	18.0	210	77%
pepperoni				
chunk/6-oz pkg	1 oz	13.0	140	84%
pillow pack				
regular	1 oz	13.0	140	84%
turkey	17 slices	4.0	80	45%
sliced/3.5-oz pkg	15 slices	13.0	140	84%
twin/5-oz pkg	1 oz	13.0	140	84%
pickled				
hot	6 links	11.0	140	71%
smoked	6 links	11.0	140	71%
prosciutto				
primissimo	1 oz	4.5	70	58%
Spiral Cure 81	3 oz	9.0	150	54%
salami				
Genoa				
DiLusso	1 oz	9.0	120	68%
San Remo	1 oz	9.0	120	68%
sandwich maker	1 oz	11.0	120	83%
hard				
homeland	1 oz	10.0	110	82%
pillow pack	4 slices	10.0	120	75%
sandwich maker	1 oz	10.0	110	82%
smoked				
Light & Lean 97/smoked dinner links	2 oz	2.0	60	30%
kielbasa/skinless	2 oz	13.0	150	78%
summer/Old Smokehouse				
1.5-lb pkg	2 oz	18.0	200	81%
2.15-lb pkg	2 oz	18.0	200	81%
3-lb pkg	2 oz	18.0	200	81%
Vienna				
chicken	2 oz	9.0	110	74%
original	2 oz	14.0	150	84%
■ (Jimmy Dean)				
Breakfast chubs				
50% less fat	2.5 oz	14.0	180	70%
97% fat-free	2.5 oz	2.0	90	20%
Dinner sausage/smoked	2 oz	14.0	170	74%
Heat 'N Serve/regular	2 oz	19.0	200	86%
Links/skinless	2 oz	19.0	200	86%
Patties				
pre-cooked	1.9 oz	22.0	230	86%
raw	2 oz	19.0	200	86%
sage	2 oz	19.0	200	86%
Polska Kielbaska	2 oz	15.0	170	79%
Premium pork/regular	2 oz	21.0	240	79%

Food and Description	Amount	Fat Grams	Total Calories	% Fat Calories
■ (Johnsonville)				
(Note: All portions are cooked unless stated otherwise.)				
Beer City Grillers	1 link	27.0	310	????
Better w/cheddar				
light	1 link	9.0	140	58%
regular	1 link	22.0	240	83%
bratwurst				
beef				
cooked	1 link	22.0	250	79%
raw	1 link	27.0	330	74%
smoked	1 link	22.0	240	83%
beer 'n bratwurst				
cheesy	1 link	25.0	300	75%
regular	1 link	25.0	290	78%
burger	1 patty	20.0	230	78%
burger/3.0 oz grilled	1 patty	18.0	220	74%
bun brat/3.0 oz grilled	1 patty	18.0	220	74%
German	1 link	25.0	290	78%
honey & garlic	1 link	22.0	280	71%
Irish O'Garlic	1 link	25.0	290	78%
kielbasa	1 link	25.0	290	78%
lower-fat/raw	1 link	22.0	250	79%
onion	1 link	25.0	290	78%
original	1 link	25.0	290	78%
pattie/pan-fried	3.3 oz	21.0	240	79%
Polish sausage	1 link	25.0	290	78%
roasted garlic	1 link	25.0	290	78%
smoked				
light	1 link	9.0	140	58%
regular	1 link	22.0	240	83%
stadium style	1 link	22.0	250	79%
breakfast				
apple 'n cinnamon/pan-fried	3 links	16.0	190	76%
brown sugar & honey/pan-fried	3 links	15.0	190	71%
maple breakfast links/lower-fat/raw	3 links	16.0	180	80%
original				
link/pan-fried	3 links	16.0	190	76%
lower-fat/raw	3 links	16.0	180	80%
pattie/pan-fried	2 patties	15.0	180	75%
Vermont maple syrup/pan-fried				
link	3 links	16.0	190	76%
patty	2 patties	15.0	180	75%
hot links				
beef	1 link	20.0	230	78%
regular	1 link	20.0	230	78%
Italian				
hot	1 link	25.0	290	90%
mild	1 link	25.0	290	90%
pattie/pan-fried	3.3 oz	21.0	240	79%

Food and Description	Amount	Fat Grams	Total Calories	% Fat Calories
perri/raw				
hot	1 link	20.0	230	78%
sweet	1 link	20.0	230	78%
Polish				
light	1 link	9.0	140	58%
regular	1 link	22.0	240	83%
summer				
beef recipe				
regular	2 oz	15.0	180	75%
sliced	13 slices	15.0	180	75%
garlic recipe				
regular	2 oz	15.0	180	75%
sliced	13 slices	15.0	180	75%
Old World recipe	2 oz	16.0	190	76%
original recipe				
regular	2 oz	15.0	180	75%
sliced	13 slices	15.0	180	75%
Swisswurst	1 link	22.0	240	83%
■ (Jones Dairy Farm)				
all natural				
brown & serve				
light	1 link	4.0	60	60%
maple	2 links	18.0	190	85%
golden brown	1 patty	14.0	150	84%
beef	1 link	6.0	75	72%
mild	2 links	18.0	190	85%
pork/light	1 link	4.0	55	65%
spicy	2 links	18.0	190	85%
little pork sausages	3 links	17.0	190	81%
original/chub	2 oz	21.0	230	82%
pork & rice links/Light	2 oz	11.0	130	76%
scrapple	1.5 oz	6.0	90	60%
■ (Kahn's)				
bratwurst	1 sausage	17.0	190	81%
kielbasa/bun size Polska	1 sausage	17.0	190	81%
salami				
beef				
8-oz pkg	1 slice	6.0	70	77%
family pack	1 slice	5.0	60	75%
cooked/8-oz pkg	1 slice	4.0	60	60%
cotto/family pack	1 slice	3.0	45	60%
■ (Libby's)				
Vienna				
chicken	3 links	8.0	100	72%
meat/regular or w/BBQ sauce	3 links	12.0	130	83%
■ (Louis Rich)				
turkey sausage				
ground/hot	2.5 oz	8.0	120	19%
Polska kielbasa	2 oz	5.0	90	50%

Food and Description	Amount	Fat Grams	Total Calories	% Fat Calories
smoked/original	2 oz	5.0	90	50%
	2.5 oz	8.0	120	60%
salami				
cooked/sliced	1 slice	2.5	40	56%
cotto/sliced	1 slice	2.5	40	56%
■ (Mr. Turkey)				
Breakfast sausage	2.5 oz	9.0	130	62%
Hearty Blend				
Polish kielbasa	1 oz	6.0	70	77%
smoked	1 oz	6.0	70	77%
Polish Kielbasa	1 oz	3.0	45	60%
smoked				
hot	1 oz	3.0	45	60%
Italian	1 oz	3.0	45	60%
original	1 oz	3.0	45	60%
turkey salami				
regular	2 oz	7.0	100	63%
variety pack	1 slice	3.0	50	54%
■ (Oscar Mayer)				
New England	2 slices	2.5	60	38%
pepperoni	15 slices	13.0	140	84%
pork links/cooked	2 links	15.0	170	79%
salami				
cotto				
beef	2 slices	7.0	90	70%
pork, chicken, & beef	2 slices	9.0	110	74%
for beer	3 slices	9.0	110	74%
Genoa	3 slices	9.0	100	81%
hard				
Deli-Thin	4 slices	11.0	130	76%
regular	3 slices	9.0	100	81%
Machiaeh/beef	2 slices	10.0	120	75%
Smokies				
beef smokies	1 link	11.0	120	83%
cheese smokies	1 link	12.0	130	83%
links sausage	1 link	12.0	130	83%
little cheese	6 links	16.0	180	80%
little links sausage	6 links	15.0	170	79%
summer/Thuringer cervelat				
beef	2 slices	12.0	140	77%
other	2 slices	13.0	140	84%
■ (Owens)				
Bratwurst/cooked				
beer	1 link	21.0	270	70%
Italian	1 link	21.0	270	70%
original	1 link	21.0	270	70%
Fresh pork sausage				
hot	2 oz	18.0	210	77%
hot link	1 link	20.0	230	78%

Food and Description	Amount	Fat Grams	Total Calories	% Fat Calories
maple	2 oz	17.0	210	73%
mild	2 oz	18.0	210	77%
Italian	2 oz	17.0	210	73%
regular	2 oz	18.0	210	77%
smoked	2 oz	16.0	170	85%
special seasoning	2 oz	18.0	210	77%
Pan-fried				
links				
maple	3 links	14.0	170	74%
small casing	3 links	16.0	190	76%
patties				
pan-ready	2 patties	21.0	240	79%
■ (Perdue)				
turkey sausage				
breakfast/links/cooked	1 link	6.0	100	54%
fresh/seasoned				
link				
roasted garlic & parsley	1 link	9.0	150	54%
Romano cheese	1 link	9.0	150	54%
sweet Italian	1 link	9.0	140	58%
rope				
roasted garlic & parsley	2 oz	6.0	110	49%
Romano cheese	2 oz	6.0	110	49%
sweet Italian	2 oz	6.0	100	54%
Italian/2-oz link	1 link	6.0	94	57%
■ (Schwan's)				
bratwurst	1 link	23.0	260	80%
Italian	2 oz	12.0	160	68%
Polish	1 link	19.0	220	78%
Pork/fully cooked				
links	3 links	20.0	220	90%
country sausage patties	1 patty	22.0	230	86%
summer	2 oz	13.0	160	73%
■ (Shelton's)				
turkey sausage				
Italian links	1 link	16.0	160	90%
original				
links	1 link	14.0	140	90%
patties/2 oz	1 patty	11.0	140	71%
■ (The Turkey Store)				
turkey sausage				
bratwurst/lean	3 oz	8.0	140	51%
breakfast links				
hot	2 oz	9.0	140	51%
maple syrup	2 oz	9.0	140	51%
mild	2 oz	9.0	140	51%
breakfast patties				
apple cinnamon	2.3 oz	12.0	160	68%
hot	2.3 oz	12.0	150	72%
maple syrup	2.3 oz	11.0	140	71%

Food and Description	Amount	Fat Grams	Total Calories	% Fat Calories
mild	2 oz	11.0	140	71%
	2.3 oz	10.0	160	56%
w/smoked bacon	2.3 oz	12.0	150	72%
Italian/lean				
hot				
links	3 oz	8.0	140	51%
rope	2.5 oz	7.0	110	57%
sweet				
links	3 oz	8.0	140	51%
rope	2.5 oz	7.0	110	57%
Polish				
links	3 oz	8.0	140	51%
rope	2.5 oz	7.0	110	57%
smoked seasoned	3 oz	8.0	140	51%

SAUSAGE DISH (See also BREAKFAST SANDWICH; FROZEN DINNER/ENTRÉE; SAUSAGE)

Food and Description	Amount	Fat Grams	Total Calories	% Fat Calories
(Mary Kitchen) sausage hash	1 cup	27.0	410	59%

SAUSAGE STICK (See JERKY STICKS & STRIPS)

SAUSAGE SUBSTITUTE (See VEGETARIAN FOODS)

Food and Description	Amount	Fat Grams	Total Calories	% Fat Calories
SAVORY/ground	1 tsp	–	4	–

SCALLION/GREEN ONION/SPRING ONION (See also ONION)

Food and Description	Amount	Fat Grams	Total Calories	% Fat Calories
fresh				
chopped	½ cup	–	15	–
(Dole)	1 Tbs	–	2	–
w/tops	5 large	–	10	–

SCALLOP (See also SEAFOOD ENTRÉE/DINNER)

Food and Description	Amount	Fat Grams	Total Calories	% Fat Calories
fresh				
breaded & fried/~½ oz each	2 scallops	3.0	67	40%
raw	3 oz	0.6	75	7%
frozen				
(Contessa)	4 oz	–	90	–
(Crystal Isle)	3 oz	1.0	150	6%
imitation				
(Louis Kemp) scallop delights/bay style	13 pieces	–	80	–

SCONE (See also ROLL)

Food and Description	Amount	Fat Grams	Total Calories	% Fat Calories
(Health Valley) Healthy Scones/fat-free				
cinnamon raisin	1 scone	–	180	–
cranberry orange	1 scone	–	180	–
mountain blueberry	1 scone	–	180	–
pineapple banana	1 scone	–	180	–
homemade/USDA Standard Home Recipe				
apricot	1 scone	7.0	230	27%
cheese	1 scone	9.0	185	44%
plain	1 scone	7.0	180	35%
(Krusteaz) mix/prepared				
scone mix				
apple cinnamon	1 scone	13.0	300	39%
blueberry	1 scone	13.0	280	42%
carrot raisin spice	1 scone	13.0	300	39%
cranberry orange	1 scone	13.0	280	42%

Food and Description	Amount	Fat Grams	Total Calories	% Fat Calories
maple pecan	1 scone	15.0	290	47%
scone & shortcake	1 scone	9.0	180	45%
SCOTCH (See LIQUOR, DISTILLED)				
SCOTCH BROTH (See SOUP)				
SCRAPPLE				
generic	1 oz	4.0	61	59%
(Jones Dairy Farm) country style	1.5 oz	6.0	90	60%
SCROD (See SEAFOOD ENTRÉE/DINNER)				
SCUP /raw	3 oz	2.0	90	20%
SEA BASS (See also SEAFOOD ENTRÉE/DINNER)				
fresh				
breaded & fried	3 oz	7.0	176	36%
cooked-dry heat	3 oz	2.0	105	17%
raw	3 oz	1.7	82	19%
frozen				
(Mirabel) Chilean/boneless-skinless	4 oz	21.0	250	76%
SEA SALT	1 tsp	–	–	–
SEA TROUT /raw	3 oz	3.0	88	31%
SEA VEGETABLE (See SEAWEED)				
SEAFOOD CHOWDER (See SOUP)				
SEAFOOD ENTRÉE/DINNER (See also FROZEN ENTRÉE/DINNER; PASTA ENTRÉE/DINNER; individual listings)				
■ CANNED				
generic/crab cakes	4.5 oz	13.0	252	46%
(Gorton's)				
cod cakes	4 oz	0.5	100	5%
crunchy fried clams	3 oz	17.0	260	59%
(Port Clyde)				
Fish Steaks				
w/Louisiana hot sauce	3.75 oz can	9.0	150	54%
w/mustard sauce	3.75 oz can	7.0	140	45%
w/soybean oil				
drained	3.3 oz can	17.0	220	70%
& hot chilies/drained	3.3 oz can	8.0	155	46%
■ FROZEN				
(Arctic Ice) herb & garlic	2 pieces	16.0	280	51%
(American Seafoods International)				
Alaska Pollack				
Bake'N Broil/Golden broil				
Tail-r-cut	4 oz	8.0	160	45%
Batter'N Brew				
fillets	1 piece	5.0	130	35%
fish fries	3 pieces	8.0	200	36%
Bold & Zesty				
Italian breaded				
Fishfries	3 pieces	12.0	220	49%
triangle nuggets	3 nuggets	10.0	170	53%
wedges	1 piece	10.0	150	60%
Bold Oriental Tempura fishfries	2 pieces	5.0	140	32%
Breaded precooked				

Food and Description	Amount	Fat Grams	Total Calories	% Fat Calories
fish sticks	3 fish sticks	8.0	180	40%
rectangle	3 oz	7.0	150	42%
	3.6 oz	9.0	180	45%
Bunch O'Crunch/minced				
nuggets	6 nuggets	11.0	210	47%
sticks	5 sticks	13.0	230	51%
Crumb Topped cuts				
Cajun	1 piece	9.0	170	48%
golden broil	1 piece	12.0	200	54%
homestyle herb	1 piece	8.0	160	45%
Italiano	1 piece	8.0	170	42%
seafood-style	1 piece	10.0	180	50%
Crunch				
Ole'/wedge	1 portion	12.0	230	47%
potatoes				
fish fries	3 pieces	16.0	260	55%
nuggets	4 nuggets	16.0	250	58%
wedge	1 piece	13.0	220	53%
tortilla				
fish fries	3 pieces	12.0	200	54%
triangle nuggets	3 pieces	8.0	170	42%
wedge	1 portion	10.0	190	47%
English cut glazed	4 oz	1.0	90	10%
English style/batter dipt				
wedge	4 oz	11.0	200	50%
Fillettes				
seasoned crunchy				
fillet shaped	3 oz	1.0	120	8%
tail shaped	4 oz	1.0	160	6%
FishFries				
country style	3 pieces	1.0	180	5%
reduced-fat/Oven Crispy	3 pieces	3.0	160	17%
Santa Fe style	3 pieces	1.0	160	6%
seasoned	3 pieces	10.0	210	43%
Southern cornmeal	3 pieces	4.0	160	23%
Oven Crispy				
nuggets	3 nuggets	9.0	160	51%
	4 nuggets	16.0	240	40%
wedge	3 oz	6.0	140	39%
	3.6 oz	8.0	170	42%
Portions				
Dijon dill crumb	1 piece	13.0	200	59%
lemon pepper crumb	1 piece	13.0	210	56%
lemon herb glaze	1 piece	7.0	150	42%
mustard glaze	1 piece	3.5	130	24%
pepper glaze	1 piece	8.0	170	42%
Reduced-Fat/Oven crispy wedge	3.5 oz	3.0	140	19%
Southern Fry fillets	4 oz	13.0	240	49%
Zesty Buffalo Battered				
Fishfries	2 pieces	11.0	190	52%

Food and Description	Amount	Fat Grams	Total Calories	% Fat Calories
triangle nuggets	3 nuggets	8.0	150	48%
wedges	1 piece	5.0	140	26%
Catfish nuggets/southern cornmeal	3 pieces	8.0	180	40%
Cod				
Bake'N Broil/Golden Broil				
Tali-r-cut	3 oz	6.0	120	45%
	4.5 oz	9.0	170	48%
Batter'N Brew	1 piece	5.0	140	32%
breaded/pre-cooked				
rectangles	3 oz	7.0	160	39%
minced rectangles	4 oz	9.0	180	45%
Bunch O'Crunch/minced				
nuggets	6 nuggets	11.0	210	47%
portions	4 oz	15.0	270	50%
sticks	5 sticks	15.0	230	59%
English cut glazed/raw-unbreaded	4 oz	1.0	90	10%
English style/batter dipt				
Boston cut	3 oz	8.0	160	45%
wedge	3 oz	8.0	160	45%
Fillets				
gourmet breaded original	3 oz	0.5	100	5%
seasoned crunch				
shaped	3 oz	1.0	110	8%
tail-shaped	4 oz	1.0	90	10%
tender crisp/original	4 oz	1.0	130	7%
Fish Sticks/breaded pre-cooked				
minced	3 fish sticks	8.0	160	45%
regular	3 fish sticks	9.0	160	51%
Oven Crispy				
minced				
nuggets	3 nuggets	9.0	160	51%
sticks	4 fish sticks	14.0	270	47%
rectangles	1 piece	9.0	190	43%
prime cut loins	3 oz	0.5	70	6%
	4 oz	1.0	90	10%
	5 oz	1.0	110	8%
	6 oz	1.0	130	7%
raw/breaded				
rectangles	3 oz	1.0	120	8%
	4 oz	1.5	160	8%
squares	1 piece	1.5	120	11%
Tail-r-cut	4 oz	1.5	160	8%
	5⅓ oz	2.0	220	8%
Southern Fry fillets	4 oz	15.0	270	50%
Tails	1 serving	1.0	110	81%
Flounder				
raw/breaded				
fillets	4 oz	1.5	140	10%
Great Silver Smelt				
English style/batter dipt wedge	4 oz	9.0	190	43%

Food and Description	Amount	Fat Grams	Total Calories	% Fat Calories
Oven crispy/minced				
Nuggets	3 nuggets	12.0	210	51%
wedges	3 oz	10.0	210	43%
	3.6 oz	12.0	250	43%
Haddock				
raw/breaded				
rectangles	3 oz	1.0	120	8%
squares	4 oz	1.5	180	8%
Tail-r-cut	4 oz	1.0	140	6%
Salmon				
Sides				
skin on-boned	4 oz	11.0	180	55%
smoked/pre-sliced	2 oz	5.0	90	50%
superior cut				
skinless boned	4 oz	11.0	180	55%
	5 oz	14.0	240	53%
	6 oz	16.0	290	50%
	7 oz	19.0	340	50%
	8 oz	22.0	390	51%
Specialty Items				
Alaska Pollock fully cooked breaded square	2.5 oz	7.0	140	45%
crabmeat stuffing	3 oz	5.0	140	32%
fish cakes	2 oz	9.0	210	39%
lemon pepper crumb prime cut cod loins	6 oz	9.0	270	30%
lemon pepper Easy Grill Alaska Pollock/tail-r-cut	4 oz	2.0	90	20%
Neptune burger	3 oz	7.0	160	39%
Whiting				
breaded pre-cooked				
fish sticks	3 fish sticks	9.0	170	48%
nuggets	3 nuggets	10.0	220	41%
rectangles	3 oz	8.0	150	48%
	3.6 oz	9.0	180	45%
English style/batter dipped wedge	3 oz	8.0	160	45%
Oven crispy				
wedges	3 oz	8.0	170	42%
	3.6 oz	10.0	200	45%
raw/breaded				
Rectangles	3 oz	2.0	130	14%
	3.6 oz	10.0	200	45%
(Contessa)				
shrimp				
cooked				
shell on	3 oz	–	60	–
shelled	3 oz	–	40	–
uncooked	4 oz	–	80	–
shrimp & linguini	2 cups	3.0	300	9%
shrimp stir-fry	2¼ cup	–	150	–

Food and Description	Amount	Fat Grams	Total Calories	% Fat Calories
generic				
cod fillets/crunchy/microwaveable	1 fillet	22.0	330	60%
fish cakes				
bite-size	5 pieces	11.0	165	60%
large	1 piece	11.0	165	60%
fish sticks/4" x 2" x ½"	1 stick	3.0	75	36%
(Gorton's)				
fish fillet tenders				
crunchy whole	4 oz	14.0	250	50%
extra crunchy	4 oz	12.0	270	40%
fish fillets				
baked				
au gratin	½ pkg	5.0	130	35%
broccoli & cheddar	½ pkg	5.0	130	35%
garlic butter crumb	½ pkg	9.0	170	48%
primavera	½ pkg	5.0	120	38%
battered				
lemon pepper	⅓ pkg	18.0	270	60%
country style/southern fried	⅓ pkg	14.0	230	55%
crunchy				
garlic & herb	⅓ pkg	11.0	220	45%
lemon herb	⅙ pkg	11.0	220	45%
Parmesan	⅓ pkg	15.0	260	52%
ranch	⅓ pkg	13.0	240	49%
grilled				
Caesar Parmesan	½ pkg	5.0	110	41%
Cajun blackened	½ pkg	6.0	120	45%
Lemon butter	½ pkg	6.0	120	45%
fish portions/value pack				
batter-dipped	1 portion	11.0	170	58%
breaded/crunchy	1 portion	12.0	180	60%
fish sticks				
breaded/value pack				
mini	13 sticks	14.0	230	55%
regular	8 sticks	12.0	210	51%
(Mrs. Paul's)				
Battered				
hearty size fish fillets	3.5 oz	10.0	200	45%
fish				
fillet	2.5 oz	8.0	150	48%
tenders	4 pieces	17.0	280	55%
Breaded				
Country cornmeal fillets	1 fillet	11.0	180	55%
fish				
fillets	2 fillets	18.0	280	58%
sticks	6 sticks	14.0	250	50%
strips	4 pieces	18.0	310	52%
hearty size fish sticks	5 sticks	17.0	300	51%
Grilled				
Fillets/4 oz				
Cajun	1 fillet	6.0	130	42%

Food and Description	Amount	Fat Grams	Total Calories	% Fat Calories
garlic butter	1 fillet	6.0	130	42%
lemon pepper	1 fillet	6.0	130	42%
salmon/3.28 oz				
creamy dill	1 fillet	2.5	90	25%
honey mustard	1 fillet	2.5	90	25%
Healthy Selects (breaded/baked)				
fillets/2.78 oz				
garlic herb	1 fillet	2.0	130	14%
lemon pepper	1 fillet	2.0	130	14%
original	1 fillet	2.0	130	14%
fish sticks	6 sticks	3.0	190	14%
Premium Fillets				
cod	1 fillet/4.28 oz	14.0	260	48%
flounder	1 fillet/6 oz	9.0	170	48%
haddock	1 fillet/8.6 oz	12.0	240	45%
Specialty Items				
cheese & crap poppers	4 poppers	16.0	320	45%
clams/fried	18 pieces	12.0	250	43%
deviled crab cakes				
mini	6 cakes	12.0	220	49%
regular	1 cake	10.0	180	50%
fish cakes	2 cakes	10.0	210	43%
scallops/fried	13 pieces	7.0	220	29%
shrimp				
butterfly	7 shrimp	14.0	270	47%
scampi	16 shrimp	1.0	80	11%
stuffed	3 shrimp	13.0	290	40%
(Oven Poppers)				
cod stuffed w/broccoli & cheese	1 piece	6.0	150	36%
sole				
stuffed w/crab	1 piece	13.0	250	47%
stuffed w/garlic shrimp & almonds	1 piece	13.0	250	47%
(Schwan's)				
Breaded seafood				
blue hake	3 oz	9.0	180	45%
catfish fingers/raw	4 oz	4.5	190	21%
cod				
Battercrisp	2 oz piece	7.0	120	53%
nuggets	6 nuggets	10.0	200	45%
haddock				
squares	4 oz	7.0	190	33%
sticks	3 sticks	5.0	140	32%
halibut fillets	4 oz	4.5	130	31%
ocean perch	4 oz	2.0	90	20%
orange roughy	4 oz	1.5	80	17%
seafood legs/fancy	3.5 oz	0.5	100	5%
scrod/New England style	5 oz	13.0	230	51%
Seafood Specialties				
clam strips/breaded	½ cup/3 oz	13.0	270	43%
salmon burger/gourmet smoked	4 oz	1.0	90	10%

Food and Description	Amount	Fat Grams	Total Calories	% Fat Calories
shrimp				
fantail/breaded	4 oz	2.0	240	8%
gourmet medium	4 oz	2.5	140	9%
jumbo cooked	3 oz	1.0	70	13%
oven-ready/breaded	3 oz	8.0	240	30%
pieces/breaded	4 oz	2.0	230	8%
Unbreaded				
blue hake loins	4 oz	–	70	–
Alaskan				
cod	4 oz	0.5	90	5%
perch	4 oz	2.0	90	90%
salmon fillets/no-bone	4 oz	2.0	100	18%
(Sea Pak) shrimp				
butterfly	4 oz	1.0	140	6%
jumbo butterfly/breaded	3 oz	9.0	200	41%
popcorn	3 oz	12.0	210	51%
poppers	20 pieces	12.0	210	51%
(Van de Kamp's)				
Battered Items				
Fillets				
fish	1 fillet	10.0	170	53%
haddock	2 fillets	12.0	240	45%
halibut	3 fillets	10.0	220	41%
ocean perch	2 fillets	13.0	240	49%
fish				
portions	1 portion	9.0	160	51%
tenders	4 pieces	17.0	290	53%
Breaded Items				
fillets				
fish	2 fillets	17.0	260	59%
fish sticks				
mini	13 sticks	14.0	250	50%
regular	6 sticks	17.0	290	53%
snack/value	6 sticks	15.0	260	52%
fish strips	4 pieces	14.0	270	47%
Hearty Size fish fillets	1 fillet	10.0	150	60%
portions	3 portions	24.0	360	60%
Crisp & Healthy/breaded & baked				
fillets				
garlic & herb	2 fillets	3.0	170	16%
lemon pepper	2 fillets	3.0	170	16%
regular/plain	2 fillets	3.0	170	16%
fish sticks	6 sticks	3.0	190	14%
Grilled Items/3.75 oz fillets				
garlic butter	1 fillet	6.0	120	45%
lemon butter	1 fillet	6.0	120	45%
lemon pepper	1 fillet	6.0	120	45%
Premium Breaded Items/fillets				
cod	4 oz fillet	11.0	230	43%
flounder	4 oz fillet	11.0	230	43%

Food and Description	Amount	Fat Grams	Total Calories	% Fat Calories
haddock	4 oz fillet	11.0	230	43%
Specialty Items				
cheese & crab peppers	4 poppers	16.0	320	45%
clams/fried	18 pieces	12.0	250	43%
crab cakes	1 cake	9.0	170	48%
shrimp				
butterfly	7 shrimp	15.0	300	45%
popcorn	20 shrimp	12.0	270	40%
scampi	16 shrimp	1.0	80	11%
stuffed	3 shrimp	13.0	290	40%

■ **HOMEMADE**

USDA Standard Home Recipe (Note: Homemade dishes were not made with low-fat substitute ingredients. The amount of fat and calories may vary, depending on the type and amount of certain ingredients used.)

Food and Description	Amount	Fat Grams	Total Calories	% Fat Calories
clam fritter/~ 1.5 oz	1 fritter	6.0	124	44%
crab				
deviled	½ cup	12.0	185	58%
stuffed	½ cup	4.0	86	42%
crab cake/fried in margarine/4 oz	1 cake	11.0	205	48%
fish cake/fried	1 regular or 5 bite-size	5.0	105	43%
fish loaf	~5 oz	5.6	186	27%
jambalaya	1 cup	6.7	250	24%
lobster Newburg	~6.5 oz	35.0	455	69%
oyster stew	1 cup	15.0	233	58%
oysters Rockefeller	4 oysters	2.7	90	27%
paella w/saffron rice, seafood, & vegetables	~8 oz	11.0	350	28%
salmon cake	3.5 oz	15.0	248	54%
salmon casserole	1 cup	35.0	555	57%
salmon patty	3.5 oz	12.0	239	45%
salmon-rice loaf	6 oz	8.0	212	34%
seafood Creole w/rice	1 cup	8.7	300	26%
seafood curry	⅔ cup	11.5	232	45%
seafood gumbo	5 oz	1.0	48	19%
seafood salad	3½ oz	10.0	160	56%
shrimp salad	¾ cup	12.0	210	51%
tuna patty	3 oz	3.0	80	34%

■ **MIX** (Note: The amount of fat and calories in dishes prepared from boxed mixes may vary slightly depending on the fat and calorie content of the seafood used in preparation.)

(Betty Crocker) Tuna Helper (prepared data is for regular recipe only)

Food and Description	Amount	Fat Grams	Total Calories	% Fat Calories
au gratin				
mix only	½ cup	3.5	190	17%
prepared	1 cup	11.0	300	33%
cheesy broccoli				
mix only	⅔ cup	3.5	200	16%
prepared	1 cup	9.0	290	28%
cheesy pasta				
mix only	¾ cup	3.0	170	16%

Food and Description	Amount	Fat Grams	Total Calories	% Fat Calories
prepared	1 cup	9.0	290	28%
creamy broccoli				
mix only	⅔ cup	4.5	190	21%
prepared	1 cup	12.0	310	35%
creamy pasta				
mix only	¾ cup	6.0	190	28%
prepared	1 cup	13.0	300	39%
fettuccine Alfredo				
mix only	¾ cup	3.5	170	19%
prepared	1 cup	14.0	310	41%
garden cheddar				
mix only	⅔ cup	3.5	190	17%
prepared	1 cup	11.0	290	34%
pasta salad				
mix only	⅓ cup	0.5	120	4%
prepared	⅔ cup	27.0	380	64%
tetrazzini				
mix only	½ cup	2.5	180	13%
prepared	1 cup	12.0	300	36%
tuna melt				
mix only	¾ cup	4.5	180	23%
prepared	1 cup	13.0	300	39%
tuna pot pie				
mix only	½ cup	20.0	340	53%
prepared	⅕ pie	24.0	440	49%
tuna Romanoff				
mix only	⅔ cup	3.0	210	13%
prepared	1 cup	8.0	280	26%

SEASONINGS (*See also* ASIAN FOOD/SAUCES & SEASONINGS; BAKE & FRY MIX; GRAVY; MARINADE; MEXICAN FOOD; SAUCE; individual listings)
(NOTE: Unless stated otherwise, data are for seasoning or seasoning mix only.)

Food and Description	Amount	Fat Grams	Total Calories	% Fat Calories
(Accent)				
flavor enhancer	⅛ tsp	–	–	–
Sa-son				
con ajo cebolla	¼ tsp	–	–	–
con azatran	¼ tsp	–	–	–
con culantro	¼ tsp	–	–	–
original	¼ tsp	–	–	–
(Adolph's)				
chili mix	~1 Tbs	–	60	–
meat				
seasoned	¼ tsp	–	–	–
un-seasoned	¼ tsp	–	–	–
stir fry teriyaki	~2 Tbs	–	30	–
(Andre Prost) A Taste Of Thai				
chorizo ancho seasoning	1 Tbs	–	5	–
green curry				
base mix	1 tsp	1.5	15	90%
dinner kit	3.5 oz	7.0	91	69%
lemon grass hearts	1 piece	–	–	–

Food and Description	Amount	Fat Grams	Total Calories	% Fat Calories
mussaman curry				
base mix	1 tsp	1.5	20	68%
dinner kit	3.5 oz	6.0	102	53%
panang curry				
base mix	1 tsp	2.0	25	72%
dinner kit	3.5 oz	8.0	105	69%
red chili peppers/minced	1 tsp	–	–	–
red curry				
base mix	1 tsp	1.5	20	68%
dinner kit	3.5 oz	7.0	94	67%
spicy chicken & rice dinner mix	¼ pkg	–	15	–
Thai peanut bake seasoning mix	¼ pkg	1.5	45	30%
yellow curry				
base mix	1 tsp	3.0	30	90%
dinner kit	3.5 oz	9.0	113	72%
(Betty Crocker) Potato Shakers				
crispy cheddar fries	3 tsp	1.0	25	36%
original	3 tsp	0.5	30	15%
Parmesan	3 tsp	1.0	30	30%
seasoned fries	3 tsp	–	20	–
zesty cheddar	3 tsp	1.5	30	45%
(Cavender's) All Purpose Greek	¼ tsp	–	–	–
(Chi~Chi's) seasoning mix	1 tsp	–	10	–
(Durkee)				
garlic bread sprinkles	½ tsp	–	–	–
roasting bag				
au jus	⅛ pkg	–	10	–
barbecue chicken	⅙ pkg	–	30	–
beef stew	⅒ pkg	–	15	–
chicken	⅙ pkg	–	20	–
country chicken	⅙ pkg	1.5	35	39%
lemon butter fish	¼ pkg	0.5	30	15%
meat loaf	⅛ pkg	–	15	–
onion pot roast	⅙ pkg	–	25	–
pork	⅙ pkg	–	25	–
pot roast	⅙ pkg	–	15	–
spareribs	⅐ pkg	–	25	–
Swiss steak	⅑ pkg	–	10	–
seasoning packet				
beef fajita/"easy"	⅙ pkg	–	15	–
beef stew	⅑ pkg	–	–	–
beef teriyaki/"easy"	⅕ pkg	1.0	30	30%
burrito	⅒ pkg	1.0	35	26%
chicken cacciatore/"easy"	⅒ pkg	–	10	–
chicken mushroom/easy'	⅛ pkg	–	15	–
fried rice	¼ pkg	–	15	–
ground beef	¼ pkg	–	25	–
Italian meatball	⅛ pkg	–	20	–
lemon pepper dill fish/"easy"	⅙ pkg	0.5	20	9%
meat loaf	⅑ pkg	–	20	–

Food and Description	Amount	Fat Grams	Total Calories	% Fat Calories
Mexican salsa chicken/"easy"	1/10 pkg	–	10	–
pasta salad	1/6 pkg	–	10	–
sloppy joe	1/6 pkg	–	20	–
stroganoff	1/8 pkg	–	10	–
sweet & sour chicken/"easy"	1/9 pkg	–	20	–
tomato basil fish/"easy"	1/7 pkg	–	15	–
(French's)				
roasting bag				
au jus	1/8 pkg	<1.0	10	45%
chicken	1/5 pkg	<1.0	25	18%
lemon butter fish	1/4 pkg	<1.0	25	18%
meatloaf	1/6 pkg	<1.0	25	18%
onion pot roast	1/8 pkg	<1.0	18	25%
pork	1/6 pkg	<1.0	25	18%
pot roast	1/8 pkg	<1.0	18	25%
Swiss steak	1/6 pkg	<1.0	20	23%
seasonings				
beef stew	1/9 pkg	–	5	–
Chili-O				
mild	1/5 pkg	0.5	30	15%
onion	1/5 pkg	–	40	–
original	1/5 pkg	–	30	–
Texas stile	1/3 pkg	1.0	45	20%
fajita	1/5 pkg	1.0	82	11%
meat marinade	1/8 pkg	–	10	–
meat loaf	1/8 pkg	–	20	–
sloppy joe	1/8 pkg	–	16	–
stroganoff	1/4 pkg	2.0	45	40%
zesty pasta	1/5 pkg	–	20	–
(Knorr) recipe mix				
beef stew w/wine	1/6 pkg	1.0	40	23%
chicken Dijonne	1/6 pkg	1.0	30	30%
goulash beef stew	1/6 pkg	1.0	40	23%
sauerbraten	1/6 pkg	1.0	35	26%
(Lawry's)				
bacon onion	1 tsp	–	10	–
burrito	1/4 pkg	–	35	–
chili	1/5 pkg	0.5	25	18%
fajitas	1/8 pkg	–	15	–
garlic pepper	1/4 tsp	–	2	–
garlic powder w/parsley	1 tsp	–	12	–
garlic salt	1 tsp	–	4	–
lemon pepper	1 tsp	–	6	–
marinade				
teriyaki BBQ for steak, chicken, & fish	1/16 pkg	–	20	–
tenderizing beef	1/12 pkg	–	–	–
weekday gourmet/London broil	1/4 pkg	–	10	–
minced onion	1 tsp	–	7	–
pepper/seasoned	1 tsp	–	4	–

Food and Description	Amount	Fat Grams	Total Calories	% Fat Calories
pinch of herbs	1 tsp	0.5	9	50%
salt/seasoned				
hot 'n spicy	1 tsp	–	3	–
lite	1 tsp	–	8	–
plain	1 tsp	–	4	–
salt free	1 tsp	–	3	–
salt free 17	1 tsp	–	10	–
taco				
chicken	¼ pkt	–	20	–
original				
1 oz. pkg	⅙ pkg	–	15	–
2.5 oz pkg	1/12 pkg	–	20	–
(McCormick/Schilling)				
Bag 'N Season				
beef stew	1 tsp	–	15	–
Buffalo wings	1 Tbs	–	30	–
chicken	1 Tbs	–	20	–
country chicken	2 tsp	1.0	25	36%
meat loaf	2 tsp	–	15	–
pork chops	2 tsp	–	15	–
pot roast	1 Tbs	–	10	–
spareribs	1 Tbs	–	30	–
Swiss steak	1 tsp	–	15	–
turkey w/gravy	1 tsp	–	15	–
gourmet spices				
arrowroot	1½ Tbs	–	40	–
beef flavor base	1 tsp	–	–	–
Bon Appetit	¼ tsp	–	–	–
char-grill seasoning	¼ tsp	–	–	–
chicken flavor base	1 tsp	2.0	35	51%
cinnamon sugar	1 tsp	–	15	–
ginger/crystallized	¼ tsp	–	–	–
lemon & pepper	¼ tsp	–	–	–
season pepper medley	¼ tsp	–	2	–
vanilla flavored powder	¼ tsp	–	2	–
vegetable delight	½ tsp	–	–	–
Grill Mates				
Montreal	¼ tsp	–	–	–
Montreal chicken & fish	¼ tsp	–	–	–
spicy Montreal steak	¼ tsp	–	–	–
International Blends				
Chinese 5 spice	½ tsp	–	–	–
herb de Provence	½ tsp	–	–	–
Thai	½ tsp	–	–	–
rice seasonings				
Creole	⅔ Tbs	–	20	–
curry	1 Tbs	1.0	25	36%
Japanese	1½ Tbs	1.5	50	27%
saffron	1 Tbs	–	25	–
Spanish	1½ Tbs	–	45	–

Food and Description	Amount	Fat Grams	Total Calories	% Fat Calories
Rotisserie Recipe				
herb & spice	2 tsp	–	15	–
tangy barbecue	2 tsp	–	20	–
salt-free blends				
all purpose	¼ tsp	–	–	–
garlic & herb	¼ tsp	–	–	–
lemon & pepper	¼ tsp	–	–	–
onion & herb	¼ tsp	–	–	–
spicy	¼ tsp	–	–	–
seasoning blends				
beef stew	2 tsp	–	15	–
beef stroganoff	2 tsp	–	15	–
burrito	1 tsp	0.5	25	18%
Cajun	½ tsp	–	–	–
Caribbean jerk	¼ tsp	–	–	–
celery salt	¼ tsp	–	–	–
cheese sauce	4 tsp	2.0	40	45%
chili				
hot	¼ pkg	1.0	40	23%
mild	¼ pkg	–	30	–
original	¼ pkg	0.5	30	15%
citrus pepper	¼ tsp	–	–	–
Creole	¼ tsp	–	–	–
fajita	¼ tsp	–	1	–
garlic, minced-wet/California style	1 tsp	0.5	15	30%
garlic & parsley salt	¼ tsp	–	–	–
garlic bread sprinkle	½ tsp	1.0	10	90%
garlic pepper				
California style	¼ tsp	–	–	–
regular	¼ tsp	–	3	–
garlic salt				
California style	¼ tsp	–	–	–
regular	¼ tsp	–	–	–
garlic spread				
garlic & herb	½ Tbs	4.5	45	90%
regular	½ Tbs	4.0	45	80%
hamburger	¼ tsp	–	–	–
herb chicken	¼ tsp	–	–	–
homestyle	¼ tsp	–	–	–
imitation butter-flavored salt	¼ tsp	–	–	–
lemon herb	½ tsp	–	–	–
lemon pepper/California style	½ tsp	–	5	–
meat loaf	1 tsp	–	15	–
meat marinade	1 tsp	–	15	–
mesquite chicken	¼ tsp	–	2	–
old bay	½ tsp	–	–	–
onion salt/California style	¼ tsp	–	–	–
pork seasoing	½ tsp	–	–	–
rotisserie chicken	¼ tsp	–	–	–
sloppy joe	⅛ pkg	–	15	–

Food and Description	Amount	Fat Grams	Total Calories	% Fat Calories
taco				
chicken	¼ pkg	–	25	–
mild	⅙ pkg	–	20	–
spice blends				
barbecue seasoning	½ tsp	–	–	–
Best O'Butter butter salt	¼ tsp	–	–	–
broiled steak seasoning	¼ tsp	–	–	–
California garlic pepper	¼ tsp	–	–	–
Caribbean Jerk	¼ tsp	–	–	–
Chesapeake Bay seafood seasoning	¼ tsp	–	–	–
chicken seasoning				
fried	½ tsp	–	–	–
herb classic	¼ tsp	–	–	–
mesquite	¼ tsp	–	–	–
rotisserie	¼ tsp	–	–	–
fajita	¼ tsp	–	–	–
garlic bread sprinkle	½ tsp	1.0	10	90%
lemon herb	½ tsp	–	–	–
meat tenderizer				
non-seasoned	¼ tsp	–	–	–
seasoned	¼ tsp	–	–	–
Mexican	½ tsp	–	–	–
Salad Supreme	¼ tsp	–	–	–
Season All				
garlic	¼ tsp	–	–	–
lite	¼ tsp	–	–	–
original	¼ tsp	–	–	–
peppered	¼ tsp	–	–	–
spicy	¼ tsp	–	–	–
Szechuan pepper	¼ tsp	–	–	–
vegetable supreme	¼ tsp	–	–	–
Thai seasoning	½ tsp	–	–	–
(Mrs. Dash)				
extra spicy	1 tsp	–	12	–
garlic & herb	1 tsp	–	12	–
lemon & herb	1 tsp	–	12	–
low pepper	1 tsp	–	12	–
original	1 tsp	–	12	–
table blend	1 tsp	–	12	–
(Molly McButter)				
cheese-flavor sprinkles	½ tsp	–	5	–
sour cream-flavor sprinkles	½ tsp	–	5	–
(NewMenu) Tofumate				
breakfast scramble	¼ pkg	–	15	–
eggless salad	¼ pkg	–	15	–
Mandarin stir-fry	¼ pkg	–	30	–
Szechwan stir-fry	¼ pkg	–	25	–
Texas taco	¼ pkg	–	15	–
(Nile Spice)				
Cleopatra's Secret	⅛ tsp	–	–	–

Food and Description	Amount	Fat Grams	Total Calories	% Fat Calories
desert spice	⅛ tsp	–	–	–
ginger curry	⅛ tsp	–	–	–
maya maize popcorn	½ tsp	–	–	–
Nile spice	⅛ tsp	–	–	–
seasoning of garlic	⅛ tsp	–	–	–
spicy lemon pepper	⅛ tsp	–	–	–
(Old El Paso) seasoning mix				
burrito	2 tsp	–	20	–
enchilada	2 tsp	–	10	–
chili	1 Tbs	0.5	25	18%
taco				
less sodium	2 tsp	–	20	–
regular	2 tsp	–	20	–
(Produce Partners) vegetable seasonings				
oven potato fries	1 Tbs	1.0	30	30%
potato toppers	1 Tbs	1.0	35	26%
roasted potatoes				
cheddar	1 Tbs	1.5	35	39%
Italian herb	2 tsp	1.5	30	45%
onion	2 tsp	1.0	30	30%
(Shake & Bake)				
Oven Fry seasoned coating mix				
chicken/extra crispy	⅛ pouch	1.0	60	15%
chicken or pork/homestyle	⅛ pouch	1.0	40	23%
pork/extra crispy	⅛ pouch	1.5	60	23%
Perfect Potatoes seasoning mix/dry mix only				
crispy cheddar	⅙ pkt	2.0	30	60%
herb & garlic	⅙ pkt	–	20	–
home fries	⅙ pkt	–	20	–
Parmesan peppercorn	⅙ pkt	1.0	25	36%
savory onion	⅙ pkt	–	10	–
seasoned coating mixture				
buffalo wings	⅒ pkt	1.0	40	23%
country mild recipe	⅛ pouch	2.0	35	51%
for chicken/original recipe	⅛ pouch	1.0	40	23%
for chicken or pork				
classic Italian	⅛ pkt	0.5	40	11%
hot & spicy	⅛ pkt	1.0	40	23%
for fish/original	⅛ pouch	1.5	80	17%
for pork/original recipe	⅛ pouch	0.5	45	10%
seasoning & coating mixture glaze				
barbecue chicken or pork	⅛ pouch	1.0	45	20%
honey mustard chicken or pork	⅛ pouch	1.0	45	20%
tangy honey chicken or pork	⅛ pouch	1.0	45	20%
(Smart Seas)				
butter sprinkles	¾ tsp	–	–	–
cheese sprinkles	½ tsp	–	–	–
garlic w/Italian herb	½ tsp	–	–	–
garlic w/parsley	¼ tsp	–	–	–
pepper & herb	¾ tsp	–	–	–

Food and Description	Amount	Fat Grams	Total Calories	% Fat Calories
steak spice	½ tsp	–	–	–
(Sun Bird) dry mix only				
beef & broccoli	¾ Tbs	–	20	–
fried rice	½ Tbs	–	10	–
hot & spicy Szechwan	2 Tbs	–	15	–
lemon chicken stir-fry	½ Tbs	–	10	–
teriyaki	½ Tbs	–	10	–
(Taco Bell) Home Originals/dry mix only				
chicken fajita	~1 Tbs	–	25	–
taco	~2 tsp	–	20	–
(Tone's) Oriental five-spice seasoning	1 tsp	–	10	–
SEAWEED				
agar				
dried	3 oz	<1.0	260	2%
(Eden)	1 Tbs	–	10	–
raw	3 oz	<1.0	23	20%
arame/(Eden)	½ cup	–	30	–
kelp/raw	3 oz	0.6	37	15%
kombu	3-½" sheet	–	10	–
laver/Nori				
dried	3 oz	<1.0	30	9%
(Eden) sushi nori sea vegetable	1 sheet	–	10	–
raw	3 oz	<1.0	31	15%
spirulina				
dried	3 oz	6.6	249	24%
raw	3 oz	<1.0	22	21%
wakame				
(Eden)	½ cup	–	25	–
raw	3 oz	<1.0	40	11%
SELTZER WATER (See SOFT DRINK; WATER)				
SEMOLINA (See also FLOUR)				
enriched	½ cup	0.5	310	1%
unenriched	½ cup	<1.0	110	2%
whole-grain	1 cup	2.0	600	3%
SESAME BUTTER/TAHINI				
(Arrowhead Mills) organic tahini	2 Tbs	19.0	190	90%
(Erewhon)				
butter	2 Tbs	17.0	190	81%
tahini	2 Tbs	17.0	170	90%
(Casbah) sauce mix/prepared	¼ cup	13.0	160	73%
generic	1 oz	15.0	169	80%
paste	1 Tbs	8.0	95	76%
tahini	2 Tbs	16.0	180	80%
toasted	2 Tbs	20.0	200	90%
(Kettle) Roaster Fresh	2 Tbs	15.0	170	79%
(Westbrae) organic				
mid-Eastern	2 Tbs	19.0	220	78%
natural	2 Tbs	19.0	220	78%
raw	2 Tbs	19.0	220	78%
toasted	2 Tbs	19.0	220	78%

Food and Description	Amount	Fat Grams	Total Calories	% Fat Calories
SESAME FLOUR (*See* FLOUR)				
SESAME SEEDS				
dried/ground	1 tsp	–	5	–
kernels				
(Arrowhead Mills) mechanically hulled	¼ cup	20.0	210	86%
generic				
dried	1 Tbs	4.0	47	77%
toasted	1 oz	13.6	161	76%
	1 cup	80.0	873	82%
whole				
(Arrowhead Mills) brown	¼ cup	20.0	200	90%
generic				
dried	1 Tbs	4.5	52	78%
roasted & toasted	1 oz	13.6	161	76%
(McCormick/Schilling) untoasted	¼ tsp	0.4	5	72%
SHAD, AMERICAN				
cooked-dry heat	3 oz	15.0	215	63%
raw	3 oz	12.0	170	63%
SHALLOT				
freeze-dried	1 Tbs	–	3	–
	¼ cup	–	13	–
	1 oz	–	100	–
fresh/raw/chopped	1 Tbs	–	7	–
SHARK				
batter-dipped & fried	3 oz	11.8	194	55%
raw	3 oz	3.8	111	31%
SHEEPSHEAD				
cooked-dry heat	3 oz	1.0	107	8%
raw	3 oz	2.0	92	20%
SHELLIE BEAN				
canned	½ cup	–	37	–
sprouted				
(La Choy)	1 cup	–	10	–
SHERBET (*See also* FRUIT ICES, BARS, & POPS)				
(Baskin-Robbins)				
blue raspberry	½ cup	1.5	120	11%
	reg scoop	2.0	160	11%
orange	½ cup	1.5	120	11%
	reg scoop	2.0	160	11%
rainbow	½ cup	1.5	120	11%
	reg scoop	2.0	160	11%
tangerine pineapple	½ cup	1.0	120	8%
(Borden) orange	½ cup	1.0	110	8%
(Breyers) Natural				
orange	½ cup	1.5	130	10%
rainbow	½ cup	1.5	130	10%
raspberry	½ cup	1.5	130	10%
(Dreyer's)				
berry rainbow	½ cup	1.0	130	7%

Food and Description	Amount	Fat Grams	Total Calories	% Fat Calories
raspberry chocolate swirl	½ cup	1.5	130	10%
orange vanilla swirl	½ cup	2.0	120	15%
Swiss orange	½ cup	3.0	150	18%
tropical rainbow	½ cup	1.0	130	7%
(Edy's)				
berry rainbow	½ cup	1.0	130	7%
orange vanilla swirl	½ cup	2.0	120	15%
raspberry chocolate swirl	½ cup	1.5	130	10%
strawberry kiwi	½ cup	1.0	120	8%
Swiss orange	½ cup	3.0	150	18%
tropical rainbow	½ cup	1.0	130	7%
(Knudsen) 3-gallon tub				
orange	½ cup	1.0	130	7%
rainbow	½ cup	1.0	120	8%
(Pet) orange	½ cup	1.0	130	7%
(Schwan's)				
orange	½ cup	1.0	120	8%
rainbow	½ cup	1.0	120	8%

SHORTENING, VEGETABLE (*See also* FAT; LARD; OIL; SHORTENING SUBSTITUTE)
(NOTE: All brands of vegetable shortening contain the same amount of calories and fat, just as all types of vegetable oil do. Because of the flexibility manufacturers are given in rounding off nutritional data, it may appear that one product has slightly fewer calories or less fat than another, but don't be fooled: They all get 100% of their calories from fat.)

(Crisco) regular or butter flavor	1 Tbs	12.0	110	100%
	1 cup	205.0	1845	100%
generic/soybean &/or cottonseed	1 Tbs	13.0	113	100%
	1 cup	205.0	1812	100%
(Snowdrift)	1 Tbs	12.0	110	100%
(Wesson)	1 Tbs	12.0	100	100%

SHORTENING SUBSTITUTE

(Plumlite) Just Like Shortenin	1⅔ Tbs	–	70	–
(Wonderslim) fat & egg substitute	¼ cup	–	35	–

SHOYU/SOY SAUCE (*See* ASIAN FOOD/SAUCES & SEASONINGS; SAUCE)
SHRIMP (*See also* ASIAN FOOD; FROZEN ENTRÉE/DINNER; SEAFOOD ENTRÉE/DINNER; SHRIMP, IMITATION; SHRIMP PASTE)
canned

(Chicken of the Sea)				
deveined				
medium	2 oz	–	45	–
small	2 oz	–	45	–
medium	2 oz	0.5	45	10%
small	2 oz	0.5	45	10%
tiny	2 oz	0.5	45	10%
(Crown Prince) tiny/peeled	½ can	–	60	–
generic/mixed species/drained	4 large	1.8	102	15%
	1 cup	3.0	155	17%
(S&W) deveined				
medium	¼ cup	–	45	–
small	¼ cup	–	45	–

Food and Description	Amount	Fat Grams	Total Calories	% Fat Calories
dried	1 oz	0.8	82	9%
fresh				
breaded & fried	4 large	3.7	73	45%
	3 oz	10.0	206	44%
cooked-moist heat	4 large	–	22	–
	3 oz	0.9	84	10%
raw	3 oz	1.0	90	10%
SHRIMP, IMITATION				
from surimi	3 oz	1.0	86	10%
SHRIMP PASTE	3 oz	8.0	155	47%
SHRIMP SOUP, CREAM OF (*See* SOUP)				
SIM-SIM (*See* SESAME SEEDS)				
SMELT (*See also* SEAFOOD ENTRÉE/DINNER)				
rainbow				
breaded & fried	3 oz	10.6	214	45%
cooked-dry heat	3 oz	2.6	106	22%
raw	3 oz	2.0	83	22%
SMOKED SALMON (*See* SALMON; SALMON SPREAD; SEAFOOD ENTRÉE/DINNER)				
SMOKED SAUSAGE (*See* SAUSAGE)				
SNACK BAR (*See* CANDY; GRANOLA/GRANOLA-TYPE BAR)				
SNACK CAKE (*See* CAKE, SNACK; PASTRY; POPCORN BARS & CAKES; RICE CAKES)				
SNACK CRACKER (*See* CRACKER)				
SNACK MIX (*See* SNACKS)				
SNACKS (*See also* FRUIT SNACK; MEXICAN FOOD; NUTS, MIXED; POPCORN; POPCORN BARS & CAKES; POTATO CHIPS & SNACKS; PRETZELS; RICE CAKES; TORTILLA CHIPS)				
(Baken-ets)				
bbq	1 oz	5.0	70	64%
hot n' spicy	1 oz	5.0	70	64%
hot n' spicy cracklins	1 oz	5.0	70	64%
regular	1 oz	5.0	80	56%
regular cracklins	1 oz	6.0	80	68%
(Barbara's) natural snacks				
cheese puffs				
bakes	1½ cup	11.0	160	62%
jalapeño	¾ cup	9.0	150	54%
original	¾ cup	10.0	150	60%
onion zings				
cheese	1 oz	7.0	140	45%
ranch	1 oz	6.0	130	42%
thangs				
major corn	1 oz	3.0	120	23%
wild ranch	1 oz	3.0	120	23%
sassy salsa	1 oz	3.0	120	23%
(Betty Crocker)				
Chex Mix				
bold party blend	½ cup	6.0	140	39%
	1.75 oz pouch	9.0	220	37%
cheddar cheese	½ cup	5.0	140	32%
	1.75 oz pouch	9.0	220	37%

Food and Description	Amount	Fat Grams	Total Calories	% Fat Calories
hot'n spicy	⅔ cup	4.5	130	31%
	1.75 oz pouch	7.0	210	30%
nacho fiesta	⅔ cup	3.5	120	26%
	1.75 oz pouch	6.0	200	27%
peanut lovers	½ cup	6.0	140	39%
	1.75 oz pouch	9.0	210	39%
traditional	⅔ cup	4.0	130	28%
	1.75 oz pouch	7.0	210	30%
Dunkaroos				
chocolate chip w/chocolate frosting	1 serving	4.5	120	34%
cinnamon graham w/vanilla frosting	1 serving	4.5	130	31%
cookies'n creme w/vanilla frosting	1 serving	4.5	120	34%
Fruit by the Foot				
Berry Tie Dye	1 roll	1.5	80	17%
cherry	1 roll	1.5	80	17%
Color by the Foot	1 roll	1.5	80	17%
endless Party	1 roll	1.5	80	17%
Flavor wave	1 roll	1.5	80	17%
Pokemon	1 roll	1.5	80	17%
strawberry	1 roll	1.5	80	17%
watermelon	1 roll	1.5	80	17%
Fruit Roll-Ups				
cherry	1 roll	0.5	50	9%
Crazy colors	1 roll	0.5	50	9%
Double fruity	1 roll	0.5	50	9%
Fun'n games				
regular pouch	1 roll	0.5	50	9%
XL pouch	2 rolls	1.5	130	10%
Galaxy blast	1 roll	0.5	50	9%
Hot colors	1 roll	0.5	50	9%
Peel 'n build				
regular pouch	1 roll	0.5	50	9%
XL pouch	2 rolls	1.5	130	10%
strawberry				
Mini handouts	2 rolls	1.0	80	11%
regular pouch	1 roll	0.5	50	9%
SL pouch	2 rolls	1.5	130	10%
Stretchy faces	1 roll	0.5	50	9%
Fruit Snacks				
Bugs bunny	1 pouch	–	80	–
Hawaiian punch	1 pouch	–	80	–
Lucky charms	1 pouch	–	80	–
Pokemon	1 pouch	–	80	–
Scooby Doo!	1 pouch	–	80	–
Shark Bites	1 pouch	–	80	–
Trix	1 pouch	–	80	–
Golden Graham Treats				
marshmallow graham w/mini marshmallows	1 bar	2.0	90	20%
peanut butter chocolate	1 bar	3.5	90	35%

Food and Description	Amount	Fat Grams	Total Calories	% Fat Calories
S'mores				
chocolate chunk	1 bar	2.5	90	25%
chocolate chunk/king size	1 bar	5.0	190	24%
(Bugles)				
baked				
cheddar cheese	1 oz	3.5	130	24%
original	1 oz	3.5	130	24%
(Cheetos)				
crunchy	1 oz	10.0	160	56%
curls	1 oz	10.0	150	60%
flamin' hot	1 oz	9.0	150	54%
hot puff rods	1 oz	10.0	160	56%
jumbo puffs	1 oz	10.0	160	56%
puffs	1 oz	10.0	160	56%
puffed balls	1 oz	10.0	150	60%
puffs	1 oz	10.0	160	56%
Zig Zags	1 oz	11.0	170	58%
(Chex Mix) (See (Betty Crocker) in this section)				
Cornnuts (See (Frito Lay) in this section)				
(Cracker Jack) (See POPCORN)				
(Crunch & Munch) (See POPCORN)				
(Featherweight) cheese curls	1 oz	7.0	140	45%
(Fisher) Snack Mixes				
Nuts & Crunchies				
golden crisp	1 oz	7.0	140	45%
honey crunch	1 oz	6.0	140	39%
Nuts & Fruits				
California-style	1 oz	8.0	140	51%
trail-style	1 oz	11.0	150	66%
Snack 'N Serve Bowl/fiesta mix	1 oz	7.0	140	45%
(Flavor Tree)				
party mix/sesame snack blend	1 oz	13.0	180	65%
sesame sticks				
garlic	1 oz	11.0	170	58%
original	1 oz	12.0	170	64%
(Frito Lay)				
Cornnuts				
barbecue	1 oz	4.0	120	30%
nacho cheese	1 oz	4.0	120	30%
Funyuns onion-flavored rings	1 oz	7.0	140	45%
Munchos	1 oz	10.0	160	56%
(Funyuns) (See (Frito Lay) in this section)				
(Gardetto's)				
Light'n Crispy				
sour cream & onion	½ cup	4.0	130	28%
special Italian recipe	½ cup	6.0	150	36%
sweet & savory barbecue	½ cup	6.0	150	36%
Snack mixes				
cheddar & sour cream	½ cup	3.0	130	21%
deli-style mustard	½ cup	2.0	130	14%

Food and Description	Amount	Fat Grams	Total Calories	% Fat Calories
Snack-ens				
original recipe	½ cup	8.0	160	45%
reduced fat	½ cup	5.0	140	32%
(Golden Graham Treats) (See (Betty Cocker) in this section)				
(Hain) carrot chips				
barbecue	1 oz	8.0	140	51%
plain				
no salt added	1 oz	9.0	150	54%
regular	1 oz	9.0	150	54%
(Health Valley) Cheddar Lites				
original	¾ oz	2.0	40	45%
w/green onion	¾ oz	2.0	40	45%
(Keebler) Sunshine Cheez It				
Party Mix				
nacho	½ cup	4.5	130	31%
original	½ cup	5.0	140	32%
reduced fat	½ cup	3.0	130	21%
single serve	1.75 oz pkg	9.0	230	35%
Snack Mix				
big crunch	¾ cup	6.0	110	49%
double cheese	¾ cup	5.0	110	41%
get nutty	½ cup	9.0	150	54%
original	½ cup	4.5	130	31%
(Kellogg's) Snack 'Ums/baked				
Big Boomin' Pops	1 cup	–	120	–
Big Rollin' Froot Loops	1¼ cup	1.0	120	8%
Rice Krispies Treats Krunch	1 cup	1.5	130	10%
(Lance)				
cheese balls	1 oz	8.0	150	48%
	1¾ oz	14.0	260	48%
crunchy cheese twists	1⅛ oz	14.0	190	66%
hot fries	⅞ oz	10.0	140	64%
onion rings	⅞ oz	6.0	120	45%
	1 oz	10.0	210	43%
pork skins				
BBQ	1 oz	9.0	140	58%
plain	1 oz	10.0	150	60%
(Max Snax) rice curls				
caramel	33 pieces	3.0	135	20%
cheese & tomato	33 pieces	5.0	160	28%
garlic & basil	35 pieces	4.0	130	26%
nacho cheddar	35 pieces	4.0	140	26%
sour cream & onion	35 pieces	5.0	140	32%
white cheddar	35 pieces	5.0	140	32%
(Michael Season's)				
Ultimate cheese puffs				
cheddar cheese	1 oz	13.0	180	65%
white cheddar	1 oz	13.0	180	65%
(Munchos) (See (Frito Lay) in this section.)				
(Nabisco) Doo Dads snack mix/original recipe	1 oz	7.0	150	42%

Food and Description	Amount	Fat Grams	Total Calories	% Fat Calories
(New York Style)				
bagel chip mix				
fat-free	1 oz	–	100	–
original	1 oz	3.5	120	26%
pita chips/toasted garlic	1 oz	4.0	140	26%
snack mix/oven baked fat-free	1 oz	–	100	–
(Pacific Grain) Gourmet Puffs				
cheese	1 oz	–	110	–
ranch	1 oz	–	110	–
(Pepperidge Farm) Goldfish cheddar				
snack mix	1 oz	7.0	160	37%
(Planter's)				
Cheez Balls	1 oz	10.0	150	60%
Cheez Curls	1 oz	10.0	150	60%
	1.2 oz pkg	12.0	190	57%
(Poppycock)	½ cup	10.0	180	50%
(Skinny Haven) Skinny Munchies				
chocolate fudge	0.5 oz	2.0	66	27%
nacho cheese	0.5 oz	2.0	59	31%
smoky Bar B Q	0.5 oz	2.0	59	31%
toasted onion	0.5 oz	2.0	59	31%
(Snyder's)				
cheese twist	1 oz	12.0	170	64%
Kruncheez cheese fries	1¼ oz	10.0	200	45%
onion toasters	1 oz	10.0	180	50%
pork skins				
barbeque fried	1 oz	4.0	80	45%
fried	1 oz	4.0	80	45%
(Spicers) crunchy diet snacks				
barbecue	1 oz	5.0	100	45%
cheddar	1 oz	5.0	100	45%
chocolate	1 oz	4.0	100	36%
natural	1 oz	4.0	100	36%
sour cream & onion	1 oz	5.0	100	45%
(SunChips)				
French onion	1 oz	7.0	140	45%
harvest cheddar	1 oz	6.0	140	39%
original	1 oz	6.0	140	39%
(Super Snax)				
hot & spicy	½ cup	7.0	140	45%
oriental	½ cup	1.5	110	12%
original	½ cup	5.0	140	32%
(Ultra Slim Fast) cheese curls	1 oz	3.0	110	25%
(Weight Watchers) Smart Snackers				
cheese curls	0.5 oz	3.0	70	39%
(Wise)				
Corn snacks/cheese-flavored				
Dizzy Doodles	1 oz	9.0	150	54%
Doodle Heads	1 oz	9.0	150	54%

Food and Description	Amount	Fat Grams	Total Calories	% Fat Calories
Doodles/crunchy				
original	1 oz	9.0	150	54%
reduced-fat	1 oz	4.5	130	31%
Doodles/puffed				
original	1 oz	8.0	150	48%
reduced-fat	1 oz	4.0	120	30%
onion-flavored rings	1 oz	6.0	140	39%
SNAIL/ESCARGOT				
canned				
(Reese) Maurice precooked/ French helix	6 pieces	1.0	45	20%
fresh				
cooked-moist heat	3 oz	1.0	230	4%
raw	3 oz	<1.0	117	4%
SNAP BEAN (*See* GREEN BEAN)				
SNAPPER				
cooked-dry heat	3 oz	1.5	110	12%
raw	3 oz	1.0	85	11%
SNOW PEA				
fresh/cooked	½ cup	–	35	–
frozen				
(Birds Eye) deluxe	⅔ cup	–	35	–
(C&W) microwaveable box				
baby pod peas	⅔ cup	–	40	–
baby pod peas w/water chestnuts	⅔ cup	–	40	–
(La Choy) snow pea pods	½ pkg	–	35	–
SOCKEYE (*See* SALMON)				
SODA (*See* COCKTAIL MIXER; SOFT DRINK; SPORTS DRINK)				
SOFT DRINK (*See also* FRUIT PUNCH; SOFT DRINK MIX; SPORTS DRINK; TEA; individual juice drink listings)				
(A&W)				
cream soda				
diet	8 fl oz	–	–	–
regular	8 fl oz	–	110	–
root beer				
diet	8 fl oz	–	–	–
regular	8 fl oz	–	110	–
(All Sport) w/vitamins				
black citrus	8 fl oz	–	70	–
blue ice	8 fl oz	–	70	–
cherry slam	8 fl oz	–	70	–
fruit punch	8 fl oz	–	70	–
grape	8 fl oz	–	70	–
lemon-lime	8 fl oz	–	70	–
orange	8 fl oz	–	70	–
raspberry burst	8 fl oz	–	70	–
watermelon	8 fl oz	–	70	–
(Arizona) Cowboy Cocktail				
grape kiwi	8 fl oz	–	120	–
kiwi strawberry	8 fl oz	–	120	–
Mucho Mango	8 fl oz	–	100	–

Food and Description	Amount	Fat Grams	Total Calories	% Fat Calories
strawberry punch	8 fl oz	–	120	–
(Barq's)				
creme soda				
red				
diet	8 fl oz	–	3.7	–
regular	8 fl oz	–	115	–
vanilla				
diet	8 fl oz	–	1.4	–
regular	8 fl oz	–	112	–
root beer				
diet	8 fl oz	–.	1.3	–
regular	8 fl oz	–	111	–
(Blue Sky)				
Genseng/Premium				
citrus squeeze	12 fl oz	–	170	–
cola	12 fl oz	–	170	–
cranberry-raspberry	12 fl oz	–	160	–
creme soda	12 fl oz	–	150	–
ginger ale	12 fl oz	–	150	–
lemon ginger	12 fl oz	–	130	–
orange-ginger	12 fl oz	–	150	–
root beer	12 fl oz	–	180	–
very berry creme	12 fl oz	–	150	–
Natural				
black cherry	12 fl oz	–	150	–
cherry cola	12 fl oz	–	140	–
cherry lemon lime	12 fl oz	–	160	–
cherry vanilla creme	12 fl oz	–	180	–
cola	12 fl oz	–	170	–
Dr. Becker	12 fl oz	–	150	–
Grape	12 fl oz	–	140	–
grapefruit	12 fl oz	–	150	–
Jamaican ginger ale	12 fl oz	–	150	–
lemon lime	12 fl oz	–	140	–
orange creme	12 fl oz	–	180	–
raspberry	12 fl oz	–	180	–
root beer	12 fl oz	–	170	–
truly orange	12 fl oz	–	150	–
Organic				
black cherry cherish	12 fl oz	–	150	–
ginger ale	12 fl oz	–	160	–
new century cola	12 fl oz	–	160	–
orange divine	12 fl oz	–	180	–
prime lime cream	12 fl oz	–	160	–
root beer encore	12 fl oz	–	180	–
(Canada Dry)				
birch beer				
brown	8 fl oz	–	110	–
clear	8 fl oz	–	110	–
bitter lemon	8 fl oz	–	100	–

Food and Description	Amount	Fat Grams	Total Calories	% Fat Calories
Black Cherry Wish	8 fl oz	–	120	–
Cactus Cooler soda	8 fl oz	–	110	–
California strawberry soda	8 fl oz	–	100	–
club soda				
regular	8 fl oz	–	–	–
sodium-free	8 fl oz	–	–	–
collins mixer	8 fl oz	–	90	–
Concord grape soda	8 fl oz	–	110	–
ginger ale				
cherry				
diet	8 fl oz	–	–	–
regular	8 fl oz	–	100	–
cranberry				
diet	8 fl oz	–	–	–
regular	8 fl oz	–	90	–
golden	8 fl oz	–	90	–
lemon				
diet	8 fl oz	–	–	–
regular	8 fl oz	–	90	–
plain				
diet	8 fl oz	–	–	–
regular	8 fl oz	–	80	–
half & half	8 fl oz	–	100	–
hi spot	8 fl oz	–	100	–
Island lime	8 fl oz	–	120	–
lemon sour	8 fl oz	–	90	–
peach soda	8 fl oz	–	110	–
pineapple soda	8 fl oz	–	100	–
seltzer				
cherry	8 fl oz	–	–	–
cranberry lime	8 fl oz	–	–	–
lemon lime	8 fl oz	–	–	–
Mandarin orange	8 fl oz	–	–	–
Peach	8 fl oz	–	–	–
pink grapefruit	8 fl oz	–	–	–
raspberry	8 fl oz	–	–	–
raspberry lime	8 fl oz	–	–	–
strawberry	8 fl oz	–	–	–
tropical	8 fl oz	–	–	–
sour mixer	8 fl oz	–	80	–
Sunripe orange soda	8 fl oz	–	110	–
Tahitian treat soda	8 fl oz	–	150	–
vanilla cream soda/brown or clear	8 fl oz	–	110	–
wild cherry soda	8 fl oz	–	110	–
(Canfield's)				
cherry fudge soda	12 fl oz	–	–	–
chocolate fudge soda	12 fl oz	–	–	–
(Clearly Canadian)				
apple	8 fl oz	–	80	–
blackberry	8 fl oz	–	100	–

Food and Description	Amount	Fat Grams	Total Calories	% Fat Calories
cherry	8 fl oz	–	90	–
cranberry	8 fl oz	–	90	–
loganberry	8 fl oz	–	90	–
peach	8 fl oz	–	90	–
raspberry	8 fl oz	–	80	–
strawberry	8 fl oz	–	80	–
(Coca-Cola)				
Coca-Cola				
cherry				
diet	8 fl oz	–	1	–
regular	8 fl oz	–	104	–
Citra	8 fl oz	–	91	–
classic				
caffeine-free	8 fl oz	–	97	–
regular	8 fl oz	–	97	–
Coke II	8 fl oz	–	105	–
Diet Coke				
caffeine-free	8 fl oz	–	1	–
regular	8 fl oz	–	1	–
Fanta				
grape	8 fl oz	–	117	–
orange	8 fl oz	–	118	–
Fresca	8 fl oz	–	2	–
Mello Yello				
diet	8 fl oz	–	3	–
regular	8 fl oz	–	118	–
Minute Maid				
black cherry soda	8 fl oz	–	110	–
blueberry	8 fl oz	–	110	–
fruit punch/carbonated	8 fl oz	–	113	–
grape soda	8 fl oz	–	113	–
grapefruit soda	8 fl oz	–	108	–
lemonade	8 fl oz	–	106	–
orange soda				
diet	8 fl oz	–	2	–
regular	8 fl oz	–	118	–
peach soda	8 fl oz	–	110	–
pineapple soda	8 fl oz	–	109	–
strawberry soda	8 fl oz	–	113	–
Mr. Pibb				
diet	8 fl oz	–	1	–
regular	8 fl oz	–	97	–
Sprite				
diet	8 fl oz	–	3	–
regular	8 fl oz	–	96	–
Surge	8 fl oz	–	116	–
Tab	8 fl oz	–	1	–
(Crush)				
cherry	8 fl oz	–	120	–
fruity red	8 fl oz	–	120	–

Food and Description	Amount	Fat Grams	Total Calories	% Fat Calories
grape	8 fl oz	–	120	–
orange				
diet	8 fl oz	–	10	–
regular	8 fl oz	–	120	–
peach	8 fl oz	–	120	–
pineapple	8 fl oz	–	120	–
strawberry	8 fl oz	–	110	–
tropical punch	8 fl oz	–	120	–
(Diet Rite)				
black cherry soda	8 fl oz	–	2	–
cola	8 fl oz	–	1	–
fruit punch	8 fl oz	–	2	–
golden peach soda	8 fl oz	–	2	–
key lime soda	8 fl oz	–	7	–
pink grapefruit soda	8 fl oz	–	2	–
red raspberry soda	8 fl oz	–	3	–
tangerine soda	8 fl oz	–	2	–
white grape soda	8 fl oz	–	1	–
(Dr. Pepper)				
diet				
caffeine-free	12 fl oz	–	–	–
regular	12 fl oz	–	–	–
regular				
caffeine-free	12 fl oz	–	160	–
regular	12 fl oz	–	160	–
(Fruitworks)				
apple raspberry	12 fl oz	–	160	–
guava berry	12 fl oz	–	170	–
passion orange	12 fl oz	–	160	–
peach papaya	12 fl oz	–	170	–
pink lemonade	12 fl oz	–	170	–
strawberry melon	12 fl oz	–	160	–
tangerine citrus	12 fl oz	–	150	–
(Hansen's) natural				
cherry	12 fl oz	–	120	–
orange	12 fl oz	–	130	–
raspberry	12 fl oz	–	130	–
strawberry	12 fl oz	–	130	–
(Health Valley)				
ginger ale	12 fl oz	1.0	153	6%
root beer/old fashioned	12 fl oz	1.0	120	8%
sarsaparilla	12 fl oz	1.0	153	6%
wild berry	12 fl oz	1.0	142	6%
(Hershey's) chocolate	8 fl oz	1.0	120	8%
(Hires)				
cream soda				
diet	8 fl oz	–	–	–
regular	8 fl oz	–	130	–
root beer				
diet	8 fl oz	–	–	–

Food and Description	Amount	Fat Grams	Total Calories	% Fat Calories
regular	8 fl oz	–	130	–
(IBC)				
black cherry	12 fl oz	–	160	
cherry cola	12 fl oz	–	160	–
cream soda				
diet	12 fl oz	–	–	–
regular	12 fl oz	–	190	–
root beer				
diet	12 fl oz	–	–	–
regular	12 fl oz	–	180	–
(Jolt) cola	12 fl oz	–	150	–
(Kool-Aid)				
Bursts				
cherry	6.75 fl oz	–	100	–
grape	6.75 fl oz	–	100	–
Great Bluedini	6.75 fl oz	–	100	–
Incrediberry	6.75 fl oz	–	100	–
Kickin' kiwi-lime	6.75 fl oz	–	100	–
Oh yeah orange-pineapple	6.75 fl oz	–	100	–
Slammin' strawberry-kiwi	6.75 fl oz	–	100	–
orange punch	6.75 fl oz	–	100	–
tropical punch	6.75 fl oz	–	100	–
Crystal Light/low-calorie				
cranberry breeze	8 fl oz	–	5	–
fruit punch	8 fl oz	–	5	–
orange-strawberry-banana	8 fl oz	–	5	–
kiwi-strawberry	8 fl oz	–	5	–
Splash				
blue raspberry	8 fl oz	–	120	–
cherry	8 fl oz	–	110	–
grape berry punch	8 fl oz	–	120	–
kiwi-strawberry	8 fl oz	–	110	–
tropical punch	8 fl oz	–	120	–
watermelon	8 fl oz	–	110	–
(Mountain Dew)				
diet				
caffeine-free	12 fl oz	–	–	–
regular	12 fl oz	–	–	–
regular				
caffeine-free	12 fl oz	–	170	–
regular	12 fl oz	–	170	–
(Mug)				
cream soda				
diet	12 fl oz	–	5	–
regular	12 fl oz	–	170	–
root beer				
diet	12 fl oz	–	–	–
regular	12 fl oz	–	160	–
(Nehi)				
cream	8 fl oz	–	120	–

Food and Description	Amount	Fat Grams	Total Calories	% Fat Calories
fruit punch	8 fl oz	–	120	–
ginger ale	8 fl oz	–	90	–
grape	8 fl oz	–	120	–
orange	8 fl oz	–	130	–
peach	8 fl oz	–	130	–
pineapple	8 fl oz	–	130	–
root beer	8 fl oz	–	120	–
strawberry	8 fl oz	–	120	–
(Pepsi)				
crystal	12 fl oz	–	150	–
diet				
caffeine-free	12 fl oz	–	–	–
regular	12 fl oz	–	–	–
Pepsi 1	12 fl oz	–	1	–
regular				
caffeine-free	12 fl oz	–	150	–
regular	12 fl oz	–	150	–
wild cherry				
diet	12 fl oz	–	–	–
regular	12 fl oz	–	160	–
(Royal Crown)				
cherry cola	8 fl oz	–	110	–
cola				
diet				
caffeine-free	8 fl oz	–	–	–
regular	8 fl oz	–	–	–
regular				
caffeine-free	8 fl oz	–	110	–
regular	8 fl oz	–	110	–
(Schweppes)				
bitter lemon	8 fl oz	–	110	–
club soda				
regular	8 fl oz	–	–	–
sodium-free	8 fl oz	–	–	–
collins mixer	8 fl oz	–	90	–
ginger ale				
grape				
diet	8 fl oz	–	2	–
dry				
diet	8 fl oz	–	–	–
regular	8 fl oz	–	90	–
regular	8 fl oz	–	100	–
plain				
diet	8 fl oz	–	–	–
regular	8 fl oz	–	90	–
raspberry				
diet	8 fl oz	–	–	–
regular	8 fl oz	–	90	–
ginger beer	8 fl oz	–	90	–
grape soda	8 fl oz	–	120	–

Food and Description	Amount	Fat Grams	Total Calories	% Fat Calories
grapefruit soda	8 fl oz	–	100	–
lemon sour	8 fl oz	–	100	–
lemon-lime soda	8 fl oz	–	90	–
seltzer				
black cherry	8 fl oz	–	–	–
lemon	8 fl oz	–	–	–
lime	8 fl oz	–	–	–
orange	8 fl oz	–	–	–
pink grapefruit	8 fl oz	–	–	–
wild raspberry	–	–	–	–
tonic water				
cranberry	8 fl oz	–	80	–
plain				
diet	8 fl oz	–	–	–
regular	8 fl oz	–	80	–
(7-Up)				
cherry				
diet	12 fl oz	–	–	–
regular	12 fl oz	–	160	–
regular				
diet	12 fl oz	–	–	–
regular	12 fl oz	–	160	–
(Shasta)				
birch beer/diet	12 fl oz	–	4	–
black cherry	12 fl oz	–	170	–
cherry cola	12 fl oz	–	160	–
citrus mist	12 fl oz	–	170	–
club soda	12 fl oz	–	–	–
cola				
diet	12 fl oz	–	–	–
free	12 fl oz	–	160	–
regular	12 fl oz	–	160	–
creme				
diet	12 fl oz	–	–	–
regular	12 fl oz	–	190	–
Doc Shasta				
diet	12 fl oz	–	–	–
regular	12 fl oz	–	160	–
fruit punch	12 fl oz	–	200	–
ginger ale	12 fl oz	–	130	–
grape	12 fl oz	–	190	–
kiwi strawberry	12 fl oz	–	170	–
lemon lime	12 fl oz	–	150	–
orange	12 fl oz	–	200	–
peach	12 fl oz	–	170	–
pineapple	12 f oz	–	200	–
raspberry creme	12 fl oz	–	170	–
red pop	12 fl oz	–	170	–
root beer	12 fl oz	–	170	–
strawberry	12 fl oz	–	190	–

Food and Description	Amount	Fat Grams	Total Calories	% Fat Calories
strawberry-peach	12 fl oz	–	170	–
(Sioux City) sarsaparilla				
bottled	12 fl oz	–	110	–
canned	16 fl oz	–	170	–
(Slice)				
cherry lime	12 fl oz	–	160	–
cherry spice	12 fl oz	–	150	–
cola				
diet	12 fl oz	–	–	–
regular	12 fl oz	–	160	–
Dr. Slice	12 fl oz	–	140	–
fruit punch	12 fl oz	–	190	–
grape soda	12 fl oz	–	190	–
lemon lime soda				
diet	12 fl oz	–	–	–
regular	12 fl oz	–	150	–
orange soda				
diet	12 fl oz	–	–	–
w/caffeine	12 fl oz	–	170	–
w/o caffeine	12 fl oz	–	190	–
pineapple soda	12 fl oz	–	190	–
red	12 fl oz	–	190	–
strawberry soda	12 fl oz	–	170	–
(Snapple)16 oz. sodas				
cherry-lime Rickey	8 fl oz	–	110	–
creme D'vanilla	8 fl oz	–		
French cherry	8 fl oz	–	120	–
true root beer	8 fl oz	–	110	–
(Squirt)				
original				
diet	8 fl oz	–	–	–
regular	12 fl oz	–	150	–
ruby red				
diet	8 fl oz	–	–	–
regular	8 fl oz	–	110	–
(Stewarts)				
country orange n' cream	12 fl oz	–	190	–
cream ale	12 fl oz	–	180	–
ginger beer	12 fl oz	–	200	–
root beer				
diet	12 fl oz	–	–	–
original	12 fl oz	–	160	–
(Storm)				
light	12 fl oz	–	–	–
regular	12 fl oz	–	140	–
(Sun Drop)				
cherry	12 fl oz	–	180	–
regular				
diet	12 fl oz	–	4	–
regular	12 fl oz	–	200	–

Food and Description	Amount	Fat Grams	Total Calories	% Fat Calories
(Sunkist)				
cherry	8 fl oz	–	130	–
citrus				
diet	8 fl oz	–	–	–
regular	8 fl oz	–	90	–
fruit punch	8 fl oz	–	120	–
grape	8 fl oz	–	130	–
lemonade				
diet sparkling	8 fl oz	–	–	–
regular	8 fl oz	–	120	–
orange				
diet	8 fl oz	–	–	–
regular	8 fl oz	–	130	–
peach	8 fl oz	–	110	–
pineapple	8 fl oz	–	120	–
strawberry	8 fl oz	–	120	–
(Vernor's) Ginger Soda				
diet	8 fl oz	–	–	–
regular	8 fl oz	–	100	–
(Welch's) sparkling sodas				
apple	8 fl oz	–	200	–
fruit punch	8 fl oz	–	210	–
grape	8 fl oz	–	130	–
lemonade	8 fl oz	–	110	–
orange	8 fl oz	–	120	–
peach	8 fl oz	–	130	–
pineapple	8 fl oz	–	130	–
strawberry	8 fl oz	–	120	–
tropical punch	8 fl oz	–	130	–
(Winks) Wink II	8 fl oz	–	110	–
(Yoo-Hoo) chocolate	12 fl oz	1.5	180	8%

SOFT DRINK MIX (*See also* FRUIT PUNCH; SOFT DRINK; SPORTS DRINK; individual fruit drink listings)

Food and Description	Amount	Fat Grams	Total Calories	% Fat Calories
(Crystal Light)/prepared				
citrus blend	8 fl oz	–	5	–
cranberry breeze	8 fl oz	–	5	–
fruit punch	8 fl oz	–	5	–
lemon-lime	8 fl oz	–	5	–
passion fruit-pineapple	8 fl oz	–	5	–
pineapple-orange	8 fl oz	–	5	–
raspberry ice	8 fl oz	–	5	–
strawberry-kiwi	8 fl oz	–	5	–
watermelon-strawberry	8 fl oz	–	5	–
(Kool-Aid)				
Sugar sweetened/prepared w/water	8 fl oz	–	60	–
Sugar-Free/Low calorie/all flavors/ prepared w/water	8 fl oz	–	5	–
Unsweetened/prepared w/sugar & water/all flavors				
cherry	8 fl oz	–	100	–
grape	8 fl oz	–	100	–

Food and Description	Amount	Fat Grams	Total Calories	% Fat Calories
grape berry splash	8 fl oz	–	100	–
kickin' kiwi-lime	8 fl oz	–	100	–
man-o-mango berry	8 fl oz	–	100	–
oh yeah orange-pineapple	8 fl oz	–	100	–
orange	8 fl oz	–	100	–
pina-pineapple	8 fl oz	–	100	–
raspberry	8 fl oz	–	100	–
roarin'raspberry-cranberry	8 fl oz	–	100	–
slammin' strawberry-kiwi	8 fl oz	–	100	–
strawberry	8 fl oz	–	100	–
tropical punch	8 fl oz	–	100	–
watermelon-cherry	8 fl oz	–	100	–

SOLE (See also FROZEN ENTRÉE/DINNER; SEAFOOD ENTRÉE/DINNER)

baked w/butter	3 oz	6.0	120	45%
cooked-dry heat	3 oz	1.0	105	91%
raw	3 oz	1.0	80	11%

SORBET (See FRUIT ICES, BARS. & POPS; SHERBET)

SORGHUM /whole-grain	1 cup	6.0	650	8%

SORGHUM SYRUP

cane & maple	1 Tbs	–	53	–
	1 cup	–	794	–
regular	1 Tbs	–	53	–
	1 cup	–	848	–
table blend	1 Tbs	–	59	–
	1 cup	–	941	–

SORREL (See DOCK)

SOUP

(NOTE: Unless stated otherwise, condensed soups were prepared as directed with water. If prepared with milk, whole milk was used unless noted otherwise. If you use reduced-fat, low-fat, or skim milk, refer to the Quick Reference-Milk, below, to adjust your fat and calorie data. Ready-to-serve soups were heated as directed with no added liquid.)

QUICK REFERENCE: MILK	Amount	Fat Grams	Total Calories	% Fat Calories
Skim/fat-free	¼ cup	–	23	–
	½ cup	–	45	–
1% fat/light	¼ cup	0.5	26	17%
	½ cup	1.0	55	16%
2% fat/reduced fat	¼ cup	1.0	31	29%
	½ cup	2.5	61	37%
Whole	¼ cup	2.0	38	47%
	½ cup	4.0	75	48%

■ CANNED

(Anderson's) split pea/ready-to-serve	1 cup	–	130	–
(Andre Prost) A Taste of Thai/ready-to-serve				
chili pepper lemon grass tom yum	1 cup	2.5	45	50%

Food and Description	Amount	Fat Grams	Total Calories	% Fat Calories
coconut ginger tom ka	1 cup	5.0	100	45%
lemon grass basil poh taek	1 cup	0.5	35	13%
(Baxters) ready-to-serve				
asparagus, cream of	1 cup	10.0	150	60%
country garden/99% fat-free	1 cup	0.5	70	6%
lobster bisque	1 cup	6.0	120	45%
minestrone/99% fat-free	1 cup	1.0	80	11%
onion/99% fat-free	1 cup	0.5	70	6%
potato & leek/100% fat-free	1 cup	–	60	–
royal gam soup	1 cup	2.5	90	25%
tomato & brown lentil/100% fat-free	1 cup	–	120	–
(Campbell's)				
Condensed/unprepared				
Healthy Request				
bean w/ham & bacon	½ cup	2.0	150	11%
chicken, cream of	½ cup	2.0	70	26%
chicken & broccoli, cream of	½ cup	2.5	80	28%
chicken & stars	½ cup	2.0	70	26%
chicken noodle	½ cup	2.0	70	26%
chicken vegetable	½ cup	2.0	80	23%
chicken w/rice	½ cup	2.5	60	38%
cream of broccoli	½ cup	2.0	70	26%
cream of celery	½ cup	2.0	70	26%
cream of chicken	½ cup	2.0	70	26%
cream of chicken & broccoli	½ cup	2.5	80	28%
hearty pasta & vegetables	½ cup	1.0	90	10%
minestrone	½ cup	1.0	90	10%
mushroom, cream of	½ cup	2.5	70	32%
tomato	½ cup	1.5	90	15%
vegetable	½ cup	1.0	90	10%
vegetable beef	½ cup	2.0	80	23%
Original soups				
American recipe/unprepared/chicken vegetable				
regular	½ cup	2.0	80	23%
Southwest style	½ cup	1.5	110	12%
bean w/bacon	½ cup	5.0	180	25%
beef broth/double rich double strength	½ cup	–	15	–
beef noodle	½ cup	2.5	70	32%
beef soup w/vegetables & barley	½ cup	2.0	80	23%
beef mushroom	½ cup	3.0	70	39%
black bean	½ cup	2.0	110	16%
broccoli cheese	½ cup	7.0	110	57%
California style vegetable	½ cup	1.0	60	15%
cheddar cheese	½ cup	4.0	90	40%
chicken alphabet w/vegetables	½ cup	2.0	80	23%
chicken & stars	½ cup	2.0	70	26%
chicken broth soup	½ cup	2.0	30	60%
chicken dumplings	½ cup	3.0	80	34%

Food and Description	Amount	Fat Grams	Total Calories	% Fat Calories
chicken gumbo	½ cup	1.5	60	23%
chicken noodle o's	½ cup	3.0	80	34%
chicken noodle	½ cup	2.0	70	26%
chicken rice	½ cup	2.5	70	32%
chicken vegetable	½ cup	2.0	80	23%
chicken w/white & wild rice	½ cup	2.0	70	26%
consommé	½ cup	–	25	–
cream of asparagus	½ cup	3.5	90	35%
cream of broccoli				
98% fat-free	½ cup	3.0	80	34%
original	½ cup	6.0	100	54%
cream of broccoli cheese/98% fat-free	½ cup	3.0	80	34%
cream of celery				
98% fat-free	½ cup	3.5	80	39%
original	½ cup	7.0	110	57%
cream of chicken & broccoli	½ cup	8.0	120	60%
cream of chicken mushroom	½ cup	9.0	130	62%
cream of chicken				
98% fat-free	½ cup	3.0	80	34%
original	½ cup	6.0	130	42%
cream of chicken w/herbs	½ cup	4.0	80	45%
cream of mushroom				
98% fat-free	½ cup	3.0	70	39%
original	½ cup	7.0	110	57%
cream of mushroom w/roasted garlic	½ cup	2.5	70	32%
cream of onion	½ cup	6.0	110	49%
cream of potato	½ cup	3.0	90	30%
cream of shrimp	½ cup	7.0	100	63%
creamy chicken noodle	½ cup	7.0	130	48%
curly chicken noodle	½ cup	2.5	80	28%
double noodle	½ cup	2.5	100	23%
fiesta chili beef w/beans	½ cup	5.0	170	26%
fiesta nacho cheese	½ cup	8.0	140	51%
French onion	½ cup	2.5	70	32%
golden mushroom	½ cup	3.0	80	34%
green pea	½ cup	3.0	180	15%
hearty vegetable w/pasta	½ cup	1.0	90	10%
homestyle chicken noodle	½ cup	2.5	70	32%
Italian tomato w/basil & oregano	½ cup	0.5	100	5%
Manhattan style clam chowder	½ cup	0.5	60	8%
minestrone	½ cup	1.5	90	15%
New England clam chowder	½ cup	2.5	90	25%
old fashioned				
tomato rice	½ cup	2.0	120	15%
vegetable	½ cup	2.5	70	32%
oyster stew	½ cup	6.0	90	60%
pepperpot	½ cup	5.0	100	45%
Rugrats pasta w/chicken in chicken broth	½ cup	1.5	60	23%

Food and Description	Amount	Fat Grams	Total Calories	% Fat Calories
scotch broth soup	½ cup	3.0	80	34%
souper stars	½ cup	1.5	50	27%
split pea w/ham	½ cup	3.5	180	18%
tomato	½ cup	–	80	–
tomato bisque	½ cup	3.0	130	21%
turkey noodle	½ cup	2.5	60	38%
turkey vegetable	½ cup	2.5	80	28%
vegetable	½ cup	0.5	80	6%
vegetable beef	½ cup	1.0	80	23%
vegetarian vegetable	½ cup	1.0	90	10%
won ton	½ cup	1.0	45	20%
Ready-To-Serve				
Chunky				
baked potato w/bacon bits & chives	1 cup	7.0	170	37%
baked potato w/cheddar & bacon bits	1 cup	8.0	180	40%
baked potato w/steak & cheese	1 cup	9.0	200	41%
bean'n ham	1 cup	2.0	190	9%
beef pasta	1 cup	3.0	140	19%
beef w/country vegetables	1 can	5.0	190	24%
	1 cup	4.0	150	24%
chicken broccoli & cheese potato	1 can	15.0	250	54%
	1 cup	12.0	200	54%
chicken corn chowder	1 can	19.0	310	55%
	1 cup	15.0	250	54%
chicken mushroom chowder	1 cup	12.0	210	51%
chicken noodle/classic	1 cup	3.0	130	21%
	1 can	4.0	160	223%
chicken w/pasta & mushrooms	1 cup	4.0	120	30%
chili beef w/beans	1 can	7.0	300	21%
hearty bean 'n ham	1 cup	2.0	190	9%
hearty chicken w/vegetables	1 cup	2.0	90	20%
hearty vegetables w/pasta	1 cup	3.0	130	21%
minestrone	1 cup	5.0	140	32%
mushroom, cream of	1 cup	13.0	170	69%
Manhattan clam chowder	1 can	4.0	170	21%
	1 cup	4.0	130	28%
New England clam chowder	1 can	18.0	300	54%
	1 cup	15.0	240	56%
old-fashioned chicken	1 cup	3.0	130	21%
old-fashioned potato ham chowder	1 cup	14.0	220	57%
old-fashioned vegetable beef	1 can	6.0	180	30%
	1 cup	5.0	150	30%
pepper steak	1 cup	3.0	130	21%
savory chicken w/rice (white & wild)	1 cup	3.0	140	19%
sirloin burger w/country vegetables	1 can	11.0	250	40%
	1 cup	9.0	210	39%
spicy chicken & vegetables	1 cup	1.0	90	10%
split pea 'n ham	1 cup	3.0	190	14%
steak & potato	1 can	5.0	190	24%

Food and Description	Amount	Fat Grams	Total Calories	% Fat Calories
	1 cup	4.0	150	24%
tomato cheese ravioli w/vegetables	1 cup	3.0	150	18%
vegetable	1 can	5.0	160	28%
	1 cup	4.0	130	28%
Healthy Request				
chicken broth	1 cup	–	20	–
chicken vegetable	1 cup	2.0	110	16%
creamy potato w/roasted garlic	1 cup	2.5	110	20%
Hearty				
chicken corn chowder	1 cup	3.0	250	18%
chicken noodle	1 cup	3.0	100	27%
chicken rice	1 cup	2.5	110	20%
minestrone	1 cup	2.0	120	15%
tomato ravioli w/vegetables	1 cup	2.5	140	16%
vegetable	1 cup	1.0	100	9%
vegetable beef	1 cup	2.5	140	16%
New England clam chowder	1 cup	3.0	120	23%
Southwestern vegetable w/black beans	1 cup	1.0	140	6%
split pea w/ham	1 cup	1.5	170	8%
Home Cookin'				
bean & ham	1 cup	2.0	180	10%
chicken & pasta w/roasted garlic	1 cup	3.0	120	23%
chicken & rice	1 can	2.0	140	13%
	1 cup	1.0	100	9%
chicken w/egg noodles	1 can	2.0	110	16%
	1 cup	2.0	90	20%
country mushroom rice	1 cup	0.5	90	5%
country vegetable	1 can	1.5	140	10%
	1 cup	1.5	110	12%
creamy potato w/roasted garlic	1 cup	9.0	180	45%
fiesta vegetable	1 cup	3.0	140	19%
Italian style chicken	1 cup	1.5	130	10%
minestrone				
Old World	1 cup	1.0	120	8%
Tuscany style	1 cup	9.0	190	43%
mushroom, cream of				
98% fat-free	1 cup	2.0	80	23%
original	1 cup	13.0	170	69%
New England clam chowder				
98% fat-free	1 cup	3.0	110	25%
original	1 can	16.0	240	60%
	1 cup	13.0	190	62%
Oriental noodles w/vegetables	1 cup	1.0	100	9%
salsa bean				
savory lentil	1 cup	1.0	130	7%
split pea w/ham	1 cup	1.5	170	8%
tomato garden	1 cup	0.5	100	5%
vegetable beef	1 cup	2.5	120	19%
Low-sodium/single can soups				

Food and Description	Amount	Fat Grams	Total Calories	% Fat Calories
chicken broth	1 can	2.0	40	45%
chicken noodle	1 can	5.0	170	26%
chunky vegetable beef	1 can	4.5	160	25%
cream of mushroom	1 can	14.0	200	63%
split pea	1 can	4.0	240	15%
tomato w/tomato pieces	1 can	6.0	170	32%
Simply Home soups				
chicken & pasta	1 cup	1.0	90	10%
chicken noodle	1 cup	1.0	80	11%
chicken w/white & wild rice	1 cup	1.0	100	9%
minestrone	1 cup	1.5	110	12%
vegetable beef w/pasta	1 cup	1.5	120	11%
vegetable garden	1 cup	0.5	110	4%
Tomato soups				
creamy	1 cup	1.5	130	10%
traditional tomato	1 cup	0.5	100	5%
(College Inn) broth/ready-to-serve				
beef	1 cup	–	16	–
chicken				
lower salt	1 cup	2.0	20	90%
regular	1 cup	3.0	35	77%
(Doxsee) New England clam chowder/condensed				
prepared w/skim milk	1 cup	2.0	130	14%
Generic				
Condensed/prepared as indicated				
asparagus, cream of				
prepared w/milk	1 cup	9.0	170	48%
prepared w/water	1 cup	4.0	87	41%
black bean	1 cup	1.5	116	12%
black turtle bean	1 cup	–	218	–
bean w/franks	1 cup	7.0	187	34%
beef broth/prepared w/water	1 cup	1.0	19	47%
beef consommé				
prepared w/water	1 cup	–	25	–
unprepared	10.5 oz	–	71	–
beef mushroom	1 cup	3.0	73	37%
celery, cream of				
prepared w/milk	1 cup	9.7	165	53%
prepared w/water	1 cup	5.6	90	56%
unprepared	10.75 oz	14.0	219	58%
cheese				
prepared w/milk	1 cup	14.6	230	57%
prepared w/water	1 cup	10.5	155	61%
unprepared	11 oz	25.0	377	60%
chicken, cream of/prepared w/water	1 cup	5.0	110	41%
chicken broth				
prepared w/water	1 cup	1.0	39	13%
unprepared	10.75 oz	3.0	94	29%
chicken mushroom	1 cup	9.0	132	61%
chicken noodle	1 cup	1.0	53	17%
chili beef				

Food and Description	Amount	Fat Grams	Total Calories	% Fat Calories
prepared w/water	1 cup	6.6	169	35%
unprepared	11.25 oz	16.0	411	35%
green pea				
prepared w/milk	1 cup	7.0	239	26%
prepared w/water	1 cup	2.9	164	16%
leek	1 cup	2.0	70	26%
mushroom, cream of				
prepared w/milk	1 cup	13.6	203	60%
prepared w/water	1 cup	9.0	129	63%
unprepared	10.75 oz	23.0	313	66%
mushroom barley	2 cup	2.0	73	25%
mushroom w/beef stock	1 cup	4.0	85	42%
nacho cheese/prepared w/milk	1 cup	12.0	180	60%
onion				
prepared w/water	1 cup	1.7	57	27%
unprepared	10.5 oz	4.0	138	26%
oyster stew/prepared w/milk	1 cup	9.0	140	58%
pepper pot/unprepared	10.5 oz	11.0	251	39%
Scotch broth/unprepared	10.5 oz	6.0	195	28%
shrimp, cream of				
prepared w/milk	1 cup	10.0	160	56%
unprepared	10.75 oz	13.0	219	55%
stockpot				
prepared w/water	1 cup	3.9	100	35%
unprepared	11 oz	9.0	242	34%
tomato/prepared w/water	1 cup	2.0	100	18%
vichyssoise	1 cup	6.0	148	37%
Ready-To-Serve				
beef broth	1 cup	0.5	16	28%
	14 oz	1.0	27	33%
chicken noodle w/meatballs	1 cup	3.6	99	33%
	20 oz	8.0	227	32%
chicken vegetable				
chunky	9.5 oz	6.0	170	32%
regular	9.5 oz	4.8	167	26%
chunky turkey	1 cup	4.0	136	27%
crab	1 cup	1.5	76	18%
escarole	1 cup	2.0	27	67%
gazpacho	1 cup	2.0	57	32%
	13 oz	3.0	87	31%
lentil w/ham	1 cup	2.8	140	18%
	13 oz	6.0	320	17%
Manhattan clam chowder	1 cup	3.0	133	21%
minestrone				
regular	1 cup	2.0	80	23%
w/Italian sausage	1.5 oz	8.0	169	43%
(Gold's) Ready-to-serve				
borscht				
low-cal	1 cup	–	20	–
original	1 cup	–	100	–

Food and Description	Amount	Fat Grams	Total Calories	% Fat Calories
schav	1 cup	–	25	–
(Gorton's)				
New England clam chowder				
Condensed/unprepared	½ cup	1.0	70	13%
Ready-to-serve	1 cup	6.0	140	39%
(Hain) Ready-To-Serve				
chicken				
broth				
no salt added	8.75 oz	5.0	60	75%
regular	8.75 oz	6.0	70	77%
noodle				
no salt added	9.5 oz	4.0	120	30%
regular	9.5 oz	4.0	120	30%
creamy mushroom	9.25 oz	4.0	110	33%
Italian vegetable pasta				
low-sodium	9.5 oz	6.0	140	39%
regular	9.5 oz	5.0	160	28%
minestrone				
no salt added	9.5 oz	4.0	160	23%
regular	9.5 oz	2.0	170	11%
mushroom barley	9.5 oz	2.0	100	18%
New England clam chowder	9.5 oz	4.0	180	20%
split pea				
no salt added	9.5 oz	1.0	170	5%
regular	9.5 oz	1.0	170	5%
turkey rice				
no salt added	9.5 oz	4.0	120	30%
regular	9.5 oz	3.0	100	27%
vegetable				
broth				
low sodium	9.5 oz	–	40	–
regular	9.5 oz	–	45	–
chicken				
no salt added	9.5 oz	4.0	130	28%
regular	9.5 oz	4.0	120	30%
split pea				
no salt added	9.5 oz	1.0	170	5%
regular	9.5 oz	1.0	170	5%
vegetarian				
lentil				
no salt added	9.5 oz	3.0	160	17%
regular	9.5 oz	3.0	160	17%
original				
no salt added	9.5 oz	5.0	150	30%
regular	9.5 oz	4.0	140	26%
(Health Valley) Ready-To-Serve				
beef broth				
fat-free	7.5 oz	–	15	–
no salt added	7.5 oz	–	10	–
regular	7.5 oz	–	10	–

Food and Description	Amount	Fat Grams	Total Calories	% Fat Calories
black bean & vegetable				
no salt added	7.5 oz	2.0	150	12%
regular	7.5 oz	2.0	150	12%
chicken broth				
fat-free	7.5 oz	–	25	–
no salt added	7.5 oz	2.0	35	51%
regular	7.5 oz	2.0	35	51%
chicken noodle/99% fat-free	7.5 oz	2.0	130	14%
chicken rice/99% fat free	7.5 oz	2.0	130	14%
chunky				
chicken vegetable	7.5 oz	2.0	125	14%
five bean vegetable				
no salt added	7.5 oz	2.0	110	16%
regular	7.5 oz	2.0	110	16%
vegetable chicken/no salt added	7.5 oz	2.0	125	14%
corn & vegetable/fat-free	7.5 oz	–	70	–
5 bean vegetable/fat free	7.5 oz	–	140	–
14 garden vegetable/fat-free	7.5 oz	–	80	–
green split pea				
no salt added	7.5 oz	–	180	
regular	7.5 oz	–	180	
lentil & carrots				
99% fat free	7.5 oz	1.0	100	9%
no salt added	7.5 oz	4.0	220	16%
regular	7.5 oz	4.0	220	16%
Manhattan clam chowder				
no salt added	7.5 oz	2.0	110	16%
regular	7.5 oz	2.0	110	16%
minestrone				
no salt added	7.5 oz	3.0	130	21%
regular	7.5 oz	3.0	130	21%
mushroom barley				
no salt added	7.5 oz	2.0	100	18%
regular	7.5 oz	2.0	100	18%
potato leek				
fat free	7.5 oz	–	70	–
no salt added	7.5 oz	2.0	130	14%
regular	7.5 oz	2.0	130	14%
tomato				
fat-free	7.5 oz	–	80	–
no salt added	7.5 oz	3.0	130	21%
regular	7.5 oz	3.0	130	21%
vegetable				
no salt added	7.5 oz	1.0	110	8%
regular	7.5 oz	1.0	110	8%
vegetable broth/fat-free	7.5 oz	–	20	–
(Healthy Choice) Ready-To-Serve				
bean & ham	1 cup	–	184	–
bean & pasta	1 cup	1.5	100	14%
beef & potato	1 cup	2.0	120	15%

Food and Description	Amount	Fat Grams	Total Calories	% Fat Calories
chicken				
cream of				
w/mushrooms	1 cup	2.0	130	14%
w/vegetables	1 cup	2.0	130	14%
hearty	1 cup	3.0	130	21%
chicken corn chowder	1 cup	3.0	176	15%
chicken noodle	1 cup	2.0	120	15%
chicken w/rice	1 cup	2.0	100	18%
chili beef	1 cup	1.5	165	8%
clam chowder	1 cup	1.0	120	8%
country vegetable	1 cup	–	100	–
creamy potato	1 cup	2.0	120	15%
fiesta chicken	1 cup	1.0	90	10%
lentil	1 cup	1.0	145	6%
minestrone	1 cup	1.0	110	8%
mushroom, cream of	1 cup	1.0	80	11%
old-fashioned chicken noodle	1 cup	3.0	140	19%
split pea & ham	1 cup	2.0	170	11%
tomato garden	1 cup	2.0	110	16%
turkey w/wild rice	1 cup	2.0	90	20%
vegetable				
clam	1 cup	0.5	80	9%
country	1 cup	1.0	105	9%
garden	1 cup	1.0	120	8%
vegetable beef	1 cup	1.0	130	7%
zesty gumbo	1 cup	1.5	90	15%
(Jake's) clam chowder/condensed	⅔ cup	11.0	200	50%
(Manischewitz) Ready-To-Serve				
borscht				
low-cal	1 cup	–	25	–
original w/beets	1 cup	–	90	–
chicken rice	1 cup	–	45	–
chicken vegetable	1 cup	–	55	–
schav	1 cup	–	10	–
split pea	1 cup	–	135	–
vegetable	1 cup	–	65	–
(Mother's) Borscht/Ready-To-Serve				
low-cal	1 cup	–	25	–
old fashioned	1 cup	–	100	–
(Old El Paso) Ready-To-Serve				
black bean w/bacon	1 cup	2.0	160	11%
chicken vegetable	1 cup	3.0	110	25%
chicken w/rice	1 cup	3.0	90	30%
garden vegetable	1 cup	3.0	110	25%
hearty beef	1 cup	3.0	120	23%
hearty chicken noodle	1 cup	3.0	110	25%
(Pritikin) condensed/prepared				
chicken & rice	1 cup	1.0	80	11%
chicken broth	1 cup	–	10	–

Food and Description	Amount	Fat Grams	Total Calories	% Fat Calories
chicken pasta	1 cup	–	80	–
lentil	1 cup	–	130	–
minestrone	1 cup	–	90	–
split pea	1 cup	0.5	180	3%
three bean chili	½ cup	0.5	90	5%
vegetable				
hearty	1 cup	0.5	90	5%
vegetarian	1 cup	–	100	–
vegetable broth	1 cup	–	10	–
(Progresso) Ready-To-Serve				
99% Fat-Free Soups				
beef barley	1 cup	2.0	130	14%
beef vegetable	1 cup	2.0	160	11%
chicken noodle	1 cup	1.5	90	15%
chicken rice w/vegetables	1 cup	2.0	110	16%
creamy chicken broccoli	1 cup	2.0	90	20%
lentil	1 cup	1.5	130	10%
minestrone	1 cup	1.0	110	8%
New England clam chowder	1 cup	1.5	110	12%
roasted chicken w/Italian style vegetables	1 cup	1.5	90	15%
roasted chicken w/wild rice	1 cup	1.5	90	15%
split pea	1 cup	1.5	170	8%
tomato garden vegetable	1 cup	1.5	100	14%
vegetable	1 cup	1.0	70	13%
white cheddar potato	1 cup	1.5	100	14%
Regular Soups				
basil rotini tomato	1 cup	1.5	120	11%
bean & ham	1 cup	2.0	160	11%
beef barley	1 cup	4.0	130	28%
beef minestrone	1 cup	3.0	140	19%
cheese & herb tortellini tomato	1 cup	3.0	140	19%
chickarina	1 cup	5.0	130	35%
chicken				
barley	1 cup	1.5	110	12%
broth	1 cup	1.5	20	68%
creamy cheddar	1 cup	9.0	210	39%
hearty	10.5 oz	2.5	120	19%
homestyle w/vegetables	1 cup	1.5	90	15%
minestrone	1 cup	1.5	110	12%
vegetable	1 cup	1.5	90	15%
chicken & wild rice	1 cup	1.5	100	14%
chicken noodle	1 cup	2.0	90	20%
chicken rice w/vegetables	1 cup	2.0	90	20%
clam chowder				
Manhattan	1 cup	2.0	110	16%
New England	1 cup	10.0	190	47%
creamy tomato garlic	1 cup	6.0	150	36%
escarole in chicken broth	1 cup	1.0	25	36%
French onion	1 cup	1.5	50	27%

Food and Description	Amount	Fat Grams	Total Calories	% Fat Calories
green split pea	1 cup	3.0	170	16%
hearty				
black bean	1 cup	1.5	170	8%
chicken & rotini	1 cup	1.5	90	15%
penne in chicken broth	1 cup	1.0	80	11%
herb & rotini vegetable	1 cup	1.0	100	9%
herb & shell minestrone	1 cup	1.5	120	11%
lentil	1 cup	2.0	140	13%
macaroni & bean	1 cup	4.0	160	23%
minestrone				
beef	1 cup	3.0	140	19%
chicken	1 cup	3.5	120	26%
Parmesan	1 cup	2.5	100	23%
regular	1 cup	2.0	120	15%
mushroom, cream of	1 cup	8.0	140	51%
oregano penne Italian style vegetable	1 cup	2.0	90	20%
peppercorn penne vegetable	1 cup	2.0	110	16%
potato broccoli & cheese	1 cup	6.0	160	34%
potato ham & cheese	1 cup	7.0	170	37%
roasted				
garlic & lentil	1 cup	1.5	120	11%
potato garlic	1 cup	9.0	180	45%
roasted chicken				
garden herb	1 cup	1.5	70	19%
Italiano	1 cup	1.5	80	17%
rotini	1 cup	1.5	80	17%
Southwestern style corn chowder	1 cup	7.0	200	32%
spicy chicken & penne	1 cup	1.5	110	12%
split pea w/ham	1 cup	4.0	150	24%
tomato basil	1 cup	2.0	100	18%
tomato vegetable Italiano	1 cup	2.0	90	20%
tortellini chicken broth	1 cup	2.0	70	26%
turkey noodle	1 cup	1.5	90	15%
turkey rice w/ vegetables	1 cup	1.0	110	8%
vegetable	1 cup	1.0	90	10%
vegetarian vegetable	1 cup	0.5	100	5%
zesty herb tomato	1 cup	3.5	130	24%
(Rokeach)				
Condensed/prepared as directed				
mushroom barley	1 cup	–	85	–
split pea w/egg barley	1 cup	0.5	130	3%
Ready-To-Serve				
borscht				
diet	1 cup	–	30	–
no salt	1 cup	–	100	–
regular	1 cup	–	100	–
(ShariAnn's) Organic Ready-To-Serve				
cream of tomato	1 cup	–	80	–

Food and Description	Amount	Fat Grams	Total Calories	% Fat Calories
French green lentil	1 cup	–	130	–
French onion	1 cup	–	60	–
great plains split pea	1 cup	–	150	–
Indian black bean	1 cup	1.0	150	6%
Italian white bean	1 cup	–	170	–
minestrone	1 cup	2.5	120	19%
potato & cheddar	1 cup	2.5	100	23%
spicy Mexican bean	1 cup	–	210	–
tomato w/red bell pepper	1 cup	–	100	–
tomato w/roasted garlic	1 cup	–	50	–
vegetable barley	1 cup	1.5	100	14%
(Shelton's) Ready-To-Serve				
black bean & chicken	1 cup	4.0	170	21%
chicken				
broth				
fat-free	1 cup	–	10	–
original	1 cup	2.5	35	64%
noodle	1 cup	2.0	80	23%
rice	1 cup	1.0	90	10%
tortilla	1 cup	1.5	110	12%
vegetable	1 cup	2.0	150	12%
turkey meatball	1 cup	3.0	90	30%
(Snow's) condensed/prepared w/whole milk				
New England clam chowder	7.5 oz	6.0	140	39%
	½ cup	1.5	80	17%
New England corn chowder	7.5 oz	6.0	150	36%
New England fish chowder	7.5 oz	6.0	130	42%
New England seafood chowder	7.5 oz	6.0	130	42%
(Swanson) broth/Ready-To-Serve				
beef				
clear	1 cup	1.0	20	45%
chicken				
clear/box	1 cup	0.5	10	45%
fat-free Natural Goodness	1 cup	–	15	–
original	1 cup	0.5	20	23%
w/Italian herbs	1 cup	0.5	20	23%
w/onion	1 cup	0.5	25	18%
w/roasted garlic	1 cup	0.5	20	23%
Vegetable/clear	1 cup	1.0	20	45%
(Weight Watchers) Ready-To-Serve				
chicken & rice	10.5 oz	2.0	110	16%
chicken noodle	10.5 oz	2.0	150	12%
minestrone	10.5 oz	2.0	130	14%
vegetable	10.5 oz	1.0	130	7%
(Westbrae) Soups of the World/Ready-To-Serve				
Alabama black bean	1 cup	–	80	–
Great Plains savory bean	1 cup	–	70	–
Old World split pea	1 cup	–	110	–
rich Mediterranean lentil	1 cup	–	100	–
Santa Fe vegetable	1 cup	–	120	–

Food and Description	Amount	Fat Grams	Total Calories	% Fat Calories
(Wolfgang Puck's) Ready-To-Serve				
chicken pot pie	1 cup	10.0	180	50%
creamy chicken	1 cup	12.0	210	51%
creamy country chicken	1 cup	12.0	210	51%
old fashioned beef barley	1 cup	4.5	140	29%
old world minestrone	1 cup	7.0	180	35%
roast chicken w/pasta & mushrooms	1 cup	5.0	130	35%
spicy 7 bean w/Italian sausage	1 cup	11.0	230	43%
thick country potato	1 cup	12.0	200	54%
turkey w/egg noodles	1 cup	6.0	140	39%
■ DEHYDRATED/(MIX OR CUBE) & MICROWAVEABLE				
(Andre Prost) A Taste of Thai				
chili pepper/prepared	1 cup	2.0	40	45%
tangy coconut ginger/mix only	2 tsp	1.0	15	60%
(Aunt Patsy's Pantry)				
island black bean				
mix only	1 serving	<1.0	126	4%
prepared	1 serving	3.5	202	16%
13-bean bouillabaisse				
mix only	1 serving	<1.0	99	5%
prepared	1 serving	3.0	174	16%
(Arrowhead Mills) mix only				
7 beans & barley/homestyle	¼ cup	–	170	–
(Bag O'Beans) mix only				
lentil & pea	¼ cup	0.5	170	3%
minestrone blend	¼ cup	0.5	150	3%
(Bean Cuisine)				
Santa Fe corn chowder				
mix only	1 serving	<1.0	112	4%
prepared	1 serving	4.5	179	23%
thick as fog split pea				
mix only	1 serving	<1.0	116	4%
prepared	1 serving	4.5	189	21%
ultima pasta & E fagioli				
mix only	1 serving	<1.0	117	4%
prepared	1 serving	3.0	179	15%
(Bear Creek) Soup mix/prepared				
cheddar broccoli	1 cup	5.0	170	26%
creamy chicken	1 cup	2.0	140	13%
damn good chili	1 cup	1.0	160	6%
minestrone	1 cup	1.0	100	9%
navy bean	1 cup	1.0	110	8%
potato	1 cup	4.0	160	23%
(Borden)				
beef bouillon/reduced sodium	1 cube	–	5	–
	1 tsp	–	5	–
chicken bouillon/reduced sodium	1 cube	–	5	–
	1 tsp	–	5	–
homestyle chicken-flavored noodle	¼ pkt	1.5	70	19%
Ronco natural	⅛ pkg	0.5	90	5%

Food and Description	Amount	Fat Grams	Total Calories	% Fat Calories
(Campbell's)				
Soup Mix/prepared				
chicken noodle	1 cup	1.5	90	15%
noodle	1 cup	1.5	100	14%
onion	1 cup	–	20	–
Soup-To-Go/microwaveable				
chicken rice	1 container	1.5	140	10%
garden vegetable	1 container	1.0	130	7%
hearty chicken noodle	1 container	1.5	100	14%
vegetable beef w/pasta	1 container	1.5	130	10%
(Fantastic Foods) dry mix only				
Big Soup Noodle Bowls				
hot & sour	1.2 oz	2.5	140	16%
miso w/tofu	1 oz	1.0	110	8%
sesame miso	0.9 oz	1.0	100	9%
spicy Thai	1.1 oz	1.0	120	8%
Creamy Soups				
asparagus	1.2 oz	2.5	130	17%
broccoli cheddar	1.4 oz	3.0	160	17%
corn & potato chowder	1.6 oz	2.0	170	11%
garlic mushroom	1.5 oz	3.0	160	17%
potato leek	1.1 oz	2.0	120	15%
Hearty Soups				
cha-cha chili	2.4 oz	2.0	250	7%
country lentil	2.3 oz	2.0	250	7%
couscous with lentils	2.3 oz	1.5	230	6%
five bean	2.3 oz	1.5	240	6%
jumpin' black bean	2.2 oz	1.5	230	6%
minestrone	1.5 oz	2.0	170	11%
split pea	2.0 oz	1.0	220	4%
vegetable barley	1.5 oz	0.5	150	3%
Ramen Noodle Cups				
chicken free	1.5 oz	0.5	140	3%
vegetable				
curry	1.5 oz	1.0	140	6%
miso	1.3 oz	1.0	130	7%
tomato	1.5 oz	1.0	150	6%
generic				
asparagus, cream of/2.2-oz pkg	1 pkg	7.0	234	27%
beef broth/cubed				
mix only	1 cube	–	8	–
prepared	1 cup	–	8	–
beef noodle/prepared	1 cup	0.8	41	17%
cauliflower/0.7-oz pkg				
mix only	1 pkg	1.7	68	23%
prepared	1 cup	1.7	68	23%
celery, cream of/0.6-oz pkg	1 pkg	1.6	63	23%
chicken, cream of/0.6-oz pkg				
mix only	1 pkg	4.0	80	35%
prepared	1 cup	5.0	107	42%

Food and Description	Amount	Fat Grams	Total Calories	% Fat Calories
chicken broth				
consommé				
mix only	1 pkg	0.8	16	45%
prepared	1 cup	1.0	21	43%
cubed				
mix only	1 cube	–	8	–
prepared	1 cup	–	8	–
chicken rice/prepared	1 cup	1.0	60	15%
chicken vegetable/prepared	1 cup	0.8	49	15%
clam chowder/prepared				
Manhattan	1 cup	1.6	65	22%
New England	1 cup	3.7	95	35%
consommé w/gelatin/2-oz pkg				
mix only	1 pkg	–	77	–
prepared	1 cup	–	17	–
mushroom	1 cup	4.9	96	46%
onion/mix only	1 pkg	0.5	35	13%
onion mushroom/mix only	1 pkg	0.5	80	6%
oxtail/prepared	1 cup	2.6	71	32%
pea, green or split/prepared	1 cup	1.6	133	11%
tomato/0.7-oz pkg				
mix only	1 pkg	2.0	77	23%
prepared	1 cup	2.0	102	18%
tomato vegetable/ 1.4-oz pkg				
mix only	1 pkg	2.0	125	14%
prepared	1 cup	0.9	55	14%
vegetable, cream of/prepared	1 cup	5.7	105	49%
vegetable beef/prepared	1 cup	1.0	53	17%
(G. Washington) seasoning & broth				
brown				
kosher				
mix only	1 pkg	–	45	–
prepared	1 serving	–	5	–
regular				
mix only	1 pkg	–	45	–
prepared	1 serving	–	5	–
golden				
kosher				
mix only	1 pkg	–	45	–
prepared	1 serving	–	5	–
regular				
mix only	1 pkg	–	45	–
prepared	1 serving	–	5	–
onion				
mix only	1 pkg	–	95	–
prepared	1 serving	–	10	–
vegetable				
mix only	1 pkg	–	95	–
prepared	1 serving	–	10	–

Food and Description	Amount	Fat Grams	Total Calories	% Fat Calories
(Goodman's) prepared				
matzo ball & soup				
50% less sodium	1 cup	1.0	50	18%
regular	1 cup	1.0	40	23%
noodleman				
low-sodium	1 cup	1.0	50	18%
regular	1 cup	1.0	45	20%
onion				
low-sodium	1 cup	1.0	30	30%
regular	1 cup	1.0	30	30%
(Hain) Savory soup mix/prepared				
cheese	¾ cup	16.0	250	58%
lentil	¾ cup	2.0	130	14%
minestrone	¾ cup	1.0	110	8%
mushroom	¾ cup	15.0	210	64%
onion	¾ cup	2.0	50	36%
potato leek	¾ cup	18.0	260	62%
split pea	¾ cup	10.0	310	29%
tomato	¾ cup	14.0	220	57%
vegetable	¾ cup	1.0	80	11%
(Health Valley) cups/prepared				
Fat-Free				
chicken flavored noodle w/vegetables	1 cup	–	110	–
chili mild black bean	1 cup	–	120	–
corn chowder w/tomatoes	1 cup	–	100	–
creamy potato w/broccoli	1 cup	–	80	–
garden split pea w/carrots	1 cup	–	130	–
lentil w/couscous	1 cup	–	130	–
pasta Italiano	1 cup	–	140	–
pasta Parmesan	1 cup	–	100	–
spicy black bean w/couscous	1 cup	–	130	–
zesty black bean w/rice	1 cup	–	110	–
Low-Fat				
shiitake mushroom rice	1 cup	1.5	140	10%
(Herb-Ox)				
bouillon cube				
beef	1 cube	–	5	–
chicken	1 cube	–	5	–
vegetable	1 cube	–	5	–
instant bouillon				
beef	1 tsp	–	5	–
chicken	1 tsp	–	5	–
instant broth/seasoning				
beef				
low-sodium	1 pkg	–	10	–
regular	1 pkg	–	5	–
chicken				
low-sodium	1 pkg	–	10	–
regular	1 pkg	–	5	–

Food and Description	Amount	Fat Grams	Total Calories	% Fat Calories
liquid				
beef	2 tsp	–	20	–
chicken	2 tsp	–	15	–
(Hormel) Micro Cup Soups				
bean & ham soup	1 cup	4.0	190	19%
beef vegetable	1 cup	1.0	90	10%
broccoli cheese w/ham	1 cup	13.0	170	69%
chicken & rice	1 cup	3.0	110	25%
chicken noodle	1 cup	2.5	110	20%
New England clam chowder	1 cup	5.0	130	35%
potato cheese w/ ham	1 cup	13.0	190	62%
(Imagine) Natural/low-fat/prepared				
creamy broccoli	1 cup	1.5	70	19%
creamy butternut squash	1 cup	2.0	120	90%
creamy mushroom	1 cup	3.0	80	34%
creamy potato leek	1 cup	2.5	90	25%
creamy sweet corn	1 cup	3.0	100	27%
creamy tomato	1 cup	1.5	90	15%
no-chicken broth	1 cup	1.0	35	26%
vegetable broth	1 cup	1.0	45	20%
zesty gazpacho	1 cup	–	60	–
(Just Delicious) Gourmet Foods soups mixes/prepared				
Albondigas	1 cup	–	25	–
barley beef	1 cup	–	120	–
black bean chili	1 cup	–	60	–
black beans & rice	1 cup	–	123	–
broccoli cheese	1 cup	1.0	20	45%
champion red lentil	1 cup	–	110	–
chicken vegetable	1 cup	–	120	–
chicken, rice, & curry spice	1 cup	–	60	–
corn chowder	1 cup	–	45	–
15 bean	1 cup	–	100	–
gourmet minestrone	1 cup	–	30	–
Jamaican black bean	1 cup	–	60	–
lentil chili	1 cup	–	110	–
lima bean	1 cup	–	50	–
navy bean	1 cup	0.5	120	4%
pinto bean	1 cup	–	18	–
potato	1 cup	–	25	–
potato cheese	1 cup	1.0	25	36%
red beans & rice	1 cup	–	120	–
seafood chowder	1 cup	–	40	–
sour cream, onion, & potato	1 cup	0.5	25	18%
split pea	1 cup	0.5	150	3%
tortilla	1 cup	–	60	–
vegetarian vegetable	1 cup	–	100	–
white bean chili	1 cup	–	120	–
(Knorr)				
bouillon cube/½ cube-prepared				
beef	1 cup	1.0	15	60%

Food and Description	Amount	Fat Grams	Total Calories	% Fat Calories
chicken	1 cup	1.0	15	60%
fish	1 cup	1.0	15	60%
pumpkin	1 cup	0.5	5	90%
pumpkin & ham	1 cup	0.5	5	90%
shrimp	1 cup	1.5	20	68%
tomato w/chicken	1 cup	1.0	15	60%
vegetarian vegetable	1 cup	1.0	10	90%
concentrated broth				
beef	1/12 container	–	15	–
chicken	1/12 container	–	5	–
Savory Soups/mix only				
creamy chicken w/rice	3 Tbs	2.5	90	25%
chicken noodle	3 Tbs	1.5	70	19%
Mediterranean style minestrone	3 Tbs	2.0	100	18%
Soup, Dip, and Recipe mix/mix only				
broccoli, cream of	3 Tbs	2.5	70	32%
French onion	2 Tbs	1.0	35	26%
hot & sour	2 Tbs	1.5	45	30%
leek	2 Tbs	2.5	70	32%
pasta w/chicken	1/4 pkg	1.0	80	11%
spaghetti style pasta	1/4 pkg	1.0	80	11%
spinach/cream of	2 Tbs	2.5	70	32%
roasted garlic	3 Tbs	1.5	80	17%
spring vegetable	2 Tbs	–	25	–
tomato beef (oxtail hearty)	2 Tbs	2.0	60	30%
vegetable	2 Tbs	0.5	30	15%
Tasty Breaks Soup cups/prepared				
black bean	1 cup	0.5	130	3%
chicken				
noodle	1 cup	2.5	130	17%
vegetable	1 cup	1.5	120	11%
corn chowder	1 cup	3.0	140	19%
hearty lentil	1 cup	1.0	200	5%
navy bean	1 cup	0.5	130	3%
potato leek	1 cup	2.5	130	17%
split pea	1 cup	0.5	150	3%
(Lipton)				
Cup-A-Soup/mix only				
chicken				
cream of	1 pkg	2.0	70	26%
supreme/hearty	1 pkg	4.0	90	40%
chicken noodle				
country style hearty	1 pkg	1.0	60	15%
w/chicken meat	1 pkg	1.0	50	18%
green pea	1 pkg	1.0	80	11%
tomato	1 pkg	2.0	90	20%
vegetable/spring	1 pkg	1.0	45	20%
Recipe Secrets/mix only				
herb				
fiesta w/red pepper	1 Tbs	–	30	

Food and Description	Amount	Fat Grams	Total Calories	% Fat Calories
golden, w/lemon	2 Tbs	1.0	35	26%
Italian, w/tomato	2 Tbs	1.0	40	235
w/garlic/savory	1 Tbs	–	30	–
mushroom/beefy	1½ Tbs	–	35	–
onion				
beefy	1 Tbs	0.5	25	18%
golden	2 Tbs	1.5	60	23%
mushroom	2 Tbs	1.0	35	26%
regular	1 Tbs	–	20	–
vegetable	2 Tbs	–	30	–
Soup Secrets /mix only				
chicken noodle	3 Tbs	2.0	80	23%
chicken w/pasta & beans	3 Tbs	2.0	110	16%
country chicken w/pasta & herbs	3 Tbs	2.0	100	18%
extra noodle	3 Tbs	2.0	90	20%
giggle noodle	2 Tbs	2.0	70	26%
minestrone	3 Tbs	1.0	110	8%
noodle w/real chicken	2 Tbs	2.0	60	30%
noodle w/vegetables/hearty	3 Tbs	2.0	70	26%
spiral pasta w/chicken broth	2 Tbs	1.0	60	15%
(MBT) Romanoff				
beef				
low-sodium	1 pkt	–	15	–
regular	1 pkt	–	15	–
chicken				
low-sodium	1 pkt	–	15	–
regular	1 pkt	–	15	–
onion broth & dip	1 pkt	–	15	–
vegetable	1 pkt	–	10	–
(Maggi) boullion				
cubes				
beef	1 cube	–	5	–
chicken	1 cube	–	5	–
vegetable	1 cube	–	5	–
instant				
beef	1 tsp	–	5	–
chicken	1 tsp	–	5	–
(Manischewitz)				
Mrs. Manischewitz's Soup Cup				
black bean	1 cup	1.0	200	5%
chicken & rice	1 cup	1.0	130	7%
lentil/hearty	1 cup	1.0	140	6%
regular/mix only				
matzo ball	1 Tbs	0.5	40	11%
minestrone	¼ pkg	–	150	–
split pea	⅕ pkg	–	110	–
vegetable w/mushroom	⅕ pkg	–	120	–
(Marachun) cup/prepared				
Instant Lunch				
beef	1 container	12.0	290	37%

Food and Description	Amount	Fat Grams	Total Calories	% Fat Calories
California vegetable	1 container	11.0	260	62%
cheddar cheese	1 container	16.0	340	42%
chicken	1 container	12.0	280	39%
chili piquin & shrimp	1 container	12.0	280	39%
creamy chicken	1 container	13.0	290	40%
creamy pesto	1 container	15.0	340	40%
picante chicken	1 container	12.0	280	39%
pork	1 container	12.0	280	39%
tomato w/vegetables	1 container	12.0	290	37%
shrimp	1 container	12.0	290	37%
Instant Wonton				
chicken	1 container	12.0	200	54%
shrimp	1 container	12.0	200	54%
Ramen Oriental Noodle Soup				
beef	½ pkt	8.0	190	38%
chicken w/mushrooms	½ pkt	7.0	190	33%
creamy chicken	½ pkt	9.0	200	41%
roast				
beef	½ pkt	8.0	190	38%
chicken	½ pkt	8.0	190	38%
tomato	½ pkt	8.0	200	36%
(Mayacamas) prepared				
Instant Soupbreak				
black bean	6 oz	<1.0	75	6%
garden pea	6 oz	<1.0	75	6%
New England clam	6 oz	<1.0	75	6%
potato leek	6 oz	<1.0	75	6%
regular				
avgholemono	6 oz	<1.0	60	8%
black bean	6 oz	<1.0	60	8%
broccoli	6 oz	<1.0	70	6%
dark mushroom	6 oz	<1.0	60	8%
French onion	6 oz	<1.0	45	10%
garden pea	6 oz	<1.0	50	9%
lentil	6 oz	<1.0	70	6%
minestrone	6 oz	<1.0	70	6%
mulligatawny	6 oz	<1.0	60	8%
potato leek	6 oz	<1.0	60	7%
senegalese	6 oz	<1.0	55	8%
tomato	6 oz	<1.0	50	9%
(Mrs. Grass) mix only				
chicken w/rice	¼ pkg	1.0	80	11%
homestyle chicken	¼ pkg	1.5	70	19%
noodle				
beef flavored	¼ pkg	1.0	70	13%
chicken flavored	¼ pkg	1.5	60	23%
onion				
mushroom	⅓ pkg	1.0	60	15%
reduced sodium	¼ pkg	–	35	–
regular soup & dip	¼ pkg	0.5	35	13%

Food and Description	Amount	Fat Grams	Total Calories	% Fat Calories
vegetable soup & dip/homestyle	¼ pkg	–	35	–
(Nile Spice) Homestyle cup mix/prepared				
black bean	1 container	2.0	190	9%
chicken vegetable	1 container	2.0	120	15%
lentil	1 container	1.0	180	10%
minestrone	1 container	2.0	160	11%
red beans & rice	1 container	2.0	190	9%
split pea	1 container	2.0	200	9%
sweet corn chowder	1 container	3.0	120	23%
(Nissin) mix only				
Top Ramen				
beef				
picante	½ pkg	7.0	180	35%
regular				
low-fat	½ pkg	1.0	150	6%
original	½ pkg	7.0	190	33%
chicken				
Cajun	½ pkg	7.0	180	35%
low-fat	½ pkg	1.0	150	6%
mushroom	½ pkg	7.0	190	33%
original	½ pkg	7.0	180	35%
teriyaki	½ pkg	7.0	190	33%
chile	½ pkg	8.0	190	38%
garden vegetable	½ pkg	7.0	190	33%
Oriental				
low-fat	½ pkg	1.0	150	6%
original	½ pkg	7.0	190	33%
pork	½ pkg	7.0	190	33%
shrimp	½ pkg	7.0	190	33%
Cup O'Noodles				
beef				
hot sauce	2.25 oz	14.0	290	43%
onion	2.25 oz	14.0	300	42%
chicken				
creamy	2.25 oz	13.0	300	39%
hot sauce	3 oz	13.0	300	39%
mushroom	2.25 oz	13.0	300	39%
regular	3.oz	14.0	300	42%
spicy	2.25 oz	14.0	300	42%
teriyaki	2.25 oz	14.0	300	42%
pork	2.25 oz	12.0	290	37%
shrimp	2.25 oz	14.0	300	42%
vegetable/garden	2.25 oz	12.0	290	37%
(Old Bay) mix only				
crab, cream of	2 Tbs	2.5	70	32%
Maryland crab	1⅓ Tbs	–	50	–
(Pritikin) instant soup cups/prepared				
black bean	10 oz	1.0	200	5%
chicken vegetable	10 oz	–	100	–
minestrone	10 oz	0.5	130	3%

Food and Description	Amount	Fat Grams	Total Calories	% Fat Calories
potato broccoli	10 oz	–	110	–
split pea	10 oz	0.5	140	3%
vegetarian chili	10 oz	1.0	160	6%
(Produce Partners) mix only				
broccoli, cream of	1⅓ Tbs	–	35	–
cheddar cheese broccoli	2 Tbs	3.0	70	39%
French onion	1 Tbs	–	40	–
potato, cream of	1 Tbs	–	25	–
vegetable/garden	1⅓ Tbs	–	40	–
(Swanson) broth/mix only				
beef	1 cube	1.0	20	45%
chicken	1 cube	2.0	30	60%
Oriental	1 cube	–	15	–
vegetable	1 cube	1.0	20	45%
(Ultra Slim Fast) prepared				
beef noodle	6 oz	<1.0	45	10%
chicken noodle	6 oz	<1.0	45	10%
creamy				
broccoli	6 oz	<1.0	75	6%
chicken leek	6 oz	<1.0	50	9%
potato leek	6 oz	<1.0	80	6%
tomato	6 oz	<1.0	60	8%
hearty				
onion	6 oz	<1.0	45	10%
vegetable	6 oz	<1.0	50	9%
(Union Foods)				
Noodles/block				
beef	½ pkg	8.0	190	38%
chicken	½ pkg	8.0	190	38%
chicken mushroom	½ pkg	8.0	190	38%
creamy chicken	½ pkg	8.0	190	38%
French onion	½ pkg	8.0	190	38%
hot & spicy	½ pkg	8.0	190	38%
oriental	½ pkg	8.0	190	38%
picante shrimp	½ pkg	8.0	190	38%
pork	½ pkg	8.0	190	38%
shrimp	½ pkg	8.0	190	38%
vegetable beef	½ pkg	8.0	190	38%
SMACK/cup Ramen				
beef	1 pkg	16.0	310	46%
chicken				
Cajun	1 pkg	16.0	310	46%
creamy	1 pkg	17.0	320	48%
mushroom	1 pkg	15.0	300	45%
original	1 pkg	17.0	320	48%
French onion	1 pkg	15.0	300	45%
Shrimp				
original	1 pkg	17.0	320	48%
picante	1 pkg	15.0	310	44%
vegetable beef	1 pkg	16.0	310	46%

Food and Description	Amount	Fat Grams	Total Calories	% Fat Calories
(Weight Watchers) broth				
beef broth	1 pkt	–	10	–
chicken broth	1 pkt	–	10	–
(Westbrae) mix only				
brown rice	½ pkg	0.5	140	3%
buckwheat	½ pkg	0.5	140	3%
carrot	⅓ pkg	1.0	100	9%
curry	½ pkg	0.5	140	3%
5 spice	½ pkg	0.5	140	3%
green tea	½ pkg	1.0	140	6%
miso	½ pkg	0.5	140	3%
mushroom	½ pkg	0.5	140	3%
seaweed	½ pkg	0.5	140	3%
spinach	½ pkg	0.5	140	3%
(Wyler's)				
bouillon cube				
beef	1 cube	–	5	–
chicken	1 cube	–	5	–
instant bouillon/Shakers				
beef				
& French onion flavor	1 tsp	–	5	–
regular	1 tsp	–	5	–
chicken				
& garlic herb	1 tsp	–	5	–
regular				
w/parsley	1 tsp	–	5	–
w/o parsley	1 tsp	–	5	–
southwest & herb flavor	1 tsp	–	5	–
very low sodium	1 tsp	–	10	–
vegetable	1 tsp	–	5	–
instant broth				
beef	1 pkt	–	15	–
chicken				
regular	1 pkt	–	15	–
low-sodium	1 pkt	–	15	–
Soup Starter/mix only				
beef vegetable	⅛ container	0.5	90	5%
chicken noodle	⅛ container	0.5	80	6%
■ FROZEN OR REFRIGERATED				
(Schwan's)				
Boston clam chowder	1 cup	8.0	190	38%
chicken noodle	1 cup	3.0	150	18%
(Stock Pot)				
clam chowder/concentrated				
prepared w/whole milk	1 cup	9.5	200	43%
unprepared	⅓ cup	4.0	100	36%
seafood gumbo	1 cup	5.0	130	35%
(Tabatchnick)				
barley mushroom				
no salt	7.5 oz	–	70	–
regular	7.5 oz	–	70	–

Food and Description	Amount	Fat Grams	Total Calories	% Fat Calories
broccoli, cream of	7.5 oz	4.0	90	40%
cabbage	7.5 oz	–	60	–
chicken				
New York	7.5 oz	–	35	–
w/dumplings	7.5 oz	2.0	70	26%
corn chowder	7.5 oz	6.0	150	36%
minestrone	7.5 oz	1.0	150	6%
pea				
no salt	7.5 oz	1.5	180	8%
regular	7.5 oz	1.5	180	8%
potato				
New England	7.5 oz	6.0	150	36%
old fashioned	7.5 oz	–	70	–
spinach, cream of	7.5 oz	4.0	90	40%
vegetable				
no salt	7.5 oz	1.0	110	8%
regular	7.5 oz	1.0	110	8%
Wisconsin cheddar vegetable	7.5 oz	9.0	140	58%
Yankee bean	7.5 oz	2.0	160	11%
■ **HOMEMADE**				
USDA Standard Home Recipe				
black turtle bean	1 cup	1.0	240	4%
Brunswick stew	1 cup	5.0	230	20%
corn & cheese chowder	1 cup	16.0	287	50%
gazpacho	1 cup	–	50	–
Greek	1 cup	2.5	85	27%
hot & sour	1 cup	2.0	75	24%
pasta e fagioli	1 cup	4.5	195	42%
potato	1 cup	12.0	201	54%
ratatouille	1 cup	23.0	265	78%
vegetable	1 cup	–	70	–
vegetable beef	1 cup	25.0	320	70%
won ton	1 cup	3.0	205	13%
SOUR CREAM (*See also* DIP; SAUCE; SEASONINGS; SOUR CREAM SUBSTITUTE)				
(Alta Dena) premium	1 Tbs	6.0	60	90%
(Breakstone)				
sour cream				
fat-free	2 Tbs	–	35	–
original	2 Tbs	5.0	60	75%
sour half & half	2 Tbs	3.5	45	70%
(Friendship)				
lite	2 Tbs	3.0	35	77%
original	2 Tbs	5.0	60	75%
generic				
cultured	1 Tbs	2.5	26	86%
	1 cup	42.0	450	84%
nondairy	1 Tbs	2.8	30	83%
	1 cup	45.0	480	84%
(Heluva Good Cheese)				
fat-free	2 Tbs	–	20	–

Food and Description	Amount	Fat Grams	Total Calories	% Fat Calories
light	2 Tbs	3.0	40	68%
original	2 Tbs	5.0	60	75%
(Kemps)				
sour cream				
cultured	1 oz	5.0	60	75%
lite	1 oz	2.0	30	6%
regular	1 cup	42.0	450	84%
w/chives	1 oz	5.0	60	75%
Tator Topper/lite	1 oz	2.0	30	6%
(Knudsen)				
fat-free	2 Tbs	–	35	–
Hampshire	2 Tbs	6.0	60	90%
light	2 Tbs	2.5	40	56%
(Land O'Lakes)				
sour cream				
lite				
plain	2 Tbs	2.0	40	45%
w/chives	2 Tbs	2.0	40	45%
no-fat	2 Tbs	–	30	–
regular	1 Tbs	3.0	30	90%
sour half & half	1 Tbs	2.0	25	72%
(Real Dairy) fat-free	2 Tbs	–	20	–
SOUR CREAM SUBSTITUTE (See also SEASONINGS)				
(Chivo)	2 Tbs	5.0	50	90%
(Dean's) Sour Delite	2 Tbs	5.0	50	90%
(Formagg) fat-free sour cream alternative	2 Tbs	–	30	–
generic				
non-butterfat	1 oz	4.0	42	86%
	1 cup	39.0	417	84%
nondairy	1 oz	6.0	60	90%
	1 cup	45.0	480	84%
(IMO)				
fat-free	2 Tbs	–	20	–
original	2 Tbs	5.0	50	90%
(Land O'Lakes) light dairy blend	1 Tbs	1.0	20	45%
(Pet)	1 Tbs	2.0	25	72%
(Soymage) sour cream alternative	2 Tbs	3.0	40	68%
(Tofutti) Sour Supreme/Better Than Sour Cream				
cherries n' berries	2 Tbs	5.0	50	90%
guacamole	2 Tbs	5.0	50	90%
plain	2 Tbs	5.0	50	90%
salsa	2 Tbs	5.0	50	90%
SOURSOP /fresh				
pieces	1 cup	1.0	150	6%
whole	1 medium	2.0	420	4%
SOY CHEESE (See CHEESE ALTERNATIVE/IMITATION)				
SOY FLOUR (See FLOUR)				
SOY NUTS (See SOYBEAN)				
SOY PROTEIN				
concentrate	1 oz		92	–

Food and Description	Amount	Fat Grams	Total Calories	% Fat Calories
isolate				
w/potassium	1 oz	1.0	96	9%
w/sodium	1 oz	1.0	96	9%
SOY SAUCE (See ASIAN FOOD/SAUCES & SEASONINGS; SAUCE)				
SOYBEAN				
dried				
(Arrowhead Mills)	¼ cup	8.0	170	42%
generic				
boiled-drained	½ cup	8.0	150	48%
dry-roasted	½ cup	18.6	387	43%
raw	½ cup	18.5	390	43%
roasted/salted or unsalted	1 oz	6.8	129	47%
	½ cup	21.8	405	48%
roasted & toasted	1 oz	6.8	129	47%
(Nature's Select) dry-roasted	¾ oz	4.0	90	40%
frozen				
(C&W) soybeans/edamae-in the pod	½ cup	1.0	60	15%
green				
boiled-drained	½ cup	6.0	130	42%
raw				
shelled	½ cup	9.0	190	43%
unshelled	4 oz	4.0	90	40%
kernels/whole/roasted & toasted	1 oz	7.0	130	48%
	1 cup	26.0	490	48%
sprouted				
raw	10 sprouts	0.5	15	30%
	½ cup	2.3	45	46%
steamed	½ cup	2.0	40	45%
stir-fried in vegetable oil	3 oz	6.0	105	51%
SOYBEAN CURD (See TOFU; TOFU FROZEN DESSERTS; VEGETARIAN FOODS)				
SOYBEAN OIL (See OIL)				
SOYBEAN PASTE (See MISO)				
SOYMILK (See also BABY/INFANT FORMULA)				
dry				
(Loma Linda) Soyagen/prepared				
all-purpose	¼ cup	6.0	130	42%
carob	¼ cup	6.0	130	42%
no sucrose	¼ cup	6.0	130	42%
(Worthington) Soyamel	1 oz	7.0	130	49%
liquid				
(Eden)				
Edenblend/original	8 fl oz	3.0	120	23%
Edensoy				
carob	8 fl oz	4.0	150	24%
original				
extra	8 fl oz	4.0	130	28%
regular	8 fl oz	4.0	135	27%
vanilla				
extra	8 fl oz	3.0	150	18%
regular	8 fl oz	3.0	150	18%

Food and Description	Amount	Fat Grams	Total Calories	% Fat Calories
generic	1 cup	4.6	80	52%
(Health Valley) Soy Moo	1 cup	6.0	120	45%
(Imagine)				
Power Dream Natural energy drink				
vanilla/mix prepared	11 fl oz	5.0	250	18%
Soy Dream				
carob	8 fl oz	4.0	210	17%
chocolate enriched	8 fl oz	3.5	210	15%
original				
enriched	8 fl oz	4.0	130	28%
regular	8 fl oz	4.0	130	28%
vanilla				
enriched	8 fl oz	4.0	150	24%
regular	8 fl oz	4.0	150	24%
(Vitasoy)				
carob supreme	8 fl oz	6.0	210	26%
cocoa				
light	8 fl oz	2.0	130	14%
rich	8 fl oz	6.0	210	26%
original				
creamy	8 fl oz	7.0	160	39%
light	8 fl oz	2.0	90	20%
vanilla				
delite	8 fl oz	6.0	190	28%
light	8 fl oz	2.0	110	16%
(Westsoy)				
almond				
lite 1%	6 fl oz	4.0	160	23%
natural	6 fl oz	11.0	250	40%
carob/plus	8 fl oz	5.0	160	28%
cocoa-flavored/lite 1%	8 fl oz	2.0	140	13%
malted				
plain				
lite 1%	6 fl oz	3.0	160	17%
natural	6 fl oz	11.0	270	37%
vanilla/natural	6 fl oz	11.0	250	40%
plain				
lite 1%	8 fl oz	2.0	100	18%
natural				
regular	8 fl oz	5.0	150	30%
unsweetened	8 fl oz	5.0	100	45%
plus	8 fl oz	5.0	150	30%
vanilla				
lite 1%	8 fl oz	2.0	110	16%
natural	8 fl oz	2.5	120	19%
plus	8 fl oz	5.0	150	30%
(White Wave) Silk soy milk				
chocolate	1 cup	2.5	90	25%
plain	1 cup	2.5	108	21%
vanilla	1 cup	3.0	90	30%

Food and Description	Amount	Fat Grams	Total Calories	% Fat Calories

SPAETZLE (*See* DUMPLING MIX)
SPAGHETTI (*See* PASTA)
SPAGHETTI DINNER (*See* FROZEN ENTRÉE/DINNER; PASTA ENTRÉE/DINNER; VEGETARIAN FOODS)
SPAGHETTI SAUCE (*See* SAUCE)
SPANISH FOOD (*See* FROZEN ENTRÉE/DINNER; MEXICAN FOOD; RICE; RICE DISH; VEGETARIAN FOODS)
SPICES (*See* SEASONINGS; individual listings)
SPINACH

Food and Description	Amount	Fat Grams	Total Calories	% Fat Calories
canned				
(Bush's Best) chopped	½ cup	–	25	–
(Del Monte)				
chopped	½ cup	–	30	–
no salt added	½ cup	–	30	–
whole leaf	½ cup	–	30	–
(Freshlike)				
cut	½ cup	–	30	–
w/o salt	½ cup	–	30	–
w/o salt or sugar	½ cup	–	30	–
(S&W)	½ cup	–	30	–
(Stokely)	½ cup	–	30	–
(Veg-All) cut	½ cup	–	30	–
fresh				
boiled	½ cup	–	21	–
raw				
chopped	½ cup	–	6	–
(Dole)	3 oz	–	10	–
frozen				
(Birds Eye)				
chopped	3.3 oz	–	20	–
cut leaf	1 cup	–	20	–
whole leaf	3.3 oz	–	20	–
(C&W)				
chopped	⅓ cup	–	20	–
whole leaf	⅓ cup	–	20	–
(Cascadian Farm) chopped	⅓ cup	–	20	–
(Freshlike) cut	3.3 oz	–	20	–
generic				
chopped	1 cup	<1.0	40	11%
	10 oz	1.0	70	13%
(Green Giant)				
cut leaf	¾ cup	–	15	–
Harvest Fresh	½ cup	0.5	30	15%
(Pictsweet) leaf	½ cup	–	30	–
(Veg-All) cut	3.3 oz	–	20	–
SPINACH, NEW ZEALAND /fresh				
boiled	½ cup	–	12	–
raw	1 lb	1.0	86	11%

SPINACH DISH (*See also* FROZEN ENTRÉE/DINNER; VEGETABLES, MIXED; VEGETARIAN FOODS)

Food and Description	Amount	Fat Grams	Total Calories	% Fat Calories
Frozen				
(Bird's Eye) creamed	½ cup	7.0	100	63%
(Green Giant)				
creamed	½ cup	3.0	80	34%
cut leaf in butter sauce	½ cup	1.0	35	26%
homemade/USDA Standard Home Recipe				
spinach quiche	~5 oz	26.0	337	69%
spinach soufflé/made w/whole milk, butter, & cheese	1 cup	18.0	218	74%
SPIRULINA (*See* SEAWEED)				
SPLIT PEA (*See* PEA)				
SPOONBREAD (*See* BREAD)				
SPORTS DRINK				
bottled or canned				
(All Sport)				
black citrus	8 fl oz	–	70	–
blue ice	8 fl oz	–	70	–
cherry slam	8 fl oz	–	70	–
fruit punch	8 fl oz	–	70	–
grape	8 fl oz	–	70	–
lemon-lime	8 fl oz	–	70	–
orange	8 fl oz	–	70	–
raspberry burst	8 fl oz	–	70	–
watermelon	8 fl oz	–	70	–
(GatorAde) Thirst Quencher				
original				
citrus cooler	8 fl oz	–	50	–
cool blue raspberry	8 fl oz	–	50	–
grape	8 fl oz	–	50	–
lemon ice	8 fl oz	–	50	–
lemon-lime	8 fl oz	–	50	–
orange	8 fl oz	–	50	–
tropical burst	8 fl oz	–	50	–
watermelon	8 fl oz	–	50	–
sports bottle				
cherry rush	8 fl oz	–	50	–
citrus cooler	8 fl oz	–	50	–
cool blue raspberry	8 fl oz	–	50	–
fruit punch	8 fl oz	–	50	–
lemon ice	8 fl oz	–	50	–
lemon-lime	8 fl oz	–	50	–
strawberry kiwi	8 fl oz	–	50	–
wild apple	8 fl oz	–	50	–
(Powerade)				
fruit punch	8 fl oz	–	72	–
grape	8 fl oz	–	73	–
lemon-lime	8 fl oz	–	72	–
Mountain Blast	8 fl oz	–	73	–
orange	8 fl oz	–	72	–

Food and Description	Amount	Fat Grams	Total Calories	% Fat Calories
(Snapple) WhipperSnapple				
power berry	10 fl oz	–	160	–
power citrus	10 fl oz	–	150	–
(10-K)				
fruit punch	8 fl oz	–	60	–
lemon-lime	8 fl oz	–	60	–
orange	8 fl oz	–	60	–
SPOT FISH /fresh				
cooked-dry heat	3 oz	4.0	134	27%
raw	2.25-oz fillet	2.5	80	28%
	3 oz	3.0	105	26%
SPRING ONION (See SCALLION)				
SQUAB/PIGEON				
raw				
breast meat only	~4 oz	4.6	135	30%
giblets	3 oz	6.0	132	41%
meat & skin	~7 oz	47.5	590	72%
meat only	~6 oz	12.6	239	47%
SQUASH				
acorn/fresh				
baked	½ cup	–	57	–
boiled-mashed	½ cup	–	41	–
banana/fresh/baked	8 oz	1.0	145	6%
butternut				
fresh				
baked	½ cup	–	41	–
boiled-mashed	½ cup	–	50	–
frozen				
generic	½ cup	–	47	–
(Southland)	½ cup	–	45	–
cocozelle				
fresh				
boiled-drained	½ cup	–	14	–
raw/sliced	½ cup	–	9	–
frozen	½ cup	–	19	–
crookneck				
fresh				
boiled-drained	½ cup	–	18	–
raw/sliced	½ cup	–	12	–
frozen	½ cup	–	24	–
hubbard/fresh				
baked/cubed	½ cup	0.6	51	11%
boiled-mashed	½ cup	0.5	37	12%
scallop/fresh				
boiled-drained	½ cup	–	14	–
boiled-drained-mashed	½ cup	–	19	–
raw/sliced	½ cup	–	12	–
spaghetti/fresh				
boiled or baked	½ cup	–	23	–
(Nature's Pasta)	½ cup	–	20	–

Food and Description	Amount	Fat Grams	Total Calories	% Fat Calories
summer/all varieties/fresh				
boiled/sliced	½ cup	–	18	–
raw/sliced	½ cup	–	13	–
winter/all varieties				
fresh				
baked/cubed	½ cup	0.6	39	14%
boiled-mashed	½ cup	0.6	39	14%
frozen				
(Birds Eye)				
cooked	½ cup	–	45	–
sliced/yellow	⅔ cup	–	15	–
zucchini				
canned				
(Del Monte) w/Italian style tomato sauce	½ cup	–	30	–
(Progresso) Italian style	½ cup	2.0	40	45%
fresh				
boiled-drained	½ cup	–	14	–
raw	½ cup	–	9	–
frozen				
(Big Valley) sliced	3.5 oz	–	12	–
(C&W) sliced	3.3 oz	–	16	–
generic	½ cup	–	19	–
(Stilwell) Qwik Krisp	6 pieces	11.0	190	52%
(Southland) sliced	3.2 oz	–	15	–
SQUASH SEEDS				
dried/hulled	1 oz	13.0	155	75%
	1 cup	63.0	747	76%
kernels/roasted	1 oz	12.0	148	73%
	1 cup	95.6	1,184	73%
whole/roasted	1 oz	5.5	127	39%
	1 cup	12.0	285	38%
SQUID				
dried	3 oz	4.6	260	16%
fresh				
breaded & fried	3 oz	6.0	149	36%
raw	3 oz	1.0	78	12%
frozen				
(Fiesta Del Mar) ras calimari	4 oz	2.0	110	16%
pickled	1 oz	–	23	–
SQUIRREL				
raw	3 oz	3.0	105	26%
roasted	3 oz	3.0	115	23%
roasted/chopped or diced	½ cup	5.0	190	24%
STAR FRUIT/CARAMBOLA				
fresh				
cubed	½ cup	–	25	–
whole	1 medium	0.5	45	10%
STEAK SAUCE (See SAUCE)				
STRAWBERRY				

Food and Description	Amount	Fat Grams	Total Calories	% Fat Calories
canned				
generic/in heavy syrup	½ cup	<1.0	120	4%
freeze-dried				
(Mountain House) prepared	¼ cup	–	45	–
fresh				
(Dole)	8 berries	–	50	–
whole	1 cup	0.5	45	9%
	1 pint	1.0	97	9%
frozen				
(Big Valley)	3.5 oz	–	35	–
(Birds Eye)				
halves				
in lite syrup	10 oz	–	120	–
in regular syrup	4.8 oz	–	120	–
whole/in lite syrup	½ cup	–	100	–
(C&W) whole	⅔ cup	–	50	–
generic				
sliced/sweetened	1 cup	<1.0	245	2%
	10 oz	0.5	275	2%
whole				
sweetened	2 cup	<1.0	200	2%
unsweetened				
thawed	3.5 oz	<1.0	50	9%
unthawed	1 cup	<1.0	52	9%

STRAWBERRY DRINK (*See also* FRUIT PUNCH; LEMONADE/LEMONADE-FLAVORED DRINK; SOFT DRINK; SOFT DRINK MIX; individual juice blend listings)

bottled, boxed, or canned				
(Betty Crocker) Squeezit/Silly Billy Strawberry	6.76 fl oz	–	110	–
(Welch's)	11.5 fl oz	–	200	–

STRAWBERRY JUICE/JUICE BLEND/JUICE DRINK (*See also* FRUIT PUNCH; SOFT DRINK MIX)

bottled, boxed, or canned				
(Chiquita)				
Calypso breeze/strawberry kiwi	8 fl oz	–	120	–
	8.45 fl oz	–	130	–
light strawberry guava	8 fl oz	–	35	–
liquid concentrate/unprepared	1.6 fl oz	–	120	–
(Kern's)				
strawberry-banana nectar	11.5 fl oz	–	220	–
strawberry-guava juice blend	8 fl oz	–	105	–
(Knudsen) strawberry juice	8 fl oz	–	140	–
(Libby's)				
Juicy Juice/strawberry pouch	4.23 fl oz	–	60	–
nectar	11.5 fl oz	–	210	–
(Snapple)				
kiwi-strawberry				
diet	8 fl oz	–	20	–
regular	8 fl oz	–	110	–
(TreeTop) strawberry, orange, banana	8 fl oz	–	120	–

Food and Description	Amount	Fat Grams	Total Calories	% Fat Calories
STUFFING/DRESSING				
(Arnold) dry				
cornbread	¾ cup	2.0	140	13%
herb seasoned	¾ cup	1.5	140	13%
sage & onion	¾ cup	1.5	140	13%
seasoned	¾ cup	1.5	140	13%
unseasoned	¾ cup	1.5	150	9%
(Brownberry) dry				
cornbread	½ cup	2.0	130	14%
herb seasoned				
cube	½ cup	1.5	130	10%
shredded	½ cup	1.5	130	10%
homestyle for turkey	1 oz	4.5	120	34%
sage & onion	¾ cup	1.5	140	13%
unseasoned bread cubes	¾ cup	1.5	140	10%
(Butterball) One-Step/prepared				
cornbread	½ cup	3.0	150	18%
seasoned	½ cup	3.0	160	17%
(Golden Grains) prepared				
chicken	½ cup	9.0	180	40%
corn bread	½ cup	9.0	180	40%
herb & butter	½ cup	9.0	180	40%
w/wild rice	½ cup	9.0	180	40%
(Kellogg's) Croutettes stuffing mix	1 cup	–	120	–
(Mrs. Manischewitz) homestyle/prepared	¾ cup	1.0	110	8%
(Oroweat) dressing				
cornbread	⅓ cup	1.0	110	8%
seasoned	⅓ cup	1.0	110	8%
(Pepperidge Farms) dry mix only				
cornbread	¾ cup	2.0	170	11%
cube				
country style	¾ cup	1.5	140	10%
original	¾ cup	1.5	140	10%
seasoned w/herbs	½ cup	1.5	170	8%
One Step				
chicken	½ cup	4.0	140	26%
turkey	½ cup	5.0	150	30%
savory herb	½ cup	5.0	150	30%
(Stove Top) prepared w/margarine				
flexible serving				
chicken	½ cup	8.0	170	42%
cornbread	½ cup	8.0	160	45%
homestyle herb	½ cup	8.0	170	42%
microwave				
chicken	½ cup	7.0	160	39%
homestyle cornbread	½ cup	7.0	160	39%
original				
beef	½ cup	9.0	180	45%

Food and Description	Amount	Fat Grams	Total Calories	% Fat Calories
chicken				
lower-sodium	½ cup	9.0	180	45%
regular	½ cup	9.0	170	48%
cornbread	½ cup	8.0	170	40%
long grain & wild rice	½ cup	9.0	180	45%
mushroom & onion	½ cup	9.0	180	45%
pork	½ cup	9.0	170	48%
San Francisco style	½ cup	9.0	170	48%
savory herbs	½ cup	9.0	170	48%
traditional sage flavor	½ cup	9.0	180	45%
turkey	½ cup	9.0	170	48%
STURGEON				
cooked-dry heat	3 oz	4.0	115	31%
raw	3 oz	3.0	90	30%
smoked	3 oz	3.7	147	23%
steamed	3 oz	4.8	135	32%
SUCCOTASH (*See also* VEGETABLES, MIXED)				
canned				
generic				
w/cream-style corn	½ cup	0.7	100	6%
w/whole kernel corn	½ cup	0.6	80	7%
(Libby) w/whole kernel corn	½ cup	0.5	90	5%
(S & W) country	½ cup	1.0	80	11%
(Seneca) w/whole kernel corn	½ cup	0.5	90	5%
(Stokely)	½ cup	–	90	–
frozen				
generic	10 oz	2.5	265	8%
(Hanover)	½ cup	–	80	–
(Pictsweet)	3.3 oz	1.0	100	9%
homemade/USDA Standard Home Recipe	½ cup	–	110	–
SUCKER, WHITE				
cooked-dry heat	3 oz	2.0	101	18%
raw	3 oz	2.0	79	22%
SUET, BEEF	1 Tbs	13.0	121	100%
SUGAR				
brown				
firmly packed	1 tsp	–	18	–
	1 Tbs	–	52	–
	1 cup	–	821	–
loosely packed	1 cup	–	541	–
maple	1 Tbs	–	52	–
	1 oz	–	99	–
turbinado				
(Hain)	1 Tbs	–	50	–
white				
cubed	1 cube	–	25	–
granulated	1 tsp	–	15	–
	1 Tbs	–	46	–
	1 cup	–	770	–

Food and Description	Amount	Fat Grams	Total Calories	% Fat Calories
powdered 10-X confectioners flavored (Domino)				
chocolate	¼ cup	–	110	–
lemon	¼ cup	–	110	–
strawberry	¼ cup	–	110	–
regular/generic	1 tsp	–	10	–
	1 Tbs	–	31	–
	1 cup	–	462	–
SUGAR APPLE/SWEETSOP				
fresh				
pulp	1 cup	0.8	235	3%
whole	1 medium	0.5	145	3%
SUGAR SUBSTITUTE				
(Equal)	1 pkt	–	–	–
	¼ tsp	–	–	–
(Estee) fructose	1 pkt	–	10	–
	1 tsp	–	15	–
(Fruit Source) sweetener & fat replacer	1 tsp	–	15	–
generic/fructose	1 tsp	–	12	–
(NutraSweet)	1 tsp	–	–	–
	1 pkt	–	4	–
(Sprinkle Sweet)	1 tsp	–	2	–
(Sucaryl)	1 tsp	–	–	–
(Sugar Twin)				
brown sugar	1 tsp	–	2	–
regular	1 tsp	–	2	–
	1 pkt	–	3	–
(Superose)	1 pkt	–	–	–
(Sweet*10)	⅛ tsp	–	–	–
(SweetLite)	1 tsp	–	12	–
(SweetMate)	1 pkt	–	3	–
(Sweet 'N Low)				
liquid	10 drops	–	–	–
powder				
brown sugar	¹⁄₁₀ tsp	–	2	–
regular	1 packet	–	4	–
	1 tsp	–	12	–
tablet	1 tablet	–	–	–
(Weight Watchers) Sweetener	1 gm	–	5	–
SUMMER SAUSAGE (*See* SAUSAGE)				
SUN-DRIED TOMATO (*See* TOMATO)				
SUNFISH/PUMPKINSEED				
fresh				
cooked-dry heat	3 oz	0.5	97	5%
raw	3 oz	0.5	76	6%
SUNFLOWER SEED BUTTER				
(Erewhon)	2 Tbs	18.0	200	81%
generic	1 Tbs	8.0	93	78%
	1 oz	13.6	165	74%

Food and Description	Amount	Fat Grams	Total Calories	% Fat Calories
(Hain)	2 Tbs	15.0	180	75%
(Kettle) Roaster fresh	2 Tbs	14.0	160	79%
SUNFLOWER SEED FLOUR (*See* FLOUR)				
SUNFLOWER SEEDS/NUTS				
(Arrowhead Mills) hulled	¼ cup	15.0	180	75%
(David)				
shelled kernels	¼ cup	17.0	200	77%
unshelled seeds	¼ cup	15.0	190	71%
(Fisher)				
dry-roasted	1 oz	14.0	170	74%
oil-roasted	1 oz	15.0	170	79%
salted in shell				
shelled kernels	1 oz	14.0	160	79%
unshelled seeds	1 oz	15.0	170	79%
(Frito-Lay)	1 oz	15.0	180	75%
generic				
dried	1 oz	14.0	162	78%
	1 cup	71.0	821	78%
dry-roasted	1 oz	14.0	165	76%
	1 cup	64.0	745	77%
oil-roasted	1 oz	16.0	175	82%
	1 cup	77.5	830	84%
oil-roasted/toasted	1 oz	16.0	176	82%
	1 cup	76.0	829	83%
(Lance)				
shelled kernels/roasted	1⅛ oz	16.0	190	76%
	¼ cup	14.0	170	74%
unshelled seeds	½ cup	11.0	140	71%
	1⅞ oz	14.0	170	74%
(Laura Scudders)				
oil-roasted	1 oz	17.0	190	81%
roasted in shell	1 oz	7.0	86	73%
(Planters)				
dry-roasted				
shelled kernels	¼ cup	17.0	190	81%
unshelled seeds				
original	¾ cup	15.0	160	84%
plain				
Munch 'N Go	0.75 oz	11.0	120	83%
regular	3.25 oz	20.0	230	78%
honey-roasted/shelled kernels	1.7 oz	22.0	280	71%
oil-roasted/shelled kernels				
BBQ				
Munch 'N Go	¼ cup	17.0	200	77%
regular	1.7 oz	25.0	290	78%
plain				
regular	1.7 oz	25.0	290	78%
	2 oz	29.0	340	77%
Munch 'N Go	¼ cup	17.0	200	77%
salted/shelled kernels	1 oz	14.0	170	74%

Food and Description	Amount	Fat Grams	Total Calories	% Fat Calories
SURIMI (*See also* CRAB, IMITATION; SEAFOOD ENTRÉE/DINNER; SHRIMP, IMITATION)				
	3 oz	0.8	84	9%
SUSHI (*See* ASIAN FOOD)				
SWAMP CABBAGE				
fresh/boiled	½ cup	–	10	–
SWEET & SOUR SAUCE (*See* ASIAN FOOD/SAUCES & SEASONINGS; SAUCE)				
SWEET POTATO (*See also* SWEET POTATO LEAVES; YAM)				
canned				
generic				
mashed	1 cup	0.5	258	2%
pieces	1 cup	<1.0	183	3%
w/syrup	1 cup	<1.0	212	2%
(Princella)				
candied	½ cup	–	240	–
in heavy syrup	½ cup	–	130	–
in light syrup	⅔ cup	0.5	160	3%
in pineapple-orange sauce	½ cup	–	210	–
in water	½ cup	–	90	–
mashed	⅔ cup	1.0	120	8%
(Royal Prince)				
candied	½ cup	1.0	210	4%
in heavy syrup	½ cup	–	130	–
in light syrup	½ cup	–	100	–
orange/pineapple	½ cup	1.0	210	4%
dried/generic				
flakes				
mix only	½ cup	<1.0	228	2%
prepared w/water	1 cup	<1.0	242	2%
fresh				
baked-mashed	½ cup	<1.0	103	4%
boiled-mashed/no skin	½ cup	0.5	172	3%
raw				
whole/5" long,/~2" dia	1 potato	<1.0	135	3%
pieces	½ cup	1.0	118	5%
frozen/generic/baked	½ cup	<1.0	88	5%
SWEET POTATO DISH				
frozen				
(Mrs. Paul's)				
candied sweet potatoes	5 oz	1.0	300	3%
candied sweets 'n apples	1¼ cup	–	270	–
homemade/USDA Standard Home Recipe				
candied sweet potatoes w/butter & brown sugar	~3.5 oz	3.0	145	19%
SWEET POTATO LEAVES/fresh				
cooked	½ cup	–	11	–
	4 oz	<1.0	40	7%
raw/chopped	½ cup	–	6	–
SWEET ROLL (*See* PASTRY)				
SWEETBREADS (*See* individual meat listings)				
SWEETENER, ARTIFICIAL (*See* SUGAR SUBSTITUTE)				

Food and Description	Amount	Fat Grams	Total Calories	% Fat Calories
SWISS CHARD (*See* CHARD)				
SWORDFISH				
fresh				
breaded & fried	3 oz	12.0	207	52%
cooked-dry heat	3 oz	4.0	132	27%
raw	3 oz	3.0	103	26%
frozen				
(Stilwell's FanSea) steaks/raw	4 oz	6.0	140	39%
SYRUP (*See* CORN SYRUP; ICE CREAM TOPPING; MAPLE SYRUP; PANCAKE & WAFFLE SYRUP; RICE SYRUP; SORGHUM SYRUP)				

T

Food and Description	Amount	Fat Grams	Total Calories	% Fat Calories
TABASCO SAUCE (*See* SAUCE)				
TABOULI/TABOULE/TABOULY				
(Casbah) mix/prepared	⅔ cup	<1.0	90	5%
(CedarLane) tabouli salad	½ cup	12.0	180	60%
(Fantastic Foods) tabouli salad/mix only	2 Tbs	–	70	–
(Near East) wheat salad mix/prepared	⅔ cup	3.0	120	23%
TACO SAUCE (*See* SAUCE)				
TAHINI (*See* SESAME BUTTER)				
TAMALE (*See* MEXICAN FOOD; FROZEN ENTRÉE/DINNER)				
TAMARIND /fresh	1 medium	–	5	–
TANGELO /fresh	1 medium	–	39	–
TANGELO JUICE /fresh	8 fl oz	–	100	–
TANGERINE (*See also* MANDARIN ORANGE)				
canned				
in juice	½ cup	–	46	–
in syrup	½ cup	–	76	–
fresh/whole	1 medium	–	37	–
(Dole)	2 medium	–	70	–
TANGERINE JUICE				
canned				
sweetened	8 fl oz	–	125	–
unsweetened	8 fl oz	–	107	–
fresh	8 fl oz	–	108	–
frozen concentrate				
generic				
prepared	8 fl oz	–	114	–
undiluted	6 oz	<1.0	345	1%

Food and Description	Amount	Fat Grams	Total Calories	% Fat Calories
(Minute Maid)	8 fl oz	–	120	–
TAPIOCA (*See also* PUDDING)				
generic				
pearl/dry	⅓ cup	–	174	–
starch	3 oz	–	300	–
(Minute)	1½ tsp	–	20	–
	3.5 oz	–	352	–
TARO				
chips (*See also* POTATO CHIPS)	10 chips	6.0	110	49%
leaves				
raw	½ cup	–	12	–
steamed	½ cup	<1.0	17	27%
root/fresh/sliced				
cooked	½ cup	–	94	–
raw	½ cup	–	56	–
shoots/fresh/sliced				
cooked	½ cup	–	10	–
raw	½ cup	–	5	–
Tahitian/fresh/sliced				
cooked	½ cup	<1.0	30	15%
raw	½ cup	1.0	25	36%
TARRAGON /ground	1 tsp	–	5	–
TARTAR SAUCE (*See* SAUCE)				
TEA				
bags				
(Bigelow)				
herbal				
almond orange	1 bag	–	–	–
apple orchard	1 bag	–	–	–
chamomile	1 bag	–	–	–
chamomile-mint	1 bag	–	–	–
cranapple	1 bag	–	–	–
fruit & almond	1 bag	–	–	–
hibiscus & rose hips	1 bag	–	–	–
I Love Lemon	1 bag	–	–	–
lemon & C	1 bag	–	–	–
mint medley	1 bag	–	–	–
orange & spice	1 bag	–	–	–
raspberry royale	1 bag	–	–	–
red raspberry	1 bag	–	–	–
sweet dreams	1 bag	–	–	–
take a break	1 bag	–	–	–
regular				
Chinese fortune	1 bag	–	–	–
cinnamon stick	1 bag	–	–	–
Constant Comment/orange spice	1 bag	–	–	–
Earl Gray				
decaffeinated	1 bag	–	–	–
regular	1 bag	–	–	–
English teatime	1 bag	–	–	–

Food and Description	Amount	Fat Grams	Total Calories	% Fat Calories
lemon lift				
decaffeinated	1 bag	–	–	–
regular	1 bag	–	–	–
plantation mint	1 bag	–	–	–
raspberry royale	1 bag	–	–	–
(Celestial Seasonings)				
herbal				
almond sunset	1 bag	–	3	–
Bengal spice	1 bag	–	5	–
chamomile	1 bag	–	2	–
cinnamon apple spice	1 bag	–	–	–
cinnamon rose	1 bag	–	–	–
country peach spice	1 bag	–	3	–
cranberry cove	1 bag	–	2	–
Emperor's choice	1 bag	–	4	–
ginseng plus	1 bag	–	3	–
Grandma's tummy mint	1 bag	–	2	–
harvest spice	1 bag	–	5	–
lemon mist	1 bag	–	3	–
lemon zinger	1 bag	–	5	–
Mandarin orange spice	1 bag	–	5	–
mellow mint	1 bag	–	2	–
mint magic	1 bag	–	1	–
orange zinger	1 bag	–	5	–
peppermint	1 bag	–	2	–
raspberry patch	1 bag	–	4	–
red zinger	1 bag	–	4	–
sleepytime	1 bag	–	–	–
spearmint	1 bag	–	5	–
strawberry fields	1 bag	–	4	–
Sunburst C	1 bag	–	3	–
tropical escape	1 bag	–	1	–
wild forest blackberry	1 bag	–	–	–
regular				
cinnamon Vienna	1 bag	–	2	–
Earl Gray extraordinary	1 bag	–	3	–
English breakfast	1 bag	–	3	–
lemon	1 bag	–	7	–
mint	1 bag	–	4	–
Morning Thunder	1 bag	–	3	–
orange spice				
decaffeinated	1 bag	–	7	–
regular	1 bag	–	7	–
organically grown	1 bag	–	12	–
raspberry	1 bag	–	7	–
(Good Earth) original herb & tea				
caffeine-free	1 bag	–	5	–
regular	1 bag	–	–	–
(Lipton)				
bedtime story	1 bag	–	–	–

Food and Description	Amount	Fat Grams	Total Calories	% Fat Calories
chamomile (100% pure)	1 bag	–	–	
cinnamon apple	1 bag	–	–	–
citrus blossom	1 bag	–	–	–
country cranberry	1 bag	–	–	–
gentle orange	1 bag	–	–	–
ginger twist	1 bag	–	–	–
golden honey lemon	1 bag	–	–	–
green	1 bag	–	–	–
lemon soother	1 bag	–	–	–
Oriental treasure	1 bag	–	–	–
plain	1 bag	–	–	–
quietly chamomile	1 bag	–	–	–
wild berry basket	1 bag	–	–	–
(Luzianne)				
decaffeinated	1 bag	–	–	–
regular	1 bag	–	–	–
(Nestea)	1 bag	–	–	–
(Tetley)				
decaffeinated	1 bag	–	–	–
regular	1 bag	–	–	–
bottled, boxed, or canned				
(Arizona Tea) iced				
lemon				
diet	8 fl oz	–	4	–
regular	8 fl oz	–	100	–
mucho mango	8 fl oz	–	100	–
raspberry	8 fl oz	–	100	–
w/ginseng	8 fl oz	–	60	–
(Lipton) iced/brisk				
green tea w/honey	8 fl oz	–	70	–
lemon				
diet	8 fl oz	–	–	–
regular	8 fl oz	–	90	–
peach				
diet	8 fl oz	–	–	–
regular	8 fl oz	–	110	–
raspberry	8 fl oz	–	110	–
sweetened w/lemon	8 fl oz	–	70	–
unsweetened/no lemon	8 fl oz	–	–	–
(Schweppes) iced	8 fl oz	–	90	–
(Snapple)				
caffeine-free	8 fl oz	–	100	–
cranberry-raspberry/diet	8 fl oz	–	10	–
just plain tea/cactus tea-unsweetened	8 fl oz	–	100	
ginseng	8 fl oz	–	80	–
green	8 fl oz	–	100	–
lemon				
decaffeinated	8 fl oz	–	100	

Food and Description	Amount	Fat Grams	Total Calories	% Fat Calories
diet	8 fl oz	–	–	–
	11.5 fl oz	–	5	–
regular	8 fl oz	–	110	–
	11.5 fl oz	–	140	–
lemonade iced tea	8 fl oz	–	110	–
lightening-ginseng black tea	8 fl oz	–	90	–
mango	8 fl oz	–	110	–
mint	8 fl oz	–	110	–
moon-green tea	8 fl oz	–	90	–
orange	8 fl oz	–	110	–
passion fruit	8 fl oz	–	110	–
peach				
diet	8 fl oz	–	–	–
regular	8 fl oz	–	100	–
	11.5 fl oz	–	150	–
raspberry				
diet	8 fl oz	–	–	–
regular	8 fl oz	–	100	–
	11.5 fl oz	–	150	–
strawberry	8 fl oz	–	100	–
sun tea				
diet	8 fl oz	–	–	–
regular	8 fl oz	–	90	–
sweet tea	8 fl oz	–	120	–
(Southwest) sun tea				
diet	12 fl oz	–	–	–
regular	12 fl oz	–	135	–
(Tropicana) fruit tea				
lemon				
diet	8 fl oz	–	15	–
regular	8 fl oz	–	100	–
peach	10 fl oz	–	140	–
	11.5 fl oz	–	160	–
raspberry				
diet	8 fl oz	–	15	–
regular	8 fl oz	–	120	–
	10 fl oz	–	140	–
	11.5 fl oz	–	160	–
tangerine	10 fl oz	–	140	–
	11.5 fl oz	–	170	–
brewed				
Russian tea	8 fl oz	–	110	–
loose				
(Lipton)	1 tsp	–	–	–
mix/instant				
(Crystal Light) mix only				
iced tea				
decaffeinated	⅛ tub	–	5	–
regular	⅛ tub	–	5	–

Food and Description	Amount	Fat Grams	Total Calories	% Fat Calories
(General Foods) prepared				
English				
breakfast creme	8 fl oz	2.0	70	26%
raspberry creme				
decaffeinated	8 fl oz	2.0	70	26%
regular	8 fl oz	2.0	70	26%
island orange creme	8 fl oz	2.0	70	26%
Viennese cinnamon creme				
decaffeinated	8 fl oz	2.0	70	26%
regular	8 fl oz	2.0	70	26%
(Lipton) prepared				
citrus	8 fl oz	–	90	–
lemon				
sugar-sweetened	8 fl oz	–	90	–
w/nutrasweet	8 fl oz	–	5	–
plain				
decaffeinated	8 fl oz	–	90	–
sugar-free/decaffeinated or regular	8 fl oz	–	–	–
w/nutrasweet	8 fl oz	–	5	–
(Maxwell House) prepared				
concentrate				
sweetened	8 fl oz	–	80	–
unsweetened	8 fl oz	–	2	–
powder	6 fl oz	–	2	–
(Natural Touch) Kaffree Roma beverage	1 rounded tsp	–	10	–
(Nestea)				
Ice Teasers				
citrus	8 fl oz	–	5	–
lemon	8 fl oz	–	5	–
orange	8 fl oz	–	5	–
tropical	8 fl oz	–	5	–
wild cherry	8 fl oz	–	5	–
regular/2 Tbs prepared				
100%				
decaffeinated	8 fl oz	–	–	–
regular	8 fl oz	–	2	–
lemon & sugar	8 fl oz	–	80	–
sugar-free lemon	8 fl oz	–	2	–
TEFF				
(Arrowhead Mills) seeds	¼ cup	1.0	160	6%
TEMPEH				
generic	½ cup	6.0	165	33%
(White Wave)				
five grain	⅓ block	4.0	140	26%
sea veggie	⅓ block	4.0	140	26%
soy	⅓ block	4.0	140	26%
soy rice	⅓ block	4.0	140	26%
wild rice	⅓ block	4.0	140	26%

TEMPURA BATTER (*See* BAKE & FRY MIX)
TEQUILA (*See* LIQUOR, DISTILLED)

Food and Description	Amount	Fat Grams	Total Calories	% Fat Calories
TERIYAKI SAUCE (*See* SAUCE)				
TERRAPIN/baked	¾ cup	4.0	161	22%
THIRST QUENCHER (*See* SPORTS DRINK; individual flavor listings)				
THURINGER SAUSAGE (*See* SAUSAGE)				
THYME/ground	1 tsp	–	4	–
TILEFISH				
cooked-dry heat	3 oz	3.0	125	22%
raw	3 oz	2.0	80	23%
TOASTER PASTRY (*See* PASTRY, TOASTER)				
TOFU (*See also* VEGETARIAN FOODS)				
(Azumaya)				
blue label	3.5 oz	1.0	50	18%
green label	3.5 oz	2.0	70	26%
name age/fried	3.5 oz	4.0	145	25%
red label	3.5 oz	1.0	70	13%
generic				
firm/raw	¼ block	7.0	118	53%
	½ cup	11.0	183	54%
fried	~½ oz	2.6	35	67%
fuyu/salted & fermented	1 block	1.0	13	69%
koyadofu/dried-frozen	~½ oz	5.0	82	55%
Okara	½ cup	1.0	47	19%
regular/raw	¼ block	5.6	88	57%
	½ cup	5.9	94	57%
(Hinoichi)				
Chinese	4 oz	3.0	70	39%
Japanese	4 oz	2.0	60	30%
kinugoshi	4 oz	2.0	50	36%
(Mori-Nu) silken				
extra firm				
lite	3 oz	0.5	35	13%
regular	3 oz	2.0	60	30%
firm				
lite	3 oz	1.0	35	26%
regular	3 oz	3.0	50	54%
silken	3 oz	2.5	50	45%
(Nasoya)				
extra firm	3 oz	5.0	90	50%
firm	3 oz	4.0	80	45%
5 spice/Chinese	3 oz	4.0	70	51%
French herb	3 oz	4.0	70	51%
silken	3 oz	2.0	50	36%
soft	3 oz	3.0	60	45%
(Tree of Life)				
ground				
hot & spicy	3 oz	4.0	60	60%
original	3 oz	4.0	60	60%
savory garlic	3 oz	4.0	60	60%
smoked				
hot'n spicy	3 oz	5.0	120	38%

Food and Description	Amount	Fat Grams	Total Calories	% Fat Calories
original	3 oz	6.0	120	45%
(White Wave)				
flavored				
Italian	2 oz	6.0	120	45%
Mexican	2 oz	6.0	120	45%
Oriental	2 oz	6.0	120	45%
Thai	2 oz	6.0	120	45%
unflavored				
extra firm style	3 oz	6.0	90	60%
organic				
firm	3 oz	6.0	90	60%
soft	3 oz	6.0	90	60%
TOFU DAIRY YOGURT				
(White Wave) Silk dairyless				
apricot-mango	1 container	2.0	150	12%
banana-strawberry	1 container	2.0	150	12%
blueberry	1 container	2.0	150	12%
cappuccino	1 container	2.0	150	12%
key lime	1 container	2.0	150	12%
lemon	1 container	2.0	150	12%
lemon-kiwi	1 container	2.0	150	12%
orange creme	1 container	2.0	150	12%
peach	1 container	2.0	150	12%
plain	1 container	2.0	150	12%
raspberry	1 container	2.0	150	12%
strawberry	1 container	2.0	150	12%
vanilla	1 container	2.0	150	12%
TOFU DISH (*See* VEGETARIAN FOODS)				
TOFU FROZEN DESSERT				
(Tofutti)				
Better Than Yogurt/low-fat				
chocolate fudge	½ cup	2.0	120	15%
coffee marshmallow	½ cup	1.0	100	9%
peach mango	½ cup	2.0	100	9%
strawberry banana	½ cup	1.0	100	9%
vanilla fudge	½ cup	2.0	120	15%
Cuties sandwiches				
chocolate	1 sandwich	5.0	130	35%
vanilla	1 sandwich	5.0	120	38%
wildberry	1 sandwich	5.0	120	38%
Dessert cakes				
chocolate cannoli	1 slice	13.0	190	62%
chocolate lovers delight	1 slice	10.0	190	47%
rock'n roll	1 slice	10.0	180	50%
sprinkle roll	1 slice	10.0	190	47%
Fruitti				
apricot mango	4 oz	–	100	–
three berry	4 oz	–	100	–
vanilla apple orchard	4 oz	–	100	–

Food and Description	Amount	Fat Grams	Total Calories	% Fat Calories
Low-fat pints				
chocolate fudge	½ cup	2.0	120	15%
coffee marshmallow	½ cup	1.0	100	9%
passion island	½ cup	1.0	100	9%
peach mango	½ cup	1.0	100	9%
strawberry-banana	½ cup	1.0	100	9%
vanilla fudge	½ cup	2.0	120	15%
Premium pints				
better pecan	4 oz	13.0	220	53%
chocolate	4 oz	11.0	180	55%
chocolate cookies	4 oz	11.0	210	47%
vanilla	4 oz	11.0	190	52%
vanilla almond bark	4 oz	13.0	210	56%
vanilla fudge	4 oz	9.0	190	43%
wildberry	4 oz	9.0	190	43%
Slices				
chocolate-covered wildberry	1 serving	10.0	180	50%
cutie pie/vanilla	1 serving	19.0	250	68%
cutie slice/chocolate	1 serving	8.0	140	51%
wildberry	1 serving	2.0	80	23%
Soft serve				
chocolate				
lite	4 oz	1.0	90	10%
regular	4 oz	4.0	190	19%
peanut butter	4 oz	4.0	190	19%
vanilla				
lite	4 oz	1.0	90	10%
regular	4 oz	4.0	190	19%
wild strawberry/lite	4 oz	1.0	90	10%
Sorbet				
chocolate	4 oz	–	90	–
coffee	4 oz	–	80	–
lemon	4 oz	–	90	–
orange peach mango	4 oz	–	90	–
raspberry	4 oz	–	80	–
strawberry	4 oz	–	80	–
Sticks				
chocolate fruitti bars	1 bar	5.0	120	38%
chocolate fudge treats	1 treat	–	30	–
crumb cake bars	1 bar	15.0	220	61%
Monkey bars/peanut butter	1 bar	13.0	220	53%
Teddy Fudge Bar	1 bar	1.0	70	13%
Sugar-free half gallons				
chocolate fudge	½ cup	–	80	–
strawberry	½ cup	–	80	–
vanilla fudge	½ cup	–	80	–
Too-Too's cookie sandwiches				
vanilla	1 sandwich	10.0	210	43%
vanilla/chocolate chip	1 sandwich	11.0	230	43%
vanilla/chocolate swirl	1 sandwich	11.0	230	43%

Food and Description	Amount	Fat Grams	Total Calories	% Fat Calories
TOMATO				
canned or jarred				
(Claussen) halves	1 oz	–	5	–
(Contadina)				
crushed	¼ cup	–	20	–
in tomato puree	¼ cup	–	20	–
w/Italian herbs	¼ cup	–	20	–
w/roasted garlic	¼ cup	–	20	–
diced				
original	½ cup	–	30	–
w/Italian herbs	½ cup	–	45	–
w/roasted garlic	½ cup	–	45	–
w/sauteed onions	½ cup	–	40	–
stewed				
Italian style	½ cup	–	35	–
original w/onions, celery, & green peppers	½ cup	–	35	–
whole/peeled	½ cup	–	25	–
(Del Monte)				
crushed				
Italian recipe	½ cup	–	45	–
original recipe	½ cup	–	45	–
w/garlic	½ cup	–	50	–
diced				
no salt added	½ cup	–	25	–
original	½ cup	–	25	–
w/basil, garlic, & oregano	½ cup	–	50	–
w/garlic & onion	½ cup	–	40	–
w/green chili peppers	½ cup	–	30	–
w/green pepper & onion	½ cup	–	40	–
w/jalapeños	½ cup	–	30	–
chunky				
chili style	½ cup	–	30	–
pasta style	½ cup	–	45	–
stewed				
Cajun recipe	½ cup	–	35	–
Italian recipe	½ cup	–	30	–
Mexican recipe	½ cup	–	35	–
original no salt added	½ cup	–	35	–
Regular	½ cup	–	35	–
wedges	½ cup	–	35	–
whole/peeled in juice	½ cup	–	25	–
(Green Giant) stewed				
classic recipe	½ cup	–	35	–
Italian recipe	½ cup	–	30	–
Mexican recipe	½ cup	–	35	–
(Hebrew National) pickled	1 oz	–	4	–
(Hunt's)				
choice				
cut	½ cup	–	22	–

Food and Description	Amount	Fat Grams	Total Calories	% Fat Calories
cut/diced				
w/green chilies	2 Tbs	–	1	–
w/roasted garlic	½ cup	–	24	–
w/Italian herb	½ cup	–	24	–
crushed				
Angela Mia	½ cup	–	27	–
original	½ cup	<1.0	30	15%
pear-shaped	½ cup	–	20	–
whole				
no salt added	2 tomatoes	<1.0	20	22%
original	2 tomatoes	–	20	–
stewed				
no salt added	½ cup	<1.0	33	8%
original	½ cup	<1.0	33	8%
whole	2 tomatoes	–	20	–
(Muir Glen) organic				
crushed w/basil	¼ cup	–	25	–
diced				
no salt added	½ cup	–	25	–
original	½ cup	–	25	–
w/basil & garlic	½ cup	–	25	–
w/garlic & onion	½ cup	–	25	–
w/green chilies	½ cup	–	25	–
w/Italian herbs	½ cup	–	25	–
ground peeled	¼ cup	–	10	–
salsa				
black bean & corn	2 Tbs	–	15	–
chipotle/medium	2 Tbs	–	15	–
fire roasted/medium	2 Tbs	–	10	–
garlic cilantro/medium	2 Tbs	–	10	–
habanero hot	2 Tbs	–	10	–
medium	2 Tbs	–	10	–
mild	2 Tbs	–	10	–
roasted garlic/medium	2 Tbs	–	10	–
stewed	½ cup	–	30	–
whole peeled				
original	½ cup	–	30	–
w/basil	½ cup	–	30	–
(Progresso)				
crushed	¼ cup	–	20	–
peeled				
Italian style	½ cup	–	20	–
whole	½ cup	–	25	–
(Rosoff's) pickled/half sour	1 oz	–	5	–
(Ro*Tel)				
diced				
extra hot	½ cup	–	25	–
Mexican fiesta	½ cup	–	30	–
Italian harvest	½ cup	–	30	–
w/green chilies	½ cup	–	20	–

Food and Description	Amount	Fat Grams	Total Calories	% Fat Calories
whole/w/green chilies	½ cup	–	20	–
(S&W)				
crushed	½ cup	–	20	–
Italian style/pear	½ cup	–	25	–
no salt	½ cup	–	35	–
ready-cut/diced				
caramelized	½ cup	–	35	–
fire-roasted	½ cup	–	35	–
Italian style	½ cup	–	25	–
Mexican recipe	½ cup	–	35	–
no salt	½ cup	–	25	–
peeled	½ cup	–	25	–
roasted garlic	½ cup	0.5	30	15%
salsa				
medium	¼ cup	–	20	–
mild	¼ cup	–	20	–
w/chipotle	¼ cup	–	20	–
w/cilantro	¼ cup	–	20	–
stewed				
Cajun	½ cup	–	35	–
Italian style	½ cup	–	35	–
original	½ cup	–	35	–
whole				
no salt	½ cup	–	20	–
(Schorr's)				
pickled	1 oz	–	4	–
stewed	½ cup	–	35	–
(Stokely)				
stewed	½ cup	–	35	–
whole	½ cup	–	25	–
fresh				
green	1 medium	–	30	–
red				
chopped or diced	1 cup	–	35	–
whole	1 medium	–	24	–
frozen				
(C&W) vine-ripened tomatoes/diced	¾ cup	–	20	–
sun-dried				
generic				
in oil	1 piece	1.0	6	–
	1 cup	15.0	235	57%
plain	1 piece	–	5	–
	1 cup	2.0	140	3%
(Sonoma)				
bits	2-3 tsp	–	15	–
halves	2-3 halves	–	15	–
julienne	7-9 pieces	–	15	–
pickled spice medley/oil drained	1 Tbs	4.0	50	72%
TOMATO ASPIC /canned				
(S&W) supreme	½ cup	–	50	–

Food and Description	Amount	Fat Grams	Total Calories	% Fat Calories
TOMATO JUICE/JUICE BLEND				
(Campbell's)				
Healthy Request				
low-sodium	8 fl oz	–	50	–
regular	8 fl oz	–	50	–
original	8 fl oz	–	50	–
	11.5 fl oz	–	70	–
(Del Monte)				
from concentrate	8 fl oz	–	50	–
not from concentrate	8 fl oz	–	40	–
Snap-E-Tom/tomato & chile cocktail	6 fl oz	–	40	–
generic				
plain	6 fl oz	–	32	–
tomato & clam	5.5 fl oz	–	77	–
tomato w/beef broth	5.5 fl oz	–	60	–
(Knudsen)				
organic	8 fl oz	–	60	–
tomato garlic	8 fl oz	–	60	–
(Libby's)	6 fl oz	–	35	–
(Mott's)				
Beefamato	8 fl oz	–	80	–
Clamato	8 fl oz	–	100	–
Clamato Caesar	8 fl oz	–	100	–
(Muir Glen) organic	5.5 fl oz	–	40	–
(S&W)	5.5 fl oz	–	30	–
	8 fl oz	–	40	–
(Stokely)	4 fl oz	–	20	–
TOMATO PASTE /canned				
(Contadina)				
100% tomatoes	2 Tbs	–	30	–
Italian				
w/Italian seasonings	2 Tbs	–	35	–
w/roasted garlic	2 Tbs	–	35	–
w/tomato pesto	2 Tbs	–	35	–
(Del Monte)	2 Tbs	–	30	–
generic	½ cup	1.0	110	8%
(Hunt's)				
Italian style	2 Tbs	<1.0	30	15%
no salt added	2 Tbs	<1.0	30	15%
original	2 Tbs	<1.0	27	16%
w/garlic	2 Tbs	<1.0	28	9%
(Muir Glen) organic	2 Tbs	–	30	–
(Progresso)	2 Tbs	–	30	–
(S&W)	6 oz	–	150	–
TOMATO POWDER	4 oz	<1.0	342	1%
TOMATO PURÉE /canned				
(Contadina)	¼ cup	–	20	–
(Hunt's)	4 oz	–	45	–
(Muir Glen) organic	¼ cup	–	20	–
(Progresso)				
original	¼ cup	–	25	–

Food and Description	Amount	Fat Grams	Total Calories	% Fat Calories
thick style	¼ cup	–	20	–
(S&W)				
original	4 oz	–	60	–
w/diced tomatoes	4 oz	–	35	–
TOMATO SAUCE (*See also* MEXICAN FOOD; SAUCE)				
canned				
(Contadina)				
garlic & onion	¼ cup	–	20	–
Italian	¼ cup	–	15	–
original	¼ cup	–	15	–
thick & zesty	¼ cup	–	20	–
(Del Monte)				
original	¼ cup	–	20	–
no salt added	¼ cup	–	20	–
(Hunt's)				
ready sauce				
chunky chili	¼ cup	<1.0	21	18%
chunky Italian	¼ cup	<1.0	26	14%
chunky Mexican	¼ cup	–	21	–
chunky special	¼ cup	<1.0	21	25%
chunky tomato	¼ cup	–	15	–
country herb	¼ cup	1.0	33	27%
garlic	¼ cup	1.0	29	31%
garlic & herb	¼ cup	<1.0	26	12%
meat loaf fixins	¼ cup	<1.0	23	19%
original Italian	¼ cup	1.0	30	30%
salsa	¼ cup	–	17	–
regular				
Italian	¼ cup	1.0	32	28%
no salt added	¼ cup	–	15	–
original	¼ cup	–	15	–
w/herb	¼ cup	1.0	32	28%
(Muir Glen) organic				
chunky	¼ cup	–	20	–
no salt added	¼ cup	–	20	–
regular	¼ cup	–	20	–
(Progresso)	¼ cup	–	20	–
(S&W)				
garden				
Italian herb	¼ cup	–	35	–
mild Mexican	¼ cup	–	20	–
original	¼ cup	–	20	–
plain	¼ cup	–	20	–
TOMATO SOUP (*See* SOUP)				
TONIC WATER (*See* COCKTAIL MIXER)				
TORTELLINI (*See* PASTA)				
TORTILLA (*See* MEXICAN FOOD)				
TORTILLA CHIPS/CORN CHIPS				
(Arizona)				
original	1 oz	6.0	140	39%

Food and Description	Amount	Fat Grams	Total Calories	% Fat Calories
restaurant style	1 oz	7.0	140	45%
(Azteca) Buenitos	1 oz	7.0	140	45%
(Barbara's)				
blue corn chips				
no salt added	1 oz	7.0	140	45%
regular	1 oz	7.0	140	45%
pinta chips/salsa	1 oz	6.0	130	42%
(Borden)				
corn chips	1 oz	10.0	160	56%
Dipsy Doodles				
mesquite barbecue	1 oz	10.0	160	56%
rippled	1 oz	10.0	160	56%
Doodle Twisters				
nacho cheese	1 oz	10.0	160	56%
nacho chips/thinner crispier	1 oz	8.0	150	48%
white tortilla chips				
crispy rounds	1 oz	8.0	150	48%
quarter rounds/restaurant style	1 oz	8.0	150	48%
yellow tortilla chips				
deli chips/triangles	1 oz	8.0	150	48%
deli rounds	1 oz	8.0	150	48%
(Doritos)				
baja picante	1 oz	7.0	140	45%
cooler ranch				
3D's	1 oz	6.0	140	39%
original	1 oz	7.0	140	45%
flamin' hot	1 oz	7.0	140	45%
nacho cheesier				
3D's	1 oz	7.0	140	45%
original	1 oz	7.0	140	45%
salsa verde	1 oz	7.0	150	48%
smokey red BBQ	1 oz	7.0	150	48%
sonic sour cream	1 oz	7.0	140	45%
spicy nacho	1 oz	6.0	140	39%
taco supreme	1 oz	7.0	140	45%
toasted corn	1 oz	7.0	140	45%
zesty salsa	1 oz	7.0	140	45%
(Fritos)				
Bar-B-Q	1 oz	10.0	150	60%
cheddar & sour cream	1 oz	10.0	160	56%
chili cheese	1 oz	10.0	160	56%
choice	1 oz	10.0	160	56%
king size	1 oz	10.0	160	56%
mesquite grille BBQ	1 oz	10.0	160	56%
original	1 oz	10.0	160	56%
racerz				
honey BBQ	1 oz	11.0	160	62%
nacho cheese	1 oz	11.0	160	62%
original	1 oz	11.0	160	62%
Sabrositas				
flamin' hot	1 oz	10.0	160	56%

Food and Description	Amount	Fat Grams	Total Calories	% Fat Calories
lime'n chile	1 oz	9.0	150	54%
scoops	1 oz	10.0	160	56%
Texas grill honey BBQ	1 oz	9.0	150	54%
(Garden of Eatin')				
black bean	1 oz	7.0	150	42%
blue corn	1 oz	7.0	150	42%
jalapeño				
no salt added	1 oz	7.0	140	45%
salted	1 oz	7.0	140	45%
mini	1 oz	7.0	150	42%
red hot blues	1 oz	7.0	150	42%
(Guiltless Gourmet) baked				
blue corn/organic	1 oz	2.0	110	16%
chili lime	1 oz	2.0	110	16%
mucho nacho	1 oz	2.0	110	16%
red corn	1 oz	2.0	110	8%
spicy black bean	1 oz	2.0	110	16%
sweet white corn	1 oz	2.0	110	16%
yellow corn				
no salt	1 oz	1.0	110	8%
regular	1 oz	2.0	110	16%
(Hain)				
sesame				
no salt	1 oz	7.0	140	45%
regular	1 oz	7.0	140	45%
sesame cheese	1 oz	8.0	160	45%
taco style/no salt	1 oz	11.0	160	62%
(Kettle)				
blue corn	1 oz	6.0	140	39%
five grain yellow corn	1 oz	6.0	140	39%
Little Dippers	1 oz	6.0	140	39%
Sesame Blue Moons	1 oz	8.0	150	48%
sesame rye w/caraway	1 oz	6.0	140	39%
sweet brown rice & black bean	1 oz	6.0	120	45%
(La Famous)				
no salt	1 oz	7.0	140	45%
regular	1 oz	7.0	140	45%
(Lance)				
corn chips				
BBQ	1¼ oz	14.0	210	60%
plain	1 oz	10.0	160	56%
	1¼ oz	13.0	200	59%
	1½ oz	15.0	240	56%
tortilla chips				
nacho chips	1 oz	7.0	140	45%
nacho triangles	1 oz	7.0	140	45%
white corn round	1¼ oz	10.0	190	47%
(Laura Scudder's)				
nacho				
jalapeño strips	1 oz	7.0	150	42%

Food and Description	Amount	Fat Grams	Total Calories	% Fat Calories
triangles	1 oz	7.0	140	45%
restaurant style				
lightly salted	1 oz	7.0	140	45%
picante strips	1 oz	7.0	150	42%
(Mi Ranchito)				
restaurant style	1 oz	7.0	140	45%
traditional	1 oz	7.0	140	45%
white corn	1 oz	6.0	140	39%
(Michael Season's) organic				
blue corn				
hot & spicy	1 oz	7.0	140	45%
sesame	1 oz	9.0	150	54%
mini yellow	1 oz	6.0	140	39%
salsa/yellow corn	1 oz	6.0	140	39%
white corn/slightly salted	1 oz	6.0	140	39%
(Mission) authentic Mexican tortilla chips				
blue corn	1 oz	7.0	140	45%
rounds	1 oz	7.0	140	45%
triangles	1 oz	7.0	140	45%
tortilla strips				
regular	1 oz	7.0	140	45%
unsalted	1 oz	7.0	140	45%
(Old El Paso)				
Nachips	9 chips	8.0	150	48%
white corn	11 chips	8.0	140	51%
(Old Vienna) deli rounds				
salted	1 oz	7.0	150	42%
white corn	1 oz	6.0	140	39%
(Pringles)				
fresh roasted	1 oz	7.0	140	45%
mild nacho cheese	1 oz	7.0	140	45%
(Rancho California)				
guacamole	1 oz	7.0	155	41%
macho nacho	1 oz	7.0	150	42%
(Santitas)				
100% white corn	1 oz	6.0	130	42%
restaurant style strips	1 oz	6.0	130	42%
(Snyder's)				
corn chips				
BBQ	1½ oz	14.0	230	55%
original	1½ oz	15.0	230	54%
tortilla chips				
nacho	1 oz	3.5	130	24%
white corn	1 oz	3.0	120	23%
yellow corn				
mini	1 oz	6.0	140	39%
regular	1 oz	3.0	120	23%
unsalted	1 oz	3.0	120	23%
(Taco Bell) restaurant style	12 chips	6 0	140	39%

Food and Description	Amount	Fat Grams	Total Calories	% Fat Calories
(Tostitos)				
baked				
bite size				
cheddar quesadilla	1 oz	3.0	120	23%
original	1 oz	1.0	110	8%
salsa & cream cheese	1 oz	3.0	120	23%
cool ranch	1 oz	3.0	120	23%
original	1 oz	1.0	110	8%
unsalted	1 oz	1.0	110	8%
original				
bite-size	1 oz	8.0	140	51%
crispy rounds	1 oz	7.0	140	45%
restaurant style				
hint of lime	1 oz	6.0	140	39%
white corn	1 oz	6.0	150	36%
Santa Fe gold	1 oz	6.0	140	39%
(Tyson)				
nacho cheese	1 oz	7.0	140	45%
ranch flavor	1 oz	7.0	140	45%
traditional	1 oz	7.0	140	45%
unsalted	1 oz	7.0	140	45%
(Wise) Bravos				
crispy rounds	1 oz	8.0	150	48%
nacho nacho!	1 oz	8.0	150	48%
restaurant style	1 oz	8.0	150	48%
(Wow)				
Doritos nacho cheesier	1 oz	1.0	90	10%
Tostitos original	1 oz	1.0	90	10%

TRAIL MIX (See CEREAL; FRUIT SNACK; MIXED NUTS; SNACK MIX)
TREACLE (See MOLASSES)
TRIPE

(Armour)				
Bannersausage				
stomachs	2 oz	5.0	90	50%
tripe	2 oz	5.0	90	50%
beef tripe	3 oz	1.5	90	20%

TRITICALE (See also FLOUR)

whole-grain	1 oz	0.5	95	5%
	1 cup	4.0	645	6%

TROUT

mixed species				
cooked-dry heat	3 oz	6.5	165	35%
raw	3 oz	5.0	125	36%
rainbow				
farmed				
cooked-dry heat	3 oz	5.5	145	34%
raw	3 oz	4.0	120	30%
wild				
cooked-dry heat	3 oz	4.5	130	31%
raw	3 oz	2.6	100	23%
smoked	3 oz	3.0	153	18%

Food and Description	Amount	Fat Grams	Total Calories	% Fat Calories
sea/mixed species				
cooked-dry heat	3 oz	3.0	115	23%
raw	3 oz	2.0	90	20%
TUNA (See also SEAFOOD ENTRÉE/DINNER; TUNA DISH; VEGETARIAN FOODS)				
canned/drained				
(Bumble Bee)				
chunk light				
in oil/drained	2 oz	6.0	110	40%
in water	2 oz	0.5	60	8%
chunk white				
in oil/drained	2 oz	12.0	160	68%
in water	2 oz	2.0	70	26%
solid white				
in oil/drained	2 oz	8.0	130	55%
in water	2 oz	1.0	60	15%
(Carnation) chunk light				
in oil	2 oz	8.0	125	58%
in water	2 oz	1.0	60	15%
(Chicken Of The Sea)				
chunk light				
in canola oil	2 oz	6.0	110	49%
	2.8 oz	8.0	140	41%
in spring water				
50% less salt	2 oz	0.5	60	8%
low sodium	2 oz	0.5	60	8%
regular	2 oz	0.5	60	8%
	2.8 oz	1.0	90	10%
chunk white				
albacore/in spring water	2 oz	1.0	60	15%
low sodium	2.8 oz	1.0	90	10%
very low sodium/in spring water	2 oz	0.5	60	15%
solid light Genova tonno/	2 oz	8.0	110	65%
in olive oil	2.9 oz	12.0	130	83%
solid white				
in canola oil	2 oz	3.0	90	30%
in spring water	2 oz	1.0	70	13%
	2.9 oz	1.0	100	9%
Tonggol chunk light/in water	2 oz	0.5	60	8%
(Empress) chunk light/in water	2 oz	1.0	60	15%
(Featherweight) chunk light/in water	¼ cup	0.5	60	8%
generic				
light				
in oil	3 oz	7.0	169	37%
in water	3 oz	<1.0	111	4%
white				
in oil	2 oz	6.9	158	39%
in water	2 oz	2.0	116	16%
(S&W)				
chunk light				
in oil	2 oz	6.0	110	33%

Food and Description	Amount	Fat Grams	Total Calories	% Fat Calories
in water	2 oz	0.5	70	6%
solid white/in oil	2 oz	1.5	80	17%
(StarKist)				
chunk light				
in oil	2 oz	6.0	110	49%
	2.7 oz	8.0	140	51%
in water	2 oz	0.5	60	8%
	2.7 oz	1.0	80	11%
chunk white				
low-salt, low-fat				
in distilled water	2 oz	0.5	60	8%
	2.7 oz	0.5	80	9%
in spring water	2 oz	0.5	60	8%
	2.7 oz	0.5	70	6%
regular/in water	2 oz	1.0	60	15%
	2.8 oz	1.0	80	11%
Select Prime Light				
chunk light fillets/in spring water	2 oz	1.0	60	15%
solid light				
hickory smoke/in water	2 oz	1.0	60	15%
Gourmet's Choice/drained				
in olive oil	2 oz	12.0	160	68%
in spring water	2 oz	1.0	60	15%
Prime Catch/in water	2 oz	1.0	60	15%
	2.8 oz	1.0	80	11%
solid white				
albacore/in water	2 oz	1.0	100	9%
hickory smoke/in water	2 oz	1.0	70	13%
regular				
in oil	2 oz	3.0	90	30%
	2.8 oz	5.0	130	35%
in water	2 oz	1.0	70	13%
	2.8 oz	1.0	100	9%
fresh				
bluefin				
cooked-dry heat	3 oz	5.0	157	29%
raw	3 oz	4.0	122	30%
skipjack				
cooked-dry heat	3 oz	1.0	112	8%
raw	3 oz	1.0	88	10%
yellowfin				
cooked-dry heat	3 oz	1.0	118	8%
raw	3 oz	1.0	90	10%
TUNA DISH (See also FROZEN ENTRÉE/DINNER; SEAFOOD ENTRÉE/DINNER)				
canned				
(Libby's) The Spreadables tuna salad	⅓ cup	8.0	130	55%
frozen				
(Peter Pan) steaks/skinless-boneless/raw				
while albacore	3.5 oz	5.0	100	45%
yellowfin	3.5 oz	4.0	130	28%

Food and Description	Amount	Fat Grams	Total Calories	% Fat Calories
homemade/USDA Standard Home Recipe				
tuna patty	3 oz	3.0	80	34%
tuna salad made w/salad dressing & tuna canned in oil/no egg	1 cup	19.0	375	46%
mix/kit				
(Bumble Bee) Tuna Salad w/crackers				
fat-free				
crackers	1 pkg	2.0	90	20%
tuna salad	1 can	–	70	–
regular				
crackers	1 pkg	2.0	90	20%
tuna salad	1 can	16.0	190	76%
(Betty Crocker) Tuna Helper				
au gratin				
mix only	½ cup	3.5	190	17%
prepared	1 cup	11.0	300	33%
cheesy broccoli				
mix only	⅔ cup	3.5	200	16%
prepared	1 cup	9.0	290	28%
cheesy noodles				
mix only	⅔ cup	3.0	170	16%
prepared	1 cup	11.0	280	35%
creamy broccoli				
mix only	⅔ cup	4.5	190	21%
prepared	1 cup	12.0	310	35%
creamy pasta				
mix only	¾ cup	6.0	190	28%
prepared	1 cup	13.0	310	38%
fettuccine Alfredo				
mix only	1 cup	3.5	170	19%
prepared	1 cup	14.0	310	41%
garden cheddar				
mix only	⅔ cup	3.5	190	17%
prepared	1 cup	11.0	290	34%
pasta salad				
mix only	⅓ cup	0.5	120	4%
prepared				
low-fat recipe	⅔ cup	2.0	170	11%
regular recipe	⅔ cup	27.0	380	64%
tetrazzini				
mix only	⅔ cup	2.5	180	13%
prepared	1 cup	12.0	300	36%
tuna melt				
mix only	¾ cup	4.5	180	23%
prepared	1 cup	13.0	300	39%
tuna pot pie				
mix only	½ cup	20.0	340	53%
prepared	1 cup	24.0	440	49%
tuna Romanoff				
mix only	⅔ cup	3.0	210	13%

Food and Description	Amount	Fat Grams	Total Calories	% Fat Calories
prepared	1 cup	8.0	280	26%
(StarKist)				
Charlie's Tuna Salad Lunch Kit				
chunk light	1 kit	7.0	210	30%
chunk white	1 kit	7.0	210	30%
Tuna salad & crackers	1 kit	6.0	190	28%
TURBINADO SUGAR (See SUGAR)				
TURBOT				
cooked-dry heat	3 oz	3.0	104	26%
raw	3 oz	2.5	81	28%
TURKEY (See also FRANKFURTER; LUNCHEON MEAT; SAUSAGE)				
■ **TURKEY & TURKEY PARTS/FRESH**				
all classes				
dark meat only/roasted				
w/skin	~2 lb	93.0	1789	47%
w/o skin	~5 oz	10.0	262	34%
chopped/diced	1 cup	9.0	223	36%
giblets & organs/simmered				
giblets	~5 oz	7.0	243	26%
gizzard	~5 oz	5.6	236	21%
heart	~5 oz	8.0	257	28%
liver	~5 oz	8.0	237	30%
light meat only				
w/skin	2¼ lb	87.0	206	38%
w/o skin	~5 oz	4.5	219	19%
chopped/diced	1 cup	4.0	194	19%
meat & skin/dark & light/no giblets	~4 lb	180.6	3857	42%
or neck				
meat only/dark & light	~5 oz	7.0	238	26%
whole/including meat, skin, giblets,	~9 lb	380.0	8245	41%
& neck/roasted				
fryer/roaster/roasted				
back				
w/skin	4 oz	11.5	230	45%
w/o skin	4 oz	6.5	195	30%
breast				
w/skin	4 oz	3.6	175	19%
w/o skin	4 oz	1.0	155	6%
dark meat				
w/skin	4 oz	8.0	206	35%
w/o skin	4 oz	5.0	185	24%
chopped/diced	1 cup	6.0	227	24%
leg				
w/skin	4 oz	6.0	193	28%
w/o skin	4 oz	4.3	180	22%
light meat				
w/skin	4 oz	5.0	185	24%
w/o skin	4 oz	1.3	159	7%
chopped/diced	1 cup	1.7	195	8%

Food and Description	Amount	Fat Grams	Total Calories	% Fat Calories
wing				
w/skin	4 oz	11.2	235	43%
w/o skin	4 oz	3.9	185	19%
young hen/roasted				
back w/skin	4 oz	17.7	288	55%
breast w/skin	4 oz	9.0	220	37%
dark meat				
w/skin	4 oz	14.5	265	49%
w/o skin	4 oz	9.0	220	37%
chopped/diced	1 cup	11.0	270	37%
leg w/skin	4 oz	12.0	245	40%
light meat				
w/skin	4 oz	10.7	235	41%
w/o skin	4 oz	4.0	180	20%
chopped/diced	1 cup	5.0	225	20%
wing w/skin	4 oz	15.3	270	51%
young tom/roasted				
back w/skin	4 oz	15.5	270	52%
breast w/skin	4 oz	8.4	214	35%
dark meat				
w/skin	4 oz	12.3	245	45%
w/o skin	4 oz	8.0	210	34%
chopped/diced	1 cup	10.0	260	35%
leg w/skin	4 oz	11.0	235	42%
light meat				
w/skin	4 oz	8.7	217	36%
w/o skin	4 oz	3.3	175	17%
chopped/diced	1 cup	4.0	215	17%
wing-w/skin	4 oz	13.0	251	47%
■ TURKEY & TURKEY PARTS/FRESH, FROZEN, OR CANNED/BRAND NAME				
(Alpine Lace) breast of turkey/skinless/ oven-roasted	1 oz	–	45	–
(Armour)				
Golden Star	1 oz	4.0	50	72%
loaf	2 oz	8.0	110	65%
Turkey Selects/boneless				
breast				
roast	3 oz	5.0	120	38%
slices	3 oz	1.0	90	10%
tenderloins	3 oz	1.0	90	10%
ground	3 oz	6.0	120	45%
strips	3 oz	4.0	100	36%
(Butterball) fresh premium turkey cuts				
breast				
cutlets	1 cutlet	0.5	80	6%
medallions	4 pieces	1.0	130	7%
roast	4 oz	6.0	160	34%
strips	4 oz	1.0	120	8%
tenderloins/boneless	4 oz	1.0	120	8%

Food and Description	Amount	Fat Grams	Total Calories	% Fat Calories
burger patties	1 piece	9.0	170	48%
ground				
all white	4 oz	3.0	130	21%
regular	4 oz	10.0	180	50%
(Honeysuckle White)				
breast steaks	4 oz	2.5	120	19%
ground/white meat	4 oz	10.0	190	47%
(Hormel)				
chunk turkey/mixed	2 oz	3.0	70	39%
chunk white turkey	2 oz	1.0	60	15%
(Jennie-O) turkey roast w/gravy				
white & dark meat	4 oz	7.0	150	42%
white meat	4 oz	7.0	150	42%
(Louis Rich)				
breaded				
nuggets	4 nuggets	16.0	260	55%
patties	1 patty	13.0	220	53%
sticks	3 sticks	15.0	230	59%
ground				
bulk	4 oz	12.0	190	57%
patties/white	1 patty	10.0	170	53%
(Mr. Turkey)				
cooked				
breast quarter/oven roasted	2 oz	1.0	50	18%
diced white meat	2 oz	2.0	84	21%
smoked breast	1 oz slice	1.5	35	39%
fresh ground				
85 % fat-free	3.5 oz	16.0	210	46%
91% fat-free	3.5 oz	10.0	170	53%
(Perdue)				
Carving Classics turkey breast/pan-roasted				
braised homestyle	2 oz	2.0	70	26%
cracked pepper	2 oz	–	50	–
hickory smoked	2 oz	2.5	70	32%
skinless	2 oz	0.5	60	8%
w/skin	2 oz	2.0	70	26%
Carving turkey breast				
Cajun style	2 oz	1.0	50	18%
honey	2 oz	1.0	50	18%
honey-smoked	2 oz	–	50	
mesquite smoked	2 oz	–	50	–
oven-roasted	2 oz	2.0	70	26%
Deli turkey				
breast/oven-roasted	2 oz	1.0	50	18%
dark pastrami/hickory smoked	2 oz	3.0	70	39%
ham/hickory smoked	2 oz	2.5	60	38%
Fit'N Easy/fresh lean ground				
turkey				
cooked	3 oz	9.0	160	51%
raw	4 oz	9.0	170	48%

Food and Description	Amount	Fat Grams	Total Calories	% Fat Calories
turkey breast				
cooked	3 oz	9.0	160	51%
raw	4 oz	9.0	170	48%
turkey burgers				
cooked	3 oz	9.0	160	51%
raw	4 oz	9.0	170	48%
Fresh/cooked				
cutlets/thin sliced	2.5 oz	1.0	90	10%
drumsticks	3 oz	7.0	150	42%
thighs	3 oz	8.0	160	45%
wing				
drumettes	3 oz	9.0	180	45%
portions	3 oz	8.0	160	45%
wings	3 oz	8.0	160	45%
sausage/cooked				
breakfast	1 link/1.8 oz	7.0	100	63%
hot Italian	1 link/2.8 oz	9.0	150	54%
sweet Italian	1 link/2.4 oz	9.0	150	54%
Healthsense turkey breast/ oven-roasted	2 oz	–	60	–
(Shady Brook) fresh/raw				
cutlets	4 oz	1.0	130	7%
breast				
ground	4 oz	1.0	120	8%
split	4 oz	9.0	190	43%
whole	4 oz	9.0	190	43%
drumstick	4 oz	9.0	170	48%
ground				
85% fat-free	4 oz	15.0	220	61%
lean	4 oz	9.0	170	48%
meatloaf/lean	4 oz	7.0	150	42%
tenderloin				
mesquite	4 oz	1.0	110	8%
unseasoned	4 oz	1.0	130	7%
teriyaki	4 oz	1.0	120	8%
zesty lemon	4 oz	1.0	120	8%
thigh	4 oz	7.0	150	42%
wing	4 oz	14.0	220	57%
(Shelton's) free-range turkey/cooked-frozen				
breakfast strips/uncured	2 slices	10.0	120	75%
meatballs	1 cup	2.5	35	64%
turkey burger	1 patty	10.0	170	53%
(The Turkey Store) fresh				
breast				
Cajun style/fat-free	2 oz	–	60	–
cutlets	3 oz	1.0	90	10%
hickory smoked/fat-free	2 oz	–	60	–
patties/seasoned	4 oz	3.0	130	21%
roast	4 oz	8.0	170	42%
slices	3 oz	1.0	90	10%

Food and Description	Amount	Fat Grams	Total Calories	% Fat Calories
strips	3 oz	1.0	90	10%
tenderloins	3 oz	1.0	90	10%
burger patties				
plain	4 oz	8.0	160	45%
seasoned	4 oz	8.0	160	45%
Classic Patties				
bacon & cheese	5.3 oz	26.0	370	63%
cheese	5.3 oz	25.0	360	63%
mushroom & Swiss	5.e oz	26.0	370	63%
original	5.3 oz	25.0	340	66%
Creative Cuts				
cutlets	4 oz	1.0	120	8%
filets	4 oz	1.0	120	8%
mignons	4 oz	1.0	120	8%
strips	4 oz	1.0	120	8%
ground				
breast	4 oz	1.5	120	11%
lean	4 oz	8.0	160	45%
Italian style /lean	4 oz	10.0	190	47%
Mexican style/lean	4 oz	10.0	190	47%
Premium seasoned turkey breasts				
Cajun	2 oz	–	50	–
cracked pepper	2 oz	–	50	–
garlic pesto	2 oz	–	50	–
homestyle	2 oz	–	50	–
honey Dijon	2 oz	–	50	–
lemon pepper	2 oz	–	50	–
sun dried tomato	2 oz	–	50	–
Seasoned Cuts/boneless, skinless				
chops				
barbecue	4 oz	1.0	130	7%
garlic herb	4 oz	1.0	110	8%
hickory	4 oz	1.0	110	8%
lemon pepper	4 oz	1.0	110	8%
Italian	4 oz	1.0	120	8%
Teriyaki	4 oz	1.0	120	8%
filets				
barbecue	4 oz	1.0	140	6%
garlic herb	4 oz	1.0	120	8%
hickory	4 oz	1.0	110	8%
Italian	4 oz	1.0	110	8%
Lemon pepper	4 oz	1.0	120	8%
Teriyaki	4 oz	1.0	120	8%
Smoked turkey breasts				
honey cured	2 oz	1.0	60	15%
natural hickory smoked	2 oz	1.0	60	15%
natural hickory smoked honey cured	2 oz	1.0	60	15%
(Wampler Longacre) cooked				
Gourmet breast				
brown & glazed	1 oz	1.0	35	26%

Food and Description	Amount	Fat Grams	Total Calories	% Fat Calories
brown & roasted	1 oz	1.0	35	26%
honey-cured	1 oz	1.0	35	26%
mini	1 oz	1.0	35	26%
mini-smoked	1 oz	1.0	35	26%
plain	1 oz	1.0	35	26%
smoked	1 oz	–	30	–
Lean-Lite breast				
Deli				
plain	1 oz	1.0	35	26%
smoked	1 oz	1.0	35	26%
skinless	1 oz	–	35	–
Tenderlings				
BBQ	4 oz	–	110	–
Cajun	4 oz	–	110	–
Garlic & pepper	4 oz	–	110	–
original	4 oz	–	110	–

TURKEY ALTERNATIVE (*See* VEGETARIAN FOODS)
TURKEY BACON (*See* BACON)
TURKEY ENTRÉE/DINNER (*See also* FROZEN ENTRÉE/DINNER; PASTA ENTRÉE/DINNER)

Food and Description	Amount	Fat Grams	Total Calories	% Fat Calories
Can or microwave container				
(Dinty Moore)				
American Classics				
turkey & dressing w/gravy	1 bowl	8.0	290	25%
turkey w/potatoes	1 bowl	7.0	250	25%
Frozen				
generic				
light	2 oz	2.0	42	43%
light & dark	2 oz	2.0	42	43%
turkey roast/light & dark meat	3 oz	5.0	130	35%
	~7 oz	11.0	304	33%
turkey roll				
(Perdue) Perdue Done It!/fully cooked				
breast nuggets	3 oz	9.0	180	45%
fun shapes/turkey-shaped nuggets	3 oz	9.0	180	45%
(Schwan's) partially or fully-cooked				
gourmet turkey breast	3 oz	1.0	90	10%
turkey breast filet/unbreaded	1 filet	–	70	–
Homemade/USDA Standard Home Recipe				
scalloped turkey	~7 oz	5.6	253	20%
turkey loaf	5 oz	15.0	280	48%
turkey sticks/breaded or battered & fried	5 oz	24.0	397	54%
Ready-to-serve				
(Wampler Longacre)				
meatloaf				
Italian	4 oz	5.0	115	39%
Mexican	4 oz	5.0	115	39%
Original	4 oz	5.0	125	36%

TURKEY HAM (*See* HAM; LUNCHEON MEAT)

Food and Description	Amount	Fat Grams	Total Calories	% Fat Calories
TURKEY SAUSAGE (*See* SAUSAGE; TURKEY & TURKEY PARTS/FRESH FROZEN, OR CANNED/BRAND NAME)				
TURKEY SUBSTITUTES (*See* VEGETARIAN FOODS)				
TURMERIC /ground	1 tsp	–	8	–
TURNIP				
fresh				
boiled	½ cup	–	14	–
raw	½ cup	–	18	–
frozen	½ cup	–	26	–
TURNIP GREENS				
canned				
(Bush's Best)	½ cup	–	25	–
generic	½ cup	–	17	–
(Glory Foods)	½ cup	0.5	45	10%
(Luck's) w/diced turnips/seasoned w/pork	½ cup	1.5	35	39%
(Stokely)	½ cup	–	20	–
fresh				
boiled-drained	½ cup	–	15	–
raw	½ cup	–	7	–
frozen				
generic				
plain	½ cup	–	24	–
	10 oz	1.0	60	15%
w/diced turnips	10 oz	0.5	60	8%
(Pictsweet) w/diced turnips	3.3 oz	–	20	–
TURTLE /green				
canned	3 oz	0.6	91	6%
raw	3 oz	<1.0	76	6%

V

Food and Description	Amount	Fat Grams	Total Calories	% Fat Calories
VEAL				
(NOTE: All serving sizes are for cooked portions, unless otherwise stated. "Lean" means veal trimmed of separable fat before cooking. "Lean & fat" means untrimmed and cooked or eaten as purchased. In most cases, 4 ounces of raw veal yields approximately 3 ounces cooked.)				
chop				
lean w/bone/raw	6.5 oz	5.0	170	26%

Food and Description	Amount	Fat Grams	Total Calories	% Fat Calories
cutlet, steak				
lean/boneless/braised or broiled	3 oz	4.0	170	21%
ground/broiled	3 oz	6.0	146	37%
loin				
lean				
braised or broiled	3 oz	8.0	195	37%
roasted	3 oz	6.0	150	36%
lean & fat				
braised or broiled	3 oz	15.0	240	56%
roasted	3 oz	11.0	185	54%
organs				
brain				
braised	3 oz	8.0	120	60%
fried	3 oz	14.0	180	70%
heart/braised	3 oz	6.0	160	34%
kidney/braised	3 oz	5.0	140	32%
liver				
braised	3 oz	6.0	140	39%
fried	3 oz	10.0	210	43%
spleen/braised	3 oz	3.0	110	25%
sweetbreads/braised	3 oz	3.0	145	19%
tongue/braised	3 oz	9.0	170	48%
rib roast				
lean				
braised or broiled	3 oz	7.0	185	34%
roasted	3 oz	6.0	150	36%
lean & fat				
braised or broiled	3 oz	11.0	214	46%
roasted	3 oz	12.0	195	55%
round w/rump				
roasts & leg cutlets/lean/braised or broiled	3 oz	4.0	175	20%
sirloin				
lean				
braised or broiled	3 oz	6.0	175	31%
braised or broiled/chopped	1 cup	9.0	290	28%
roasted	3 oz	5.0	145	31%
roasted/chopped	1 cup	9.0	235	34%
lean & fat				
braised or broiled	3 oz	11.0	220	45%
braised or broiled/chopped	1 cup	18.0	355	45%
roasted	3 oz	9.0	175	46%
roasted/chopped	1 cup	15.0	285	47%
top round				
lean				
roasted	4 oz	6.0	230	23%
roasted/chopped	1 cup	5.0	210	21%
lean & fat				
braised or broiled	4 oz	6.0	230	23%
braised or broiled/chopped	1 cup	7.0	285	22%

Food and Description	Amount	Fat Grams	Total Calories	% Fat Calories
roasted	4 oz	5.0	180	25%
roasted/chopped	1 cup	7.0	225	28%

VEAL DISH (See also FROZEN ENTRÉE/DINNER)
homemade/USDA Standard Home Recipe

veal Parmigiana	~6.5 oz	20.0	351	51%
veal scallopini w/sauce	~3.5 oz	19.0	255	67%

VEGETABLE DISH (See FROZEN ENTRÉE/DINNER; VEGETARIAN FOODS; individual vegetable listings)

VEGETABLE JUICE/JUICE COCKTAIL
bottled, boxed, or canned
(Campbell's) V-8

Healthy Request	8 fl oz	–	50	–
lightly tangy	8 fl oz	–	60	–
low-sodium	8 fl oz	–	60	–
original	8 fl oz	–	50	–
	10 fl oz	–	60	–
picante	8 fl oz	–	50	–
spicy hot	8 fl oz	–	50	–
Splash				
berry blend	1 cup	–	110	–
citrus blend	1 cup	–	120	–
strawberry kiwi	1 cup	–	110	–
tropical blend	1 cup	–	110	–
(DelMonte) vegetable blended cocktail				
Snap-E-Tom/tomato & chile cocktail	6 fl oz	–	40	–
	10 fl oz	–	60	–
(Knudsen)				
Very Veggie	8 fl oz	–	50	–
Viva Vegetable	8 fl oz	–	60	–
(Mott's)	8 fl oz	–	60	–
(Muir Glen) organic				
original	5.5 fl oz	–	50	–
reduced sodium	5.5 fl oz	–	50	–
spicy	5.5 fl oz	–	50	–

VEGETABLE OIL (See COOKING SPRAY; OIL)
VEGETABLE SOUP (See SOUP)
VEGETABLES, MIXED (See also ASIAN FOOD; FROZEN ENTRÉE/DINNER; SUCCOTASH)
■ **CANNED OR JARRED**
(Allen)

green beans & potatoes	½ cup	–	35	–
okra & tomatoes	½ cup	–	25	–
okra, tomatoes, & corn	½ cup	–	30	–
(Bush's Best) mixed greens	½ cup	–	20	–
(Chun King) chow mein vegetables	⅔ cup	–	15	–
(Del Monte)				
mixed vegetables				
no salt added	½ cup	–	40	–
regular	½ cup	–	40	–
peas & carrots	½ cup	–	60	–

Food and Description	Amount	Fat Grams	Total Calories	% Fat Calories
(Freshlike)				
mixed vegetables				
no salt	½ cup	–	35	–
no salt or sugar	½ cup	–	35	–
sweet peas & carrots	½ cup	–	60	–
generic				
beets w/onions	½ cup	–	80	–
peas & carrots	½ cup	–	48	–
peas & onions	½ cup	–	30	–
(Green Giant)				
garden medley	½ cup	–	40	–
mixed vegetables	½ cup	–	60	–
peas & carrots	½ cup	–	50	–
sweet peas w/tiny pearl onions	½ cup	–	60	–
(La Choy) vegetables				
Chinese	⅔ cup	–	10	–
chop suey	½ cup	–	15	–
(LeSueur)				
early peas w/mushrooms & pearl onions	½ cup	–	60	–
(Libby's)				
mixed vegetables	½ cup	–	45	–
peas & carrots	½ cup	–	60	–
vegetables for stew	½ cup	–	45	–
(S&W)				
old fashioned harvest time mixed	½ cup	–	35	–
peas & carrots	½ cup	–	50	–
peas & onions	½ cup	–	40	–
(Seneca)				
mixed vegetables	½ cup	–	45	–
peas & carrots	½ cup	–	60	–
vegetables for stew	½ cup	–	40	–
(Stokely)				
mixed vegetables				
no salt or sugar added	½ cup	–	35	–
regular	½ cup	–	35	–
peas & carrots	½ cup	–	60	–
(Trappey)				
okra & tomatoes	½ cup	–	25	–
okra, tomatoes, & corn	½ cup	–	30	–
(Veg-All)				
Cajun	½ cup	–	50	–
hot'n spicy	½ cup	–	50	–
original	½ cup	–	40	–
(Vlasic) hot & spicy garden mix	1 oz	–	4	–
■ **FROZEN**				
(Big Valley)				
California Blend	¾ cup	–	25	–
Italian Blend	¾ cup	–	30	–

Food and Description	Amount	Fat Grams	Total Calories	% Fat Calories
Oriental Blend	¾ cup	–	25	–
stew vegetables	¾ cup	–	25	–
Winter Blend	¾ cup	–	25	–
(Birds Eye)				
Baby Blends				
baby bean & carrot blend	½ cup	–	30	–
baby broccoli blend	⅔ cup	1.5	70	19%
baby corn blend	⅔ cup	0.5	60	8%
baby corn & bean blend	¾ cup	0.5	60	8%
baby gourmet potato blend	⅔ cup	–	45	–
baby sweet pea blend/tiny tender	¾ cup	–	40	–
Baby Vegetables				
baby gold and white corn	⅔ cup	0.5	60	8%
baby sweet peas & pearl onions	⅔ cup	0.5	60	8%
Plain vegetables				
mixed	⅓ cup	–	50	–
peas & carrots	⅔ cup	–	50	–
vegetables for soup	⅔ cup	–	45	–
Sauce Vegetables/boxed				
broccoli, cauliflower, & carrots in cheese sauce	½ cup	4.0	70	51%
California style sugar snap peas, sweet peas, & carrots	½ cup	5.0	100	45%
French style broccoli, red potatoes, & carrots	⅔ cup	6.0	110	49%
gold & white corn blend	½ cup	1.0	60	15%
Italian style vegetables & bow-tie pasta	1 cup	9.0	150	54%
New England style vegetables & pasta shells	1 cup	14.0	260	48%
Oriental style vegetables	1 cup	8.0	190	38%
peas & potatoes in real cream sauce	½ cup	2.5	90	25%
rice & broccoli in cheese sauce	10 oz pkg	9.0	290	28%
radiatore pasta & vegetables	1 cup	8.0	200	36%
roasted potatoes & broccoli	⅔ cup	3.5	100	32%
roletti pasta & vegetables	1 cup	8.0	190	38%
stir fry vegetables	½ cup	4.0	60	60%
tender peas & pearl onions	⅔ cup	0.5	90	5%
white & wild rice w/green beans	1 cup	9.0	150	54%
Southern vegetables				
gumbo blend	¾ cup	–	40	–
okra & tomatoes	¾ cup	–	25	–
seasoning blend	¾ cup	–	20	–
turnip greens w/diced turnips	1 cup	–	25	–
vegetables for stew	⅔ cup	–	40	–
Stir-Fry Vegetables				
Asparagus	2 cups	0.5	90	5%
broccoli	1 cup	–	30	–
pepper	3 oz	–	25	–
sugar snap	¾ cup	–	35	–

Food and Description	Amount	Fat Grams	Total Calories	% Fat Calories
whole bean	5.4 oz	0.5	100	5%
Vegetable Blends				
broccoli & cauliflower	½ cup	–	20	–
broccoli, cauliflower, & carrots	½ cup	–	25	–
broccoli, cauliflower, & red pepper	½ cup	–	20	–
broccoli, carrots, & water chestnuts	½ cup	–	30	–
broccoli, corn, & red peppers	½ cup	–	50	–
broccoli, green beans, whole onion, & red pepper	½ cup	–	25	–
broccoli, red pepper, onion, & mushrooms	½ cup	–	25	–
brussels sprouts, cauliflower, & carrots	½ cup	–	30	–
cauliflower nuggets, carrots, & snow peapods	½ cup	–	30	–
(C&W)				
organic				
fancy mixed vegetables	¾ cup	–	60	–
regular				
baby pea pods w/water chestnuts	⅔ cup	–	40	–
corn & black bean salad	⅔ cup	–	80	–
early harvest petite peas & baby carrots	⅔ cup	–	60	–
fancy mixed vegetables	¾ cup	–	60	–
petite peas w/pearl onions	⅔ cup	–	70	–
rancho fiesta blend	⅔ cup	–	60	–
vegetable stand combinations				
broccoli florets, julienne red peppers, sugarsnap peas, & water chestnuts	1 cup	–	40	–
crisp sugar snap peas, sweet baby carrots, tender cauliflower, & hand-cut broccoli florets	1 cup	–	30	–
early harvest corn, broccoli florets, & julienne red peppers	⅔ cup	0.5	60	8%
petite peas, early harvest corn, baby carrots, & sugar snap peas	⅔ cup	0.5	60	8%
roasted Parmesan & garlic potatoes, Italian green beans, & sweet baby carrots	¾ cup	1.0	60	15%
roasted rosemary & garlic potatoes, sweet red & green peppers, & onions	¾ cup	1.5	90	15%
sugar snap peas, baby carrots cauliflower, & broccoli florets	1 cup	–	30	–
Ultimate Stir Fry	¾ cup	–	30	–
(Cascadian Farm as packaged				
California blend	⅔ cup	–	20	–
Gardener's blend	¾ cup	–	57	–

Food and Description	Amount	Fat Grams	Total Calories	% Fat Calories
hearty stew veggies	⅔ cup	–	45	–
peas & carrots	⅔ cup	–	50	–
peas & pearl onions	¾ cup	–	60	–
Santa Fe blend	¾ cup	0.5	60	8%
Stir-fry blends				
Chinese	1 cup	–	25	–
Thai	¾ cup	–	25	–
(Flav-R-Pac) as packaged				
Just add Chicken				
creamy country sage	1¼ cups	3.5	170	19%
Japanese Yakitori	2-½ cups	2.5	150	15%
Just add Hamburger/vegetable stroganoff	2-¼ cups	12.0	220	49%
vegetable stir fry				
w/asparagus	¾ cup	–	25	–
w/noodles	¾ cup	0.5	80	6%
(Freshlike) as packaged				
California blend	3.5 oz	–	30	–
Chuck wagon blend	3.5 oz	–	70	–
Italian blend	3.5 oz	–	30	–
Midwestern blend	3.5 oz	–	40	–
mixed vegetables	3.5 oz	–	70	–
Oriental blend	3.5 oz	–	25	–
vegetables for stew	3.5 oz	–	50	–
Winter blend	3.5 oz	–	95	–
(Green Giant) as packaged				
Cheese & cream sauce vegetables				
broccoli, cauliflower & carrots	⅔ cup	2.5	70	32%
Create a Meal! vegetables				
beef & broccoli stir-fry	2⅓ cups	3.5	120	26%
garlic & ginger stir-fry	1⅔ cup	1.5	130	10%
garlic herb chicken	1⅓ cup	9.0	230	35%
lo mein stir-fry	2⅓ cups	1.5	170	8%
mushroom wine chicken	1¾ cup	7.0	240	26%
sweet & sour stir-fry	1½ cups	–	180	–
Szechuan stir-fry	1¾ cups	5.0	150	30%
teriyaki stir-fry	1¾ cups	0.5	100	–5%
Create a Meal! for ground beef				
Cheesy pasta & vegetable	1¾ cup	8.0	210	34%
homestyle stew	1¼ cup	3.0	140	19%
Create a Meal! Oven-roasted				
barbecue chicken	1½ cups	0.5	170	3%
chicken & stuffing	6 oz	3.0	190	14%
garlic w/herb chicken	1¾ cup	0.5	160	3%
lemon pepper chicken	1½ cup	0.5	140	3%
Harvest Fresh/sweet peas & pearl onions	½ cup	–	50	–
Marinated, seasoned vegetables				
Southwestern style corn & roasted peppers	¾ cup	1.0	90	10%

Food and Description	Amount	Fat Grams	Total Calories	% Fat Calories
vegetables teriyaki	1¼ cup	5.0	80	56%
regular/mixed vegetables	¾ cup	–	50	–
Select American Mixtures				
broccoli, carrots, & cauliflower	⅔ cup	–	25	–
broccoli, carrots, & water chestnuts	⅔ cup	–	25	–
(Pictsweet) as packaged				
Mixed vegetables for stirfry				
California	1 cup	–	35	–
Chinese	1¼ cups	–	50	–
Singapore	1¼ cups	–	45	
Teriyaki	1¼ cups	0.5	45	10%
Premium mixed vegetables/carrots,	⅔ cup	–	50	–
green beans, & corn				
(Seneca)				
broccoli				
Italian blend	¾ cup	–	30	–
Normandy	1 cup	–	30	–
stir-fry blend	1 cup	–	30	–
mixed vegetables	⅔ cup	–	60	–
Oriental				
blend	¾ cup	–	25	–
stir-fry blend	¾ cup	–	25	–
peas & carrots	⅔ cup	–	50	–
peas & onions	⅔ cup	–	70	–
Scandinavian blend	¾ cup	–	40	–
soup mix	¾ cup	–	40	–
winter blend	1 cup	–	25	–
(Veg-All)				
mixed vegetables	3.5 oz	–	70	–
soup vegetables/potato	3.5 oz	–	50	–
stew vegetables				
5-ways	3.5 oz	–	50	–
4-ways	3.5 oz	–	55	–
vegetable blends				
country	3.5 oz	–	50	–
Scandinavian	3.5 oz	–	45	–

VEGETARIAN FOODS

(NOTE: Some of the foods listed in this category were designed to be substitutes for meat and foods traditionally made with meat, and their names may therefore reflect the items they are intended to replace. However, all products listed here are meatless.)

(Amy's)
Can or Jar

Chili				
medium				
regular	1 cup	6.0	190	28%
w/vegetables	1 cup	6.0	190	28%
spicy	1 cup	6.0	190	28%
Pasta sauces				
family marinara	½ cup	1.0	50	18%
garlic mushroom	½ cup	7.0	120	53%

Food and Description	Amount	Fat Grams	Total Calories	% Fat Calories
tomato basil	½ cup	3.0	80	34%
Soups				
black bean vegetable	1 cup	1.0	110	8%
cream of mushroom	¾ cup	9.0	120	68%
cream of tomato	1 cup	2.0	100	18%
lentil	1 cup	4.0	130	28%
minestrone	1 cup	1.5	90	15%
no chicken noodle	1 cup	3.0	90	30%
split pea	1 cup	–	100	–
Frozen				
Asian Meals				
Asian noodle stir-fry	10 oz	4.5	240	17%
Thai stir-fry	9.5 oz	11.0	270	37%
Burgers				
All American	2.5 oz	3.0	170	16%
California veggie	2.5 oz	5.0	130	35%
Chicago veggie	2.5 oz	5.0	160	28%
Texas veggie	2.5 oz	2.5	130	17%
Burritos				
bean & rice burrito				
nondairy	6 oz	6.0	270	20%
regular	6 oz	8.0	280	26%
black bean vegetable	6 oz	8.0	320	23%
breakfast	6 oz	6.0	210	26%
Desserts/apple pie	4 oz	8.0	220	33%
Entrées				
black bean vegetable enchilada	4.75 oz	4.0	130	28%
cheese enchilada	4.75 oz	12.0	210	51%
cheese lasagna	10.25 oz	11.0	310	32%
macaroni & cheese	9 oz	16.0	410	35%
macaroni & soy cheese	9 oz	14.0	360	35%
pasta primavera	9.5 oz	12.0	320	34%
ravioli w/sauce	8 oz	12.0	340	32%
tofu vegetable lasagna	9.5 oz	10.0	300	30%
vegetable lasagna	9.5 oz	10.0	300	30%
Family Size				
black bean vegetable enchilada	4.38 oz	4.0	120	30%
cheese enchilada	5 oz	13.0	240	49%
vegetable lasagna	7 oz	8.0	200	36%
Pizzas				
cheese	⅓ pizza	12.0	300	36%
mushroom & olive	⅓ pizza	9.0	250	32%
pesto w/tomato & broccoli	⅓ pizza	11.0	300	33%
roasted vegetable	⅓ pizza	8.0	270	27%
soy cheese	⅓ pizza	11.0	280	35%
spinach	⅓ pizza	11.0	320	31%
veggie combo	⅓ pizza	9.0	250	32%
Pocket Sandwiches				
broccoli & cheese	4.5 oz	10.0	270	33%
cheese pizza	4.5 oz	9.0	300	27%

Food and Description	Amount	Fat Grams	Total Calories	% Fat Calories
Mediterranean vegetables	4.5 oz	7.0	220	29%
Mexican tamale	4.5 oz	7.0	250	25%
roasted vegetables	4.5 oz	8.0	220	33%
soy cheese veggie pizza	4.5 oz	8.0	270	27%
spinach feta	4.5 oz	9.0	250	32%
vegetable pie	5 oz	9.0	300	27%
vegetarian pizza	4.5 oz	6.0	250	22%
Pot Pies				
broccoli	1 pie	22.0	430	46%
country vegetable	1 pie	16.0	370	39%
Mexican tamale	1 pie	3.0	220	12%
shepherd's	1 pie	4.0	160	23%
vegetable				
nondairy	1 pie	9.0	320	25%
regular	1 pie	19.0	420	41%
Snacks				
cheese pizza	5-6 pieces	6.0	180	30%
spinach feta	5-6 pieces	6.0	170	32%
Whole Meals				
black bean enchilada	10 oz	8.0	250	29%
cannelloni	9 oz	12.0	330	33%
cheese enchilada	9 oz	14.0	330	38%
chili & cornbread	10.5 oz	6.0	320	17%
country dinner	11 oz	12.0	380	28%
veggie loaf	10 oz	5.0	260	17%
bean & rice burrito	6 oz	5.0	250	18%
bean, rice, & cheese burrito	6 oz	8.0	280	26%
black bean burrito	6 oz	8.0	320	23%
black bean & vegetable enchilada	4.75 oz	4.0	130	28%
breakfast burrito	6 oz	5.0	230	20%
California veggie burger	2.5 oz	3.0	100	27%
cannelloni dinner	9 oz	11.0	260	38%
cheese enchilada	4.75 oz	9.0	210	39%
cheese ravioli	8 oz	12.0	340	32%
Chicago Veggie Burger	2.5 oz	5.0	160	28%
country dinner	11 oz	21.0	480	39%
enchilada dinner	10 oz	8.0	250	29%
macaroni & cheese	1 serving	19.0	450	38%
macaroni & soy cheese	1 serving	14.0	360	35%
Mexican tamale pie	1 pie	3.0	220	12%
pizza pocket	4.5 oz	9.0	290	28%
pot pies				
broccoli	1 pie	22.0	430	46%
vegetable tofu	1 pie	18.0	360	45%
shepherd's pie	1 pie	4.0	160	23%
tofu-vegetable lasagna	9.5 oz	10.0	300	30%
vegetable lasagna w/cheese	9.5 oz	10.0	300	30%
veggie loaf dinner	10 oz	5.0	260	17%
■ **(Boca Burgers)** frozen				
Chef Max's Favorite	1 burger	2.0	110	16%

Food and Description	Amount	Fat Grams	Total Calories	% Fat Calories
hint of garlic	1 patty	2.0	110	16%
original vegan	1 burger	–	80	–
■ **(Bonavita)** Vegetarian Pate/canned				
herb	1 Tbs	2.0	30	60%
garlic	1 Tbs	2.0	30	60%
green pepper	1 Tbs	2.0	30	60%
mushroom	1 Tbs	2.0	30	60%
■ **(Cascadian Farm)** frozen				
Meals For A Small Planet				
Aztec	½ bag	3.0	230	12%
Cajun	½ bag	2.0	230	8%
Indian	½ bag	4.0	250	14%
Mediterranean	½ bag	6.0	215	25%
Moroccan	½ bag	4.0	250	14%
Oriental	½ bag	7.0	260	24%
Organic Quick Starts				
South Indian curry	2¼ cups	4.0	200	18%
Southwest skillet	2¼ cups	1.5	190	7%
Teriyaki veggies & rice	2¼ cups	6.0	220	25%
Thai veggies & rice	2¼ cups	4.0	210	17%
Veggie Bowls				
Caribbean veggies & rice	1 bowl	5.0	280	16%
Cascade veggies au gratin	1 bowl	6.0	170	32%
Fiesta casserole	1 bowl	11.0	340	29%
garden calzone	1 bowl	10.0	340	26%
Japenese noodles & vegetables	1 bowl	2.5	180	13%
Madras curry	1 bowl	5.0	270	17%
New England corn chowder	1 bowl	4.0	170	21%
pasta marinara	1 bowl	3.0	180	15%
pasta primavera	1 bowl	8.0	270	27%
Szechuan rice	1 bowl	1.5	210	6%
Teriyaki rice	1 bowl	7.0	270	23%
■ **(CedarLane)** Natural Cuisine				
Frozen				
Burritos				
beans, rice, & cheese/low-fat	1 burrito	1.0	260	3%
roasted vegetable & cheese	1 burrito	8.0	330	22%
Enchiladas				
garden vegetable/low-fat	1 enchilada	1.0	135	7%
3-layer enchilada pie	5.5 oz	7.0	215	29%
Lasagna/garden vegetable/low-fat	10 oz	2.0	280	6%
Pot Pie/vegetable/less fat	1 pie	8.0	390	18%
Veggie Wraps/low-fat				
couscous & vegetable	1 wrap	3.0	220	12%
rice & vegetable teriyaki	1 wrap	3.0	280	10%
vegetarian pizza	1 wrap	3.0	220	12%
Refrigerated				
Caviar/eggplant	2 Tbs	1.0	30	30%
Dip/roasted eggplant & red pepper	2 Tbs	2.0	30	60%

Food and Description	Amount	Fat Grams	Total Calories	% Fat Calories
Pasta Salad				
Caribbean	½ cup	5.0	160	28%
Tofu Salad				
cottage style	½ cup	13.0	190	62%
egg free	½ cup	12.0	180	60%
ranchero	½ cup	8.0	140	51%
■ **(Fantastic Foods)**				
Entrées/mix				
Nature's Burger				
BBQ				
mix only	⅓ cup	1.5	170	8%
prepared	1 patty	1.5	170	8%
original				
mix only	⅛ cup	3.0	170	16%
prepared	1 patty	3.0	170	16%
Nature's Sausage/mix-prepared	2 links	1.0	70	13%
sloppy Joe	¼ cup	0.5	70	6%
taco filling	¼ cup	1.0	25	36%
tofu burger	3 Tbs	2.5	80	28%
tofu scrambler	2 Tbs	–	35	–
vegetarian chili/mix only	¼ cup	1.0	100	9%
International Dishes/mix only				
black beans/instant	⅓ cup	1.5	150	9%
falafel	¼ cup	2.0	120	15%
hummus				
original	2 Tbs	3.0	80	34%
pesto	2 Tbs	4.0	90	40%
spinach & Parmesan	2 Tbs	3.0	80	34%
tabouli	2 Tbs	–	70	–
■ **(Gardenburger)** frozen				
classic Greek	1 burger	3.0	120	23%
fire roasted vegetable	1 burger	3.0	120	23%
garden vegan	1 burger	–	140	–
hamburger style/fat-free	1 burger	–	90	–
Lifeburger/fat-free	1 burger	–	100	–
original	1 burger	3.0	130	21%
roasted garlic/fat-free	1 burger	–	90	–
Santa Fe	1 burger	2.5	130	17%
savory mushroom	1 burger	3.0	120	23%
sauteed onion/fat-free	1 burger	–	100	–
smoked cheddar	1 burger	3.0	140	19%
veggie medley	1 burger	–	100	–
■ **(Gloria's Kitchen)** frozen vegetarian entrées				
Jamaican Jerk	1 entrée	3.0	140	18%
mu shu vegetables	1 entrée	1.5	260	5%
orange peel soy chick	1 entrée	2.5	160	14%
spicy kung pau	1 entrée	2.0	150	12%
spicy Thai rice noodles	1 entrée	3.5	140	23%
tofu balls w/spaghetti	1 entrée	3.0	180	15%

Food and Description	Amount	Fat Grams	Total Calories	% Fat Calories
■ **(Green Giant)**				
frozen				
breakfast patties	2 patties	4.0	100	36%
breakfast links	3 links	5.0	110	41%
Harvest Burgers				
Italian style	1 burger	5.0	140	32%
original	1 burger	4.0	140	26%
Southwestern style	1 burger	4.0	140	26%
■ **(Health Valley)** Chicken-free/frozen				
nuggets	3 nuggets	1.0	90	10%
patties	3 oz patty	1.5	120	11%
■ **(Lightlife)**				
frozen				
Gimmie Lean				
beef	2 oz	–	70	–
sausage	2 oz	–	70	–
Grilles				
BBQ	1 patty	3.5	120	26%
lemon	1 patty	5.0	120	38%
tamari	1 patty	5.0	120	38%
Hot dogs				
Smart Deli Jumbos	1 link	–	80	–
Smart Dogs	1 link	–	40	–
Tofu Pups	1 link	2.5	60	38%
Wonderdogs	1 link	2.0	60	38%
Light Sausage	2 patties	–	80	–
Links				
Breakfast	1 link	3.0	60	45%
lean Italian	1 link	2.0	60	38%
Lightburgers				
2 pack	1 patty	–	100	–
4 pack	1 patty	2.5	120	19%
8 pack	1 patty	2.5	120	19%
Savory Seitan				
BBQ	4 oz	2.0	160	11%
teriyaki	4 oz	2.0	160	11%
Slices				
Foney baloney	3 slices	2.5	60	38%
Smart Deli/fat-free				
bologna	3 slices	–	50	–
ham style	3 slices	–	50	–
roasted turkey	3 slices	–	40	–
3-peppercorn	3 slices	–	45	–
Smart Cutlets				
salisbury steak w/mushroom gravy	4.5 oz	0.5	120	4%
seasoned chicken	4 oz	0.5	140	3%
Smart Deli Sticks/pepperoni	1 oz	–	45	–
Smart Ground				
original	⅓ cup	–	70	–
taco burrito	⅓ cup	–	60	–

Food and Description	Amount	Fat Grams	Total Calories	% Fat Calories
Tempeh				
garden vegetable	4 oz	8.0	200	36%
smokey strips	4 oz	2.5	80	28%
soy	4 oz	8.0	210	34%
3-Grain	4 oz	7.0	200	32%
wild rice	4 oz	7.0	190	33%
■ **(Loma Linda)**				
canned or dry-packed				
Big Franks				
Low-fat	1 link	3.0	80	34%
original	1 link	7.0	110	57%
chicken supreme/mix only	⅓ cup	1.0	90	10%
dinner cuts	1 slice	1.5	90	15%
fried chik'n/gravy	2 pieces	10.0	160	56%
gravy/quik/mix only				
brown	1 Tbs	–	20	–
chicken style	1 Tbs	–	20	–
country style	1 Tbs	0.5	25	18%
mushroom	1 Tbs	–	15	–
onion	1 Tbs	–	20	–
Linketts	1 link	4.5	70	58%
Little Links	2 links	6.0	90	60%
Nuteena luncheon loaf	⅜" slice	13.0	160	73%
ocean platter mix/mix only	⅓ cup	1.0	90	10%
patty mix/mix only	⅓ cup	1.0	90	10%
Redi-Burger	⅝" slice	2.5	120	19%
sandwich spread	¼ cup	4.5	80	51%
savory dinner loaf/mix only	⅓ cup	1.5	90	15%
Swiss Stake	1 piece	6.0	120	45%
Tender Bits	6 pieces	4.5	110	37%
Tender Rounds	8 pieces	5.0	120	38%
Vege-Burger	¼ cup	1.5	70	19%
Vitaburger/mix only				
chunks	¼ cup	1.0	70	13%
granules	3 Tbs	1.0	70	13%
frozen				
Chik Nwggets	5 pieces	16.0	240	60%
corn dog	1 piece	4.0	150	24%
mix				
Soyagen/mix only				
all-purpose	¼ cup	6.0	130	42%
carob	¼ cup	6.0	130	42%
no sucrose	¼ cup	6.0	130	42%
■ **(Morningstar Farms)**				
Dry				
roasted soy butter	2 Tbs	11.0	170	58%
veggie burger kits				
Garden Grille	¼ pkg	–	80	–
Southwestern	¼ pkg	–	90	–

Food and Description	Amount	Fat Grams	Total Calories	% Fat Calories
Frozen				
America's original veggie dog	1 link	0.5	80	6%
Better 'n Burgers	1 patty	–	70	–
Better 'n Eggs	¼ cup	–	20	–
breakfast links	2 links	2.5	60	38%
breakfast patties	1 patty	3.0	70	39%
breakfast sandwiches				
bagel/Scramblers/patty/cheese	1 sandwich	4.5	320	13%
English muffin/Scramblers/patty	1 sandwich	2.5	240	9%
English muffin/Scramblers/patty/cheese	1 sandwich	3.0	280	10%
breakfast strips	2 strips	4.5	60	68%
burger style recipe crumbles	⅔ cup	3.0	90	30%
Chik nuggets	4 pieces	4.0	160	23%
Chik Patties	1 patty	6.0	150	36%
deli franks	1 link	7.0	110	57%
garden grille patty	1 patty	2.5	120	19%
garden veggie patties	1 patty	2.5	100	23%
Grillers	1 patty	7.0	140	45%
ground meatless	½ cup	–	60	–
Quarter Prime Patties	1 patty	2.0	140	13%
sausage style recipe crumbles	⅔ cup	3.0	90	30%
Scramblers	¼ cup	–	35	–
spicy black bean burger	1 patty	1.0	110	8%
Refrigerated				
breakfast patties	2 patties	5.0	120	38%
Chik nuggets	4 pieces	4.0	160	23%
Garden Veggie patties	1 patty	3.5	150	21%
Quarter prime	1 patty	2.0	140	13%
spicy black bean burger	1 patty	1.0	120	8%
■ (Mudpie)				
frozen/veggi burger	1 burger	4.5	180	23%
■ (Natural Touch)				
canned/vegetarian chili	1 cup	1.0	170	5%
mix/dry mix only				
Kaffree Roma	1 rounded tsp	–	10	–
loaf	4 Tbs	0.5	100	5%
roasted soybutter	2 Tbs	11.0	170	58%
Roma Cappuccino	3 Tbs	3.0	50	54%
stroganoff	4 Tbs	3.5	90	35%
taco	3 Tbs	1.0	60	15%
Veggie Burger Kit				
original	¼ pkg	–	80	–
Southwestern	¼ pkg	–	90	–
frozen				
dinner entrée	1 patty	15.0	220	61%
garden veggie patty	1 patty	2.5	110	20%
lentil rice loaf	1" slice	9.0	170	48%
nine bean loaf	1" slice	8.0	160	45%
okra patty	1 patty	5.0	110	41%

Food and Description	Amount	Fat Grams	Total Calories	% Fat Calories
spicy black bean burger	1 patty	1.0	100	9%
Toaster Squares				
blueberry	1 serving	2.0	180	10%
date walnut	1 serving	3.0	200	14%
vegan burger	1 patty	–	70	–
vegan burger crumbles	½ cup	–	60	–
vegan sausage crumbles	½ cup	–	60	–
vege frank	1 link	6.0	100	54%
■ (Near East)				
vegetable burger mix				
broiled	1½ patties	1.5	110	12%
fried	2½ patties	15.0	230	59%
■ (NewMenu)				
refrigerated				
Vegi-Burger	1 patty	1.0	110	8%
Vegidogs	1 link	–	45	–
■ (Van's)				
frozen/eggless/dairy-free				
pancakes/multigrain	2 pancakes	1.5	180	9%
waffles				
Belgian				
original	2 waffles	4.0	160	23%
7 grain	2 waffles	3.5	150	21%
berry fresh	2 waffles	8.0	220	33%
blueberry	2 waffles	5.0	225	20%
cinnamon apple	2 waffles	5.0	220	20%
mini	2 waffles	3.5	107	29%
organic	2 waffles	4.5	190	21%
waffle heaven	2 waffles	6.0	200	27%
wheat-free/plain	2 waffles	5.0	220	20%
whole grain	2 waffles	2.0	155	12%
■ (Worthington)				
canned or dry-packed				
Chik				
diced/drained	¼ cup	–	40	–
sliced/drained	3 slices	6.0	90	60%
chili				
low-fat	1 cup	1.0	170	5%
original	1 cup	15.0	290	47%
choplets	2 slices	1.5	90	15%
corned beef meatless	4 slices	9.0	140	26%
country stew	1 cup	9.0	210	34%
cutlets	1 slice	1.0	70	13%
FriChik				
low-fat	2 pieces	3.0	80	34%
original	2 pieces	8.0	120	60%
GranBurger	3 Tbs	0.5	60	8%
Multigrain cutlets	2 slices	2.0	100	18%
Numete	⅜" slice	10.0	130	69%
Prime Stakes	1 piece	9.0	120	68%

Food and Description	Amount	Fat Grams	Total Calories	% Fat Calories
Protose	⅜" slice	7.0	130	48%
Saucettes	1 link	6.0	90	60%
Savorex	1 tsp	–	10	–
savory slices	3 slices	9.0	150	54%
sliced chik	3 slices	0.5	70	6%
Super Links	1 link	8.0	110	65%
Tuno/drained	⅓ cup	4.0	80	45%
turkee slices	3 slices	12.0	170	64%
vegetable skallops	½ cup	1.5	90	15%
vegetable steaks	2 pieces	1.5	80	17%
vegetarian burger	¼ cup	2.0	60	30%
Veja-Links				
low-fat	1 link	1.5	40	34%
original	1 link	3.0	50	54%
frozen				
beef style	⅜" slice	7.0	110	57%
Bolono	3 slices	3.5	80	39%
chicken slices	2 slices	4.5	80	23%
Chic-ketts roll	2⅜" slice	7.0	120	53%
Chik Stiks	1 piece	7.0	110	57%
corned beef meatless	4 slices	9.0	140	58%
Crispy Chik	1 patty	6.0	150	36%
dinner roast	¾" slice	12.0	180	60%
egg roll	1 piece	8.0	180	40%
fillet	2 fillets	10.0	180	50%
Fripats	1 patty	6.0	130	42%
golden croquettes	4 pieces	10.0	210	43%
Leanies	1 link	7.0	100	63%
multigrain cutlets	2 slices	2.0	100	18%
Prosage				
links	2 links	2.5	60	38%
patties	1 patty	3.0	80	34%
roll	⅝" slice	10.0	140	64%
salami meatless	3 slices	8.0	130	55%
smoked beef	6 slices	6.0	120	45%
smoked turkey meatless	3 slices	10.0	140	64%
Stakelets	1 piece	8.0	140	51%
Stripples	2 strips	4.5	60	68%
Tuno/drained	½ cup	5.0	80	68%
vegetarian egg rolls	1 roll	8.0	180	40%
Wham	2 slices	5.0	80	56%
VENISON /boneless				
cured	3 oz	5.0	151	30%
raw				
ground/antelope	3.5 oz	2.0	110	16%
lean meat	3 oz	3.0	107	25%
steak	3 oz	5.0	153	29%
stew meat				
antelope	3.5 oz	2.0	110	16%
nilgai	3.5 oz	2.0	110	16%

Food and Description	Amount	Fat Grams	Total Calories	% Fat Calories
roasted	3 oz	3.0	135	20%
stewed	3 oz	5.0	153	29%
VICHYSSOISE (*See* SOUP)				
VIENNA SAUSAGE (*See* SAUSAGE)				
VINE SPINACH				
fresh/raw	4 oz	–	22	–
VINEGAR				
(China Bowl) white rice	1 Tbs	–	–	–
generic				
cider	1 oz	–	–	–
	½ cup	–	15	–
distilled	1 Tbs	–	2	–
	1 cup	–	29	–
(Great Impressions)				
apple cider	1 Tbs	–	7	–
basil	1 Tbs	–	7	–
hot paprika	1 Tbs	–	6	–
raspberry	1 Tbs	–	7	–
(Grey Poupon)				
balsamic	1 Tbs	–	–	–
garden herb	1 Tbs	–	10	–
raspberry	1 Tbs	–	10	–
(Hain)				
apple cider/raw-unpasteurized	1 Tbs	–	2	–
cider	1 Tbs	–	2	–
(Heinz)				
apple cider	1 Tbs	–	2	–
white	1 Tbs	–	2	–
wine	1 Tbs	–	2	–
regular/gourmet decanter	1 Tbs	–	4	–
tarragon	1 Tbs	–	2	–
(Indian Summer)				
apple cider	1 Tbs	–	3	–
	1 cup	–	40	–
white	1 Tbs	–	2	–
	1 cup	–	30	–
(LuvYu)				
pineapple salad	1 Tbs	–	10	–
rice	1 Tbs	–	11	–
(Musselman's)				
apple cider	2 Tbs	–	4	–
red wine	2 Tbs	–	–	–
white	2 Tbs	–	4	–
(Nakano)	1 Tbs			
(Progresso)				
balsamic	1 Tbs	–	2	–
garlic	1 Tbs	–	2	–
red wine	1 Tbs	–	2	–
red wine distilled flavored	1 Tbs	–	2	–
white wine	1 Tbs	–	2	–

Food and Description	Amount	Fat Grams	Total Calories	% Fat Calories
(Regina) wine				
red/garlic or regular	1 oz	–	4	–
white	1 oz	–	4	–
(S&W)				
cider	1 Tbs	–	–	–
international				
garlic wine	1 Tbs	–	–	–
Italian herb	1 Tbs	–	–	–
malt ale	1 Tbs	–	–	–
red wine	1 Tbs	–	–	–
tarragon	1 Tbs	–	–	–
white distilled	1 Tbs	–	–	–
(Spectrum Naturals) organic				
brown rice	1 Tbs	–	–	–
wine				
garlic	1 Tbs	–	–	–
Italian herb	1 Tbs	–	–	–
raspberry	1 Tbs	–	10	–
red	1 Tbs	–	–	–
white	1 Tbs	–	–	–
(White House)				
apple cider	2 Tbs	–	2	–
red wine	2 Tbs	–	4	–

VODKA (*See* LIQUOR, DISTILLED)

W

Food and Description	Amount	Fat Grams	Total Calories	% Fat Calories
WAFFLE (*See also* PANCAKE/WAFFLE MIX)				
(Aunt Jemima) frozen				
blueberry	2 waffles	6.0	210	26%
buttermilk	2 waffles	6.0	200	27%
low-fat	2 waffles	1.5	160	8%
homestyle	2 waffles	6.0	200	27%
(Belgian Chef) frozen	2 waffles	2.5	140	16%
(Hungry Jack)				
apple cinnamon	2 waffles	6.0	200	27%
blueberry	2 waffles	7.0	210	30%
buttermilk	2 waffles	6.0	190	28%
homestyle	2 waffles	6.0	180	30%
wildberry	2 waffles	6.0	200	27%

Food and Description	Amount	Fat Grams	Total Calories	% Fat Calories
(Kellogg's) frozen				
Eggo				
apple cinnamon	2 waffles	7.0	200	32%
banana bread	2 waffles	6.0	190	28%
blueberry	2 waffles	7.0	200	32%
buttermilk	2 waffles	7.0	190	33%
chocolate chip	2 waffles	7.0	200	32%
cinnamon toast	2 waffles	10.0	290	31%
golden oat	2 waffles	2.5	140	16%
homestyle				
low-fat	2 waffles	2.5	160	14%
mini	4 waffles	9.0	260	31%
regular	2 waffles	7.0	190	33%
nut & honey	2 waffles	9.0	220	37%
strawberry	2 waffles	7.0	200	32%
Nutri-Grain				
low-fat				
blueberry	2 waffles	2.5	150	15%
whole wheat	2 waffles	2.5	140	16%
multi-bran	2 waffles	5.0	160	28%
whole wheat	2 waffles	5.0	170	26%
Special K	2 waffles	–	120	–
(Krusteaz)				
frozen				
Belgian	1 waffle	7.0	190	33%
golden	1 waffle	2.5	110	20%
mix/prepared				
Belgian waffle/ 7" round	1 waffle	19.0	440	39%
Supreme waffle/4x4" square	3 waffles	21.0	420	45%
(Thomas) Fresh				
blueberry	2 waffles	9.0	230	35%
buttermilk	2 waffles	8.0	220	33%
homestyle	1 waffle	4.0	110	33%
(Van's) frozen				
vegetarian-eggless & dairy-free				
Belgian				
original	2 waffles	4.0	160	23%
7 grain	2 waffles	3.5	150	21%
berry fresh	2 waffles	8.0	220	33%
blueberry	2 waffles	5.0	225	20%
cinnamon-apple	2 waffles	5.0	220	20%
mini	2 waffles	3.5	107	29%
organic	2 waffles	4.5	190	21%
waffle heaven	2 waffles	6.0	200	27%
wheat free/plain	2 waffles	5.0	220	20%
whole grain	2 waffles	2.0	155	17%

WAFFLE SYRUP (*See* MAPLE SYRUP; PANCAKE/WAFFLE SYRUP)
WAKAME (*See* SEAWEED)
WALNUT

Food and Description	Amount	Fat Grams	Total Calories	% Fat Calories
(Ann's House of Nuts) English	1 oz	18.0	180	90%

Food and Description	Amount	Fat Grams	Total Calories	% Fat Calories
(Azar) English/pieces	1 oz	19.0	190	90%
(Diamond) English				
pieces	¼ cup	19.0	190	90%
shelled	¼ cup	19.0	190	90%
(Diamond of California)				
black walnuts	¼ cup	18.0	200	81%
chopped	¼ cup	20.0	210	86%
finely diced	¼ cup	20.0	210	86%
ground	¼ cup	20.0	210	86%
halves & pieces	¼ cup	20.0	210	86%
shelled	¼ cup	20.0	210	86%
toasted walnut toping	2 Tbs	10.0	110	82%
	¼ cup	20.0	210	86%
generic				
dried				
black/shelled	1 oz	16.0	172	84%
ground	1 cup	45.0	490	83%
pieces	1 cup	71.0	760	84%
English or Persian				
pieces	1 cup	74.0	770	87%
shelled	1 oz	18.0	190	85%
(Planters)				
black	2 oz	31.0	340	82%
English or Persian				
halves				
Gold Measure	2 oz	38.0	380	90%
regular	⅓ cup	22.0	220	90%
pieces	¼ cup	20.0	190	95%
WATER (See also SOFT DRINK; COCKTAIL MIXER)				
bottled				
(Arrowhead)				
distilled	1 liter	–	–	–
drinking	1 liter	–	–	–
fluoridated	1 liter	–	–	–
spring	1 liter	–	–	–
(Canada Dry) seltzer/sparkling water	8 fl oz	–	–	–
cherry	8 fl oz	–	–	–
cranberry	8 fl oz	–	–	–
grapefruit	8 fl oz	–	–	–
lemon lime	8 fl oz	–	–	–
Mandarin orange	8 fl oz	–	–	–
peach	8 fl oz	–	–	–
raspberry	8 fl oz	–	–	–
strawberry	8 fl oz	–	–	–
tropical	8 fl oz	–	–	–
(Cascadia) sparkling water w/juice				
cherry-blackberry	6 fl oz	–	2	–
grapefruit	6 fl oz	–	2	–
guava-berry	6 fl oz	–	2	–
lemonade	6 fl oz	–	2	–

Food and Description	Amount	Fat Grams	Total Calories	% Fat Calories
(Clearly Canadian) sparkling water				
blackberry	8 fl oz	–	100	–
cherry	8 fl oz	–	90	–
cranberry	8 fl oz	–	90	–
peach	8 fl oz	–	90	–
raspberry	8 fl oz	–	80	–
(Coor's) Rocky Mountain sparkling water				
cherry	8 fl oz	–	–	–
lemon lime	8 fl oz	–	–	–
original	8 fl oz	–	–	–
(Crystal Geyser) seltzer water/light				
black cherry cider	6 fl oz	–	60	–
cranberry-raspberry	6 fl oz	–	60	–
kiwi lemonade	6 fl oz	–	60	–
natural peach	6 fl oz	–	60	–
vanilla creme	6 fl oz	–	60	–
(Evian) spring water	8 fl oz	–	–	–
generic				
pain/all types	any amount	–	–	–
seltzer water/flavored				
lemon	12 fl oz	–	–	–
lime	12 fl oz	–	–	–
orange	12 fl oz	–	–	–
strawberry	12 fl oz	–	–	–
(Perrier) mineral water with-a-twist				
lemon	12 fl oz	–	–	–
lime	12 fl oz	–	–	–
(Poland Spring) spring water	8 fl oz	–	–	–
(Polar) spring water	8 fl oz	–	–	–
(Quest) sparkling water				
black cherry	8 fl oz	–	–	–
peach	8 fl oz	–	–	–
raspberry	8 fl oz	–	–	–
red raspberry	8 fl oz	–	–	–
strawberry-kiwi	8 fl oz	–	–	–
tangerine-lemon	8 fl oz	–	–	–
tangerine-lime	8 fl oz	–	–	–
(San Francisco) sweetened seltzer				
almond cream	8 fl oz	–	100	–
black cherry	8 fl oz	–	110	–
peach	8 fl oz	–	100	–
raspberry	8 fl oz	–	110	–
(Savoir Faire) natural spring water	8 fl oz	–	–	–
(Schweppes) seltzer/sparkling water				
black cherry	8 fl oz	–	–	–
lemon	8 fl oz	–	–	–
lemon lime	8 fl oz	–	–	–
lime	8 fl oz	–	–	–
orange	8 fl oz	–	–	–
peaches & cream	8 fl oz	–	–	–
raspberry	8 fl oz	–	–	–

Food and Description	Amount	Fat Grams	Total Calories	% Fat Calories
(Water Joe) caffeine-enhanced natural artesian water	8 fl oz	–	–	–
WATER CHESTNUT (*See also* ASIAN FOOD)				
canned/sliced	½ cup	–	35	–
fresh/raw/sliced	½ cup	–	66	–
WATERCRESS /fresh/raw				
chopped	½ cup	–	2	–
whole	1 sprig	–	–	–
WATERCRESS SOUP (*See* SOUP)				
WATERMELON (*See also* WATERMELON RIND)				
fresh				
wedges/10" dia	1/16 wedge	2.0	152	12%
cubed	1 cup	0.7	50	12%
WATERMELON RIND				
(Old South)	2 cubes	–	70	–
WATERMELON SEEDS/KERNELS				
dried	1 oz	13.0	158	74%
	1 cup	51.0	602	76%
WAX BEAN				
canned				
(Del Monte) golden-cut	½ cup	–	20	–
generic	½ cup	–	25	–
(S&W) premium golden-cut	½ cup	–	20	–
(Seneca) cuts	½ cup	–	25	–
(Stokely)				
no salt or sugar	½ cup	–	20	–
regular	½ cup	–	20	–
frozen				
(Seabrook) cut	½ cup	–	25	–
WAX GOURD /fresh				
boiled	1 cup	–	23	–
raw	1 cup	–	17	–
WEAKFISH				
broiled w/butter or margarine	3 oz	9.6	177	49%
WELSH RAREBIT (*See also* FROZEN ENTRÉE/DINNER; SAUCE)				
homemade/USDA Standard Home Recipe	1 cup	32.0	415	69%
WHALE /raw	3 oz	6.0	130	42%
WHEAT (*See also* BULGUR; FLOUR; WHEAT GERM)				
(Arrowhead Mills)				
flakes	⅓ cup	0.5	110	4%
whole grain	¼ cup	1.0	160	6%
(White Wave)				
seitan	¼ pkg	–	140	–
slices/marinated	3 slices	–	60	–
strips/fajita	⅓ cup	–	60	–
WHEAT GERM (*See also* CEREAL)				
(Bob's Red Mill) natural raw	⅛ cup	1.0	52	17%
generic				
crude	¼ cup	3.0	105	26%
toasted	¼ cup	3.0	110	25%

Food and Description	Amount	Fat Grams	Total Calories	% Fat Calories
(Hodgson Mill)	2 Tbs	1.0	55	16%
(Kretschmer)				
honey crunch	2 Tbs	1.0	50	18%
plain	1⅔ Tbs	1.0	50	18%
(Mother's) toasted	2 Tbs	1.0	50	18%
(Stone-Buhr) untoasted	2 Tbs	2.0	60	30%
WHELK (*See* SNAIL)				
WHEY				
dried				
acid	1 Tbs	–	10	–
	1 cup	–	193	–
sweet	1 Tbs	–	26	–
	1 cup	–	512	–
fluid				
acid	1 Tbs	–	4	–
	1 cup	<1.0	60	8%
sweet	1 Tbs	–	4	–
	1 cup	0.7	65	10%
WHIPPED TOPPING (*See also* CREAM)				
(NOTE: Unless specified otherwise, 1 serving of mix = the amount in 2 Tbs prepared)				
(Cool Whip)				
extra creamy	2 Tbs	2.0	25	72%
Free	2 Tbs	–	15	–
lite	2 Tbs	1.0	20	45%
whipped topping/original	2 Tbs	1.5	25	54%
(Dream Whip)				
mix only	1 serving	0.5	15	30%
prepared w/2% milk	2 Tbs	1.0	20	45%
(D-Zerta) mix only	1 serving	1.0	10	100%
(Estee) mix/mix only	¾ tsp	0.5	10	45%
generic				
frozen				
nondairy	1 Tbs	0.8	11	66%
regular	1 Tbs	1.0	15	60%
powdered				
low calorie	1 Tbs	1.0	8	100%
w/whole milk	1 Tbs	–	10	–
	1 cup	10.0	150	60%
pressurized				
cream	1 Tbs	1.0	8	100%
	½ cup	7.0	75	84%
nondairy	1 Tbs	1.0	10	81%
	1 cup	16.0	185	78%
(Kraft)				
Free/fat-free	2 Tbs	–	15	–
light cream/whipped	2 Tbs	1.0	10	90%
(LaCreme) lite	2 Tbs	1.0	15	60%
(Pet) whip	2 Tbs	2.0	30	60%
(RediWhip)				
deluxe	2 Tbs	3.0	30	90%

Food and Description	Amount	Fat Grams	Total Calories	% Fat Calories
fat-free	2 Tbs	–	5	–
lite	2 Tbs	1.0	15	60%
non-dairy	2 Tbs	2.0	20	90%
real whipped				
heavy cream	2 Tbs	3.0	30	90%
light cream	2 Tbs	2.0	20	90%
(Rich's)				
nondairy				
aerosol	2 Tbs	2.0	25	72%
bowl	2 Tbs	1.5	25	54%
Richwhip				
liquid	2 Tbs	2.0	25	72%
whipped	2 Tbs	2.0	25	72%
WHISKEY (See LIQUOR, DISTILLED)				
WHITE BEAN				
canned				
generic	½ cup	–	153	–
(Goya) Spanish style	½ cup	0.5	125	4%
dried				
boiled				
regular	½ cup	–	125	–
small	½ cup	0.5	127	4%
raw				
regular	½ cup	1.0	340	30%
small	½ cup	1.5	365	4%
WHITE PERCH/raw	3 oz	3.0	100	27%
WHITE SAUCE (See SAUCE)				
WHITEFISH/mixed species				
fresh				
cooked-dry heat	3 oz	5.5	145	34%
raw	1 oz	1.7	38	39%
	3 oz	5.0	115	39%
jarred				
(Manischewitz)				
jellied				
14.5-oz jar	1 ball	2.0	60	30%
24-oz jar	1 ball	2.0	60	30%
regular				
24-oz jar	1 ball	1.5	40	34%
(Mother's)				
jellied				
12-oz jar	1 ball	<1.0	50	14%
24-oz jar	1 ball	1.0	60	15%
31-oz jar	1 ball	1.0	60	15%
regular				
12-oz jar	1 ball	<1.0	55	13%
24-oz jar	1 ball	1.0	70	13%
31-oz jar	1 ball	1.0	70	13%
smoked	1 oz	<1.0	30	6%
	3 oz	<1.0	92	7%

Food and Description	Amount	Fat Grams	Total Calories	% Fat Calories
WHITEFISH & PIKE				
jarred				
(Manischewitz)				
jelled				
14.5 oz jar	1 ball	1.5	60	23%
regular				
14.5-oz jar	1 ball	1.5	50	27%
24-oz jar	1 ball	1.5	50	27%
sweet	1 ball	1.5	70	19%
(Mother's)				
jellied in broth				
12-oz jar	1 ball	<1.0	50	14%
24-oz jar	1 ball	1.0	60	15%
31-oz jar	1 ball	1.0	60	15%
regular	1 ball	1.0	70	13%
(Rokeach) jellied	1 ball	1.0	60	15%
WHITING (See also SEAFOOD ENTRÉE/DINNER)				
breaded & fried	3 oz	9.7	171	51%
cooked-dry heat	3 oz	1.0	98	9%
raw	3 oz	1.0	77	12%
WIENER (See FRANKFURTER; FRANKFURTER, VEGETARIAN; SAUSAGE; VEGETARIAN FOODS)				
WILD CELERY (See CELERIAC)				
WINE (Note: For the calories in a 4 ounce glass of wine, simply multiply calorie figures by 4.)				
(Andre) champagne				
blush	1 fl oz	–	22	–
brut	1 fl oz	–	25	–
cold duck	1 fl oz	–	25	–
extra dry	1 fl oz	–	24	–
(Carl Jung) white/alcohol removed	1 fl oz	–	20	–
(Carlo Rossi)				
blush	1 fl oz	–	21	–
burgundy	1 fl oz	–	22	–
chablis	1 fl oz	–	21	–
paisano	1 fl oz	–	23	–
red sangria	1 fl oz	–	24	–
rhine	1 fl oz	–	21	–
vin rose	1 fl oz	–	21	–
white grenache	1 fl oz	–	20	–
(Eden Roc)				
brut	1 fl oz	–	21	–
brut rose	1 fl oz	–	22	–
extra dry	1 fl oz	–	21	–
(Gallo)				
Ernest & Julio Gallo Vineyards label				
cabernet sauvignon	1 fl oz	–	23	–
cafe zinfadel	1 fl oz	–	19	–
chardonnay	1 fl oz	–	24	–
classic Burgundy	1 fl oz	–	22	–

Food and Description	Amount	Fat Grams	Total Calories	% Fat Calories
hearty burgundy	1 fl oz	–	24	–
sauvignon blanc	1 fl oz	–	20	–
Malvasia chardonnay	1 fl oz	–	19	–
Merlot	1 fl oz	–	24	–
white grenache	1 fl oz	–	21	–
white zinfandel	1 fl oz	–	20	–
Gallo Of Sonoma				
Barbera/Barrelli Creek-'95	1 fl oz	–	25	–
Cabernet Sauvignon				
Frei Ranch Vineyards				
'92	1 fl oz	–	24	–
'93	1 fl oz	–	24	–
'94	1 fl oz	–	25	–
Sonoma City				
'94	1 fl oz	–	24	–
'95	1 fl oz	–	24	–
'96	1 fl oz	–	24	–
'97	1 fl oz	–	25	–
Stefani Vineyards				
'93	1 fl oz	–	25	–
'94	1 fl oz	–	24	–
Chardonnay				
Laguna Ranch Vineyards				
'94	1 fl oz	–	25	–
'95	1 fl oz	–	25	–
'96	1 fl oz	–	25	–
Russian River Valley				
'96	1 fl oz	–	25	–
'97	1 fl oz	–	25	–
'98	1 fl oz	–	25	–
Sonoma County/ '95	1 fl oz	–	24	–
Stevani Vineyards				
'94	1 fl oz	–	24	–
'95	1 fl oz	–	24	–
'96	1 fl oz	–	25	–
Merlot				
Frei Ranch Vineyards				
'91	1 fl oz	–	24	–
'92	1 fl oz	–	23	–
Sonoma City				
'96	1 fl oz	–	25	–
'97	1 fl oz	–	25	–
Sonoma County	1 fl oz	–	24	–
Pinot Noir/Russian River Valley				
'96	1 fl oz	–	25	–
'97	1 fl oz	–	25	–
'98	1 fl oz	–	24	–
Sangivoese/Alexander Valley-'97	1 fl oz	–	26	–
Valdiquie/Barrelli Creek Vineyards				
'94	1 fl oz	–	23	–

Food and Description	Amount	Fat Grams	Total Calories	% Fat Calories
'95	1 fl oz	–	22	–
Zinfandel				
Chiotti Vineyards/ '95	1 fl oz	–	24	–
Frei Ranch Vineyards				
'92	1 fl oz	–	24	–
'93	1 fl oz	–	26	–
'94	1 fl oz	–	26	–
'95	1 fl oz	–	25	–
Sonoma County				
'95	1 fl oz	–	25	–
'96	1 fl oz	–	25	–
'97	1 fl oz	–	27	–
Sheffield label				
sherry				
cream	1 fl oz	–	44	–
very dry	1 fl oz	–	32	–
tawny port	1 fl oz	–	45	–
Turning Leaf				
Cabernet Sauvignon				
'95	1 fl oz	–	24	–
'96	1 fl oz	–	23	–
Chardonnay				
'95	1 fl oz	–	22	–
'96	1 fl oz	–	23	–
Fume Blanc				
'95	1 fl oz	–	23	–
'96	1 fl oz	–	23	–
Johannisberg Reisling/ '96	1 fl oz	–	22	–
Merlot/ '95	1 fl oz	–	23	–
White Zinfandel/ '96	1 fl oz	–	20	–
Zinfandel				
'95	1 fl oz	–	23	–
'96	1 fl oz	–	24	–
Turning Leaf Sonoma Reserve				
Cabernet Sauvignon				
'93	1 fl oz	–	22	–
'94	1 fl oz	–	24	–
'95	1 fl oz	–	24	–
Chardonnay				
'94	1 fl oz	–	23	–
'95	1 fl oz	–	24	–
'96	1 fl oz	–	25	–
Chardonnay Fume '95	1 fl oz	–	22	–
Merlot				
'94	1 fl oz	–	22	–
'95	1 fl oz	–	24	–
'96	1 fl oz	–	24	–
Pinot Noir				
'95	1 fl oz	–	22	–
'96	1 fl oz	–	24	–

Food and Description	Amount	Fat Grams	Total Calories	% Fat Calories
Zinfandel				
'94	1 fl oz	–	23	–
'95	1 fl oz	–	24	–
'96	1 fl oz	–	24	–
general				
barbera/white	4 fl oz	–	91	–
Beaujolais-12% alcohol	4 fl oz	–	96	–
Bordeaux/red-12% alcohol	4 fl oz	–	96	–
Burgundy				
cooking	¼ cup	–	2	–
red-12% alcohol	4 fl oz	–	96	–
sparkling-12% alcohol	4 fl oz	–	116	–
white-12% alcohol	4 fl oz	–	90	–
cabernet sauvignon	4 fl oz	–	88	–
chablis	4 fl oz	–	84	–
emerald	4 fl oz	–	102	–
gold	4 fl oz	–	97	–
pink	4 fl oz	–	98	–
ruby	4 fl oz	–	104	–
champagne				
brut	4 fl oz	–	100	–
domestic	4 fl oz	–	84	–
extra dry	4 fl oz	–	105	–
pink	4 fl oz	–	98	–
chardonnay	4 fl oz	–	88	–
Chenin Blanc	4 fl oz	–	86	–
Chianti	4 fl oz	–	100	–
cold duck	4 fl oz	–	108	–
dessert	4 fl oz	–	180	–
Dubonnet	4 fl oz	–	160	–
French colombard	4 fl oz	–	88	–
Liebfraumilch-10% alcohol	4 fl oz	–	84	–
Madeira-19% alcohol	4 fl oz	–	160	–
muscatel	3.5 fl oz	–	158	–
port				
ruby-20% alcohol	4 fl oz	–	184	–
tawny-20% alcohol	4 fl oz	–	184	–
white	4 fl oz	–	172	–
Reisling-12% alcohol	4 fl oz	–	90	–
Rhine-11 % alcohol	4 fl oz	–	96	–
Rhone-12% alcohol	4 fl oz	–	96	–
rosé	4 fl oz	–	90	–
sake/saki	1.5 fl oz	–	36	–
sauternes				
cooking	¼ cup	–	2	–
dry-12% alcohol	4 fl oz	–	108	–
12% alcohol	4 fl oz	–	116	–
sauvignon blanc	4 fl oz	–	80	–
sherry				
cooking	¼ cup		20	–

Food and Description	Amount	Fat Grams	Total Calories	% Fat Calories
cream-19.5% alcohol	4 fl oz	–	200	–
dry-19% alcohol	4 fl oz	–	162	–
sweet	4 fl oz	–	165	–
sylvaner-12% alcohol	4 fl oz	–	90	–
table				
red	3.5 fl oz	–	74	–
rose	3.5 fl oz	–	73	–
white	3.5 fl oz	–	70	–
Tokay	4 fl oz	–	164	–
vermouth				
dry-17% alcohol	4 fl oz	–	136	–
sweet-17% alcohol	4 fl oz	–	180	–
wine spritzer	5 fl oz	–	61	–
zinfandel				
red	4 fl oz	–	92	–
white	4 fl oz	–	82	–
(Grey Poupon) cooking wine				
Burgundy	1 fl oz	–	20	–
sherry	1 fl oz	–	35	–
while	1 fl oz	–	20	–
(Holland House) cooking wine				
Marsala	1 fl oz	–	9	–
red	1 fl oz	–	6	–
sherry	1 fl oz	–	5	–
vermouth	1 fl oz	–	2	–
white	1 fl oz	–	2	–
(Regina) cooking wine				
Burgundy	¼ cup	–	2	–
sauternes	¼ cup	–	2	–
sherry	¼ cup	–	20	–
WINE COOLER				
(Bartles & Jaymes)				
Malt-based coolers				
berry	12 fl oz	–	210	–
black cherry	12 fl oz	–	200	–
Brazilian mist berry	12 fl oz	–	200	–
fuzzy navel	12 fl oz	–	230	–
kiwi strawberry	12 fl oz	–	214	–
margarita	12 fl oz	–	260	–
Oriental dragon fruit	12 fl oz	–	200	–
original	12 fl oz	–	190	–
peach	12 fl oz	–	210	–
pina colada	12 fl oz	–	270	–
strawberry daiquiri	12 fl oz	–	220	–
tropical	12 fl oz	–	230	–
Wine-based coolers				
berry	12 fl oz	–	220	–
Brazilian mist berry	12 fl oz	–	210	–
fuzzy navel	12 fl oz	–	250	–
kiwi strawberry	12 fl oz	–	230	–

Food and Description	Amount	Fat Grams	Total Calories	% Fat Calories
margarita	12 fl oz	–	270	–
Oriental dragon fruit (citrus wine)	12 fl oz	–	250	–
original	12 fl oz	–	200	–
strawberry daiquiri	12 fl oz	–	230	–
tropical	12 fl oz	–	240	–
(Boone's)				
country quencher	1 fl oz	–	24	–
delicious apple	1 fl oz	–	21	–
sangria	1 fl oz	–	22	–
snow creek berry	1 fl oz	–	18	–
strawberry hill	1 fl oz	–	22	–
sun peak peach	1 fl oz	–	18	–
wild island	1 fl oz	–	18	–
generic	7 fl oz	–	100	–
	12 fl oz	–	192	–
WINGED BEAN				
cooked	½ cup	5.0	126	36%
raw	½ cup	15.0	375	36%
WOLFFISH				
Atlantic/fresh				
cooked-dry heat	3 oz	2.0	105	17%
raw	3 oz	2.0	80	23%

WON TON (*See* ASIAN FOOD)
WON TON SOUP (*See* SOUP)
WON TON WRAPPER (*See* ASIAN FOOD)
WORCESTERSHIRE SAUCE (*See* SAUCE)

Y

Food and Description	Amount	Fat Grams	Total Calories	% Fat Calories
YAM (*See also* SWEET POTATO)				
canned				
(Bruce's)				
candied	½ cup	–	170	–
cut or whole	½ cup	1.0	140	6%
mashed	½ cup	1.0	130	7%
(Bush's Best)	½ cup	–	120	–
generic				
in heavy syrup	½ cup	–	120	–
in light syrup	½ cup	–	110	–
mashed	½ cup	–	90	–
w/pineapple-orange sauce	½ cup	–	190	–

Food and Description	Amount	Fat Grams	Total Calories	% Fat Calories
(S&W) candied/old-fashioned	½ cup	–	170	–
(Trappey's) golden/whole in heavy syrup	½ cup	–	130	–
fresh				
Hawaii/mountain				
cooked/cubed	½ cup	–	59	–
raw				
cubed	½ cup	–	46	–
whole/ 8¼" long/2½" dia	1 yam	0.5	280	2%
regular				
boiled or baked/cubed	1 cup	–	158	–
raw/cubed	1 cup	–	177	–
YAM BEAN-TUBER (*See* JICAMA)				
YARDLONG BEAN				
dried				
boiled	½ cup	<1.0	100	4%
raw	½ cup	1.0	290	3%
fresh				
boiled/drained/sliced	½ cup	–	25	–
raw/sliced	½ cup	–	22	–
YEAST				
baker's				
(Fleischmann's)				
active dry & rapid rise/packet or jar	¼ oz	–	20	–
fresh active	0.6 oz	–	15	–
household	0.5 oz	–	15	–
generic/active dry				
compressed	1 oz	1.0	24	38%
powdered	1 oz	0.5	80	6%
(Red Star)				
active dry	¼ oz	–	15	–
	4 Tbs	–	45	–
flakes	3 Tbs	–	45	–
brewer's				
generic	1 Tbs	–	25	–
	1 oz	–	80	–
(Louis Laboratories)	2 Tbs	1.0	114	8%
torula	1 oz	–	79	–
YELLOWEYE BEAN				
canned				
(B&M) baked	½ cup	2.0	170	11%
dried				
(Bean Cuisine)	½ cup	1.0	115	8%
YELLOWTAIL				
mixed species/fresh				
cooked-dry heat	3 oz	5.5	160	31%
raw	3 oz	4.5	125	32%
YOGURT, DAIRY				
(Alta Dena)				
black cherry	1 cup		200	

Food and Description	Amount	Fat Grams	Total Calories	% Fat Calories
mixed berries	1 cup	–	190	–
peach	1 cup	–	210	–
piña colada	1 cup	–	220	–
raspberry	1 cup	–	190	–
vanilla	1 cup	–	180	–
(Breyers)				
Blended low-fat/1% milkfat				
blueberry	4.4 oz	1.0	130	7%
peach	4.4 oz	1.0	130	7%
strawberry	4.4 oz	1.0	130	7%
Light/Non-fat				
apple pie a la mode	8 oz	–	120	–
berry bananc split	8 oz	–	120	–
black cherry jubilee	8 oz	–	120	–
blueberries'N Cream-flavored	8 oz	–	120	–
cherry bon-bon-flavored	8 oz	–	120	–
cherry vanilla cream-flavored	8 oz	–	120	–
classic strawberry	8 oz	–	120	–
key lime pie	8 oz	–	120	–
lemon chiffon	8 oz	–	120	–
peaches'N cream-flavored	8 oz	–	120	–
raspberries'N cream-flavored	8 oz	–	120	–
strawberry cheesecake-flavored	8 oz	–	120	–
Low-fat/1% milkfat				
black cherry	8 oz	2.5	240	9%
blueberry	8 oz	2.5	230	10%
mixed berry	8 oz	2.5	230	10%
peach	8 oz	2.5	240	9%
pineapple	8 oz	2.5	240	9%
red raspberry	8 oz	2.5	230	10%
strawberry	8 oz	2.5	230	10%
strawberry-banana	8 oz	2.5	240	9%
vanilla	8 oz	3.0	220	12%
Smooth & Creamy lowfat/1% milkfat				
apple cobbler	8 oz	2.0	230	8%
black cherry parfait	4.4 oz	1.0	130	7%
	8 oz	2.0	240	8%
blueberries'N cream-flavored	4.4 oz	1.0	130	7%
	8 oz	2.0	240	8%
classic strawberry	4.4 oz	1.0	130	7%
	8 oz	2.0	230	8%
orange vanilla cream-flavored	8 oz	2.0	230	8%
peaches'N cream-flavored	4.4 oz	1.0	130	7%
	8 oz	2.0	230	8%
raspberries'N cream-flavored	8 oz	2.0	230	8%
strawberry banana split	8 oz	2.0	240	8%
strawberry cheesecake	8 oz	2.0	240	8%
(Brown Cow Farm)				
cherry vanilla	8 oz	8.0	230	31%
plain	8 oz	10.0	170	53%

Food and Description	Amount	Fat Grams	Total Calories	% Fat Calories
raspberry	8 oz	8.0	230	31%
strawberry	8 oz	8.0	230	31%
vanilla	8 oz	9.0	210	39%
(Colombo)				
Fat-free				
apples 'n spice	8 oz	–	200	–
apricot	8 oz	–	200	–
banana-strawberry	8 oz	–	220	–
black cherry parfait	8 oz	–	200	–
blackberry burst	8 oz	–	200	–
blueberry	8 oz	–	200	–
cherry	8 oz	–	200	–
fruit burst	8 oz	–	200	–
peach	8 oz	–	200	–
plain	8 oz	–	100	–
raspberry	8 oz	–	200	–
strawberry	8 oz	–	200	–
strawberry kiwi	8 oz	–	200	–
strawberry pineapple orange	8 oz	–	200	–
vanilla	8 oz	–	160	–
white chocolate raspberry	8 oz	–	200	–
Light 100				
blueberry	8 oz	–	100	–
cherry vanilla	8 oz	–	100	–
key lime pie	8 oz	–	100	–
lemon meringue	8 oz	–	100	–
mixed berries	8 oz	–	100	–
peach	8 oz	–	100	–
raspberry	8 oz	–	100	–
raspberry lemonade	8 oz	–	100	–
strawberry	8 oz	–	100	–
strawberry banana	8 oz	–	100	–
strawberry colada	8 oz	–	100	–
vanilla	8 oz	–	100	–
Low-Fat				
blueberry	8 oz	3.0	200	14%
plain	8 oz	4.0	130	28%
raspberry	8 oz	3.0	200	14%
strawberry				
8 oz container	8 oz	3.0	200	14%
32 oz container	8 oz	4.0	180	20%
vanilla	8 oz	3.5	180	18%
(Crowley)				
Non-Fat				
banana creme	8 oz	1.5	130	10%
black cherry	8 oz	1.5	130	10%
blueberry	8 oz	1.5	130	10%
cappuccino	8 oz	1.5	130	10%
cherry vanilla	8 oz	1.5	130	10%
lemon	8 oz	1.5	130	10%

Food and Description	Amount	Fat Grams	Total Calories	% Fat Calories
mixed berry	8 oz	1.5	130	10%
peach	8 oz	1.5	130	10%
raspberry	8 oz	1.5	130	10%
strawberry	8 oz	1.5	130	10%
strawberry banana	8 oz	1.5	130	10%
key lime pie	8 oz	1.5	130	10%
pina colada	8 oz	1.5	130	10%
plain	8 oz	1.5	130	10%
vanilla	8 oz	1.5	130	10%
white chocolate raspberry	8 oz	1.5	130	10%
Swiss Style				
black cherry	8 oz	2.5	240	9%
blueberry	8 oz	2.5	240	9%
cherry vanilla	8 oz	2.5	240	9%
lemon	8 oz	2.5	240	9%
key lime pie	8 oz	2.5	240	9%
orange creme	8 oz	2.5	240	9%
pina colada	8 oz	2.5	240	9%
pineapple cherry	8 oz	2.5	240	9%
plain	8 oz	2.5	240	9%
raspberry	8 oz	2.5	240	9%
strawberry	8 oz	2.5	240	9%
strawberry banana	8 oz	2.5	240	9%
vanilla	8 oz	2.4	240	9%
(Dannon)				
Blended				
blueberry	4 oz	–	100	–
cherry	4 oz	–	100	–
peach	4 oz	–	100	–
raspberry	4 oz	–	100	–
strawberry	4 oz	–	100	–
strawberry-banana	4 oz	–	100	–
Danimals/low-fat				
cherry	4.4 oz	0.5	110	4%
strawberry	4.4 oz	0.5	110	4%
strawberry banana	4.4 oz	0.5	110	4%
tropical punch	4.4 oz	0.5	120	4%
wild raspberry	4.4 oz	0.5	110	4%
vanilla	4.4 oz	0.5	110	4%
Dannon Sprinkl'ins/low-fat				
Magic crystals				
vanilla w/cherry crystals	1 container	1.0	120	8%
vanilla w/orange crystals	1 container	1.0	120	8%
Rainbow sprinklins				
cherry vanilla	1 container	1.0	130	7%
strawberry	1 container	1.0	130	7%
strawberry banana vanilla	1 container	1.0	130	7%
Double Delights/lowfat w/toppings				
Bavarian creme w/raspberry	6 oz	1.0	170	5%

Food and Description	Amount	Fat Grams	Total Calories	% Fat Calories
blueberry French vanilla	6 oz	1.0	170	5%
cheesecake				
cherry	6 oz	1.0	180	5%
chocolate	6 oz	1.0	170	5%
strawberry	6 oz	1.0	170	5%
lemon meringue pie	6 oz	1.0	180	5%
Fruit on the bottom/low-fat				
apple cinnamon	8 oz	2.0	210	9%
blueberry	4 oz	1.0	110	8%
	8 oz	2.0	220	8%
boysenberry	8 oz	2.0	210	9%
cherry	8 oz	2.0	220	8%
French vanilla				
raspberry	8 oz	3.0	240	11%
strawberry	8 oz	3.0	240	11%
mixed berry	4 oz	1.0	110	8%
	8 oz	2.0	210	9%
peach	4 oz	1.0	110	8%
	8 oz	2.0	210	9%
raspberry	8 oz	2.0	210	9%
strawberry	4 oz	1.0	110	8%
	8 oz	2.0	210	9%
strawberry-banana	8 oz	2.0	240	8%
tropical peach	8 oz	3.0	250	11%
Light/nonfat				
banana cream pie	8 oz	–	120	–
blackberry pie	8 oz	–	120	–
blueberry	8 oz	–	120	–
cappuccino	8 oz	–	120	–
cherry vanilla	8 oz	–	120	–
coconut cream pie	8 oz	–	120	–
creme caramel	8 oz	–	120	–
lemon chiffon	8 oz	–	120	–
orange mango	8 oz	–	120	–
peach	8 oz	–	120	–
raspberry	8 oz	–	120	–
strawberry	8 oz	–	120	–
strawberry-banana	8 oz	–	120	–
strawberry-kiwi	8 oz	–	120	–
tangerine chiffon	8 oz	–	120	–
tropical fruit	8 oz	–	120	–
vanilla	8 oz	–	120	–
white chocolate raspberry	8 oz	–	120	–
Light 'n Crunchy				
caramel apple crunch	8 oz	0.5	170	3%
cookies 'n cream	8 oz	–	160	–
raspberry w/granola	8 oz	0.5	170	3%
generic				
lowfat				
coffee or vanilla	4 oz	1.0	100	9%

Food and Description	Amount	Fat Grams	Total Calories	% Fat Calories
fruit flavors	4 oz	1.0	115	8%
plain	4 oz	2.0	75	24%
nonfat	4 oz	–	65	–
whole-milk	4 oz	4.0	70	51%
(Horizon) Organic fat-free				
blueberry	¾ cup	–	130	–
cherry	¾ cup	–	130	–
strawberry	¾ cup	–	130	–
strawberry banana	¾ cup	–	130	–
(Jell-O) Low-fat/2% milkfat				
cherry	4.4 oz	1.0	130	7%
grape	4.4 oz	1.0	130	7%
raspberry	4.4 oz	1.0	130	7%
tropical berry twist	4.4 oz	1.0	130	7%
tropical punch	4.4 oz	1.0	130	7%
watermelon	4.4 oz	1.0	130	7%
wild berry	4.4 oz	1.0	130	7%
strawberry	4.4 oz	1.0	130	7%
(La Yogurt)				
French Style				
banana	6 oz	3.0	180	15%
blueberry				
non-fat	6 oz	–	70	–
original	6 oz	3.0	180	15%
cherry				
non-fat	6 oz	–	70	–
original	6 oz	3.0	180	15%
cherry vanilla	6 oz	3.0	180	15%
guava	6 oz	3.0	180	15%
key lime	6 oz	3.0	180	15%
mango	6 oz	3.0	180	15%
mixed berry	6 oz	3.0	180	15%
peach	6 oz	3.0	180	15%
piña colada	6 oz	3.0	180	15%
raspberry				
non-fat	6 oz	–	70	–
original	6 oz	3.0	180	15%
strawberry				
non-fat	6 oz	–	70	–
original	6 oz	3.0	180	15%
strawberry fruit cup	6 oz	4.0	190	19%
strawberry-banana				
non-fat	6 oz	–	70	–
original	6 oz	3.0	180	15%
tropical orange	6 oz	3.0	180	15%
vanilla	6 oz	3.0	170	16%
Latin Style				
banana	6 oz	3.0	190	14%
guava	6 oz	3.0	190	14%
mango	6 oz	3.0	190	14%

Food and Description	Amount	Fat Grams	Total Calories	% Fat Calories
papaya	6 oz	3.0	190	14%
passion fruit	6 oz	3.0	190	14%
(Light 'n Lively)				
Free/Non-fat				
blueberry	4.4 oz	–	70	–
peach	4.4 oz	–	70	–
strawberry	4.4 oz	–	70	–
strawberry banana cream	4.4 oz	–	70	–
strawberry fruit cup	4.4 oz	–	70	–
low-fat/1 % milk fat				
blueberry	4.4 oz	1.0	130	7%
peach	4.4 oz	1.0	130	7%
pineapple	4.4 oz	1.0	130	7%
red raspberry	4.4 oz	1.0	120	8%
strawberry	4.4 oz	1.0	130	7%
strawberry banana	4.4 oz	1.0	130	7%
strawberry fruit cup	4.4 oz	1.0	130	7%
(Mountain High)				
Fat-free				
black cherry	6 oz	–	120	–
blueberry	6 oz	–	120	–
cherry	6 oz	–	120	–
key lime	6 oz	–	120	–
plain	6 oz	–	110	–
raspberry	6 oz	–	120	–
strawberry	6 oz	–	120	–
strawberry-banana	6 oz	–	120	–
vanilla	1 cup	–	170	–
Low-fat/vanilla	1 cup	2.0	200	9%
Original/plain	1 cup	8.0	190	38%
(New Country) low-fat				
apple crisp	6 oz	2.0	150	12%
blueberry supreme	6 oz	2.0	150	12%
cherry supreme	6 oz	2.0	150	12%
French vanilla	6 oz	2.0	150	12%
fruit crunch	6 oz	2.0	150	12%
Hawaiian salad	6 oz	2.0	150	12%
lemon supreme	6 oz	2.0	150	12%
mixed berries	6 oz	2.0	150	12%
orange supreme	6 oz	2.0	150	12%
peaches 'n cream	6 oz	2.0	150	12%
raspberry supreme	6 oz	2.0	150	12%
strawberry fruit cup	6 oz	2.0	150	12%
strawberry supreme	6 oz	2.0	150	12%
strawberry-banana supreme	6 oz	2.0	150	12%
(TCBY)				
light				
black cherry	8 oz	–	100	–
blueberry	8 oz	–	100	
strawberry	8 oz	–	100	
strawberry-banana	8 oz	–	100	

Food and Description	Amount	Fat Grams	Total Calories	% Fat Calories
low-fat				
blueberry	8 oz	2.0	220	8%
cherry-vanilla	8 oz	2.0	220	8%
peach	8 oz	2.0	220	8%
raspberry	8 oz	2.0	220	8%
strawberry	8 oz	2.0	220	8%
strawberry-banana	8 oz	2.0	220	8%
(Weight Watchers) Ultimate 90				
blueberries 'n creme	1 cup	–	90	–
cappuccino	1 cup	–	90	–
cherries jubilee	1 cup	–	90	–
cranberry raspberry	1 cup	–	90	–
lemon chiffon	1 cup	–	90	–
peach	1 cup	–	90	–
plain	1 cup	–	90	–
raspberries 'n creme	1 cup	–	90	–
strawberry	1 cup	–	90	–
strawberry-banana	1 cup	–	90	–
vanilla	1 cup	–	90	–
(Yoplait)				
Custard style				
banana	6 oz	3.5	190	17%
blueberry	6 oz	3.5	190	17%
cherry vanilla	6 oz	3.5	190	17%
key lime pie	6 oz	3.5	190	17%
lemon	6 oz	3.5	190	17%
peaches'n cream	4 oz	2.0	120	15%
	6 oz	3.5	190	17%
raspberry	4 oz	2.0	120	15%
raspberry cheesecake	6 oz	3.5	190	17%
strawberry	4 oz	2.0	120	15%
	6 oz	3.5	190	17%
strawberry banana	4 oz	2.0	120	15%
	6 oz	3.5	190	17%
strawberry vanilla	4 oz	2.0	120	15%
vanilla	6 oz	3.5	190	17%
Go-Gurt				
berry blue	2¼ oz	2.0	70	26%
cherry	2¼ oz	2.0	70	26%
cotton candy	2¼ oz	2.0	70	26%
punch	2¼ oz	2.0	70	26%
raspberry	2¼ oz	2.0	70	26%
strawberry	2¼ oz	2.0	70	26%
strawberry banana	2¼ oz	2.0	70	26%
strawberry kiwi	2¼ oz	2.0	70	26%
watermelon	2¼ oz	2.0	70	26%
Light				
apricot mango	6 oz	–	90	–
banana cream pie	6 oz	–	90	–
berries'n cream	6 oz	–	90	–

Food and Description	Amount	Fat Grams	Total Calories	% Fat Calories
blueberry	6 oz	–	90	–
Boston cream pie	6 oz	–	90	–
cherry	6 oz	–	90	–
key lime pie	6 oz	–	90	–
lemon cream pie	6 oz	–	90	–
peach	6 oz	–	90	–
raspberry	6 oz	–	90	–
raspberry peach melba	6 oz	–	90	–
strawberry	6 oz	–	90	–
strawberry banana	6 oz	–	90	–
strawberry orange banana	6 oz	–	90	–
white chocolate strawberry	6 oz	–	90	–
Original/99% fat free				
banana	6 oz	1.5	170	8%
blueberry	6 oz	1.5	170	8%
boysenberry	6 oz	1.5	170	8%
cherry	6 oz	1.5	170	8%
coconut cream pie	6 oz	3.0	190	14%
French vanilla	6 oz	1.5	170	8%
harvest peach	4 oz	1.0	110	8%
	6 oz	1.5	170	8%
key lime pie	6 oz	1.5	170	8%
lemon	6 oz	1.5	180	8%
Mandarin orange	6 oz	1.5	170	8%
mixed berry	4 oz	1.0	110	8%
	6 oz	1.5	170	8%
orange creme	6 oz	1.5	170	8%
pineapple	6 oz	1.5	170	8%
raspberry	4 oz	1.0	110	8%
	6 oz	1.5	170	8%
raspberry lemonade	6 oz	1.5	170	8%
strawberry	4 oz	1.0	110	8%
	6 oz	1.5	170	8%
strawberry-banana	4 oz	1.0	110	8%
	6 oz	1.5	170	8%
strawberry cheesecake	6 oz	1.5	170	8%
strawberry kiwi	6 oz	1.5	170	8%
strawberry mango	6 oz	1.5	170	8%
tropical peach	6 oz	1.5	170	8%
vanilla	6 oz	1.0	170	5%
white chocolate raspberry	6 oz	1.0	170	5%
Trix				
cotton candy	4 oz	1.5	120	11%
raspberry rainbow	4 oz	1.5	120	11%
strawberry banana bash	4 oz	1.5	120	11%
strawberry kiwi	4 oz	1.5	120	11%
strawberry punch	4 oz	1.5	120	11%
triple cherry	4 oz	1.5	120	11%
watermelon burst	4 oz	1.5	120	11%
wild berry blue	4 oz	1.5	120	11%

Food and Description	Amount	Fat Grams	Total Calories	% Fat Calories
YOGURT, FROZEN				
■ BARS & NOVELTIES				
(Ben & Jerry's) Cherry Garcia pop	1 pop	13.0	250	47%
(Cascadian Farm) Organic				
blackberry	1 bar	1.0	80	11%
chocolate	1 bar	1.5	80	17%
vanilla	1 bar	1.0	80	11%
(Haagen-Dazs) raspberry & vanilla bar	1 bar	–	90	–
■ REGULAR & SOFT-SERVE/CARTON OR PACKAGE				
(Baskin-Robbins) Yogurt Gone Crazy				
Maui brownie madness	½ cup	3.0	140	19%
perils of praline	½ cup	3.0	140	19%
raspberry cheese Louise	½ cup	3.0	130	21%
(Ben & Jerry's)				
Cherry Garcia				
chocolate	½ cup	4.0	190	19%
original	½ cup	3.0	170	16%
chocolate chip cookie dough	½ cup	4.5	200	20%
chocolate fudge brownie	½ cup	2.5	190	12%
chocolate Heath bar crunch	½ cup	6.0	210	26%
Chunky Monkey	½ cup	6.0	200	27%
Ooey Gooey Cake	½ cup	3.5	190	17%
(Breyers) All Natural				
chocolate	½ cup	3.0	130	21%
strawberry	½ cup	2.5	120	19%
vanilla	½ cup	3.0	120	23%
vanilla/chocolate/strawberry	½ cup	2.5	120	19%
(Cascadian Farm) Organic				
chocolate	½ cup	3.0	90	30%
harvest berry	½ cup	2.0	120	15%
lemon chiffon	½ cup	2.0	120	15%
mocha fudge	½ cup	2.0	120	15%
raspberry/chocolate swirl	½ cup	2.0	110	16%
vanilla	½ cup	3.0	130	21%
(Columbo) Soft Serve				
Low-Fat				
old world chocolate	½ cup	2.0	110	16%
peanut butter	½ cup	2.5	120	19%
strawberry	½ cup	1.5	110	12%
vanilla				
French	½ cup	1.5	110	12%
original	½ cup	1.5	110	12%
simply	½ cup	1.5	110	12%
Non-fat				
Alpine strawberry	½ cup	–	100	–
banana	½ cup	–	100	–
black cherry	½ cup	–	100	–
butter nut toffee	½ cup	–	100	–
butter pecan	½ cup	–	100	–
cappuccino	½ cup	–	100	–
cheesecake	½ cup	–	100	–

Food and Description	Amount	Fat Grams	Total Calories	% Fat Calories
cherry vanilla	½ cup	–	100	–
coconut cooler	½ cup	–	100	–
cookies'n cream	½ cup	–	120	–
country pumpkin	½ cup	–	100	–
double Dutch chocolate	½ cup	–	100	–
eggnog	½ cup	–	100	–
frango mint chocolate	½ cup	–	100	–
German chocolate fudge	½ cup	–	110	–
Grandma's apple pie	½ cup	–	100	–
honey-almond	½ cup	–	100	–
Irish creme	½ cup	–	100	–
mocha madness	½ cup	–	100	–
Swiss chocolate almond	½ cup	–	100	–
vanilla	½ cup	–	100	
Slender Sensations				
amaretto	½ cup	–	60	–
chocolate	½ cup	–	70	–
raspberry	½ cup	–	60	–
strawberry	½ cup	–	60	–
strawberry banana	½ cup	–	60	–
vanilla	½ cup	–	60	–
(Dannon) Soft				
Fat-free				
blueberry pie	½ cup	–	100	–
cappuccino	½ cup	–	100	–
chocolate	½ cup	–	100	–
French vanilla	½ cup	–	100	–
New York cheese cake	½ cup	–	100	–
orange	½ cup	–	100	–
peach	½ cup	–	100	–
praline pecan	½ cup	–	100	–
red raspberry	½ cup	–	100	–
strawberry	½ cup	–	100	–
vanilla	½ cup	–	100	–
white chocolate mousse	½ cup	–	100	–
Low-fat				
chocolate	½ cup	3.0	120	23%
peanut butter	½ cup	3.0	120	23%
vanilla	½ cup	2.0	110	16%
(Dreyer's)				
fat-free				
black cherry vanilla swirl	½ cup	–	90	–
caramel praline crunch	½ cup	–	100	–
chocolate fudge	½ cup	–	100	–
coffee fudge sundae	½ cup	–	100	–
vanilla	½ cup	–	90	–
vanilla chocolate swirl	½ cup	–	90	–
regular				
Bananafana	½ cup	4.0	120	30%
Carmel Fudge Cosmo	½ cup	4.0	140	26%
cookies 'n cream	½ cup	3.0	110	25%

Food and Description	Amount	Fat Grams	Total Calories	% Fat Calories
Heath Toffee Crunch	½ cup	4.0	120	30%
Hokey Pokey	½ cup	4.5	140	29%
Mumbo jumbo	½ cup	3.0	120	23%
ultimate tin roof sundae	½ cup	4.0	130	28%
vanilla	½ cup	2.5	100	23%
(Edys)				
fat-free				
black cherry vanilla swirl	½ cup	–	90	–
caramel praline crunch	½ cup	–	100	–
chocolate fudge	½ cup	–	100	–
coffee fudge sundae	½ cup	–	100	–
vanilla	½ cup	–	90	–
vanilla chocolate swirl	½ cup	–	90	–
regular				
Bananafana	½ cup	4.0	120	30%
Carmel Fudge Cosmo	½ cup	4.0	140	26%
cookies 'n cream	½ cup	3.0	110	25%
Heath Toffee Crunch	½ cup	4.0	120	30%
Hokey Pokey	½ cup	4.5	140	29%
Mumbo jumbo	½ cup	3.0	120	23%
ultimate tin roof sundae	½ cup	4.0	130	28%
vanilla	½ cup	2.5	100	23%
(Elan)				
caramel almond praline	½ cup	4.0	150	24%
chocolate	½ cup	3.0	130	21%
chocolate almond	½ cup	6.0	160	34%
coffee	½ cup	3.0	130	21%
peach	½ cup	3.0	130	21%
rum raisin	½ cup	3.0	135	20%
strawberry	½ cup	3.0	125	22%
vanilla	½ cup	3.0	130	21%
(Friendly's)				
apple Bettie	½ cup	3.0	140	19%
fabulous fudge swirl	½ cup	3.0	140	19%
strawberry cheesecake blast	½ cup	4.0	140	26%
toffee almond crunch	½ cup	5.0	160	28%
(Haagen-Dazs) pints				
Low-fat				
Dulce de Leche	½ cup	2.5	190	12%
Non-fat				
chocolate	½ cup	–	140	–
coffee	½ cup	–	140	–
raspberry swirl	½ cup	–	130	–
strawberry	½ cup	–	140	–
vanilla	½ cup	–	140	–
vanilla fudge	½ cup	–	160	–
Soft Serve/at shops-Non-fat				
chocolate	½ cup	–	110	–
chocolate mousse	½ cup	–	80	–
coffee	½ cup	–	110	–
strawberry	½ cup	–	110	–

Food and Description	Amount	Fat Grams	Total Calories	% Fat Calories
vanilla	½ cup	–	110	–
vanilla mousse	½ cup	–	70	–
white chocolate	½ cup	–	110	–
(Hood)				
Nonfat				
caramel & brownie sundae	½ cup	–	120	–
chocolate marshmallow	½ cup	–	110	–
double raspberry	½ cup	–	120	–
mocha fudge	½ cup	–	120	–
peach cobbler A la mode	½ cup	–	110	–
strawberry	½ cup	–	100	–
vanilla	½ cup	–	120	–
vanilla fudge	½ cup	–	120	–
Regular				
Bavarian truffle & twist	½ cup	4.0	150	24%
coffee toffee chunk sundae	½ cup	4.0	150	24%
cookies & cream	½ cup	4.0	140	26%
Grandma's raisin oatmeal cookie dough	½ cup	3.0	140	19%
mixed berry swirl	½ cup	2.0	120	15%
vanilla Swiss almond sundae	½ cup	4.0	150	24%
(Kemp's)				
Nonfat				
chocolate	½ cup	–	110	–
cookies 'n cream	½ cup	–	120	–
fudge marble	½ cup	–	110	–
mint fudge	½ cup	–	110	–
peach	½ cup	–	90	–
rocky road	½ cup	–	130	–
strawberry	½ cup	–	90	–
strawberry shortcake	½ cup	–	100	–
vanilla	½ cup	–	110	–
Regular/praline caramel	½ cup	4.0	150	24%
Sundae topper				
chocolate chip cookie dough	½ cup	4.0	140	50%
Heath Bar Crunch	½ cup	4.0	140	50%
(Miss Karen's) gourmet				
Low-fat				
chocolate	½ cup	5.0	160	28%
premium	½ cup	3.0	120	23%
original	½ cup	2.0	90	20%
Nonfat				
chocolate temptation	½ cup	–	110	–
original	½ cup	–	80	–
select/no sugar added	½ cup	–	80	–
vanilla bean	½ cup	–	100	–
(Schwan's) premium lowfat				
black cherry	½ cup	2.5	120	19%
chocolate	½ cup	3.0	120	23%
chocolate fudge brownie	½ cup	3.0	130	21%
glacier bay lemon	½ cup	3.0	130	21%

Food and Description	Amount	Fat Grams	Total Calories	% Fat Calories
vanilla	½ cup	3.0	110	25%
wild berry	½ cup	1.5	120	11%
(TCBY)				
Soft-Serve/all flavors				
96% Fat-Free	½ cup	3.0	130	21%
Nonfat	½ cup	–	110	–
Nonfat/no sugar added	½ cup	–	80	–
(Turkey Hill)				
Nonfat				
chocolate cherry cordial	½ cup	–	100	–
chocolate marshmallow	½ cup	–	130	–
coffee cappuccino	½ cup	–	110	–
mint cookie'n cream	½ cup	–	110	–
raspberry chocolate bliss	½ cup	–	110	–
Southern lemon pie	½ cup	–	110	–
Regular				
chocolate cherry cordial	½ cup	3.0	130	21%
chocolate chip cookie dough	½ cup	5.0	140	32%
death by chocolate	½ cup	4.0	150	24%
tin roof sundae	½ cup	5.0	140	32%
YOGURT BAR (*See* CANDY; YOGURT, FROZEN)				
YOGURT DRINK				
(Dannon) Danimals drinkable				
cherry	3.1 fl oz	1.5	90	15%
raspberry	3.1 fl oz	1.5	90	15%
strawberry	3.1 fl oz	1.5	90	15%
tropical punch	3.1 fl oz	1.5	90	15%
(Yogloo) all flavors	10 fl oz	–	170	–
(Yonique) low-fat				
banana	6 fl oz	1.5	130	10%
mango	6 fl oz	1.5	130	10%
peach	6 fl oz	2.0	170	11%
strawberry	6 fl oz	2.0	190	9%

Z

Food and Description	Amount	Fat Grams	Total Calories	% Fat Calories
ZABAGLIONE (*See* CUSTARD)				
ZUCCHINI (*See* SQUASH)				
ZWIEBACK (*See* BABY FOOD; COOKIE)				

FAST FOOD

Food and Description	Amount	Fat Grams	Total Calories	% Fat Calories
GENERAL (USDA averages derived from several restaurant chains)				
■ **BREAKFAST**				
biscuit/plain	1 biscuit	13.0	276	42%
croissant				
w/egg, cheese, & bacon	1 croissant	28.0	413	6 %
w/egg, cheese, & ham	1 croissant	33.6	475	64%
w/egg, cheese, & sausage	1 croissant	38.0	524	65%
w/egg & cheese	1 croissant	24.7	369	60%
Danish				
cheese	1 Danish	24.6	353	63%
cinnamon	1 Danish	16.7	349	43%
fruit	1 Danish	15.9	335	43%
egg/scrambled	2 eggs	15.0	200	68%
English muffin				
w/butter	1 muffin	5.8	189	27%
w/cheese & sausage	1 muffin	24.0	394	55%
w/egg. cheese & Canadian bacon	1 muffin	19.8	383	46%
w/egg, cheese & sausage	1 muffin	30.9	487	57%
French toast w/butter	2 slices	18.8	356	47%
French toast stick	5 sticks	29.0	479	55%
omelet/ham & cheese	2 egg	17.7	255	52%
pancakes w/syrup & butter	3 pancakes	14.0	519	24%
potatoes/hash brown	½ cup	9.0	151	54%
sausage	1 patty	8.0	100	72%
■ **BURGERS, HOT DOGS, & BEEF**				
(NOTE: A regular meat patty = 2 oz; large = 4 oz [¼ lb]. Single burgers contain 1 patty; double burgers contain 2 patties; triple burgers contain 3 patties. All burgers and hot dogs are served on appropriate size buns. Items marked with an asterisk [*] do not include condiments or garnishes such as pickle, catsup, lettuce, onions, tomato, mustard, or mayonnaise-type dressing.)				
cheeseburger				
large patty/w/bacon				
double	1 burger	43.7	706	56%
single	1 burger	36.8	609	60%
regular patty/double	1 burger	28.0	457	55%
cheeseburger*				
large patty				
single	1 burger	33.0	608	49%
triple	1 burger	51.0	796	57%

Food and Description	Amount	Fat Grams	Total Calories	% Fat Calories
regular patty				
single	1 burger	15.0	320	42%
double/double bun	1 burger	21.6	461	42%
corn dog*	1 corn dog	18.9	460	37%
hamburger				
large patty				
single	1 burger	27.0	511	48%
triple	1 burger	41.0	693	53%
regular patty				
single	1 burger	13.0	279	42%
double	1 burger	32.0	576	50%
hamburger*				
large patty/single	1 burger	22.9	400	52%
regular patty				
double	1 burger	27.9	544	46%
single	1 burger	11.8	275	39%
hotdog*				
plain	1 hot dog	14.5	242	54%
w/chili	1 hot dog	17.5	324	49%
roast beef on bun*				
plain				
regular	1 sandwich	13.8	346	36%
super	1 sandwich	28.0	620	41%
w/cheese*	1 sandwich	18.0	402	40%

■ CHICKEN, EGG, HAM, & SEAFOOD

(NOTE: Items marked with an asterisk [*] do not include condiments or garnishes such as pickle, catsup, lettuce, onions, tomato, mustard, or mayonnaise-type dressing.)

Food and Description	Amount	Fat Grams	Total Calories	% Fat Calories
chicken/breaded & fried				
dark meat	2 pieces	26.7	430	56%
wing & breast	2 pieces	29.5	494	54%
chicken fillet sandwich*				
plain	1 sandwich	29.0	515	51%
w/cheese	1 sandwich	38.8	632	55%
chicken nuggets				
plain	1 piece	3.0	48	55%
	6 pieces	17.7	290	55%
w/barbecue sauce	6 pieces	18.0	330	49%
w/honey	6 pieces	17.5	329	48%
w/mustard sauce	6 pieces	18.9	323	53%
w/sweet & sour sauce	6 pieces	18.0	346	47%
clams/breaded & fried	¾ cup	26.0	451	52%
crab/soft shell/fried	1 serving	17.9	334	48%
crab cake				
baked	1 cake	1.0	88	10%
fried	1 cake	18.8	290	58%
fish fillet/battered or breaded & fried	1 fillet	11.0	211	47%
fish fillet sandwich*				
plain	1 sandwich	22.8	431	48%
w/tartar sauce & cheese	1 sandwich	28.6	524	49%
ham, egg, & cheese on bun*	1 sandwich	16.0	348	41%

Food and Description	Amount	Fat Grams	Total Calories	% Fat Calories
ham & cheese on bun*	1 sandwich	15.0	353	38%
oysters/battered or breaded & fried	6 pieces	17.9	368	44%
scallops/breaded & fried	6 pieces	19.0	386	44%
shrimp/breaded & fried	6-8 pieces	24.9	454	49%
■ **CONDIMENTS** (*See also* Salad & Salad Bar Items in this section)				
butter/ ½-oz pkt	1 pkt	11.0	100	100%
catsup/ ¼-oz pkt	1 pkt	–	3	–
half & half/ ½-oz pkt	1 pkt	1.6	18	80%
honey/ ½-oz pkt	1 pkt	–	43	–
jelly/ ¾-oz pkt	1 pkt	–	58	–
lemon ½-oz pkt	1 pkt	–	3	–
lettuce	2 leaves	–	2	–
mayonnaise/ ⅖-oz pkt	1 pkt	9.0	81	100%
mustard/ ⅕-oz pkt	1 pkt	–	4	–
nondairy creamer/ ⅖-oz pkt	1 pkt	3.5	55	57%
onion	2 slices	–	7	–
pickle	2 slices	–	2	–
sugar	1 pkt	–	25	–
sugar substitute	1 pkt	–	4	–
syrup/ 1½-oz pkt	1 pkt	–	122	–
tartar sauce/ ½-oz pkt	1 pkt	8.0	74	97%
tomato	1 slice	–	5	–
■ **DESSERT**				
brownie	1 brownie	10.0	243	37%
fried pie	1 pie	14.0	266	47%
ice cream cone				
chocolate-dipped	1 small	7.0	150	42%
	1 medium	13.0	300	39%
	1 large	20.0	450	40%
plain	1 small	3.0	110	25%
	1 medium	7.0	230	27%
	1 large	10.0	340	27%
ice cream sandwich	1 sandwich	4.0	140	26%
ice milk/soft serve w/cone	1 oz	6.0	164	33%
sundae				
caramel	1 sundae	9.0	303	27%
hot fudge	1 sundae	8.6	284	27%
strawberry	1 sundae	7.9	269	26%
■ **MEXICAN FOOD**				
burrito				
bean	2 burritos	13.5	448	27%
bean & cheese	2 burritos	11.7	377	28%
bean & chili peppers	2 burritos	14.7	413	32%
bean & meat	2 burritos	17.8	508	32%
bean, cheese, & beef	2 burritos	13.0	331	35%
beef	2 burritos	20.8	523	36%
beef & chili peppers	2 burritos	16.5	426	35%
beef, cheese, & chili peppers	2 burritos	24.8	634	35%
chili con carne	1 cup	8.0	254	28%

Food and Description	Amount	Fat Grams	Total Calories	% Fat Calories
chimichanga				
beef	1 piece	19.7	425	42%
beet & cheese	1 piece	23.5	443	48%
beet & red chili peppers	1 piece	19.0	424	40%
beef, cheese, & red chili peppers	1 piece	17.6	364	43%
enchilada				
cheese, beef, & beans	1 enchilada	16.0	344	42%
cheese & beef	1 enchilada	17.6	324	49%
cheese & sour cream	1 enchilada	18.9	320	53%
frijoles/cheese	1 cup	7.8	226	31%
nachos				
cheese	6-8 pieces	19.0	345	49%
cheese & jalapeño pepper	6-8 pieces	34.0	607	50%
cheese, ground beef, beans & jalapeño pepper	6-8 pieces	30.7	568	49%
cinnamon & sugar	6-8 pieces	36.0	592	55%
taco	1 small	20.6	370	50%
	1 large	31.6	569	50%
taco salad/lettuce, tomato, chili sauce, ground beef, cheese, & taco shell	1½ cups	14.8	279	47%
w/chili con carne	1½ cups	13.0	288	41%
tostada				
bean, beef, & cheese	1 tostada	16.9	334	46%
bean & cheese	1 tostada	9.9	223	40%
beef, cheese, & guacamole	2 tostadas	23.0	360	58%
beef & cheese	1 tostada	16.0	315	46%
■ SALAD & SALAD BAR ITEMS				
alfalfa sprouts	1 oz	–	10	–
bacon bits	2 Tbs	3.0	54	50%
broccoli	~2 oz	–	6	–
carrots	~2 oz	–	12	–
cauliflower	~ 2 oz	–	14	–
cheese				
cheddar/shredded	3 Tbs	7.0	84	75%
cottage	½ cup	5.0	117	39%
mozzarella	1 oz	7.0	90	70%
Parmesan	3 Tbs	4.5	70	58%
Chef's salad w/cheese, turkey, ham, & egg	1½ cups.	16.0	267	54%
coleslaw	½ cup	8.0	90	80%
croutons	18 pieces	1.0	35	26%
cucumber/sliced	3 slices	–	2	–
egg/hard-cooked/chopped	2 Tbs	2.0	30	60%
garbanzo beans	1 Tbs	–	11	–
green peas	½ cup	–	60	–
lettuce	½ cup	–	5	–
mushroom/pieces	¼ cup	–	6	–
onion	2 Tbs	–	4	–
green pepper	2 Tbs	–	4	–
salad dressing (Note: 2 oz of dressing = 4 level Tbs)				
blue cheese/ 2½-oz pkt	1 pkt	34.0	342	90%

Food and Description	Amount	Fat Grams	Total Calories	% Fat Calories
French/ 2-oz pkt	1 pkt	20.6	228	81%
Italian/ 2-oz pkt	1 pkt	34.0	326	94%
low-calorie/ 2-oz pkt	1 pkt	2.0	50	36%
Oriental/ 2-oz pkt	1 pkt	1.0	102	9%
Thousand Island/ 2½-oz pkt	1 pkt	39.0	396	89%
wine vinegar	1 Tbs	–	2	–
tossed salad w/lettuce, tomato, radishes carrots, cabbage, cucumber, & green pepper				
plain/no dressing	1½ cups	–	32	–
w/cheese & egg	1½ cups	5.8	102	51%
w/chicken	1½ cups	2.0	105	17%
w/pasta & seafood	1½ cups	20.9	380	49%
w/shrimp	1½ cups	2.0	107	17%
tomato	1 oz	–	6	–

■ SANDWICHES

(NOTE: Unless otherwise stated, regular sandwiches are on sliced whole wheat bread w/average portions. Subs are on rolls, 6 to 8 inches long [8 to 12 ounces].)

Food and Description	Amount	Fat Grams	Total Calories	% Fat Calories
regular				
bacon, lettuce, & tomato	1 sandwich	16.0	290	50%
bologna/plain	1 sandwich	16.0	305	47%
chicken/sliced w/lettuce	1 sandwich	15.0	310	44%
chicken salad	1 sandwich	20.0	255	71%
club/chicken, bacon, & tomato	1 sandwich	26.0	570	41%
corned beef/plain	1 sandwich	10.0	296	30%
cream cheese & jelly	1 sandwich	16.0	370	39%
egg salad	1 sandwich	13.0	285	41%
ham/plain	1 sandwich	16.0	285	51%
ham & Swiss	1 sandwich	24.0	390	55%
ham salad	1 sandwich	17.0	321	48%
liverwurst/plain	1 sandwich	12.0	260	42%
peanut butter	1 sandwich	20.0	350	51%
peanut butter & jelly	1 sandwich	15.0	385	35%
roast beef/hot w/gravy	1 sandwich	25.0	421	53%
roast pork/hot w/gravy	1 sandwich	31.0	503	56%
steak/sirloin/lean & fat/3 oz	1 sandwich	12.0	325	33%
tuna salad	1 sandwich	14.0	275	46%
turkey/plain	1 sandwich	19.0	400	43%
subs/heroes				
roast beef, lettuce, tomato, & mayonnaise	1 sandwich	13.0	411	28%
salami, ham, cheese, lettuce, tomato, & onion	1 sandwich	18.6	456	37%
tuna salad	1 sandwich	28.0	584	43%

■ SIDE ORDERS (See also Salad & Salad Bar Items in this section)

Food and Description	Amount	Fat Grams	Total Calories	% Fat Calories
baked potato				
w/cheese	1 potato	28.7	475	54%
w/cheese & bacon	1 potato	25.9	451	52%
w/cheese sauce & broccoli	1 potato	21.0	402	47%
w/cheese sauce & chili	1 potato	21.9	481	41%
w/sour cream & chives	1 potato	22.0	394	50%
chili	1 cup	9.0	268	30%

Food and Description	Amount	Fat Grams	Total Calories	% Fat Calories
coleslaw	¾ cup	11.0	147	67%
corn on the cob				
plain	1 ear	1.0	125	7%
w/butter	1 ear	3.0	155	17%
French fries				
fried in beef tallow	regular	12.0	237	46%
	large	18.5	358	47%
fried in beef tallow & vegetable oil	regular	12.0	237	46%
	large	18.5	358	47%
fried in vegetable oil	regular	12.0	235	46%
	large	18.5	355	47%
hushpuppies	5 pieces	12.0	256	41%
macaroni salad w/mayonnaise	½ cup	6.0	168	32%
mashed potatoes w/whole milk				
& margarine	⅓ cup	1.0	66	13%
onion rings	8-9 pieces	15.5	175	80%
potato chips	10 chips	7.0	105	60%
	1 oz	10.0	148	61%
potato salad	⅓ cup	5.7	108	48%
Waldorf salad	½ cup	5.0	90	50%

ARBY'S

■ BEVERAGES

coffee	8 fl oz	–	–	–
hot chocolate	8 fl oz	1.0	110	8%
iced tea	16 fl oz	–	–	–
milk/2% reduced fat	8 fl oz	5.0	120	38%
orange juice	10 fl oz	–	140	–
shakes				
chocolate	10.3 oz	9.0	390	21%
jamocha	10.3 oz	9.0	380	21%
strawberry	10.3 oz	9.0	380	21%
vanilla	10.3 oz	9.0	380	21%

■ BREAKFAST

bacon	2 strips	7.0	90	70%
biscuit w/margarine	1 biscuit	16.0	270	53%
croissant	1 croissant	16.0	260	55%
egg/scrambled	1 egg	5.0	70	64%
French Toastix	6 stix	17.0	370	41%
ham	1.5 oz	3.0	50	54%
maple syrup	1.5 oz	–	220	–
sausage	1 patty	19.0	200	86%
Swiss cheese slice	0.5 oz	3.0	45	60%

■ CONDIMENTS (*See also* Salads & Related Items in this section)

Arby's sauce	½ oz	–	15	–
BBQ sauce	1 oz	–	40	–
beef stock aus jus	2 oz	–	10	–
Bronco Berry Sauce	1.5 oz	–	90	–
German mustard packet	1 pkt	–	5	–
honey mustard	1 oz	12.0	130	99%
Horsey Sauce packet	1 pkt	5.0	60	75%

Food and Description	Amount	Fat Grams	Total Calories	% Fat Calories
ketchup	1 pkt	–	10	–
marinara sauce	1.5 oz	1.5	35	39%
mayonnaise				
light	1 pkt	2.0	20	90%
regular	1 pkt	10.0	86	100%
Tangy Southwest Sauce	1.52 oz	25.0	250	90%
■ DESSERT				
turnovers				
apple	1 turnover	14.0	360	35%
cherry	1 turnover	14.0	350	36%
■ SALADS/SALAD DRESSINGS				
salad				
garden salad/light grilled	1 serving	5.0	280	16%
roast chicken salad/light	1 serving	5.0	200	23%
side salad	1 serving	3.0	90	30%
salad dressing				
bleu cheese dressing	2.5 oz	39.0	390	90%
buttermilk ranch dressing/reduced				
calorie	2 oz	–	50	–
honey French dressing	2.5 oz	27.0	350	69%
Italian dressing/reduced calorie	2.19 oz	1.0	20	45%
thousand island dressing	2.5 oz	33.0	350	85%
■ SANDWICHES				
Chicken				
bacon'N Swiss	1 sandwich	30.0	610	44%
breast fillet	1 sandwich	28.0	560	45%
cordon bleu	1 sandwich	34.0	650	47%
grilled deluxe	1 sandwich	16.0	420	34%
light				
grilled chicken	1 sandwich	5.0	280	16%
roast chicken deluxe	1 sandwich	5.0	260	17%
roast club	1 sandwich	29.0	540	48%
roast deluxe				
light	1 sandwich	6.0	276	20%
regular	1 sandwich	22.0	433	46%
Fish Fillet	1 sandwich	27.0	540	45%
Roast beef				
Arby Q	1 sandwich	15.0	380	36%
Arby's melt w/cheddar	1 sandwich	19.0	380	45%
Beef'N cheddar	1 sandwich	28.0	510	49%
Big Montana	1 sandwich	40.0	720	50%
original				
giant	1 sandwich	28.0	550	46%
junior	1 sandwich	16.0	340	42%
regular	1 sandwich	20.0	400	45%
super	1 sandwich	27.0	530	46%
Sub Sandwiches				
French dip	1 sandwich	22.0	490	40%
hot ham 'N Swiss	1 sandwich	31.0	570	49%
Italian	1 sandwich	54.0	800	61%

Food and Description	Amount	Fat Grams	Total Calories	% Fat Calories
Philly beef 'N Swiss	1 sandwich	48.0	780	55%
roast beef	1 sandwich	49.0	770	57%
turkey	1 sandwich	39.0	670	52%
Turkey/Light Roast Deluxe	1 sandwich	5.0	230	20%
■ SIDE ORDERS				
Baked potato				
broccoli 'N cheddar	1 potato	25.0	550	41%
chicken broccoli	1 potato	47.0	830	51%
cool ranch	1 potato	23.0	500	41%
deluxe	1 potato	31.0	610	46%
jalapeño	1 potato	36.0	660	49%
Philly chicken	1 potato	53.0	880	54%
plain w/butter and sour cream	1 potato	24.0	500	43%
Chicken finger				
meal	1 meal	47.0	880	48%
snack	1 snack	32.0	610	47%
Curly fries				
cheddar	6 oz	25.0	450	50%
regular	small	16.0	320	45%
	medium	19.0	380	45%
	large	30.0	600	45%
Homestyle fries	medium	19.0	420	41%
	large	29.0	630	41%
Jalapeño Bites	3.9 oz	21.0	330	57%
Mozzarella sticks	4.8 oz	29.0	470	56%
Onion petals	4 oz	24.0	410	53%
Potato cakes	2 cakes	14.0	220	57%
AU BON PAIN				
■ BAGEL SPREADS & BAGELS/Sourdough				
Bagel Spreads				
Lite cream cheese				
honey walnut	2 oz	11.0	150	66%
plain	2 oz	8.0	100	72%
raspberry	2 oz	7.0	130	48%
sun-dried tomato	2 oz	8.0	120	60%
vanilla hazelnut	2 oz	11.0	140	71%
veggie	2 oz	11.0	130	76%
Regular cream cheese				
plain	2 oz	18.0	180	90%
Bagels				
Asiago cheese	1 bagel	6.0	380	14%
cheddar & scallion	1 bagel	7.0	310	20%
cinnamon raisin	1 bagel	1.0	390	2%
cranberry walnut	1 bagel	4.0	460	8%
Dutch apple w/walnut streusel	1 bagel	5.0	350	13%
everything	1 bagel	2.5	360	6%
focaccia	1 bagel	4.5	330	12%
honey 9 grain	1 bagel	2.0	360	5%
jalapeño double cheddar	1 bagel	3.5	290	11%
onion	1 bagel	1.0	360	3%

Food and Description	Amount	Fat Grams	Total Calories	% Fat Calories
plain	1 bagel	1.0	350	4%
poppy seed	1 bagel	3.5	380	8%
sesame	1 bagel	4.0	380	9%
wild blueberry	1 bagel	1.5	380	4%
■ BEVERAGES				
apple cider/hot	8 oz	–	120	–
cappuccino/iced	1 small	4.0	110	33%
	1 medium	6.0	150	36%
	1 large	10.0	270	33%
malt shoppe blast/frozen wilch drink	16 oz	9.0	460	18%
mocha blast/frozen				
blender	16 oz	3.0	320	8%
	24 oz	4.0	480	8%
wilch drink	16 oz	7.0	350	18%
strawberry banana split blast/				
frozen wilch drink	16 oz	5.0	280	16%
tea/iced				
peach	small	–	90	–
	medium	–	130	–
	large	–	170	–
■ BREADS & LOAVES				
baguette	1 slice	1.0	130	7%
braided roll	1 roll	11.0	370	27%
bread bowl	1 bowl	3.0	680	4%
bread stick/rosemary-garlic	1 stick	2.5	180	13%
country white loaf	1 slice	0.5	130	3%
four grain	1 slice	1.5	170	8%
French	1 slice	1.0	300	3%
hearth roll	1 roll	2.0	200	9%
hearth/four grain	1 slice	3.0	290	9%
multigrain loaf	1 slice	1.5	140	10%
Parisienne loaf	1 slice	–	130	–
petit pain roll	1 roll	1.0	210	4%
pita bread/wrap	½ wrap	–	130	–
tomato herb loaf	1 slice	1.0	130	7%
■ COOKIE BARS & COOKIES				
Cookie Bars				
Mochaccino	1 bar	24.0	404	53%
Oreo	1 bar	29.0	550	47%
7-layer bar	1 bar	10.0	300	30%
walnut fudge brownie	1 bar	18.0	380	43%
Cookies				
chocolate chip	1 cookie	13.0	280	42%
English toffee	1 cookie	6.0	200	27%
gingerbread man	1 cookie	8.0	300	24%
holiday brownie nut fudge	1 cookie	14.0	260	46%
holiday tree cookie w/icing	1 cookie	3.5	200	16%
oatmeal raisin	1 cookie	10.0	250	36%
shortbread				
chocolate dipped	1 cookie	27.0	410	59%

Food and Description	Amount	Fat Grams	Total Calories	% Fat Calories
plain	1 cookie	25.0	390	58%
red sugar heart	1 cookie	22.0	350	57%
■ CROISSANTS				
dessert				
almond	1 croissant	38.0	570	60%
apple	1 croissant	10.0	280	32%
chocolate	1 croissant	23.0	440	47%
cinnamon raisin	1 croissant	5.0	340	13%
plain	1 croissant	6.0	250	22%
raspberry cheese	1 croissant	11.0	340	29%
strawberry cheese	1 croissant	19.0	370	46%
sweet cheese	1 croissant	14.0	350	36%
filled/hot				
ham & cheese	1 croissant	10.0	330	27%
spinach & cheese	1 croissant	9.0	240	34%
■ FRUIT & YOGURT				
Fruit Cup/fresh	8 oz	0.5	90	5%
	10 oz	1.0	110	8%
Yogurt				
blueberry				
w/fresh berries	8.5 oz	2.5	210	11%
w/granola	8 oz	3.5	230	14%
plain				
w/fresh berries	8.5 oz	2.5	210	11%
w/granola	8.0 oz	3.5	230	14%
strawberry				
w/fresh berries	8.5 oz	2.5	210	11%
w/granola	8.0 oz	3.5	230	14%
■ MUFFINS				
gourmet				
blueberry	1 muffin	15.0	410	33%
carrot walnut	1 muffin	23.0	480	43%
chocolate chip	1 muffin	20.0	490	37%
corn	1 muffin	18.0	470	34%
pumpkin w/streusel topping	1 muffin	18.0	470	34%
raisin bran	1 muffin	11.0	390	25%
low-fat				
chocolate cake	1 muffin	3.0	290	9%
triple berry	1 muffin	3.0	270	10%
■ PASTRY				
cinnamon roll	1 roll	15.0	340	13%
Danish				
lemon swirl	1 Danish	11.0	360	28
sweet cheese	1 Danish	18.0	420	39%
pecan roll	1 roll	28.0	730	35%
strudel				
apple	1 piece	26.0	490	48%
cherry	1 piece	26.0	490	48%
■ SALAD DRESSINGS & SALADS				
Salad dressing				
bleu cheese	3 oz	41.0	410	90%

Food and Description	Amount	Fat Grams	Total Calories	% Fat Calories
buttermilk ranch	3 oz	32.0	310	93%
Caesar	3 oz	39.0	380	92%
Greek	3 oz	50.0	440	100%
honey mustard/lite	3 oz	17.0	280	55%
Italian/Lite	3 oz	20.0	230	78%
lemon basil vinaigrette	3 oz	32.0	330	87%
mandarin orange	3 oz	33.0	380	78%
sesame French	3 oz	30.0	370	73%
Thai peanut	2 oz	6.0	130	48%
tomato basil/fat-free	3 oz	–	70	–
Salads				
Caesar salad	1 serving	10.0	270	33%
chef	1 serving	26.0	390	60%
chicken				
Caesar salad	1 serving	11.0	360	28%
Oriental	1 serving	4.0	270	13%
pesto	1 serving	11.0	230	43%
tarragon w/almonds	1 serving	23.0	470	44%
field green, gorgonzola & roasted walnuts	1 serving	34.0	400	77%
garden salad	1 small	1.0	100	9%
	1 large	1.5	160	8%
mozzarella & roasted red pepper	1 serving	18.0	340	48%
Thai chicken salad	1 serving	8.0	330	22%
tuna salad	1 serving	27.0	490	50%
■ SANDWICH FILLINGS				
(Note: Data are for fillings only; bread is not included)				
cheese				
cheddar	½ portion	14.0	170	74%
provolone	½ portion	11.0	150	66%
Swiss	½ portion	12.0	160	68%
chicken				
grilled	1 portion	1.6	140	10%
tarragon	1 portion	17.0	240	64%
country ham	1 portion	7.0	150	42%
roast beef	1 portion	4.5	140	29%
tuna salad	1 portion	29.0	360	73%
turkey breast	1 portion	1.0	120	8%
■ SANDWICHES & WRAPS				
Breakfast				
egg on a bagel				
plain	1 sandwich	5.0	500	9%
w/bacon	1 sandwich	12.0	580	19%
w/bacon & cheese	1 sandwich	19.0	660	26%
w/cheese	1 sandwich	12.0	580	19%
Fresh sandwiches				
chicken				
Arizona chicken	1 sandwich	33.0	720	41%
grilled w/mozzarella focaccia	1 sandwich	20.0	910	20%
honey Dijon chicken salad	1 sandwich	18.0	730	22%

Food and Description	Amount	Fat Grams	Total Calories	% Fat Calories
Of-Cha-Cha-Cha	1 sandwich	5.0	260	17%
Thai	1 sandwich	6.0	420	13%
mozzarella, tomato, & pesto	1 sandwich	30.0	650	42%
turkey/hot-roasted club	1 sandwich	50.0	950	47%
Wraps				
chicken Caesar	1 wrap	31.0	630	44%
fields & feta	1 wrap	17.0	560	27%
honey smoked turkey	1 wrap	7.0	540	12%
roast beef & brie	1 wrap	39.0	770	46%
Southwestern tuna	1 wrap	64.0	950	61%
■ SCONES				
blueberry	1 scone	23.0	430	48%
cinnamon	1 scone	17.0	440	35%
cranberry almond orange	1 scone	18.0	480	34%
orange w/icing	1 scone	15.0	430	31%
sour cream lemon	1 scone	8.0	390	18%
■ SOUP				
artichoke portabella w/chicken	12 oz	18.0	270	60%
	16 oz	25.0	370	61%
Asiago				
cheese bisque	8 oz	16.0	230	63%
	12 oz	25.0	370	61%
	16 oz	32.0	460	63%
tomato lentil	8 oz	2.0	120	15%
	12 oz	3.0	180	15%
	16 oz	4.0	240	15%
beef barley	8 oz	2.0	75	24%
	12 oz	3.0	112	24%
	16 oz	4.0	150	24%
broccoli, cream of	8 oz	18.0	220	74%
	12 oz	28.0	330	76%
	16 oz	37.0	440	76%
chicken noodle	8 oz	1.5	80	17%
	12 oz	2.0	120	15%
	16 oz	2.5	170	13%
chili/Southwest tortilla	8 oz	7.0	150	42%
	12 oz	10.0	230	39%
	14 oz	13.0	300	39%
clam chowder	8 oz	19.0	270	63%
	12 oz	29.0	400	65%
	16 oz	39.0	540	65%
corn chowder	8 oz	16.0	260	55%
	12 oz	24.0	380	57%
	16 oz	33.0	530	56%
curry chicken	8 oz	5.0	110	41%
	12 oz	8.0	160	45%
	16 oz	10.0	220	41%
forest mushroom bisque w/chicken	8 oz	6.0	130	42%
	12 oz	9.0	200	41%
	16 oz	12.0	250	43%

Food and Description	Amount	Fat Grams	Total Calories	% Fat Calories
garden vegetable	8 oz	–	30	–
	12 oz	–	45	–
	16 oz	–	60	–
lobster bisque	12 oz	30.0	460	59%
	16 oz	37.0	580	57%
mushroom orzo	8 oz	1.5	60	23%
	12 oz	2.5	90	25%
	16 oz	3.5	130	24%
tomato Florentine	8 oz	1.0	60	15%
	12 oz	2.0	90	20%
	16 oz	2.0	120	15%
tomato tortellini	8 oz	1.0	55	16%
	12 oz	1.5	83	16%
	16 oz	2.0	110	16%
vegetable bisque/roasted	8 oz	11.0	210	47%
	12 oz	18.0	340	48%
	16 oz	23.0	430	48%
vegetarian/corn & green chile bisque	8 oz	10.0	190	47%
	12 oz	16.0	300	48%
	16 oz	20.0	380	47%
BAGELNOSH				
Bagel				
cinnamon-raisin	1 bagel	1.0	353	3%
oatbran	1 bagel	2.0	341	5%
plain	1 bagel	1.0	330	3%
pumpernickel	1 bagel	1.0	349	3%
sesame	1 bagel	2.0	340	5%
whole wheat	1 bagel	2.0	348	5%
BLIMPIE				
■ SANDWICHES				
Blimpie best	1 sandwich	13.0	410	29%
cheese trio	1 sandwich	23.0	510	41%
club	1 sandwich	13.0	450	26%
5 meatball	1 sandwich	22.0	500	40%
grilled chicken	1 sandwich	9.0	400	20%
grilled chicken salad	1 sandwich	12.0	350	31%
ham & Swiss	1 sandwich	13.0	400	29%
ham, salami, & provolone	1 sandwich	28.0	590	43%
roast beef	1 sandwich	4.5	340	12%
steak & cheese	1 sandwich	26.0	550	43%
tuna	1 sandwich	32.0	570	51%
turkey	1 sandwich	4.5	320	13%
BOSTON MARKET				
■ BAKED GOODS				
brownie	1 piece	27.0	450	54%
chocolate chip cookie	1 cookie	17.0	340	45%
cinnamon apple pie	⅓ pie	23.0	390	53%
cornbread	1 loaf	6.0	200	27%
■ ENTRÉES				
chicken pot pie	1 pie	46.0	780	53%

Food and Description	Amount	Fat Grams	Total Calories	% Fat Calories
chunky chicken salad	¾ cup	27.0	370	66%
ham/Boston Hearth	5 oz	9.0	210	39%
meat loaf				
w/chunky tomato sauce	8 oz	18.0	370	44%
w/brown gravy	7 oz	22.0	390	51%
roast chicken				
¼ chicken				
dark meat				
skinless	1 serving	10.0	190	47%
w/skin	1 serving	21.0	320	59%
white meat				
skinless, w/o wing	1 serving	4.0	170	21%
w/skin & wing	1 serving	12.0	280	39%
½ chicken w/skin	1 serving	33.0	590	50%
southwestern savory chicken	1 serving	15.0	400	34%
tabasco BBQ				
drumstick	1 drumstick	6.0	130	42%
wings	1 wing	7.0	110	57%
teriyaki chicken/¼ chicken				
dark w/skin	1 serving	21.0	380	50%
white w/skin	1 serving	12.0	340	32%
triple topped chicken	1 serving	22.0	470	42%
turkey breast rotisserie/skinless	5 oz	1.0	170	5%
■ SALADS				
Caesar				
Chicken	12 oz salad	45.0	650	62%
entrée	10 oz salad	42.0	510	92%
side	4 oz salad	17.0	200	77%
w/o dressing	8 oz salad	12.0	230	47%
Tossed/individual				
w/Caesar dressing	1 salad	31.0	380	73%
w/fat-free ranch	1 salad	2.5	160	14%
w/Old Venice dressing	1 salad	27.0	340	71%
■ SANDWICHES				
chicken				
BBQ	1 sandwich	9.0	540	15%
plain	1 sandwich	4.5	430	9%
w/cheese & sauce	1 sandwich	33.0	750	40%
chicken salad	1 sandwich	30.0	680	39%
ham				
plain	1 sandwich	8.0	440	16%
w/cheese & sauce	1 sandwich	34.0	750	41%
ham & turkey club				
plain	1 sandwich	6.0	430	13%
w/cheese & sauce	1 sandwich			
meat loaf				
plain	1 sandwich	21.0	690	27%
w/cheese	1 sandwich	33.0	860	35%
pastry sandwich				
BBQ chicken	1 sandwich	39.0	640	55%

Food and Description	Amount	Fat Grams	Total Calories	% Fat Calories
ham & cheddar	1 sandwich	41.0	640	58%
Italian chicken	1 sandwich	41.0	630	59%
w/broccoli, chicken, & cheddar	1 sandwich	47.0	690	61%
turkey				
club	1 sandwich	26.0	650	36%
open-faced	1 meal	12.0	500	22%
plain	1 sandwich	3.5	400	8%
w/cheese & sauce	1 sandwich	28.0	710	35%
■ SIDE DISHES				
Cold				
Caesar side salad	4 oz	17.0	200	77%
chunky cinnamon apple sauce	¾ cup	–	250	–
coleslaw	¾ cup	19.0	300	57%
coyote bean salad	¾ cup	9.0	190	43%
cranberry relish	¾ cup	5.0	370	12%
fruit salad	¾ cup	0.5	70	6%
old-fashioned potato salad	¾ cup	24.0	340	64%
Hot				
baked sweet potato	1 potato	7.0	460	14%
BBQ baked beans	¾ cup	5.0	270	17%
black beans & rice	1 cup	10.0	300	30%
broccoli cauliflower au gratin	¾ cup	11.0	200	50%
broccoli w/red peppers	¾ cup	3.5	60	53%
broccoli rice casserole	¾ cup	12.0	240	45%
butternut squash	¾ cup	6.0	160	34%
chicken gravy	1 oz	1.0	15	60%
creamed spinach	¾ cup	20.0	260	69%
green bean casserole	¾ cup	9.0	130	62%
green beans	¾ cup	6.0	80	68%
honey-glazed carrots	¾ cup	15.0	280	48%
hot cinnamon apples	¾ cup	4.5	250	16%
macaroni & cheese	¾ cup	11.0	280	35%
mashed potatoes				
homestyle w/gravy	¾ cup	10.0	210	43%
plain	⅔ cup	9.0	190	43%
new potatoes/low-fat	¾ cup	2.5	130	17%
oven roasted potato planks/low-fat	5 planks	5.0	180	25%
red beans & rice/low-fat	1 cup	5.0	260	28%
rice pilaf	⅔ cup	5.0	180	25%
savory stuffing	¾ cup	12.0	310	35%
squash casserole	3 cup	24.0	330	65%
steamed vegetables/low-fat	⅔ cup	0.5	35	13%
sweet potato casserole	¾ cup	18.0	280	58%
whole kernel corn	¾ cup	4.0	180	20%
zucchini marinara	¾ cup	3.0	60	45%
■ SOUPS				
chicken chili	1 cup	7.0	220	29%
chicken noodle	1 cup	4.5	130	31%
chicken tortilla	1 cup	11.0	220	45%

Food and Description	Amount	Fat Grams	Total Calories	% Fat Calories
potato	1 cup	16.0	270	53%
tomato bisque	1 cup	23.0	280	74%
BURGER KING				
■ BEVERAGES				
Coca-Cola				
classic	1 medium	–	280	–
Diet Coke	1 medium	–	1	–
coffee	1 serving	–	5	–
milk 2% reduced fat	1 serving	5.0	130	42%
orange juice	1 serving	–	140	–
shakes				
chocolate shake				
regular	1 small	7.0	330	19%
	1 medium	10.0	440	20%
syrup added	1 small	7.0	390	16%
	1 medium	10.0	570	16%
strawberry shake/syrup added	1 small	7.0	390	16%
	1 medium	9.0	550	15%
vanilla shake	1 small	7.0	330	19%
	1 medium	5.0	430	10%
Sprite	1 medium	–	260	–
■ BREAKFAST				
biscuit				
bacon, egg, & cheese	1 biscuit	21.0	380	50%
plain	1 biscuit	15.0	300	45%
sausage	1 biscuit	33.0	490	61%
sausage, egg, & cheese	1 biscuit	43.0	620	62%
cini-minis-w/o icing	4 rolls	23.0	440	47%
Croissan'wich				
w/sausage & cheese	1 sandwich	35.0	450	70%
w/sausage, egg, & cheese	1 sandwich	41.0	530	70%
French toast sticks	1 serving	23.0	440	47%
hash browns	small	15.0	240	56%
	large	26.0	410	57%
■ BURGERS				
bacon cheeseburger				
double	1 burger	38.0	620	55%
regular	1 burger	22.0	400	50%
Big King Sandwich	1 burger	42.0	640	59%
cheeseburger				
double				
plain	1 burger	36.0	580	56%
regular	1 burger	19.0	360	48%
hamburger/regular	1 burger	15.0	320	42%
Whopper				
Double sandwich				
w/mayo	1 burger	59.0	920	58%
w/o mayo	1 burger	31.0	600	47%
Double w/cheese sandwich				
w/mayo	1 burger	67.0	1010	60%

Food and Description	Amount	Fat Grams	Total Calories	% Fat Calories
w/o mayo	1 burger	50.0	850	53%
original sandwich				
plain	1 burger	31.0	600	47%
w/cheese	1 burger	48.0	760	57%
original w/cheese sandwich				
w/mayo	1 burger	40.0	660	55%
w/o mayo	1 burger	23.0	510	41%
Whopper Jr. sandwich				
w/mayo	1 burger	24.0	400	54%
w/o mayo	1 burger	15.0	320	42%
Whopper Jr. w/cheese sandwich				
w/mayo	1 burger	28.0	450	56%
w/o mayo	1 burger	19.0	370	46%
■ CHICKEN & FISH				
Chicken				
sandwich				
BK Broiler				
w/mayo	1 sandwich	26.0	530	44%
w/o mayo	1 sandwich	9.0	370	22%
chick'N crisp				
w/mayo	1 sandwich	27.0	460	53%
w/o mayo	1 sandwich	16.0	360	40%
regular				
w/mayo	1 sandwich	43.0	710	55%
w/o mayo	1 sandwich	20.0	500	36%
Tenders	4 pieces	11.0	180	55%
	5 pieces	14.0	230	55%
	8 pieces	22.0	350	57%
Fish sandwich/BK Big Fish	1 sandwich	43.0	720	54%
■ CONDIMENTS & COMPONENTS				
A.M. Express				
grape jam	1 serving	–	30	–
Land O'Lakes whipped classic blend	1 serving	7.0	65	98%
strawberry jam	1 serving	–	30	–
bacon	3 pieces	3.0	40	68%
Bull's Eye barbecue sauce	1 Tbs	–	20	–
Buns				
hamburger/regular	1 bun	2.0	130	14%
Whopper	1 bun	4.0	220	16%
butter blend/Land O'Lakes Whipped Classic Blend	1 serving	7.0	65	100%
catsup	1 Tbs	–	15	–
cheese/processed American	¾ oz	8.0	90	80%
dipping sauce/1-oz serving				
barbecue	1 serving	–	35	–
honey-flavored	1 serving	–	90	–
honey mustard	1 serving	6.0	90	60%
ranch	1 serving	17.0	170	90%
sweet & sour	1 serving	–	45	–
ham	1.2 oz	1.0	35	26%

Food and Description	Amount	Fat Grams	Total Calories	% Fat Calories
King sauce	½ oz	7.0	70	90%
lettuce	1 piece	–	–	–
mayonnaise	2 Tbs	23.0	210	99%
mustard	1 serving	–	–	–
patty				
BK Broiler chicken breast patty	1 patty	4.0	140	26%
hamburger/regular	1 patty	13.0	170	69%
Whopper	1 patty	19.0	250	68%
pickle	1 serving	–	–	–
tartar sauce	1.5 oz	29.0	260	100%
tomato	1 oz	–	5	–
vanilla icing for Cini-minis	1 oz	3.0	110	25%
■ **DESSERT**				
Dutch apple pie	1 pie	15.0	300	45%
■ **SIDE ORDERS**				
French fries				
salted	small	13.0	250	56%
	medium	21.0	400	47%
	king-size	30.0	590	46%
unsalted	small	13.0	250	56%
	medium	21.0	400	47%
	king-size	30.0	590	46%
onion rings	medium	19.0	380	45%
	king size	30.0	600	45%

CAPTAIN D'S
■ CAPTAIN'S BROILER

Food and Description	Amount	Fat Grams	Total Calories	% Fat Calories
Meals				
chicken				
lunch	1 meal	9.0	503	16%
platter	1 meal	10.0	802	11%
sandwich	1 sandwich	19.0	450	38%
fish & chicken				
lunch	1 meal	8.0	478	15%
platter	1 meal	10.0	777	12%
fish				
lunch	1 meal	7.0	435	14%
platter	1 meal	7.0	734	9%
shrimp				
lunch	1 meal	7.0	421	15%
platter	1 meal	8.0	720	10%
stuffed crab	1 serving	7.0	90	70%
■ **CONDIMENTS**				
cocktail sauce	side portion	–	34	–
	bulk portion	1.0	135	7%
creamer/nondairy	1 serving	1.0	14	64%
margarine	1 serving	12.0	102	100%
salad dressing				
blue cheese	1 packet	11.7	105	100%
French	1 packet	10.7	110	88%
Italian/light	1 serving	0.5	16	28%

Food and Description	Amount	Fat Grams	Total Calories	% Fat Calories
ranch	1 packet	10.0	92	98%
sour cream/imitation	1 serving	3.0	30	70%
sugar	1 packet	–	13	–
sweet & sour sauce	side portion	–	50	–
	bulk portion	–	205	–
tartar sauce	side portion	7.0	78	81%
	bulk portion	27.0	300	81%
■ **DESSERT**				
Cake				
carrot cake	1 piece	22.8	434	47%
cheesecake	1 piece	31.0	420	66%
chocolate cake	1 piece	10.0	305	30%
Pie				
lemon pie	1 piece	10.0	351	26%
pecan pie	1 piece	20.0	460	39%
■ **SANDWICH**				
broiled chicken	1 serving	18.5	451	37%
■ **SIDE ORDERS**				
Side Dishes				
baked potato	1 potato	–	278	–
beans				
green	1 serving	2.0	45	40%
white	1 serving	1.0	125	7%
breadstick	1 breadstick	4.0	113	32%
coleslaw	1 serving	12.0	160	68%
	1 pint	47.0	635	67%
crackers	4 pieces	1.0	50	18%
cracklins	1 oz serving	17.0	220	70%
French fries	1 serving	10.0	300	30%
fried okra	1 serving	15.6	300	47%
hushpuppy	1 piece	4.0	125	29%
	5 pieces	20.0	625	29%
rice	1 serving	–	124	
salad/dinner	1 serving	–	20	–
vegetable medley	1 serving	1.0	36	25%
CARL'S JR.				
■ **BEVERAGES**				
Barq's Root Beer	16 fl oz	–	220	–
Coca-Cola				
classic	16 fl oz	–	200	–
Diet Coke	16 fl oz	–	–	–
coffee	12 fl oz	–	5	–
Dr. Pepper	16 fl oz	–	200	–
hot chocolate	12 fl oz	2.0	110	16%
iced tea	1 regular	–	5	–
milk/1% low-fat	10 fl oz	3.0	150	18%
Minute Maid				
lemonade/original style	16 fl oz	–	190	–
orange soda	16 fl oz	–	210	–
orange juice	10 fl oz	–	140	–

Food and Description	Amount	Fat Grams	Total Calories	% Fat Calories
raspberry Nestea	16 fl oz	–	160	–
7-Up/diet	16 fl oz	–	–	–
shakes				
chocolate shake	13.5 fl oz	7.0	390	16%
strawberry shake	13.5 fl oz	7.0	400	16%
vanilla shake	13.5 fl oz	8.0	330	22%
Sprite	16 fl oz	–	190	–
■ BREAKFAST				
bacon	2 strips	4.0	50	72%
breakfast burrito	1 burrito	30.0	480	56%
breakfast quesadilla	1 quesadilla	16.0	310	46%
eggs/scrambled	1 serving	11.0	160	62%
English muffin w/margarine	1 muffin	9.0	210	39%
French toast dips	1 serving	20.0	370	49%
sausage	1 patty	19.0	200	86%
sunrise sandwich/no bacon or sausage	1 sandwich	21.0	360	53%
■ BURGERS				
cheeseburger/Western bacon				
double	1 burger	49.0	900	49%
regular	1 burger	30.0	650	42%
hamburger				
Famous Star	1 burger	32.0	580	50%
junior	1 burger	13.0	330	35%
Super Star	1 burger	46.0	790	52%
■ CHICKEN & FISH SANDWICHES				
chicken sandwich				
BBQ	1 sandwich	3.0	280	10%
Bacon Swiss crispy	1 sandwich	36.0	590	55%
chicken club	1 sandwich	22.0	460	43%
Ranch crispy	1 sandwich	29.0	590	44%
Santa Fe	1 sandwich	31.0	510	55%
fish sandwich/Carl's Catch	1 sandwich	27.0	510	48%
■ CONDIMENTS (See also Salad Bar)				
BBQ sauce	1 oz	–	50	–
cheese				
American	1 slice	5.0	60	75%
Swiss	1 slice	3.5	50	63%
grape jelly	1 Tbs	–	35	–
honey sauce	1 oz	–	90	–
mustard sauce	1 oz	0.5	45	10%
salsa	1 oz	–	10	–
strawberry jam	1 Tbs	–	35	–
sweet 'n sour sauce	1 oz	–	50	–
table syrup	1 oz	–	90	–
■ DESSERTS				
cheese Danish	1 Danish	22.0	400	50%
cheesecake/strawberry swirl	1 piece	17.0	290	53%
chocolate cake	1 piece	10.0	300	30%
chocolate chip cookie	1 serving	19.0	370	46%

Food and Description	Amount	Fat Grams	Total Calories	% Fat Calories
■ POTATOES				
bacon & cheese	1 serving	29.0	630	41%
broccoli & cheese	1 serving	21.0	530	36%
plain	1 serving	–	290	–
sour cream & chive	1 serving	14.0	430	29%
■ SALAD BAR				
breadsticks	1 serving	0.5	35	13%
croutons	1 serving	1.0	35	26%
Salad Dressing				
Fat-free				
French	2 oz	–	60	–
Italian	2 oz	–	15	–
regular				
blue cheese	2 oz	35.0	320	98%
house	2 oz	22.0	220	90%
Thousand Island	2 oz	23.0	230	90%
Salads To Go				
charbroiled chicken	1 serving	7.0	200	32%
garden salad	1 serving	2.5	50	45%
■ SIDE ORDERS				
chicken stars	1 serving	19.0	280	61%
criscut fries	1 serving	24.0	410	53%
French fries	1 serving	14.0	290	43%
hash brown nuggets	1 serving	21.0	330	57%
onion rings	1 serving	21.0	430	44%
zucchini	1 serving	19.0	340	50%
CHICK-FIL-A				
■ BEVERAGES				
Coca-Cola				
classic	9 fl oz	–	110	–
Diet Coke	9 fl oz	–	1	–
iced tea				
sweetened	9 fl oz	–	150	–
unsweetened	9 fl oz	–	–	–
lemonade				
diet	9 fl oz	–	5	–
regular	9 fl oz	–	90	–
■ CHICKEN				
chicken salad sandwich on wheat bread	1 sandwich	5.0	320	14%
Chik-fil-A				
chargrilled				
club/no dressing	1 sandwich	12.0	390	28%
sandwich/regular	1 sandwich	3.0	280	10%
original sandwich	1 sandwich	9.0	290	28%
Chik-fil-A original				
Chick-n Strips	4 pieces	8.0	230	31%
nuggets	8 pieces	14.0	290	43%
■ DESSERT				
cheesecake/plain	1 slice	21.0	300	63%
fudge brownie w/nuts	1 brownie	16.0	350	41%

Food and Description	Amount	Fat Grams	Total Calories	% Fat Calories
ice cream				
cone	1 small	4.0	140	26%
cup	1 small	10.0	350	26%
lemon pie	1 slice	22.0	280	71%
■ **DIPPING SAUCES**				
barbecue	1 pkg	–	45	–
Dijon honey mustard	1 pkg	5.0	60	90%
honey mustard	1 pkg	–	45	–
Polynesian	1 pkg	6.0	110	49%
■ **SALADS, SALAD DRESSINGS, & SOUP**				
Salad dressings				
basil vinaigrette	1 pkg	26.0	250	94%
blue cheese	1 pkg	24.0	230	94%
buttermilk ranch	1 pkg	24.0	220	98%
honey Dijon mustard/fat-free	1 pkg	0.5	70	6%
house	1 pkg	17.0	190	81%
spicy	1 pkg	22.0	210	94%
thousand island	1 pkg	20.0	210	86%
Salads				
chargrilled chicken garden salad	1 serving	5.0	190	24%
chicken Caesar salad	1 serving	10.0	230	39%
Chick-fil-A Chick-n Strips salad	1 serving	17.0	370	41%
tossed salad	1 serving	4.5	80	51%
Soup/hearty breast of chicken	1 cup	1.0	110	8%
■ **SIDE ORDERS** (*See also* Salads in this section)				
carrot & raisin salad	1 serving	2.0	150	12%
coleslaw	1 serving	6.0	130	42%
waffle potato fries				
salted	small	10.0	290	31%
unsalted	small	10.0	290	31%
CHILI'S/Guiltless Grilled Selections				
chicken				
pita	1 pita	9.0	597	14%
platter	1 meal	9.0	563	14%
salad w/dressing	1 salad	5.0	272	17%
sandwich	1 sandwich	8.0	527	14%
veggie pasta				
plain	1 meal	13.0	680	17%
w/chicken	1 meal	15.0	786	17%
CHURCH'S CHICKEN				
■ **CHICKEN**				
breast	2.8 oz	12.4	200	56%
leg	2 oz	9.0	140	58%
tender strip	1.1 oz	4.0	80	45%
thigh	2.8 oz	16.0	230	63%
wing	3.1 oz	16.0	250	58%
■ **DESSERT**				
apple pie	1 piece	12.3	280	39%
■ **SIDE ORDERS**				
biscuit	1 biscuit	16.4	250	59%

Food and Description	Amount	Fat Grams	Total Calories	% Fat Calories
Cajun rice	1 serving	7.0	130	48%
coleslaw	1 serving	5.5	92	54%
com on the cob	1 piece	3.2	139	21%
French fries	1 serving	10.5	210	45%
okra	1 serving	16.0	210	69%
potatoes & gravy	1 serving	3.3	90	33%
COUSINS SUBS				
■ **DESSERTS**				
Cookies				
chocolate chip	1 cookie	11.0	210	47%
cranberry walnut	1 cookie	8.4	187	40%
■ **SUBS**				
Cold Subs				
BLT				
w/mayo	½ sub	39.8	593	60%
w/o mayo	½ sub	13.5	337	36%
cheese				
w/mayo	½ sub	46.3	664	63%
w/o mayo	½ sub	20.1	427	42%
club				
w/mayo	½ sub	45.4	730	56%
w/o mayo	½ sub	19.2	494	35%
cold veggie	½ sub	11.0	360	28%
ham	½ sub	34.3	547	56%
ham & cheese				
w/mayo	½ sub	40.1	622	58%
w/o mayo	½ sub	13.8	386	32%
Italian				
Cappacolla & cheese	½ sub	33.9	567	54%
Cappacolla & Genoa	½ sub	35.5	567	56%
Cousins' Special	½ sub	48.6	731	59%
Genoa & cheese	½ sub	44.5	668	60%
regular	½ sub	40.0	622	58%
roast beef	½ sub	34.8	598	52%
seafood w/crab	½ sub	33.6	555	54%
tuna salad				
w/added mayo on bread	½ sub	54.3	756	65%
w/o added mayo on bread	½ sub	28.0	500	50%
turkey	½ sub	34.8	561	56%
Cold Subs/lower fat w/o mayo				
ham	½ sub	8.0	311	23%
roast beef	½ sub	8.5	361	21%
turkey	½ sub	8.5	325	24%
Hot Subs				
cheese steak	½ sub	17.0	470	33%
chicken breast	½ sub	31.8	556	51%
double cheese steak	½ sub	26.0	550	43%
gyro	½ sub	23.0	550	38%
Italian sausage	½ sub	57.5	816	63%
meatball & cheese	½ sub	43.3	685	57%

Food and Description	Amount	Fat Grams	Total Calories	% Fat Calories
pepperoni melt				
w/mayo	½ sub	46.1	702	59%
w/o mayo	½ sub	19.8	466	38%
Philly cheese steak	½ sub	23.0	510	41%
steak	½ sub	12.0	425	25%
veggie	½ sub	14.3	380	34%
Hot Subs/lower fat w/o mayo				
chicken breast	½ sub	5.5	320	15%
Kids Subs				
cheeseburger	½ sub	16.7	290	52%
hot dog	½ sub	16.7	290	52%
Mini Subs				
cheese				
w/mayo	½ sub	24.7	354	63%
w/o mayo	½ sub	10.7	228	42%
Cousins' Special	½ sub	14.0	290	43%
ham	½ sub	18.3	292	56$
ham & cheese	½ sub	21.4	332	58%
meatball w/cheese	½ sub	23.1	365	57%
seafood w/crab	½ sub	17.9	296	54%
turkey	½ sub	18.5	299	56%
tuna salad				
w/added mayo on bread	½ sub	37.0	495	67%
w/o added mayo on bread	½ sub	16.0	290	50%
Mini Subs/lower fat w/o mayo				
ham	½ sub	4.3	167	23%
ham & cheese	½ sub	7.4	206	32%
turkey	½ sub	4.4	172	23%
■ SALADS, SAUCE, & SOUPS				
Salads				
Italian	1 salad	17.9	288	56%
tuna	1 salad	19.9	306	59%
Salads/lower fat & calories				
chef	1 salad	7.9	194	37%
garden	1 salad	5.9	136	39%
seafood	1 salad	5.9	176	30%
side	1 salad	4.2	71	53%
Sauce/Tzatziki	1 serving	4.0	50	72%
Soups				
cheese	regular	14.0	210	60%
	large	22.0	330	60%
cheese broccoli	regular	10.5	166	57%
	large	16.5	261	57%
chicken w/wild rice	regular	10.5	184	51%
	large	16.5	289	51%
chili	large	13.8	344	36%
cream of potato	large	12.4	261	43%
Soups/lower fat & calories				
chicken noodle	regular	2.6	105	22%
	large	4.1	165	22%

Food and Description	Amount	Fat Grams	Total Calories	% Fat Calories
chili	regular	8.8	219	36%
clam chowder	regular	5.3	158	30%
	large	8.3	248	30%
cream of potato	regular	7.9	166	43%
red beans & rice	regular	1.3	114	10%
	large	2.1	179	11%
tomato basil	regular	2.6	88	27%
	large	4.1	138	27%
vegetable beef	regular	1.3	70	17%
	large	2.1	110	17%
■ SIDE ORDERS				
bacon strips	3 strips	4.0	50	72%
bread				
Italian	1 oz	2.0	85	21%
wheat	1 oz	2.0	85	21%
chips				
plain	5 oz	15.0	230	59%
sour cream	5 oz	14.0	230	55%
French fries	small	12.8	275	42%
	medium	18.7	400	42%
	large	24.5	525	42%
pepperoni	6 slices	6.0	70	77%
DAIRY QUEEN				
■ BEVERAGES				
DQ Glacier Smoothy/strawberry-banana	1 serving	14.0	670	19%
Hot chocolate/frozen	1 serving	35.0	860	37%
Malt/chocolate	small	16.0	650	22%
	medium	22.0	880	23%
Misty Slush	small	–	220	–
	medium	–	290	–
Shakes/chocolate	small	15.0	560	24%
	medium	20.0	770	23%
■ BURGERS & HOT DOGS				
Hamburger/DQ homestyle				
double				
deluxe				
plain	1 burger	17.0	340	45%
w/bacon & cheese	1 burger	36.0	610	53%
w/cheese	1 burger	31.0	540	52%
single				
plain	1 burger	12.0	290	37%
w/cheese	1 burger	17.0	340	45%
Ultimate	1 burger	43.0	670	58%
Hotdog				
chili n' cheese	1 hot dog	21.0	330	57%
plain	1 hot dog	14.0	240	53%
■ CHICKEN & STEAK				
Chicken				
grilled breast fillet sandwich	1 sandwich	10.0	310	24%
Strip Basket	1 basket	50.0	1000	45%

Food and Description	Amount	Fat Grams	Total Calories	% Fat Calories
Steak/The Great Steakmelt Basket	1 basket	37.0	750	44%
■ **FROZEN DESSERT SPECIALTIES**				
banana split	1 serving	12.0	510	21%
Blizzard				
chocolate chip cookie dough	small	24.0	660	33%
	medium	36.0	950	34%
chocolate sandwich cookie	small	18.0	520	31%
	medium	23.0	640	32%
Breeze (see "frozen yogurt" in this listing)				
Buster Bar	1 bar	28.0	450	56%
Chocolate Rock Treat	1 serving	38.0	730	47%
cone				
chocolate	small	8.0	240	30%
	regular	11.0	340	29%
chocolate-dipped	small	17.0	340	45%
	medium	24.0	490	44%
vanilla	small	7.0	230	27%
	medium	9.0	330	25%
	large	12.0	410	26%
Dilly Bar/chocolate	1 bar	13.0	210	56%
DQ				
Cake/undecorated				
frozen 8" round	⅛ cake	13.0	370	32%
layered 8" round	⅛ cake	12.0	330	33%
Freeze/lemon	½ cup	–	80	–
fudge bar/no sugar added	1 bar	–	50	–
sandwich	1 sandwich	5.0	150	30%
soft serve				
Chocolate	½ cup	5.0	150	30%
vanilla	½ cup	4.5	140	29%
Treatzza Pizza				
Heath	⅛ pizza	7.0	180	35%
M & M's	⅛ pizza	7.0	190	33%
vanilla orange bar/no sugar added	1 bar	–	60	–
frozen yogurt				
Breeze				
Heath	small	10.0	170	53%
	medium	18.0	710	23%
strawberry	small	0.5	320	1%
	medium	1.0	460	2%
cone				
	medium	1.0	260	3%
cup				
DQ non-fat	½ cup	–	100	–
regular	medium	0.5	230	3%
strawberry sundae	medium	0.5	280	2%
Pecan Mudslide Treat	1 serving	30.0	650	42%
Peanut Buster parfait	1 serving	31.0	730	38%
Starkiss	1 serving	–	80	–
strawberry shortcake	1serving	14.0	430	29%

Food and Description	Amount	Fat Grams	Total Calories	% Fat Calories
sundae				
chocolate sundae	small	7.0	280	23%
	medium	10.0	400	23%
■ SIDE ORDERS				
French fries	small	18.0	350	46%
	medium	23.0	440	47%
lettuce	1 piece	–	2	–
onion rings	1 serving	16.0	320	45%
tomato	1 slice	–	3	–
DEL TACO				
■ BEVERAGES				
Coca-Cola				
classic	1 small	–	120	–
	1 medium	–	150	–
	1 large	–	230	–
	1 best value	–	320	–
Diet Coke	1 small	–	–	–
	1 medium	–	–	–
	1 large	–	5	–
	1 best value	–	10	–
coffee	1 regular	–	–	
iced tea	1 small	–	–	–
	1 medium	–	–	–
	1 large	–	5	–
	1 best value	–	10	–
milk/1% low-fat	1 regular	3.0	130	21%
Mr. Pibb	1 small	–	120	–
	1 medium	–	150	–
	1 large	–	230	–
	1 best value	–	320	–
orange juice	1 regular	–	140	–
shakes				
chocolate	1 small	12.0	520	21%
	1 large	16.0	680	21%
strawberry	1 small	6.0	410	13%
	1 large	8.0	540	13%
vanilla	1 small	7.0	420	15%
	1 large	10.0	550	16%
Sprite	1 small	–	110	–
	1 medium	–	140	–
	1 large	–	230	–
	1 best value	–	310	–
■ BURGERS				
cheeseburger				
Del cheeseburger				
single	1 burger	25.0	430	52%
double	1 burger	35.0	560	56%
regular	1 burger	13.0	330	35%

Food and Description	Amount	Fat Grams	Total Calories	% Fat Calories
■ **BREAKFAST**				
bacon	1 slices	4.0	50	72%
burritos				
egg & cheese	1 burrito	24.0	450	48%
Macho bacon & egg	1 burrito	60.0	1030	52%
regular breakfast	1 burrito	11.0	250	40%
steak & egg	1 burrito	34.0	580	53%
Quesadillas				
bacon & egg	1 quesadilla	23.0	450	46%
■ **BURRITOS**				
beef				
Del Beef				
regular	1 burrito	30.0	550	49%
deluxe	1 burrito	33.0	590	50%
macho	1 burrito	62.0	1170	48%
chicken				
Del Classic	1 burrito	36.0	560	58%
spicy	1 burrito	16.0	480	30%
Works	1 burrito	23.0	520	40%
combination				
deluxe	1 burrito	25.0	570	39%
macho	1 burrito	44.0	1050	38%
regular	1 burrito	22.0	530	37%
green				
bean & cheese	1 burrito	8.0	280	26%
half pound	1 burrito	12.0	430	25%
red				
bean & cheese	1 burrito	8.0	270	27%
half pound	1 burrito	12.0	430	25%
Steak Works	1 burrito	31.0	590	47%
Veggie Works	1 burrito	18.0	490	33%
■ **CONDIMENTS** American cheese	1 slice	4.0	53	68%
guacamole	1 oz	6.0	60	90%
hot sauce	1 pouch	–	<1	–
nacho cheese sauce	1 serving	8.0	100	72%
salsa	2 oz	–	15	–
sour dream	1 oz	6.0	60	90%
■ **GET A LOT MEALS**				
#1 Combo burrito, fries, drink	1 meal	44.0	1020	30%
#2 Del Classic chicken burrito, fries, drink	1 meal	59.0	1050	51%
#3 Chicken quesadilla, fries, drink	1 meal	54.0	1070	45%
#4 Two chicken soft tacos, fries, drink	1 meal	46.0	910	45%
#5 Deluxe Del beef burrito, fries, drink	1 meal	56.0	1080	47%
#6 Two tacos, quesadilla, drink	1 meal	47.0	960	44%
#7 Macho combo burrito, fries, drink	1 meal	67.0	1540	39%
#8 Two Big Fat Tacos, fries, drink	1 meal	45.0	1130	36%
#9 Double Del cheeseburger, fries, drink	1 meal	58.0	1050	50%
■ **QUESADILLAS**				
chicken/regular	1 quesadilla	31.0	580	48%
plain	1 quesadilla	12.0	257	42%

Food and Description	Amount	Fat Grams	Total Calories	% Fat Calories
regular	1 quesadilla	27.0	500	49%
Spicy Jack	1 quesadilla	12.0	254	43%
chicken	1 quesadilla	30.0	570	47%
regular	1 quesadilla	26.0	490	48%
■ SALADS				
chicken salad/deluxe	1 serving	34.0	730	42%
taco salad/deluxe	1 serving	40.0	780	46%
tostada	1 tostada	9.0	210	39%
■ SIDE ORDERS (See also Salads & Dressing in this section)				
Beans'N cheese cup	1 serving	3.0	260	10%
fries				
regular	small	14.0	210	60%
	medium	23.0	350	59%
	large	32.0	490	59%
chili cheese				
deluxe	1 serving	49.0	710	62%
regular	1 serving	46.0	670	62%
nachos				
Nacho Nachos	1 serving	63.0	1100	52%
regular	1 serving	24.0	380	57%
rice cup	1 serving	2.0	140	13%
■ TACOS				
Big Fat Taco				
Chicken	1 taco	13.0	340	34%
Crispy Chicken	1 taco	38.0	620	55%
Steak	1 taco	19.0	390	44%
Taco	1 taco	11.0	320	31%
Chicken/soft	1 taco	11.0	197	50%
Taco				
regular	1 taco	10.0	160	56%
soft	1 taco	8.0	160	45%
Ultimate Taco	1 taco	17.0	260	59%
DENNY'S				
■ APPETIZERS, ENTRÉES, & SIDES				
Appetizers				
buffalo				
chicken strips	5 strips	42.0	734	51%
wings	12 wings	54.0	856	57%
chicken strips	5 strips	33.0	720	41%
chili cheese fries	1 serving	44.0	816	49%
mozzarella sticks	8 sticks	41.0	710	52%
sampler	1 serving	80.0	1405	51%
smothered cheese fries	1 serving	48.0	767	56%
Entrées				
Beef				
chicken-fried steak	1 serving	17.0	265	58%
pot roast dinner w/gravy	1 serving	11.0	292	34%
sirloin steak dinner	1 serving	21.0	271	70%
steak & shrimp dinner	1 serving	42.0	645	59%
T-bone steak dinner	1 serving	50.0	642	70%

Food and Description	Amount	Fat Grams	Total Calories	% Fat Calories
Chicken				
Charleston dinner	1 serving	18.0	327	50%
pot pie	1 pie	55.0	1065	46%
pot pie dinner	1 serving	55.0	1065	46%
grilled dinner	1 serving	4.0	130	28%
grilled stir-fry	1 serving	10.0	864	10%
strips	1 serving	25.0	635	35%
Seafood				
grilled Alaskan salmon dinner	1 meal	4.0	210	17%
Mandarin glazed salmon	1 meal	20.0	616	29%
Shrimp dinner/fried	1 meal	32.0	558	52%
Vegetable stir fry	1 meal	9.0	429	19%
Sides				
applesauce/Mussleman's	1 serving	–	60	–
baked potato/plain w/skin	1 potato	–	220	–
bread stuffing/plain	1 serving	1.0	100	18%
broccoli in butter sauce	1 serving	2.0	50	36%
carrots in honey glaze	1 serving	3.0	80	34%
corn in butter sauce	1 serving	4.0	120	30%
cottage cheese	1 serving	3.0	72	38%
fries				
French/unsalted	1 serving	14.0	323	30%
seasoned	1 serving	12.0	261	41%
green beans w/bacon	1 serving	4.0	60	60%
green peas in butter sauce	1 serving	18.0	100	18%
mashed potatoes/plain	1 serving	1.0	105	9%
mushrooms, grilled	1 serving	–	14	–
onion rings	1 serving	23.0	381	54%
tomatoes/sliced	3 slices	–	13	–
vegetable rice pilaf	1 serving	1.0	85	11%
■ **BEVERAGES**				
Coffee/flavored				
French vanilla	8 fl oz	1.0	76	12%
hazelnut	8 fl oz	1.0	66	14%
Irish cream	8 fl oz	1.0	73	12%
Hot chocolate	8 fl oz	2.0	90	20%
Iced tea/raspberry/sweetened	16 fl oz	–	78	–
Juice				
apple	10 oz	–	126	–
grapefruit	10 oz	–	115	–
orange	10 oz	–	126	–
tomato	10 oz	–	56	–
Juice Drink/orange, strawberry, banana	10 oz	–	137	–
Lemonade	16 oz	–	150	–
Milk				
2%/white	10 oz	6.0	151	36%
whole/chocolate	10 oz	9.0	235	34%
■ **BREAKFAST**				
applesauce, Musselman's	3 oz	–	65	–

Food and Description	Amount	Fat Grams	Total Calories	% Fat Calories
bacon				
peppered	4 strips	13.0	175	67%
regular	4 strips	18.0	162	100%
bagel	1 bagel	1.0	235	4%
banana				
strawberry medley	1 serving	1.0	108	8%
whole	1 banana	–	110	–
biscuit				
bittered	1 serving	11.0	272	36%
w/sausage gravy	1 serving	21.0	398	47%
buttermilk pancakes				
plain	3 pancakes	7.0	491	13%
w/2 oz syrup	3 pancakes	7.0	650	10%
w/1 Tbs whipped butter	3 pancakes	14.0	555	23%
w/2 oz syrup & 1 Tbs whipped butter	3 pancakes	14.0	715	18%
cantaloupe	¼ melon	–	32	–
cereal, Kellogg's/dry	1 serving	–	100	–
chicken fried steak & eggs-w/o bread	1 serving	36.0	430	75%
cream cheese	1 oz	10.0	100	90%
egg	1 egg	10.0	120	75%
Egg Beaters/egg substitute	1 serving	5.0	71	63%
eggs Benedict/add choice of potatoes or grits	1 serving	46.0	695	60%
English muffin/no butter or margarine	1 muffin	1.0	125	7%
French toast/add topping, syrup, or margarine				
cinnamon swirl	1 serving	49.0	1030	43%
regular	1 serving	24.0	507	43%
fruit mix	3 oz serving	–	36	–
grapefruit	½ fruit	–	60	–
grapes	1 serving	–	55	–
grits	1 serving	–	80	–
ham/grilled slice	1 serving	3.0	94	29%
hashed browns				
covered	1 serving	23.0	318	65%
covered & smothered	1 serving	26.0	359	65%
doubled, covered, & smothered	1 serving	26.0	460	51%
honeydew	¼ melon	–	31	–
Moons Over My Hammy/add choice of potato or grits	1 meal	48.0	807	54%
Oatmeal				
N' Fixins-w/o bread	1 serving	6.0	460	12%
Quaker	1 serving	2.0	100	18%
Omelettes-w/o bread				
Farmer's	1 serving	51.0	650	71%
Ham 'N'Cheddar	1 serving	45.0	581	70%
Ultimate	1 serving	47.0	564	75%
Veggie-cheese	1 serving	39.0	480	73%
potato pancakes	1 serving	27.0	530	46%
potatoes/country fried	1 serving	35.0	515	61%

Food and Description	Amount	Fat Grams	Total Calories	% Fat Calories
sausage				
links	4 links	32.0	354	81%
patties	2 patties	28.0	300	84%
sirloin steak & eggs-w/o bread	1 serving	49.0	622	74%
Skillet Meals				
Big Texas Chicken Fajita Skillet	1 serving	70.0	1,217	52%
Meat Lover's Skillet-w/o bread	1 serving	93.0	1,147	73%
Slam Meals				
All-American	1 meal	62.0	712	78%
Cinnamon Swirl/add topping or syrup & margarine	1 meal	78.0	1,105	64%
Country	1 meal	66.0	1,000	59%
Farmer's	1 meal	80.0	1,200	60%
French	1 meal	71.0	1,029	62%
Lumberjack/add topping or syrup & margarine	1 meal	70.0	1,259	50%
Original Grand	1 meal	50.0	795	57%
Play It Again Slam/add topping or syrup & margarine	1 meal	75.0	1,192	57%
Sausage Lover's	1 meal	68.0	960	64%
Scram-w/o bread	1 meal	62.0	740	75%
Slim Slam/add topping	1 meal	12.0	495	22%
Southern	1 meal	84.0	1,065	71%
steak & eggs	1 serving	51.0	800	57%
syrup				
blueberry-flavored	~3 Tbs	–	102	–
maple-flavored	~3 Tbs	–	143	–
sugar-free maple-flavored	~3 Tbs	–	23	–
strawberry-flavored	~3 Tbs	–	91	–
T-bone steak & eggs-w/o bread	1 serving	77.0	991	90%
toast/no butter	1 piece	1.0	90	10%
toppings				
blueberry	3 oz	–	106	–
cherry	3 oz	–	86	–
strawberry	3 oz	1.0	115	8%
tortillas, flour & salsa	1 serving	8.0	281	26%
waffle/add topping, syrup, & margarine	1 waffle	21.0	304	62%
Whipped				
cream	1 dollop	2.0	23	78%
margarine	1 Tbs	10.0	87	100%
■ BURGERS/add French fries or substitute & condiments				
bacon-cheddar	1 burger	52.0	875	53%
Big Texas BBQ	1 burger	51.0	872	53%
Buffalo chicken	1 burger	45.0	803	50%
Classic				
plain	1 burger	40.0	673	53%
w/cheese	1 burger	53.0	836	57%
Denny burger	1 burger	25.0	485	46%
Double Decker	1 burger	80.0	1,247	58%
Garden	1 burger	33.0	665	45%

Food and Description	Amount	Fat Grams	Total Calories	% Fat Calories
Garlic mushroom Swiss	1 burger	51.0	872	53%
■ CONDIMENTS				
BBQ sauce	1.5 oz	1.0	47	19%
gravy				
brown	2 Tbs	–	13	–
chicken	2 Tbs	0.5	14	32%
country	2 Tbs	1.0	17	53%
guacamole	1.5 oz	6.0	74	73%
herb toast	2 oz	11.0	170	58%
marinara sauce	1.5 oz	2.0	48	38%
salsa	2 oz	–	10	–
sour cream	1.5 oz	9.0	91	89%
tartar sauce	1.5 oz	24.0	230	94%
■ DESSERT/pie servings are ⅙ of a pie				
Banana				
royale	1 serving	25.0	548	41%
split	1 serving	43.0	894	43%
Butterfinger Blender Blaster	13 oz	38.0	768	45%
Cake				
chocolate layer	1 slice	12.0	275	39%
hot fudge	1 slice	35.0	620	51%
Floats				
cola	12 fl oz	10.0	280	32%
rootbeer	12 fl oz	10.0	280	32%
Milkshakes				
malted-vanilla/chocolate	12 fl oz	26.0	583	40%
regular-vanilla/chocolate	12 fl oz	26.0	560	42%
Pie				
apple pie				
Dutch				
traditional	1 slice	19.0	440	39%
cheesecake pie-w/o topping	1 slice	27.0	470	52%
cherry pie	1 slice	25.0	630	36%
chocolate				
peanut butter pie	1 slice	39.0	653	54%
silk	1 slice	43.0	650	60%
Key lime pie	1 slice	27.0	600	41%
Oreo Cookies & Creme	1 slice	30.0	590	46%
Sherbet/rainbow	½ cup	1.5	120	11%
Sundaes				
Butterfinger Hot Fudge	1 serving	38.0	780	44%
double scoop	1 serving	27.0	375	65%
single scoop/Delicious Dip	1 serving	14.0	188	67%
Toppings				
blueberry	2 oz	–	71	–
cherry	2 oz	–	57	–
chocolate	2 oz	25.0	317	71%
fudge	2 oz	10.0	210	44%
nut	1 tsp	4.0	42	86%
strawberry	2 oz	1.0	77	12%

Food and Description	Amount	Fat Grams	Total Calories	% Fat Calories
whipped cream	2 bs	2.0	23	78%
Yogurt/lowfat chocolate chip	½ cup	2.0	110	16%
■ KID'S MEALS				
Burgerlicious				
plain	1 meal	17.0	296	52%
w/cheese	1 meal	20.0	341	53%
Dennysaur chicken nuggets	1 meal	13.0	190	62%
Frenchtastic Slam	1 meal	33.0	452	66%
Heads'N' Tails appetizer cracker	½ oz	3.0	70	39%
Jr.				
Blender Blaster	7 oz	18.0	370	44%
Butterfingers hot fudge sundae	1 sundae	17.0	341	45%
Junior Grand Slam	1 meal	25.0	397	57%
Pigs in a Blanket	1 meal	21.0	479	39%
Pizza Party	1 meal	15.0	400	34%
Shrimpsational basket	1 meal	16.0	291	49%
Smiley-face hotcakes				
w/meat	1 meal	22.0	463	43%
w/o meat	1 meal	9.0	344	24%
The Big Cheese	1 meal	20.0	334	54%
Wacky Waffles	1 meal	12.0	215	50%
■ SALADS & SALAD DRESSINGS				
Salads (w/o dressing, unless otherwise noted)				
buffalo chicken salad	1 serving	35.0	516	61%
Caesar salad/side-w/dressing	1 serving	26.0	362	65%
California grilled chicken salad	1 serving	12.0	277	30%
Chef's salad	1 serving	26.0	370	63%
fried chicken salad	1 serving	26.0	438	53%
garden chicken De-lite	1 serving	5.0	277	16%
grilled chicken Caesar salad-w/dressing	1 serving	41.0	600	62%
side garden salad	1 serving	4.0	113	32%
Salad dressings				
blue cheese	2 Tbs	18.0	163	100%
Caesar	2 Tbs	14.0	133	95%
French	2 Tbs	10.0	106	85%
honey mustard/fat-free	2 Tbs	–	38	–
Italian/reduced calorie	2 Tbs	8.0	72	100%
ranch	2 Tbs	11.0	110	90%
Thousand Island	2 Tbs	11.0	118	84%
■ SANDWICHES				
bacon, lettuce, & tomato	1 sandwich	46.0	634	65%
Charleston chicken	1 sandwich	32.0	632	46%
club	1 sandwich	38.0	718	48%
grilled chicken	1 sandwich	14.0	520	24%
ham & Swiss on rye	1 sandwich	31.0	533	52%
Rueben	1 sandwich	35.0	580	54%
Super Bird	1 sandwich	32.0	620	46%
turkey breast w/multigrain	1 sandwich	26.0	476	49%

Food and Description	Amount	Fat Grams	Total Calories	% Fat Calories
■ **SENIOR MEALS**				
Belgian waffle Slam	1 meal	33.0	399	74%
chicken fried steak	1 meal	18.0	341	48%
fried shrimp dinner	1 meal	16.0	291	49%
grilled chicken breast	1 meal	5.0	200	23%
omelette	1 meal	20.0	429	42%
pot roast	1 meal	6.0	160	34%
sandwiches/add fries or substitute				
grilled cheese	1 sandwich	30.0	510	53%
ham & Swiss	1 sandwich	30.0	497	54%
turkey	1 sandwich	26.0	476	49%
Triple Play	1 meal	25.0	537	42%
turkey & stuffing	1 meal	2.0	220	9%
■ **SOUP**				
broccoli, cream of	1 serving	12.0	193	56%
cheese	1 serving	23.0	293	71%
chicken noodle	1 serving	2.0	60	30%
chili w/beans	1 serving	6.0	160	34%
chili w/cheese topping	1 serving	19.0	401	43%
clam chowder	1 serving	11.0	214	46%
potato, cream of	1 serving	12.0	222	49%
split pea	1 serving	6.0	146	37%
vegetable beef	1 serving	1.0	79	11%
DOMINO'S PIZZA				
■ **BUFFALO WINGS & BREAD**				
Bread				
cheesy	1 piece	6.0	142	38%
sticks	1 piece	4.0	116	31%
Wings				
BBQ	1 average piece	2.5	50	43%
Hot	1 average piece	2.4	45	48%
■ **6" DEEP DISH PIZZA**				
Cheese	1 personal pizza	27.6	598	17%
Toppings/add to basic cheese pizza values				
anchovies	1 order	2.0	45	40%
bacon	1 order	7.0	82	77%
banana peppers	1 order	–	3	–
beef/precooked	1 order	4.0	44	82%
cheese				
cheddar	1 order	7.0	86	73%
extra	1 order	4.5	58	70%
green olives	1 order	1.0	10	90%
green peppers	1 order	–	2	–
ham	1 order	1.0	17	53%
Italian sausage	1 order	3.5	44	61%
mushrooms, fresh	1 order	–	2	–

Food and Description	Amount	Fat Grams	Total Calories	% Fat Calories
onion	1 order	–	3	–
pepperoni	1 order	4.0	49	73%
pineapple tidbits	1 order	–	3	–
ripe (black) olives	1 order	1.0	11	82%
■ 12" MEDIUM PIZZA				
Cheese				
deep dish	2 slices	22.0	482	41%
hand-tossed	2 slices	11.0	375	26%
thin crust	¼ pizza	12.0	273	40%
Toppings/add to basic cheese pizza values				
combination toppings				
America's favorite/pepperoni, sausage, mushrooms, ripe olives, extra cheese	1 order	11.0	135	73%
deluxe/green peppers, onions, pepperoni, mushrooms, sausage	1 order	7.0	90	70%
extravaganzza/green peppers, onions, pepperoni, ham, ripe olives, mushrooms, sausage, beef	1 order	12.0	153	71%
Hawaiian/ham, pineapple, extra cheese	1 order	4.5	76	53%
meatzza/pepperoni, ham, sausage, beef, extra cheese	1 order	14.9	185	72%
pepperoni/extra pepperoni & cheese	1 order	12.5	147	77%
veal/onions, green peppers, mushrooms, ripe olives, extra cheese	1 order	5.0	65	69%
single toppings				
anchovies	1 order	1.5	34	40%
bacon	1 order	8.7	102	77%
banana peppers	1 order	–	5	–
beef/pre-cooked	1 order	7.0	78	81%
cheese				
cheddar	1 order	4.7	57	74%
extra	1 order	3.8	49	70%
green olives	1 order	2.0	18	20%
green peppers	1 order	–	4	–
ham	1 order	1.0	23	39%
Italian sausage	1 order	6.0	77	70%
mushrooms, fresh	1 order	–	7	–
onion	1 order	–	5	–
pepperoni	1 order	6.5	74	79%
pineapple tidbits	1 order	–	12	–
ripe (black) olives	1 order	2.0	21	86%
■ 12" LARGE PIZZA				
Cheese	⅓ pizza	15.5	365	38%
deep dish	2 slices	30.0	677	40%
hand-tossed	2 slices	15.4	516	27%
thin crust	¼ pizza	17.0	382	40%
Toppings/add to basic cheese pizza values				

Food and Description	Amount	Fat Grams	Total Calories	% Fat Calories
combination toppings				
America's favorite/pepperoni, sausage, mushrooms, ripe olives, extra cheese	1 order	14.0	175	72%
deluxe/reen peppers, onions, mushrooms, sausage pepperoni,	1 order	8.7	112	70%
extravaganzza/green peppers, onions, pepperoni, ham, ripe olives, mushrooms, sausage, beef	1 order	14.8	190	70%
Hawaiian/ham, pineapple, extra cheese	1 order	6.0	107	50%
meatzza/pepperoni, ham, sausage, beef, extra cheese	1 order	19.0	237	72%
pepperoni/extra pepperoni & cheese	1 order	17.0	204	75%
veal/onions, green peppers, mushrooms, ripe olives, extra cheese	1 order	6.5	89	66%
single toppings				
anchovies	1 order	2.0	45	40%
bacon	1 order	13.0	153	76%
banana peppers	1 order	–	7	–
beef/pre-cooked	1 order	10.0	111	81%
cheese				
cheddar	1 order	6.0	71	76%
extra	1 order	5.4	68	71%
green olives	1 order	2.7	25	97%
green peppers	1 order	–	4	–
ham	1 order	1.0	32	28%
Italian sausage	1 order	8.7	110	71%
mushrooms, fresh	1 order	–	9	–
onion	1 order	–	7	–
pepperoni	1 order	8.7	99	79%
pineapple tidbits	1 order	–	19	–
ripe (black) olives	1 order	2.5	28	80%
DUNKIN' DONUTS (See also BAGEL; COOKIE; CROISSANT; DONUT; PASTRY)				
■ **BEVERAGES**				
Coffee				
coolatta				
w/cream	16 fl oz	22.0	410	48%
w/skim milk	16 fl oz	–	230	–
w/2%milk	16 fl oz	2.0	240	8%
w/whole milk	16 fl oz	4.0	260	14%
Dunkaccino	10 fl oz	11.0	250	40%
	14 fl oz	17.0	360	43%
	18.75 fl oz	22.0	480	41%
	20 fl oz	23.0	510	41%
hot chocolate	10 fl oz	8.0	230	31%
	14 fl oz	11.0	330	30%
	18.75 fl oz	15.0	440	31%

Food and Description	Amount	Fat Grams	Total Calories	% Fat Calories
	20 fl oz	16.0	470	31%
orange mango fruit coolatta	20 fl oz	16.0	470	31%
pink lemonade fruit collatta	16 fl oz	–	350	–
raspberry lemonade coolatta	16 fl oz	–	280	–
strawberry fruit coolatta	16 fl oz	–	280	–
vanilla coolatta	16 fl oz	7.0	450	14%
■ **CREAM CHEESE**				
chive	1 pkt	19.0	190	90%
garden vegetable	1 pkt	17.0	180	85%
lite	1 pkt	11.0	130	76%
plain	1 pkt	19.0	200	86%
salmon	1 pkt	17.0	180	85%
■ **CROISSANTS**				
USA				
almond	1 croissant	22.0	350	57%
chocolate	1 croissant	25.0	400	56%
plain	1 croissant	18.0	290	56%
■ **MUFFINS**				
apple cinnamon pecan	1 muffin	21.0	510	37%
apple n'spice	1 muffin	12.0	350	31%
apple & spice/low-fat	1 muffin	1.5	240	6%
banana/low-fat	1 muffin	1.5	250	5%
banana nut	1 muffin	15.0	360	38%
blueberry	4 oz muffin	12.0	320	34%
	6 oz muffin	17.0	490	31%
blueberry				
low-fat	1 muffin	1.5	250	5%
reduced-fat	1 muffin	12.0	450	24%
bran	1 muffin	12.0	390	28%
bran/low-fat	1 muffin	1.0	240	4%
cherry	1 muffin	12.0	340	32%
cherry/low-fat	1 muffin	1.5	250	5%
chocolate/low-fat	1 muffin	2.5	250	9%
chocolate chip	4 oz muffin	17.0	400	38%
	6 oz muffin	24.0	590	37%
chocolate hazelnut chunk	1 muffin	26.0	610	38%
corn	4 oz muffin	15.0	390	35%
	6 oz muffin	16.0	500	29%
corn				
low-fat	1 muffin	2.5	240	9%
reduced-fat	1 muffin	11.0	460	22%
cranberry orange	1 muffin	15.0	470	29%
cranberry orange/low-fat	1 muffin	1.5	240	6%
cranberry orange nut	1 muffin	15.0	350	39%
honey bran raisin	1 muffin	16.0	490	29%
lemon poppyseed	1 muffin	13.0	360	33%
oat bran	1 muffin	13.0	370	32%
■ **SANDWICHES**				
Bagel				

Food and Description	Amount	Fat Grams	Total Calories	% Fat Calories
bacon/cheddar omwich	1 sandwich	21.0	600	32%
Spanish/cheese omwich	1 sandwich	18.0	570	28%
three cheese omwich	1 sandwich	22.0	610	35%
Croissant				
breakfast				
bacon/cheddar omwich	1 sandwich	38.0	560	61%
Spanish/cheese omwich	1 sandwich	36.0	530	61%
three cheese omwich	1 sandwich	39.0	560	63%
lunch				
broccoli & cheese	1 sandwich	21.0	370	51%
chicken salad	1 sandwich	31.0	540	52%
ham & cheese	1 sandwich	32.0	710	41%
roast beef & cheese	1 sandwich	27.0	490	49%
seafood salad	1 sandwich	26.0	480	49%
tuna salad	1 sandwich	30.0	540	50%
English Muffin				
Spanish/cheese omwich	1 sandwich	18.0	370	44%
three cheese omwich	1 sandwich	22.0	400	50%
Ham/egg/cheese breakfast sandwich	1 sandwich	12.0	320	34%
■ SOUP				
beef barley	1 serving	0.5	90	5%
beef noodle	1 serving	1.0	90	10%
chicken noodle	1 serving	1.5	80	17%
chili	1 serving	6.0	170	32%
chili con carne w/beans	1 serving	15.0	300	45%
cream of broccoli	1 serving	11.0	200	50%
cream of potato	1 serving	10.0	190	47%
harvest vegetable	1 serving	2.0	80	23%
Manhattan clam chowder	1 serving	0.5	70	6%
minestrone	1 serving	1.0	100	9%
New England clam chowder	1 serving	10.0	200	45%
split pea w/ham	1 serving	9.0	190	43%
EINSTEIN BROTHERS BAGELS				
■ BAGELS				
asiago cheese	1 bagel	3.0	360	8%
chocolate chip	1 bagel	3.0	370	7%
chopped garlic	1 bagel	3.0	380	7%
chopped onion	1 bagel	1.0	330	3%
cinnamon raisin swirl	1 bagel	1.0	350	3%
cinnamon sugar	1 bagel	1.0	330	3%
cranberry	1 bagel	1.0	350	3%
dark pumpernickel	1 bagel	1.0	320	3%
egg	1 bagel	3.0	340	8%
everything	1 bagel	2.0	340	5%
honey 8-grain	1 bagel	1.0	320	3%
jalapeño	1 bagel	1.0	330	3%
lucky green	1 bagel	1.0	320	3%
marble rye	1 bagel	2.0	340	5%
nutty banana	1 bagel	3.0	360	8%

Food and Description	Amount	Fat Grams	Total Calories	% Fat Calories
peppercorn potato	1 bagel	4.0	350	10%
plain	1 bagel	1.0	320	3%
poppy dip'd	1 bagel	2.0	350	5%
potato	1 bagel	4.5	350	12%
power	1 bagel	5.0	410	11%
pumpkin	1 bagel	1.5	330	4%
salt	1 bagel	1.0	330	3%
sesame dip'd	1 bagel	5.0	380	12%
spinach herb	1 bagel	1.0	310	3%
sun-dried tomato	1 bagel	1.0	320	3%
sunflower	1 bagel	5.0	350	13%
wild blueberry	1 bagel	1.0	350	3%
■ BEVERAGES				
Coffee				
cafe latte	12 fl oz	5.0	140	32%
cappuccino				
non-fat	12 fl oz	–	60	–
regular	12 fl oz	3.5	90	35%
	16 fl oz	6.0	150	36%
espresso	regular	–	1	–
iced				
almond delight				
non-fat	12 fl oz	–	150	–
regular	16 fl oz	4.0	180	20%
Americano	8 fl oz	–	1	–
coffee	12 fl oz	–	–	–
intellccino	16 fl oz	7.0	140	45%
latte				
non-fat	16 fl oz	–	90	–
regular	16 fl oz	4.5	120	34%
mocha				
low-fat	16 fl oz	2.5	180	13%
regular	16 fl oz	6.0	210	26%
plain	12 fl oz	–	–	–
Coffee Extras				
light whipped cream	2 Tbs	2.0	30	60%
On Top reduced fat topping	2 Tbs	1.5	20	68%
Syrup				
almond	2 Tbs	–	80	–
caramel	2 Tbs	–	80	–
hazelnut	2 Tbs	–	80	–
raspberry	2 Tbs	–	–	–
sugar-free/premium				
caramel	2 Tbs	–	–	–
vanilla	2 Tbs	–	–	–
Other Beverages				
Frutopia				
fruit integration	8 fl oz	–	110	–
raspberry psychic lemonade	8 fl oz	–	110	–
strawberry passion awareness	8 fl oz	–	110	–

Food and Description	Amount	Fat Grams	Total Calories	% Fat Calories
tangerine wavelength	8 fl oz	–	110	–
the grape beyond	8 fl oz	–	110	–
hot chocolate				
lower-fat	12 fl oz	7.0	260	24%
regular	12 fl oz	11.0	290	34%
lemonade				
HiC/pink				
light	8 fl oz	–	4	–
regular	8 fl oz	–	96	–
Minute Maid original	8 fl oz	–	96	–
smoothie/mocha	10 fl oz	5.0	470	10%
steamer				
non-fat	12 fl oz	–	160	–
	16 fl oz	0.5	250	2%
regular	12 fl oz	5.0	200	23%
tea				
hot				
cinnamon apple spice	1 cup	–	–	–
Earl Grey	1 cup	–	–	–
English breakfast	1 cup	–	–	–
lemon zinger	1 cup	–	–	–
mandarin orange spice	1 cup	–	–	–
peppermint	1 cup	–	–	–
iced/Nestea				
peach	8 fl oz	–	78	–
raspberry	8 fl oz	–	78	–
southern style	8 fl oz	–	123	–
unsweetened	8 fl oz	–	1	–
■ BREAD SPECIALTY				
Bagel Shtick				
asiago	1 shtick	9.0	450	18%
cinnamon sugar	1 shtick	24.0	570	38%
everything	1 shtick	4.5	380	11%
potato	1 shtick	4.5	350	12%
sesame	1 shtick	8.0	420	17%
Baguette bread	2 oz	0.5	160	3%
Challah				
loaf	2 oz	2.5	150	15%
roll	2.75 oz	3.5	200	16%
Club Mex	1 serving	45.0	750	54%
Flat bread				
peanut sesame	1 piece	15.0	650	21%
rosemary & asiago	1 piece	9.0	520	16%
Focaccia				
cheese pizza	1 serving	11.0	500	20%
margherita	1 serving	17.0	400	38%
pepperoni pizza	1 serving	19.0	590	29%
⊐ CREAM CHEESE/Whipped				
blueberry cheesecake	2 Tbs	5.0	70	64%
cappuccino	2 Tbs	5.0	70	64%

Food and Description	Amount	Fat Grams	Total Calories	% Fat Calories
garden vegetable	2 Tbs	5.0	60	75%
honey almond	2 Tbs	5.0	70	64%
jalapeño salsa	2 Tbs	5.0	60	75%
maple raisin walnut	2 Tbs	5.0	60	75%
onion & chive	2 Tbs	6.0	70	77%
plain				
reduced-fat	2 Tbs	5.0	60	75%
regular	2 Tbs	7.0	70	90%
smoked salmon	2 Tbs	6.0	60	90%
strawberry	2 Tbs	5.0	70	64%
■ ROLL-UPS				
Albuquerque turkey	1 roll-up	33.0	690	43%
Baja shaved beef	1 roll-up	36.0	720	45%
Pacific smoked salmon	1 roll-up	31.0	590	47%
Thai noodle & vegetable	1 roll-up	21.0	630	30%
Thai noodle & vegetable w/chicken	1 roll-up	18.0	670	24%
■ SALADS & SALAD DRESSINGS				
Salad Dressings				
raspberry mustard	2 Tbs	2.0	50	36%
raspberry vinaigrette	2 Tbs	14.0	160	79%
Salads				
Asian chicken	1 serving	4.5	480	8%
broccoli poppyseed cole slaw	1 serving	9.0	150	54%
Bros. Bistro	1 serving	52.0	1050	45%
Caesar/small side	1 serving	17.0	220	70%
fresh fruit salad cup	1 serving	0.5	110	4%
harvest chicken w/rosemary & asiago flat bread	1 serving	20.0	730	25%
mind bagaling side	1 serving	18.0	220	74%
roasted chicken Caesar	1 serving	42.0	890	42%
traditional potato	½ cup	24.0	290	74%
tuna	1 serving	6.0	150	36%
■ SANDWICHES				
BBQ chicken	1 sandwich	11.0	550	18%
baguette/Our Big Hero	1 sandwich	39.0	920	38%
beef				
roast beef/deli	1 sandwich	4.0	400	9%
shaved w/smoked gouda & caramelized onion baguette	1 sandwich	40.0	930	39%
Chicago bagel dog				
asiago	1 sandwich	34.0	740	41%
chili cheese	1 sandwich	38.0	810	42%
everything	1 sandwich	34.0	730	42%
onion w/o cheese	1 sandwich	30.0	680	40%
plain w/cheese	1 sandwich	44.0	850	47%
Cobbie	1 sandwich	33.0	630	47%
egg				
original	1 sandwich	10.0	480	19%
salmon & shmear	1 sandwich	22.0	650	30%
Santa Fe	1 sandwich	24.0	650	33%

Food and Description	Amount	Fat Grams	Total Calories	% Fat Calories
egg salad				
deli	1 sandwich	18.0	560	29%
homestyle bacon	1 sandwich	19.0	580	29%
homestyle ham	1 sandwich	13.0	500	23%
homestyle sausage	1 sandwich	14.0	550	23%
ham				
deli	1 sandwich	6.0	450	12%
w/smoked gouda baguette	1 sandwich	13.0	510	23%
harvest chicken salad/deli	1 sandwich	12.0	540	20%
Holey Cow bagel	1 sandwich	50.0	900	50%
Mediterranean hummus	1 sandwich	13.0	540	22%
New York lox & bagels	1 sandwich	27.0	660	37%
roasted				
chicken & smoked gouda baguette	1 sandwich	11.0	520	19%
eggplant & red pepper w/goat cheese baguette	1 sandwich	10.0	550	16%
tuna salad/deli	1 sandwich	7.0	500	13%
turkey				
deli				
pastrami	1 sandwich	2.0	440	4%
pastrami Rueben	1 sandwich	9.0	680	8%
smoked	1 sandwich	1.5	420	3%
tasty	1 sandwich	21.0	600	32%
Veg Out	1 sandwich	13.0	490	24%
■ SOUPS				
Aztec chicken chili	1 bowl	10.0	320	28%
	1 cup	6.0	190	28%
chicken noodle	1 bowl	7.0	210	30%
	1 cup	4.5	140	29%
chicken & wild rice	1 bowl	16.0	320	45%
cream of potato	1 bowl	13.0	280	42%
	1 cup	8.0	180	40%
red beans & rice	1 bowl	–	200	–
	1 cup	–	130	–
smoked salmon corn chowder	1 bowl	12.0	300	36%
	1 cup	8.0	190	38%
tortilla	1 bowl	19.0	340	50%
	1 cup	14.0	260	48%
turkey chili w/beans	1 bowl	17.0	340	45%
	1 cup	12.0	240	45%
vegetarian black bean	1 bowl	6.0	240	23%
	1 cup	3.5	160	20%
very veggie white bean	1 bowl	10.0	270	33%
	1 cup	7.0	190	33%
zesty lentil	1 bowl	4.5	220	18%
	1 cup	2.5	130	17%
■ SWEETS				
Big brownie	1	21.0	500	38%
Buns				
pull-a-part cinnamon w/icing	1 bun	10.0	380	24%

Food and Description	Amount	Fat Grams	Total Calories	% Fat Calories
pull-a-part sticky	1 bun	13.0	470	25%
Cake				
crumb/traditional pound	1 slice	38.0	800	43%
lemon iced	1 slice	24.0	540	40%
marble	1 slice	24.0	480	45%
Cookies				
black & white	1	12.0	390	28%
chocolate chunk	1	28.0	600	42%
ginger white chocolate	1	17.0	510	30%
oatmeal raisin	1	21.0	550	34%
peanut butter	1	35.0	620	51%
sugar	1	32.0	610	47%
Muffins				
97% fat-free apple cinnamon	1	1.5	350	4%
banana nut	1	29.0	520	50%
blueberry	1	24.0	460	47%
chocolate chip	1	13.0	240	49%
lemon poppyseed/low-fat	1	7.0	370	17%
mocha chocolate chip	1	29.0	550	47%
morning harvest	1	19.0	460	37%
Scones				
lemon currant	1 scone	17.0	490	31%
whole wheat-w/fruit	1 scone	17.0	480	31%
EL POLLO LOCO				
■ **BOWLS, SALADS, & SALAD DRESSINGS**				
Polo Bowl				
regular	1 bowl	11.0	469	21%
smokey black bean	1 bowl	23.0	604	34%
Salad Bowl				
flame broiled chicken	1 bowl	13.0	357	33%
Mexican chicken Caesar	1 bowl	35.0	734	43%
Southwest chicken salad	1 bowl	31.0	529	53%
Salad Dressings				
bleu cheese	2 oz	32.0	300	96%
creamy cilantro	1.75 oz	29.0	266	98%
light Italian	2 oz	1.0	25	36%
1,000 Island	2 oz	27.0	270	90%
ranch	2 oz	39.0	350	100%
Southwest	1.75 oz	32.0	301	96%
Salads/other				
garden	1 serving	7.0	105	60%
tostada w/o shell	1 salad	11.0	304	33%
shell only	1 shell	27.0	440	55%
■ **BURRITOS**				
bean, rice, & cheese	1 burrito	16.0	503	29%
chicken				
classic	1 burrito	22.0	580	34%
lover's	1 burrito	19.0	475	36%
Mexican Caesar	1 burrito	35.0	734	43%

Food and Description	Amount	Fat Grams	Total Calories	% Fat Calories
Southwest	1 burrito	27.0	627	39%
ultimate	1 burrito	23.0	633	33%
■ **CHICKEN**/flamed broiled				
breast	1 piece	6.0	160	34%
leg	1 piece	5.0	90	50%
thigh	1 piece	12.0	180	60%
wing	1 piece	6.0	110	49%
■ **CONDIMENTS**				
avocado salsa	1 pkt	1.0	12	75%
guacamole	1 Tbs	2.0	30	60%
house salsa	1 pkt	–	6	–
jalapeño hot sauce	1 pkt	0.5	5	9%
Pico de Gallo salsa	1 pkt	0.5	11	41%
sour cream/light	1 pkt	3.0	45	60%
spicy chipotle salsa	1 pkt	–	7	–
■ **DESSERT**				
banana split	1	28.0	717	35%
churro	1 piece	11.0	179	55%
Foster's Freeze w/o cone	1 serving	5.0	180	25%
smoothies				
berry banana	11 oz	7.0	367	17%
kiwi strawberry	9.5 oz	7.0	357	18%
■ **KIDS**				
Dinosaur chicken bites	1 serving	10.4	185	51%
■ **SPECIALTIES & SIDE DISHES**				
beans				
pinto	1 serving	4.0	185	19%
smokeyblack	1 serving	16.0	306	47%
chicken taquito	1 serving	17.0	370	41%
coleslaw	1 serving	16.0	206	70%
corn cobbette/3"	1 piece	1.0	80	11%
French fries	1 serving	19.0	444	39%
gravy	1 serving	–	14	–
macaroni & cheese	1 serving	12.0	244	44%
mashed potatoes	1 serving	1.0	97	9%
potato salad	1 serving	14.0	256	49%
rice/Spanish	1 serving	3.0	130	21%
tortilla chips/unsalted	1 serving	24.0	426	51%
vegetables/fresh	1 serving	2.0	57	32%
■ **TACOS**				
chicken soft taco	1 taco	12.0	237	46%
taco al carbon	1 taco	6.0	164	33%
■ **TORTILLAS**				
corn				
4.5"	1 tortilla	0.5	32	14%
6"	1 tortilla	1.0	70	13%
flour				
6.5"	1 tortilla	3.0	90	30%
11"	1 tortilla	7.0	260	24%
spicy tomato	1 tortilla	6.0	254	21%

Food and Description	Amount	Fat Grams	Total Calories	% Fat Calories
FAZOLI'S				
▨ **DESSERT**				
cheesecake				
plain	1 serving	20.8	270	69%
w/strawberry topping	1 serving	20.8	310	60%
chocolate chocolate chip cheesecake	1 serving	21.8	298	66%
■ **ENTRÉES**				
baked ziti				
large	1 serving	25.6	748	31%
regular	1 serving	17.0	485	32%
broccoli fettucine				
large	1 serving	22.7	826	25%
regular	1 serving	15.4	563	25%
fettucine Alfredo				
large	1 serving	22.4	798	25%
regular	1 serving	15.0	535	25%
lasagna	1 serving	19.0	437	39%
meatball sub	1 serving	30.2	650	42%
ravioli				
w/meat sauce	1 serving	16.4	361	41%
w/marinara sauce	1 serving	15.2	332	41%
sampler platter	1 serving	20.8	437	43%
spaghetti				
Parmesan/baked	1 serving	25.5	697	33%
w/marinara sauce				
large	1 serving	8.3	622	12%
regular	1 serving	5.7	418	12%
w/meat sauce				
large	1 serving	11.5	675	15%
regular	1 serving	7.8	453	15%
w/meatballs				
large	1 serving	45.6	1022	40%
regular	1 serving	30.7	718	38%
■ **PIZZA**				
cheese	double slice	10.7	360	27%
combination	double slice	20.8	484	39%
pepperoni	double slice	17.0	430	36%
■ **SALADS & RELATED ITEMS**				
breadstick				
regular	1 breadstick	8.0	172	42%
dry	1 breadstick	0.8	99	7%
chicken & Ceasar salad	1 serving	15.3	537	26%
garden salad	1 serving	0.3	28	10%
salad dressing				
honey French	1 oz	14.0	160	79%
house Italian				
reduced calorie	1 oz	3.5	69	46%
regular	1 oz	15.0	138	98%
ranch	1 oz	20.0	180	100%
Thousand Island	1 oz	14.0	140	90%

Food and Description	Amount	Fat Grams	Total Calories	% Fat Calories
■ SOUP				
bean & pasta	1 serving	7.2	174	37%
minestrone	1 serving	1.3	90	13%
GODFATHER'S PIZZA				
■ GOLDEN CRUST PIZZA				
cheese				
medium	⅛ pizza	8.0	212	34%
large	¹⁄₁₀ pizza	9.0	242	33%
combo				
medium	⅛ pizza	12.0	271	40%
large	¹⁄₁₀ pizza	14.0	305	41%
■ ORIGINAL PIZZA				
cheese				
mini	¼ pizza	3.0	131	21%
medium	⅛ pizza	5.0	231	19%
large	¹⁄₁₀ pizza	6.0	258	21%
jumbo	¹⁄₁₀ pizza	9.0	382	21%
combo				
mini	¼ pizza	7.0	176	36%
medium	⅛ pizza	11.0	306	32%
large	¹⁄₁₀ pizza	12.0	338	32%
jumbo	¹⁄₁₀ pizza	18.0	503	32%
HARDEE'S				
■ BEVERAGES				
chocolate shake	1 shake	5.0	370	12%
vanilla shake	1 shake	5.0	350	13%
■ BREAKFAST				
Big Country Breakfast				
w/bacon	1 serving	43.0	740	52%
w/sausage	1 serving	61.0	930	59%
biscuits				
apple cinnamon 'n' raisin	1 serving	8.0	250	29%
bacon, egg, & cheese	1 serving	30.0	520	52%
bacon & egg	1 serving	27.0	490	50%
Biscuit 'N' Gravy	1 serving	30.0	530	51%
chicken	1 serving	27.0	590	41%
country ham	1 serving	22.0	440	45%
ham	1 serving	20.0	410	44%
ham, egg, & cheese	1 serving	27.0	500	49%
jelly	1 serving	21.0	440	43%
Made From Scratch	1 serving	21.0	390	48%
Omelet	1 serving	32.0	550	52%
rise 'n' shine	1 serving	21.0	390	48%
sausage	1 serving	36.0	550	59%
sausage & egg	1 serving	41.0	620	60%
steak	1 serving	32.0	580	50%
Frisco breakfast sandwich/ham	1 serving	22.0	450	44%
Hash Rounds	1 serving	14.0	230	55%
margarine/butter blend	1 serving	4.0	35	100%
orange juice	11 fl oz	–	140	–

Food and Description	Amount	Fat Grams	Total Calories	% Fat Calories
■ BURGERS & SANDWICHES				
Burgers				
All Star	1 burger	43.0	660	59%
Famous Star	1 burger	35.0	570	55%
Frisco	1 burger	49.0	720	61%
Monster Burger	1 burger	79.0	1060	67%
regular	1 burger	11.0	270	37%
Super Star	1 burger	53.0	790	60%
Sandwiches				
chicken fillet	1 sandwich	23.0	480	43%
Fisherman's Fillet	1 sandwich	28.0	530	48%
grilled chicken	1 sandwich	16.0	350	41%
hot dog w/condiments	1 sandwich	32.0	450	64%
hot ham'n'cheese	1 sandwich	12.0	300	36%
roast beef				
Big	1 sandwich	24.0	410	53%
regular	1 sandwich	16.0	310	46%
■ CHICKEN/Fried				
breast	1 serving	15.0	370	36%
leg	1 serving	7.0	170	37%
thigh	1 serving	15.0	330	41%
wing	1 serving	8.0	200	36%
■ DESSERT				
apple turnover	1 serving	12.0	270	40%
cool twist cone-vanilla/chocolate	1 cone	2.0	180	10%
peach cobbler	1 serving	7.0	310	20%
■ SALADS & DRESSING				
salad dressing				
French	1 pkt	–	70	–
ranch	1 pkt	29.0	290	90%
Thousand Island	1 pkt	23.0	250	83%
salads				
garden	1 serving	13.0	210	56%
grilled chicken	1 serving	3.0	150	18%
side	1 serving	–	25	–
■ SIDES				
coleslaw	4 oz	20.0	240	75%
Crispy Curls potatoes	medium	18.0	340	48%
	large	28.0	520	48%
	monster	31.0	590	47%
French fries	regular	16.0	340	42%
	large	21.0	440	43%
	monster	24.0	510	42%
gravy	1 serving	–	20	–
mashed potatoes	4 oz	–	70	–
JACK-N-THE-BOX				
■ BEVERAGES				
Barq's Root Beer	1 regular	–	180	–
Coca-Cola				
classic	1 regular	–	170	–
Diet Coke	1 regular	–	–	–

Food and Description	Amount	Fat Grams	Total Calories	% Fat Calories
coffee	1 regular	–	5	–
Dr. Pepper	1 regular	–	190	–
iced tea	1 regular	–	–	–
milk/2% reduced fat	8.5 fl oz	5.0	130	35%
Minute Maid lemonade	1 regular	–	190	–
Orange juice	6.5 fl oz	–	80	–
Shakes-w/Ice Cream				
cappuccino	1 regular	29.0	630	41%
chocolate	1 regular	27.0	630	39%
Oreo cookie	1 regular	36.0	740	44%
strawberry	1 regular	28.0	640	39%
vanilla	1 regular	31.0	610	46%
Sprite	1 regular	–	160	–
■ BREAKFAST				
bacon	1 serving	1.5	20	68%
biscuit	1 biscuit	9.0	190	43%
Breakfast Jack	1 serving	12.0	280	39%
Country Crock spread	1 serving	2.5	25	90%
French toast sticks	1 serving	20.0	420	43%
grape jelly	1 pkt	–	40	–
hash browns	1 serving	12.0	170	64%
syrup	1 pkt	–	130	–
sausage biscuit	1 biscuit	27.0	380	64%
sausage croissant	1 croissant	48.0	660	65%
sausage, egg, & cheese biscuit	1 biscuit	36.0	510	64%
scrambled egg pocket	1 pocket	21.0	430	44%
Sourdough Breakfast Sandwich	1 sandwich	24.0	450	48%
Supreme Croissant	1 croissant	34.0	530	58%
Ultimate Breakfast Sandwich	1 sandwich	34.0	600	51%
■ BURGERS & BEEF				
Cheeseburger				
bacon bacon	1 burger	50.0	760	59%
Bacon Ultimate	1 burger	71.0	1020	63%
double	1 burger	24.0	440	49%
Ultimate	1 burger	66.0	950	63%
hamburger				
regular	1 burger	9.0	250	32%
w/cheese	1 burger	13.0	300	39%
Jumbo Jack				
plain	1 burger	30.0	550	49%
w/cheese	1 burger	38.0	640	53%
Sourdough Jack	1 burger	45.0	690	59%
■ CHICKEN, FISH & MEXICAN ITEMS				
Chicken				
breast pieces	5 pieces	17.0	360	43%
sandwich				
Caesar	1 sandwich	26.0	520	45%
grilled fillet	1 sandwich	24.0	480	45%
Jack's spicy chicken	1 sandwich	29.0	570	46%
regular	1 sandwich	21.0	400	47%

Food and Description	Amount	Fat Grams	Total Calories	% Fat Calories
supreme	1 sandwich	49.0	830	53%
Fish & chips	1 serving	39.0	780	45%
Mexican				
chicken fajita pita	1 sandwich	10.0	320	28%
taco				
Monster	1 taco	17.0	270	57%
regular	1 taco	10.0	170	53%
■ CONDIMENTS				
Catsup	1 pkt	−	10	−
Cheese				
American	1 slice	4.0	45	80%
Swiss-style	1 slice	4.0	40	90%
Dipping sauce				
BBQ	1 pkt	−	45	−
buttermilk house	1 pkt	13.0	130	90%
Frank's Red Hot Buffalo	1 pkt	−	10	−
sweet & sour	1 pkt	−	45	−
tartar	1 pkt	22.0	210	90%
Hot sauce	1 pkt	−	5	−
Ketchup	1 pkt	−	10	−
Mayonnaise	1 pkt	17.0	155	99%
Mustard				
Chinese hot	1 pkt	−	5	−
regular	1 pkt	−	5	−
Salsa	1 pkt	−	10	−
Sour cream	1 pkt	6.0	60	90%
■ DESSERT				
cheesecake/plain	1 slice	18.0	320	51%
double fudge cake	1 slice	10.0	300	30%
hot apple turnover	1 turnover	18.0	340	48%
■ SALADS & RELATED ITEMS				
Croutons	1 serving	2.0	50	36%
Salad dressing				
blue cheese	1 pkt	15.0	210	64%
buttermilk house	1 pkt	30.0	290	93%
Italian/low-calorie	1 pkt	1.5	25	54%
Thousand Island	1 pkt	24.0	250	86%
Salads				
garden chicken salad	1 serving	9.0	200	41%
side salad	1 serving	3.0	50	54%
Teriyaki Bowl				
chicken	1 bowl	4.0	670	5%
soy sauce	1 pkt	−	5	−
■ SIDE ORDERS				
Bacon & cheddar potato wedges	1 serving	50.0	750	60%
Curly Fries				
chili cheese	1 serving	41.0	650	57%
seasoned	1 serving	23.0	410	50%
Egg roll	1 piece	8.0	150	48%
	3 pieces	24.0	440	49%

Food and Description	Amount	Fat Grams	Total Calories	% Fat Calories
French fries	regular	16.0	350	41%
	jumbo	20.0	430	42%
	superscoop	28.0	610	41%
Jalapeños/stuffed	3 pieces	13.0	230	51%
	7 pieces	31.0	530	53%
Onion rings	1 serving	25.0	450	50%
KENNY ROGERS ROASTERS				
■ CHICKEN & TURKEY				
¼ chicken				
dark meat				
w/skin	4.35 oz	16.7	271	55%
skinless	3.29 oz	7.3	169	39%
white meat				
w/skin	4.7 oz	10.7	244	40%
skinless	3.74 oz	2.3	144	14%
½ chicken				
w/skin	9.06 oz	27.5	515	48%
skinless	7.03 oz	9.5	313	27%
pot pie/chicken	1 pot pie	33.0	708	42%
turkey breast/sliced	4.5 oz	2.2	158	13%
■ SALADS & DRESSING				
Salad Dressings				
blue cheese	2.5 oz	39.0	370	95%
buttermilk ranch	2.5 oz	48.0	430	100%
Caesar	2.5 oz	36.0	340	95%
honey French	2.5 oz	29.0	350	75%
honey mustard	2.5 oz	28.0	320	79%
Italian/fat-free	2.5 oz	–	35	–
Thousand Island	2.5 oz	33.0	330	90%
Salads				
chicken Caesar salad	1 serving	8.7	285	27%
roasted chicken salad	1 serving	10.3	292	32%
■ SANDWICHES				
BBQ chicken pita	1 sandwich	7.2	400	16%
chicken Caesar pita	1 sandwich	34.8	606	52%
roasted chicken pita	1 sandwich	35.3	685	46%
turkey sandwich	1 sandwich	12.0	385	28%
■ SIDE ORDERS (*See also* Salads & Dressing in this section)				
baked sweet potato	1 serving	0.3	263	1%
chicken noodle soup	1 cup	1.0	55	16%
	1 bowl	2.0	90	20%
cinnamon apples	1 serving	5.0	200	23%
coleslaw	1 serving	15.5	225	62%
corn muffin	1 muffin	8.0	175	41%
corn niblets	1 serving	0.7	112	6%
corn on the cob	1 piece	0.8	68	11%
cornbread stuffing	1 serving	18.6	326	51%
creamy Parmesan spinach	1 serving	5.5	119	42%
honey baked beans	1 serving	1.0	150	6%
Italian green beans	1 serving	8.2	116	64%

Food and Description	Amount	Fat Grams	Total Calories	% Fat Calories
macaroni & cheese	1 serving	5.8	197	26%
pasta salad				
regular	1 serving	11.6	236	44%
sour cream & dill	1 serving	16.3	233	63%
potato salad	1 serving	27.3	390	63%
potatoes				
garlic parsley	1 serving	12.0	259	42%
real mashed	1 serving	14.4	295	44%
rice pilaf	1 serving	4.7	173	24%
side salad	1 serving	0.3	23	12%
steamed vegetables	1 serving	0.3	48	6%
tomato-cucumber salad	1 serving	2.2	123	16%
zucchini & squash Santa Fe	1 serving	4.5	70	58%

KENTUCKY FRIED CHICKEN

■ CHICKEN

Food and Description	Amount	Fat Grams	Total Calories	% Fat Calories
Extra Crispy				
breast	1 piece	28.0	470	54%
drumstick	1 piece	12.0	195	55%
thigh	1 piece	27.0	380	64%
wing/whole	1 piece	15.0	220	61%
Hot & spicy				
breast	1 piece	29.0	505	52%
drumstick	1 piece	10.0	175	51%
thigh	1 piece	26.0	355	66%
wing/whole	1 piece	15.0	210	64%
Nuggets & sauce				
nuggets only	3.4 oz	18.0	284	57%
sauce				
barbeque	1 oz	<1.0	35	13%
honey	1 oz	–	49	–
mustard	1 oz	<1.0	36	23%
sweet & sour	1 oz	<1.0	58	9%
Original Recipe				
breast	1 piece	24.0	400	54%
drumstick	1 piece	9.0	140	58%
thigh	1 piece	18.0	250	65%
wing/whole	1 piece	10.0	140	64%
Popcorn chicken	small	23.0	362	57%
Pot pie/chunky	1 pot pie	42.0	770	49%
Strips/crispy				
Colonel's	3 pieces	16.0	300	48%
spicy	3 pieces	15.0	335	40%
	Large	40.0	620	58%
Wings				
honey BBQ	6 pieces	38.0	607	56%
Hot	6 pieces	33.0	471	63%

■ DESSERTS

Food and Description	Amount	Fat Grams	Total Calories	% Fat Calories
Colonel's Pies				
apple	1 slice	14.0	310	41%
pecan	1 slice	23.0	490	42%

Food and Description	Amount	Fat Grams	Total Calories	% Fat Calories
strawberry creme	1 slice	15.0	280	48%
double chocolate chip cake	1 slice	16.0	320	45%
Little Bucket Parfaits				
chocolate cream	1 serving	15.0	290	47%
fudge brownie	1 serving	3.5	280	11%
lemon creme	1 serving	14.0	410	31%
strawberry shortcake	1 serving	7.0	200	7%
■ **SANDWICHES**/Chicken				
Honey BBQ flavored	1 sandwich	6.0	310	17%
Original Recipe	1 sandwich	22.0	450	44%
Tender Roast	1 sandwich	15.0	350	39%
Triple Crunch	1 sandwich	22.0	490	40%
Triple Crunch Zinger	1 sandwich	32.0	550	52%
■ **SIDE ORDERS**				
BBQ baked beans	1 serving	3.0	190	14%
buttermilk biscuit	1 biscuit	10.0	180	50%
coleslaw	1 serving	13.5	232	52%
corn on the cob	1 piece	1.5	150	9%
macaroni & cheese	1 serving	8.0	180	40%
mashed potatoes & gravy	1 serving	6.0	120	45%
potato salad	1 serving	14.0	230	55%
potato wedges	1 serving	13.0	280	42%
KOO KOO ROO				
■ **CHICKEN**				
Rotisserie				
breast & wing	1 serving	16.0	355	41%
half chicken	½ chicken	34.0	655	47%
leg & thigh	1 serving	18.0	300	54%
Original skinless flame-broiled				
Breast meat	1 serving	1.0	159	6%
breast & wing (wing portion w/skin)	1 serving	8.0	218	33%
half chicken (wing portion w/skin)	½ chicken	16.0	391	37%
leg & thigh	1 serving	8.0	173	42%
Sandwiches				
BBQ	1 sandwich	14.0	568	22%
chicken Caesar	1 sandwich	37.0	728	46%
Original chicken breast	1 sandwich	47.0	752	56%
■ **CONDIMENTS**				
Salad Dressings				
balsamic vinaigrette	2 Tbs	9.0	90	90%
BBQ	2 Tbs	–	40	–
Caesar	2 Tbs	18.0	160	100%
Chinese chicken	2 Tbs	8.0	110	65%
chopped salad	2 Tbs	7.0	100	63%
■ **SIDE DISHES**				
artichokes	1 serving	–	33	–
asparagus	1 serving	–	24	–
baby carrots	1 serving	–	73	

Food and Description	Amount	Fat Grams	Total Calories	% Fat Calories
baked yams	1 serving	–	362	–
BBQ beans	1 serving	2.0	139	13%
black beans	1 serving	2.0	139	13%
brussels sprouts	5 pieces	–	49	–
butternut squash	1 serving	–	87	–
confetti rice	1 serving	–	131	–
cracked wheat rice	1 serving	1.0	97	9%
cranberry sauce	1 oz serving	–	45	–
creamed spinach	1 serving	12.0	141	77%
cucumber salad	1 serving	–	30	–
gravy	1 serving	1.0	24	38%
green beans	1 serving	2.0	50	36%
hand-mashed potatoes	1 serving	5.0	185	24%
homemade stuffing	1 serving	9.0	189	43%
hot potatoes	1 serving	3.0	115	23%
kernel corn	1 serving	–	97	–
Koo Koo Roo slaw	1 serving	2.0	55	33%
Lavash (flatbread)	1 serving	–	94	–
lentil salad	1 serving	5.0	175	26%
macaroni & cheese	1 serving	11.0	270	37%
roasted garlic potatoes	1 serving	2.0	116	16%
roll	1 roll	1.0	107	8%
steamed vegetables	1 serving	–	33	–
tangy tomato salad	1 serving	3.0	56	48%
■ SOUPS & SALADS				
Salads				
BBQ chicken	1 salad	21.0	466	41%
Caesar				
chicken	1 salad	11.0	310	32%
original	1 salad	8.0	170	42%
chicken chop salads				
Original				
w/dressing	1 salad	39.0	864	41%
w/o dressing	1 salad	13.0	634	18%
Southwestern	1 salad	28.0	880	29%
Thai	1 salad	16.0	565	25%
Chinese chicken	1 salad	8.0	296	24%
Koo Koo Roo house	1 salad	6.0	164	33%
pasta salads				
pesto	1 salad	5.0	168	27%
Santa Fe	1 salad	6.0	206	26%
tomato basil	1 salad	2.0	108	17%
12-vegetable chopped	1 salad	1.0	78	12%
Soups				
chicken chili	1 serving	2.0	98	18%
ten vegetable soup	1 serving	3.0	121	22%
turkey dumpling	1 serving	4.0	166	22%
■ TURKEY				
Fresh Roasted carved				
pot pie	1 pie	45.0	905	45%

Food and Description	Amount	Fat Grams	Total Calories	% Fat Calories
sandwiches				
breast	1 sandwich	7.0	538	12%
½ breast	1 sandwich	4.0	269	13%
open-faced	1 sandwich	21.0	672	28%
sliced turkey				
dark meat	¼ lb	8.0	212	34%
white meat	¼ lb	1.0	153	6%
turkey dinner/hand-carved	1 dinner	21.0	705	27%
KRYSTAL				
■ BEVERAGE				
chocolate shake	16 fl oz	10.0	275	33%
■ BREAKFAST				
biscuits				
bacon	1 biscuit	17.0	306	50%
bacon, egg, & cheese	1 biscuit	26.0	423	55%
country ham	1 biscuit	17.0	334	46%
egg	1 biscuit	19.0	327	52%
gravy	1 biscuit	26.0	419	56%
plain	1 biscuit	12.0	244	44%
sausage	1 biscuit	30.0	437	62%
donuts				
iced				
chocolate	1 donut	11.0	212	47%
vanilla	1 donut	9.0	196	41%
plain	1 donut	9.0	150	54%
pancakes	3 pancakes	12.0	212	51%
Sunriser	1 serving	17.0	259	59%
■ BURGERS & HOT DOGS				
Burger Plus				
plain	1 burger	26.0	415	56%
w/cheese	1 burger	31.0	473	59%
cheeseburger				
bacon	1 burger	34.0	521	59%
cheese Krystal	1 burger	10.0	167	54%
double cheese Krystal	1 burger	18.0	337	48%
hamburger				
Big K	1 burger	35.0	540	58%
double Krystal	1 burger	14.0	277	45%
Krystal	1 burger	7.0	158	40%
Pups				
chili	1 hot dog	10.0	162	55%
chili cheese	1 hot dog	13.0	211	55%
corn	1 hot dog	14.0	214	59%
plain	1 hot dog	9.0	160	51%
■ DESSERT				
apple pie	1 slice	10.0	300	30%
lemon meringue pie	1 slice	9.0	340	24%
pecan pie	1 slice	23.0	450	46%
■ SANDWICH				
crispy crunchy chicken	1 sandwich	24.0	467	46%

Food and Description	Amount	Fat Grams	Total Calories	% Fat Calories
■ **SIDE ORDERS**				
chili	8 oz	8.0	218	33%
	12 oz	12.0	327	33%
fries				
Krys Kross				
chili cheese	1 serving	39.0	625	56%
plain	1 serving	29.0	486	54%
w/cheese	1 serving	31.0	516	54%
regular	small	13.0	262	45%
	regular	18.0	355	46%
	large	23.0	463	45%
LA SALSA FRESH MEXICAN GRILL				
Burrito/bean & cheese	1 burrito	14.0	535	24%
Sides				
black beans	1 serving	4.0	321	11%
rice	1 serving	4.0	321	11%
Tacos				
chicken				
Mexico City	1 taco	6.0	220	25%
Taco La Salsa	1 taco	10.0	300	30%
fish (Sonora style)	1 taco	9.0	225	36%
vegetarian taco	1 taco	8.0	290	28%
LITTLE CAESAR'S PIZZA				
■ **PIZZA**				
Baby Pan! Pan!	1 pizza	15.0	310	44%
By-The-Slice				
cheese only	⅛ of 14" pizza	10.0	290	31%
pepperoni	⅛ of 14" pizza	14.0	340	37%
Deep Dish/Square				
12"				
cheese only	1 slice	5.0	140	32%
pepperoni	1 slice	6.0	160	34%
14"				
cheese only	1 slice	5.0	140	32%
pepperoni	1 slice	7.0	160	39%
Round				
12"				
cheese only	1 slice	6.0	160	34%
pepperoni	1 slice	8.0	180	40%
14"				
cheese only	1 slice	6.0	170	32%
meatsa	1 slice	10.0	220	41%
pepperoni	1 slice	8.0	200	36%
supreme	1 slice	10.0	230	39%
veggie	1 slice	7.0	290	22%
16"				
cheese only	1 slice	8.0	230	31%
pepperoni	1 slice	11.0	260	38%

Food and Description	Amount	Fat Grams	Total Calories	% Fat Calories
18"				
cheese only	1 slice	8.0	240	30%
pepperoni	1 slice	11.0	270	37%
Thin Crust				
12"				
cheese only	1 slice	6.0	120	45%
pepperoni	1 slice	8.0	150	48%
14"				
cheese only	1 slice	6.0	130	42%
pepperoni	1 slice	9.0	160	51%
■ **SALADS & SIDES**				
Bread				
Crazy bread	1 slice	2.5	90	25%
Italian cheese	1 piece	6.0	120	45%
Chicken wings	1 wing	4.0	50	72%
Cinnamon Caesar stick	1 stick	9.0	340	24%
Salad dressings				
Italian				
fat-free	1.5 oz	–	25	–
regular	1.5 oz	22.0	210	94%
ranch	1.5 oz	29.0	270	97%
Salads				
antipasto salad	1 salad	7.0	130	48%
tossed side	1 salad	0.5	50	9%
Sauce/Crazy	1 serving	–	45	–
■ **SANDWICHES**				
cold/deli-style				
ham & cheese	1 sandwich	22.0	600	33%
Italian	1 sandwich	32.0	690	42%
veggie	1 sandwich	38.0	720	48%
LONG JOHN SILVER'S				
■ **BEVERAGE**				
Coke				
Diet	medium	–	–	–
regular	medium	–	270	
Dr. Pepper	medium	–	250	–
Hi-C pink lemonade	medium	–	260	–
Minute Maid lemonade	medium	–	260	–
Sprite	medium	–	260	–
■ **CONDIMENTS**				
honey mustard sauce	1 pkt	–	20	–
catsup	1 pkt	–	10	–
lettuce	1 serving	–	8	–
malt vinegar	1 pkt	–	–	–
margarine	1 tsp	4.0	35	100%
salad dressing				
French/fat-free	1 pkt	–	40	–
Italian	1 pkt	9.0	90	90%
ranch				
fat-free	1 pkt	–	40	–
regular	1 oz	18.0	170	95%

Food and Description	Amount	Fat Grams	Total Calories	% Fat Calories
Thousand Island	1 oz	10.0	120	75%
shrimp sauce	1 pkt	–	15	–
sweet & sour sauce	1 pkt	–	20	–
tartar sauce	1 pkt	3.5	40	79%
■ DESSERTS				
Pie				
banana split sundae	1 piece	17.0	300	51%
chocolate creme	1 piece	17.0	280	55%
double lemon	1 piece	18.0	350	46%
Dutch apple	1 piece	13.0	290	40%
pecan	1 piece	19.0	390	44%
pineapple creme cheesecake pie	1 piece	17.0	310	49%
strawberries 'N creme	1 piece	15.0	280	48%
■ ENTRÉES				
chicken/batter-dipped plank	1 piece	8.0	140	51%
clams\breaded	1 order	14.0	250	50%
fish				
batter-dipped				
junior	1 piece	8.0	120	60%
regular	1 piece	13.0	230	51%
country-style breaded	1 piece	10.0	200	45%
lemon crumb	2 pieces	12.0	240	45%
lemon crumb				
a-la-carte	2 fish w/rice	17.0	480	32%
Add-A-Piece	1 fish w/rice	7.0	150	42%
fish meal	1 meal	29.0	730	36%
shrimp				
battered	1 piece	2.5	45	50%
popcorn	1 serving	15.0	320	42%
■ SALADS				
Garden	1 salad	–	45	–
Grilled Chicken	1 salad	2.5	140	16%
Ocean Chef	1 salad	2.0	130	14%
side	1 salad	–	20	–
■ SANDWICHES				
chicken				
plain	1 sandwich	14.0	340	37%
w/cheese	1 sandwich	19.0	390	44%
fish				
batter-dipped/w/o sauce	1 sandwich	13.0	320	37%
plain	1 sandwich	20.0	430	42%
ultimate	1 sandwich	25.0	480	47%
w/cheese	1 sandwich	25.0	480	47%
■ SIDE ORDERS				
broccoli cheese soup	1 bowl	12.0	180	60%
cheese sticks	1 serving	9.0	160	51%
coleslaw	1 serving	7.0	170	37%
corn cobbette				
w/butter	1 piece	8.0	140	51%
w/o butter	1 piece	0.5	80	6%

Food and Description	Amount	Fat Grams	Total Calories	% Fat Calories
fries	regular	15.0	250	54%
	large	24.0	420	51%
hushpuppy	1 piece	2.5	60	38%
rice pilaf	1 serving	4.0	180	20%
side salad	1 serving	–	25	–
MACHEEZMO MOUSE				
■ **BURRITOS**				
chicken	1 burrito	11.0	580	17%
chill	1 burrito	11.0	605	16%
combo	1 burrito	12.0	630	17%
veggie	1 burrito	8.0	655	11%
■ **EL BENTO**				
deluxe	1 serving	7.0	740	9%
Kid	1 serving	1.0	235	4%
■ **ENCHILADAS**				
chicken	1 enchilada	16.0	545	26%
chili	1 enchilada	16.0	560	26%
veggie	1 enchilada	14.0	635	20%
■ **QUESADILLAS**				
Kid				
cheese	1 serving	13.0	360	33%
chicken	1 serving	15.0	430	31%
snack				
cheese	1 serving	13.0	377	31%
chicken	1 serving	15.0	450	30%
■ **OTHER MISC. MENU ITEMS**				
beans	1 oz	–	35	–
Boss Sauce	1 oz	–	30	–
broccoli	1 oz	–	4	–
cheese	1 oz	5.0	81	56%
chicken	1 oz	1.0	35	26%
chili	1 oz	1.0	43	21%
chips	1 serving	6.0	140	39%
cilantro	1 oz	–	8	–
el bento	1 serving	1.0	77	12%
enchilada sauce	1 oz	–	6	–
Famouse #5	1 serving	5.0	585	8%
fresh greens	1 oz	–	2	–
quacamole	1 oz	3.0	100	27%
marinated veggies	1 oz	<1.0	10	45%
Mexican, cheese	1 oz	8.0	100	72%
mustard dressing	1 oz	<1.0	25	18%
nacho grande	1 serving	44.0	855	46%
rice	1 oz	<1.0	45	10%
salsa	1 oz	–	4	–
sour cream	1 oz	3.0	35	77%
tortilla				
corn	2 pieces	–	90	–
flour	2.5 oz	3.0	200	14%
wheat	2.5 oz	3.0	200	14%

Food and Description	Amount	Fat Grams	Total Calories	% Fat Calories
■ RICE & BEANS				
rice, beans, salad	1 meal	<1.0	344	1%
rice, beans, broccoli	1 meal	<1.0	328	1%
■ SALADS				
chicken	1 serving	11.0	445	22%
chicken power	1 serving	1.0	275	3%
veggie power	1 serving	<1.0	200	2%
veggie taco	1 serving	14.0	655	19%
■ TACOS				
snack				
chicken	1 serving	8.0	290	25%
chili	1 serving	8.0	310	23%
veggie	1 serving	6.0	290	19%
Kid				
cheese	1 serving	5.0	285	16%
chicken	1 serving	7.0	355	18%
veggie deluxe	1 serving	6.0	665	8%
MAZZIO'S PIZZA				
■ APPETIZERS				
garlic bread w/cheese	2 slices	35.0	700	45%
meat nachos	1 serving	36.5	500	66%
■ PASTA				
chicken Parmesan	1 serving	19.0	590	29%
fettuccine Alfredo	small	28.0	440	57%
meat lasagna	small	25.0	460	49%
spaghetti	small	10.0	290	31%
■ PIZZA				
deep pan/medium				
cheese	1 slice	13.0	350	33%
combo	1 slice	18.0	410	40%
Pan sausage	1 slice	22.0	430	46%
pepperoni	1 slice	17.0	380	40%
original crust/medium				
cheese	1 slice	8.0	260	28%
combo	1 slice	13.0	320	37%
pepperoni	1 slice	11.0	280	35%
sausage	1 slice	16.0	350	41%
thin crust/medium				
cheese	1 slice	9.0	220	37%
■ SANDWICHES				
BBQ beef & cheddar	1 sandwich	24.0	580	37%
chicken & cheddar	1 sandwich	24.0	570	38%
ham & cheese	1 sandwich	39.0	790	44%
submarine/deluxe	1 sandwich	43.0	810	48%
McDONALD'S				
■ BEVERAGES				
apple juice	6 fl oz	–	80	–
Coca-Cola				
Classic	small	–	150	–
Diet Coke	small	–	–	

Food and Description	Amount	Fat Grams	Total Calories	% Fat Calories
Hi-C orange drink	small	–	160	–
milk/1% low-fat	8 fl oz	2.5	100	23%
orange juice	6 fl oz	–	80	–
shakes				
chocolate	small	9.0	360	23%
strawberry	small	9.0	360	23%
vanilla	small	9.0	360	23%
Sprite	small	–	150	–
■ BREAKFAST				
apple bran muffin/low-fat	1 muffin	3.0	300	9%
bagels				
ham & egg cheese	1 bagel	23.0	550	38%
Spanish omelet	1 bagel	38.0	690	50%
steak & egg cheese	1 bagel	31.0	660	42%
biscuits				
bacon, egg, & cheese	1 biscuit	34.0	540	57%
plain	1 biscuit	15.0	290	47%
sausage	1 biscuit	31.0	470	59%
sausage & egg	1 biscuit	37.0	550	61%
breakfast burrito	1 burrito	20.0	320	56%
cinnamon roll	1 roll	18.0	390	42%
Danish				
apple	1 Danish	15.0	340	40%
cheese	1 Danish	21.0	400	47%
Egg McMuffin	1 McMuffin	12.0	290	37%
English muffin w/spread	1 muffin	2.0	140	13%
hash brown potatoes	1 serving	8.0	130	55%
hotcakes				
plain	1 serving	8.0	340	21%
w/margarine & syrup	1 serving	17.0	600	26%
pork sausage	1 serving	16.0	170	85%
Sausage McMuffin				
regular	1 McMuffin	23.0	360	58%
w/egg	1 McMuffin	28.0	440	57%
scrambled eggs	2 eggs	11.0	160	62%
■ BURGERS				
Big Mac	1 burger	32.0	570	51%
Big Xtra!				
w/cheese	1 burger	55.0	810	61%
w/o cheese	1 burger	46.0	710	58%
cheeseburger	1 burger	13.0	320	37%
hamburger	1 burger	9.0	270	30%
Quarter Pounder				
w/cheese	1 burger	30.0	530	51%
w/o cheese	1 burger	21.0	430	44%
■ CHICKEN & FISH				
Chicken McNuggets & sauce				
McNuggets	4 pieces	11.0	190	52%
	6 pieces	17.0	290	53%
	9 pieces	25.0	430	52%

Food and Description	Amount	Fat Grams	Total Calories	% Fat Calories
sauce				
barbecue	1 pkt	–	45	–
honey	1 pkt	–	45	–
honey mustard	1 pkt	4.5	50	81%
hot mustard	1 pkt	3.5	60	46%
light mayonnaise	1 pkt	4.0	40	90%
sweet & sour	1 pkt	–	50	–
Sandwiches				
chicken				
Crispy	1 sandwich	27.0	500	49%
McChicken sandwich	1 sandwich	30.0	510	53%
McGrilled				
w/mayonnaise	1 sandwich	18.0	450	36%
w/o mayonnaise	1 sandwich	7.0	340	19%
Fillet-O-Fish sandwich	1 sandwich	26.0	470	50%
■ DESSERT				
Apple pie	1 pie	13.0	260	45%
Cookies				
chocolate chip	1 cookie	10.0	170	53%
McDonaldland	1 pkg	5.0	180	25%
Ice cream				
cone/reduced fat	1 cone	4.5	150	27%
sundaes				
hot caramel sundae	1 serving	10.0	360	25%
hot fudge	1 serving	12.0	340	32%
strawberry	1 serving	7.0	290	22%
McFlurry				
Butterfinger	1	22.0	620	32%
M & M	1	23.0	630	33%
Nestle Crunch	1	24.0	630	34%
Nuts for sundaes	1 serving	3.5	40	79%
■ SALADS & RELATED ITEMS				
Bacon bits	1 pkg	1.0	15	60%
Croutons	1 pkg	1.5	50	27%
Salad dressing				
honey mustard	1 pkg	11.0	150	66%
ranch	1 pkg	18.0	170	95%
red French/reduced-calorie	1 pkg	6.0	130	42%
Thousand Island	1 pkg	9.0	130	62%
vinaigrette/fat-free herb	1 pkg	–	30	–
Salads				
chef salad	1 salad	8.0	150	48%
garden salad	1 salad	6.0	100	54%
grilled chicken Caesar	1 salad	2.5	100	23%
side salad	1 serving	2.0	45	40%
■ SIDE ORDERS				
French fries	small	10.0	210	43%
	large	26.0	540	43%
	super size	29.0	610	43%

Food and Description	Amount	Fat Grams	Total Calories	% Fat Calories
NATHAN'S				
■ **BURGERS & SANDWICHES**				
Hamburgers				
double	1 burger	41.0	670	55%
regular	1 burger	23.0	435	48%
super	1 burger	32.0	535	54%
Sandwiches				
cheese steak	1 sandwich	26.0	485	48%
chicken				
broiled/breaded	1 sandwich	25.0	510	44%
charbroiled	1 sandwich	6.0	290	19%
salad	1 sandwich	4.0	154	23%
fillet of fish	1 sandwich	15.0	405	33%
frankfurter	1 hot dog	19.0	310	55%
pastrami	1 sandwich	12.0	325	33%
turkey	1 sandwich	2.0	270	7%
■ **PLATTERS**				
Chicken				
2 pieces	1 platter	66.0	1095	54%
4 pieces	1 platter	109.0	1790	55%
Clam/fried	1 platter	51.0	1025	45%
Fish/fillet of	1 platter	74.0	1455	46%
Shrimp/fried	1 platter	34.0	795	38%
■ **SIDES**				
French fries	1 serving	26.0	515.0	45%
Sauteed onions	1 serving	1.0	40	23%
OLIVE GARDEN				
■ **LUNCH ENTRÉES**				
capellini Pomodora	1 serving	10.0	380	24%
capellini Primavera				
w/chicken	1 serving	13.0	510	23%
w/o chicken	1 serving	7.0	350	18%
chicken Giardino	1 serving	9.0	360	23%
linguine alla Marinara	1 serving	6.0	320	17%
■ **DINNER ENTRÉES**				
capellini Pomodoro	1 serving	16.0	620	23%
capellini primavera				
w/chicken	1 serving	18.0	760	21%
w/o chicken	1 serving	12.0	600	18%
chicken Giardino	1 serving	11.0	550	18%
grilled chicken Capri	1 serving	12.0	555	19%
linguine alla Marinara	1 serving	9.0	530	15%
shrimp primavera	1 serving	12.0	725	15%
■ **OTHER ITEMS**				
apple Caramellina	1 serving	2.0	560	3%
breadstick	1 piece	1.5	140	10%
soup/minestrone	1 serving	1.0	90	10%

Food and Description	Amount	Fat Grams	Total Calories	% Fat Calories
1 POTATO 2 POTATO				
■ **POTATOES**				
Baked potatoes				
bacon				
& cheese	1 potato	47.0	660	64%
double cheeseburger	1 potato	54.0	765	64%
broccoli & cheese	1 potato	36.0	545	59%
Chicken				
BBQ cheddar & bacon	1 potato	43.0	685	56%
broccoli & cheddar/3 cheese	1 potato	37.0	590	56%
Caesar & broccoli				
Gourmet	1 potato	51.0	710	65%
Lite	1 potato	12.0	375	29%
Caribbean fajita	1 potato	1.5	270	5%
Mexican spinach soufflé/Lite	1 potato	9.0	310	26%
mushroom & roasted red peppers	1 potato	2.0	245	7%
stir-fry	1 potato	3.0	328	8%
crab & broccoli				
& cheese/Gourmet	1 potato	35.0	595	53%
DeLite	1 potato	2.5	335	7%
herb roasted vegetable	1 potato	6.0	260	21%
Mexican/Gourmet	1 potato	46.0	670	62%
Philly steak & cheese	1 potato	40.0	675	53%
veggie & herb	1 potato	2.0	243	7%
Country Skillet				
BBQ chicken, cheddar, & bacon	1 serving	57.0	890	58%
bacon, ranch, & cheddar	1 serving	74.0	1090	61%
Idaho Nachos	1 serving	61.0	1010	54%
Fries				
fresh cut	small	39.0	615	57%
	medium	49.0	765	58%
	large	78.0	1225	57%
topped				
nacho cheese	1 serving	54.0	840	58%
'n chicken tenders	1 serving	50.0	920	49%
Potato Skins				
bacon'n cheddar-w/sour cream	1 serving	53.0	975	49%
Southwestern-w/sour cream	1 serving	46.0	910	45%
Soups				
baked potato	1 serving	26.0	640	37%
broccoli & cheese potato	1 serving	29.0	665	39%
PERKINS				
■ **BREAKFAST**				
hash brown potatoes	3 oz serving	2.5	100	23%
muffins				
apple	1 muffin	24.0	543	40%
banana nut	1 muffin	29.0	586	45%
blueberry	1 muffin	23.0	506	41%
bran	1 muffin	17.0	478	32%
carrot	1 muffin	23.0	560	37%

Food and Description	Amount	Fat Grams	Total Calories	% Fat Calories
chocolate chocolate chip	1 muffin	26.0	548	43%
corn	1 muffin	17.0	683	22%
cranberry nut	1 muffin	28.0	558	45%
98% fat-free	1 muffin	1.0	495	2%
oat bran	1 muffin	16.0	513	28%
plain	1 muffin	26.0	586	40%
omelettes				
country club				
omelette only	1 serving	79.0	935	76%
w/hash browns	1 serving	82.0	1033	71%
deli ham & cheese				
omelette only	1 serving	79.0	962	74%
w/hash browns	1 serving	82.0	1063	69%
Denver w/fruit cup	1 serving	6.5	235	25%
Everything				
omelette only	1 serving	53.5	700	69%
w/hash browns	1 serving	56.0	800	63%
Granny's country				
omelette only	1 serving	81.5	940	78%
w/hash browns	1 serving	89.0	1245	64%
ham & cheese				
omelette only	1 serving	51.5	745	62%
w/hash browns	1 serving	54.0	745	65%
mushroom & cheese				
omelette only	1 serving	60.0	690	78%
w/hash browns	1 serving	62.5	788	71%
seafood w/fruit cup	1 serving	5.7	270	19%
pancakes				
buttermilk	3 pancakes	12.0	445	24%
harvest grain w/low-calorie syrup	5 pancakes	3.5	475	7%
short stack	3 pancakes	2.0	270	7%
toast w/margarine & grape jelly	1 piece	12.0	220	49%
■ DESSERT				
apple pie				
regular	1 slice	26.0	520	45%
sweetened w/Equal	1 slice	24.0	420	51%
cherry pie				
regular	1 slice	26.0	570	41%
sweetened w/Equal	1 slice	24.0	425	51%
coconut cream pie	1 slice	33.0	435	68%
French silk pie	1 slice	37.0	550	61%
lemon meringue pie	1 slice	16.0	395	36%
peanut butter brownie pie	1 slice	35.0	455	69%
pecan pie	1 slice	26.0	669	35%
■ SALADS				
chef	1 mini	11.0	215	46%
dinner/lite	1 serving	2.0	105	17%
■ SANDWICH				
vegetable pita stir-fry				
sandwich only	1 serving	9.0	305	27%

Food and Description	Amount	Fat Grams	Total Calories	% Fat Calories
w/coleslaw	1 serving	18.0	440	37%
w/coleslaw & pasta salad	1 serving	32.5	625	47%

PAPA JOHN'S PIZZA
■ PIZZA/Based on 14" pizza
Original crust

Food and Description	Amount	Fat Grams	Total Calories	% Fat Calories
All The Meats	⅛ pizza	19.0	390	44%
cheese	⅛ pizza	9.0	270	30%
garden special	⅛ pizza	10.0	290	31%
pepperoni	⅛ pizza	12.0	305	35%
sausage	⅛ pizza	14.0	335	38%
The Works	⅛ pizza	14.0	345	37%
Thin crust				
All The Meats	⅛ pizza	22.0	345	57%
cheese	⅛ pizza	12.0	225	48%
garden special	⅛ pizza	12.0	240	45%
pepperoni	⅛ pizza	15.0	260	52%
sausage	⅛ pizza	17.0	285	54%
The Works	⅛ pizza	17.0	295	52%

■ SIDE ITEMS

Food and Description	Amount	Fat Grams	Total Calories	% Fat Calories
bread sticks	1 stick	2.0	140	13%
cheese sticks	2 sticks	8.0	180	40%
sauce				
garlic	1 Tbs	8.0	75	96%
nacho cheese	1 Tbs	2.0	30	60%
pizza	1 Tbs	0.5	10	45%

PETER PIPER PIZZA
■ PIZZA
bacon

Food and Description	Amount	Fat Grams	Total Calories	% Fat Calories
Express Lunch Pizza	⅛ pizza	6.5	182	32%
extra large	1/12 pizza	10.7	311	31%
large	⅛ pizza	11.4	331	31%
medium	⅛ pizza	8.6	249	31%
small pie	⅛ pizza	7.6	217	32%
beef				
Express Lunch Pizza	⅛ pizza	5.0	165	27%
extra large	1/12 pizza	7.8	280	25%
large	⅛ pizza	8.0	296	24%
medium	⅛ pizza	6.0	222	24%
small	⅛ pizza	5.4	194	25%
black olive				
Express Lunch Pizza	⅛ pizza	4.4	157	25%
extra large	1/12 pizza	6.8	265	23%
large	⅛ pizza	7.0	279	23%
medium	⅛ pizza	5.0	209	22%
small	⅛ pizza	4.6	182	23%
cheese				
Express Lunch Pizza	⅛ pizza	4.0	152	24%
	1 pizza	15.7	608	23%
extra large	1/12 pizza	6.0	257	21%
	1 pizza	73.0	3,078	21%

Food and Description	Amount	Fat Grams	Total Calories	% Fat Calories
large	⅛ pizza	6.0	270	20%
	1 pizza	49.5	2,160	21%
medium	⅛ pizza	4.6	203	20%
	1 pizza	37.0	1,620	21%
small	⅛ pizza	4.0	177	20%
	1 pizza	24.5	1,059	21%
extra cheddar				
Express Lunch Pizza	⅛ pizza	6.0	180	30%
extra large	1/12 pizza	9.0	290	28%
large	⅛ pizza	9.0	306	26%
medium	⅛ pizza	6.4	224	26%
small	⅛ pizza	5.7	196	26%
extra mozzarella				
Express Lunch Pizza	⅛ pizza	5.5	174	28%
extra large	1/12 pizza	9.0	300	27%
large	⅛ pizza	10.0	320	28%
medium	⅛ pizza	7.0	236	27%
small	⅛ pizza	5.7	198	26%
green pepper				
Express Lunch Pizza	⅛ pizza	4.0	153	24%
extra large	1/12 pizza	6.0	259	21%
large	⅛ pizza	6.0	272	20%
medium	⅛ pizza	4.6	204	20%
small	⅛ pizza	4.0	178	20%
ham				
Express Lunch Pizza	⅛ pizza	4.0	156	23%
extra large pie	1/12 pizza	6.0	261	21%
large pie	⅛ pizza	6.4	276	21%
medium pie	⅛ pizza	4.8	207	21%
small pie	⅛ pizza	4.0	180	20%
jalapeño				
Express Lunch Pizza	⅛ pizza	4.0	153	24%
extra large	1/12 pizza	6.0	259	21%
large	⅛ pizza	6.0	266	20%
medium	⅛ pizza	4.6	205	20%
small	⅛ pizza	4.0	178	20%
mushroom				
Express Lunch Pizza	⅛ pizza	4.0	153	24%
extra large	1/12 pizza	6.0	259	21%
large	⅛ pizza	4.0	181	20%
medium	⅛ pizza	4.7	204	21%
small	⅛ pizza	4.0	178	20%
onion				
Express Lunch Pizza	⅛ pizza	4.0	153	23%
extra large	1/12 pizza	6.0	258	21%
large	⅛ pizza	6.0	271	20%
medium	⅛ pizza	4.6	204	20%
small	⅛ pizza	4.0	177	20%
pepperoni				
Express Lunch Pizza	⅛ pizza	5.5	168	29%

Food and Description	Amount	Fat Grams	Total Calories	% Fat Calories
extra large	¹⁄₁₂ pizza	8.8	284	28%
large	⅛ pizza	9.0	308	26%
medium	⅛ pizza	7.0	229	28%
small	⅛ pizza	6.0	198	27%
pineapple				
Express Lunch Pizza	⅛ pizza	4.0	154	23%
extra large	¹⁄₁₂ pizza	6.0	260	21%
large	⅛ pizza	6.0	274	20%
medium	⅛ pizza	4.7	206	21%
small	⅛ pizza	4.0	179	20%
salami				
Express Lunch Pizza	⅛ pizza	5.0	164	27%
extra large	¹⁄₁₂ pizza	7.5	273	25%
large	⅛ pizza	7.8	288	24%
medium	⅛ pizza	6.0	216	25%
small	⅛ pizza	5.0	189	24%
sausage				
Express Lunch Pizza	⅛ pizza	5.8	178	29%
extra large	¹⁄₁₂ pizza	8.0	284	25%
large	⅛ pizza	8.4	300	25%
medium	⅛ pizza	6.0	224	24%
small	⅛ pizza	5.6	197	26%
tomato				
Express Lunch Pizza	⅛ pizza	4.0	153	24%
extra large	¹⁄₁₂ pizza	6.0	257	21%
large	⅛ pizza	6.0	275	20%
medium	⅛ pizza	4.7	204	21%
small	⅛ pizza	4.0	177	20%

PICCADILLY CAFETERIA
■ BREADS

Food and Description	Amount	Fat Grams	Total Calories	% Fat Calories
corn				
Mexican corn bread	1 piece	14.0	220	57%
sticks	1 stick	10.0	165	55%
French	1 slice	2.0	132	14%
roll				
white	1 roll	2.0	130	14%
whole wheat	1 roll	1.0	117	8%

■ MAIN MENU ITEMS

Food and Description	Amount	Fat Grams	Total Calories	% Fat Calories
au Jus	1 serving	–	5	–
beans				
baby lima	1 serving	6.0	150	36%
green	1 serving	6.0	75	72%
beef				
chopped steak/fried	4 oz serving	23.0	310	67%
liver/fried	4.5 oz serving	29.0	430	61%
roast/leg	4 oz serving	18.0	310	52%
tips/braised	10 oz serving	26.0	470	50%
black-eyed peas w/pork jowls	1 serving	6.0	110	49%

Food and Description	Amount	Fat Grams	Total Calories	% Fat Calories
broccoli				
& rice au gratin	1 serving	9.0	185	44%
w/butter	1 serving	6.0	80	68%
carrots/baby w/butter	½ cup	6.0	90	60%
cauliflower w/butter	1 serving	6.0	80	68%
chicken				
baked w/o skin	¼ chicken	11.0	350	28%
teriyaki	1 seving	22.0	445	44%
teriyaki Polynesian	1 serving	27.0	535	45%
corn	1 serving	7.0	130	48%
cornbread stuffing	1 serving	9.0	165	49%
cranberry sauce	1 serving	–	65	–
eggplant/escalloped	½ cup	10.0	180	50%
fish/baked	7 oz serving	10.0	195	46%
ham/baked	1 serving	10.0	225	40%
macaroni & cheese	½ cup	11.0	320	31%
okra/smothered	1 serving	10.0	120	75%
Potatoes				
baked				
plain	1 potato	–	220	–
w/topping	1 potato	15.0	350	39%
new/boiled	½ cup	12.0	150	72%
rice/Polynesian	1 serving	6.0	140	39%
spaghetti				
baked	1 serving	10.0	255	35%
w/meatballs/baked	1 serving	5.0	110	41%
squash				
baked Italian	1 serving	3.0	75	36%
mixed yellow & zucchini	1 serving	5.0	70	64%
yellow/baked French style	1 serving	5.0	85	53%
turkey breast	3 oz serving	2.0	100	18%
■ SALADS				
broccoli salad	1 serving	20.0	200	90%
cabbage combination salad	1 serving	–	50	–
carrot & raisin salad	1 serving	23.0	320	65%
cole slaw w/cream	1 serving	18.0	185	88%
cucumber & celery salad	1 serving	6.0	85	64%
fruit salad	1 serving	1.0	60	15%
Neptune salad	1 serving	34.0	360	85%
spinach tossed salad	1 serving	6.0	90	60%
spring salad	1 bowl	–	25	–
■ SOUPS				
gumbo				
chicken	1 serving	4.0	130	29%
seafood	1 serving	2.0	100	18%
vegetable	1 serving	–	50	–
■ SWEETS				
Pies				
apple	1 slice	19.0	439	39%
chocolate cream	1 slice	25.0	512	44%

Food and Description	Amount	Fat Grams	Total Calories	% Fat Calories
custard	1 slice	18.0	412	39%
lemon chiffon	1 slice	20.0	481	37%
Cake/pound	1 slice	17.0	371	41%
Fruit				
cantaloupe	1 serving	1.0	90	10%
fresh fruit plate	1 serving	5.0	390	12%
honeydew melon	5.5 oz	–	55	–
	9 oz	–	90	–
watermelon	1 serving	1.0	100	9%
Gelatin	1 serving	4.0	130	28%
PIZZA HUT				
■ APPETIZERS				
Bread stick	1 serving	4.0	130	28%
Bread stick dipping sauce	1 serving	0.5	30	15%
Buffalo Wings				
hot	4 pieces	12.0	210	51%
mild	5 pieces	12.0	200	54%
Garlic bread	1 piece	8.0	150	48%
■ DESSERT				
apple dessert pizza	1 slice	4.5	250	16%
cherry dessert pizza	1 slice	4.5	250	16%
■ PASTA				
Cavatini				
pasta	1 serving	14.0	480	26%
Supreme pasta	1 serving	19.0	560	31%
Spaghetti				
w/marinara	1 serving	6.0	490	11%
w/meat sauce	1 serving	13.0	600	20%
w/meatballs	1 serving	24.0	850	25%
■ PIZZA				
Big New Yorker				
cheese	1 slice	16.6	393	38%
pepperoni	1 slice	16.0	380	38%
supreme	1 slice	22.3	459	44%
Hand-tossed/medium pizza				
beef	1 slice	12.0	347	31%
beef taco	1 slice	8.0	270	27%
cheese	1 slice	9.0	309	26%
chicken supreme	1 slice	6.0	291	19%
chicken taco	1 slice	11.0	290	34%
ham	1 slice	6.0	279	19%
Italian sausage	1 slice	14.0	363	35%
Meat Lover's	1 slice	15.0	376	36%
meatless taco	1 slice	8.0	250	29%
pepperoni	1 slice	8.0	301	24%
Pepperoni Lover's	1 slice	14.0	372	34%
pork topping	1 slice	12.0	342	32%
supreme	1 slice	11.0	333	30%
super supreme chicken	1 slice	12.0	359	30%
taco	1 slice	11.0	280	35%

Food and Description	Amount	Fat Grams	Total Calories	% Fat Calories
Veggie Lover's	1 slice	6.0	281	19%
Pan/medium pizza				
beef	1 slice	18.0	399	41%
beef taco	1 slice	12.0	300	36%
cheese	1 slice	15.0	361	37%
chicken supreme	1 slice	12.0	343	31%
chicken taco	1 slice	15.0	320	42%
ham	1 slice	12.0	331	33%
Italian sausage	1 slice	20.0	415	43%
Meat Lover's	1 slice	21.0	428	44%
meatless taco	1 slice	12.0	290	37%
pepperoni	1 slice	14.0	353	36%
Pepperoni Lover's	1 slice	16.0	370	39%
pork topping	1 slice	18.0	394	41%
super supreme	1 slice	18.0	401	40%
supreme	1 slice	17.0	385	40%
taco	1 slice	13.0	310	38%
Veggie Lover's	1 slice	12.0	333	32%
Personal Pan				
cheese	1 pizza	27.0	813	30%
pepperoni	1 pizza	28.0	810	31%
supreme	1 pizza	27.0	808	30%
taco	1 pizza	35.0	780	40%
Sicilian/medium pizza				
beef	1 slice	12.0	282	38%
cheese	1 slice	13.0	295	40%
chicken supreme	1 slice	10.0	269	33%
ham	1 slice	10.0	257	35%
Italian sausage	1 slice	18.0	333	49%
Meat Lover's	1 slice	18.0	344	47%
pepperoni	1 slice	13.0	227	52%
Pepperoni Lover's	1 slice	16.0	321	45%
pork topping	1 slice	16.0	314	46%
super supreme	1 slice	16.0	323	45%
supreme	1 slice	15.0	307	44%
Veggies Lover's	1 slice	10.0	252	36%
Stuffed Crust/ham/medium pizza				
beef	1 slice	22.0	466	42%
cheese	1 slice	19.0	445	38%
chicken supreme	1 slice	17.0	432	36%
ham	1 slice	22.0	404	49%
Italian sausage	1 slice	23.0	478	43%
Meat Lover's	1 slice	29.0	543	48%
pepperoni	1 slice	19.0	438	39%
Pepperoni Lover's	1 slice	26.0	525	45%
pork topping	1 slice	21.0	461	41%
super supreme	1 slice	25.0	505	45%
supreme	1 slice	23.0	487	43%
Veggie Lover's	1 slice	17.0	421	36%

Food and Description	Amount	Fat Grams	Total Calories	% Fat Calories
The Edge/medium pizza				
chicken veggie	1 slice	3.0	120	23%
meaty	1 slice	7.0	150	42%
taco	1 slice	6.0	140	39%
The Works	1 slice	5.0	140	32%
Veggie	1 slice	2.5	110	20%
Thin 'N Crispy/medium pizza				
beef	1 slice	15.0	305	44%
beef taco	1 slice	10.0	260	35%
cheese	1 slice	10.0	243	37%
chicken supreme	1 slice	7.0	232	27%
chicken taco	1 slice	12.0	260	42%
ham	1 slice	7.0	212	30%
Italian sausage	1 slice	18.0	325	50%
Meat Lover's	1 slice	19.0	339	50%
Meatless Taco	1 slice	8.0	230	31%
pepperoni	1 slice	10.0	235	38%
Pepperoni Lover's	1 slice	14.0	289	44%
pork topping	1 slice	15.0	298	45%
super supreme	1 slice	15.0	304	44%
supreme	1 slice	13.0	284	41%
taco	1 slice	11.0	260	31%
Veggie Lover's	1 slice	8.0	222	32%
■ SANDWICHES				
ham & cheese	1 sandwich	21.0	550	34%
supreme	1 sandwich	28.0	640	39%
PONDEROSA				
■ CONDIMENTS				
BBQ sauce	1 Tbs	–	25	–
cheese				
sauce	4 Tbs	2.0	52	35%
spread	1 oz	6.7	98	62%
cocktail sauce	2 Tbs	1.0	34	26%
coconut/shredded	½ oz	5.0	62	73%
gravy				
brown	4 Tbs	1.0	25	36%
turkey	4 Tbs	–	25	–
margarine				
liquid	1 Tbs	11.0	100	100%
whipped	1 Tbs	7.0	70	90%
salad dressings				
blue cheese	2 Tbs	13.0	130	90%
cole slaw	2 Tbs	14.0	150	84%
cucumber/reduced-calorie	2 Tbs	6.0	70	77%
Italian				
creamy	2 Tbs	10.0	105	86%
reduced-calorie	2 Tbs	3.0	30	90%
Parmesan pepper	2 Tbs	15.0	150	90%
ranch	2 Tbs	15.0	150	90%
salad oil	1 Tbs	14.0	120	100%

Food and Description	Amount	Fat Grams	Total Calories	% Fat Calories
sweet-'N-Tangy	2 Tbs	9.0	120	68%
thousand island	2 Tbs	10.0	115	78%
sour cream	1 Tbs	2.5	26	87%
spaghetti sauce	4 oz	4.0	110	33%
sweet & sour sauce	1 oz	<1.0	37	12%
tartar sauce	1 oz	10.5	95	100%
■ **DESSERT**				
banana pudding	1 oz	2.4	52	42%
ice milk				
chocolate	3.5 oz	2.9	152	17%
vanilla	3.5 oz	2.6	150	16%
mousse				
chocolate	1 oz	4.4	78	51%
strawberry	1 oz	4.6	74	50%
strawberry glaze	1 oz	–	37	–
topping				
caramel	1 oz	–	100	–
chocolate	1 oz	–	89	–
strawberry	1 oz	–	71	–
whipped	1 oz	6.4	80	72%
■ **ENTRÉES**/Chicken, Meat, & Fish				
chicken				
breast	1 serving	2.0	98	19%
wings	2 pieces	9.0	213	38%
fish				
baked/Bake 'n Broil	1 serving	13.0	230	51%
fried	1 serving	9.0	190	43%
fish nuggets	1 piece	1.7	31.0	49%
halibut/broiled	1 serving	2.4	170	13%
hot dog	1 hot dog	13.0	144	81%
roughy/broiled	1 serving	4.8	138	31%
salmon/broiled	1 serving	2.7	192	13%
scrod/baked	1 serving	1.0	120	8%
shrimp				
fried	7 pieces	0.5	231	2%
mini	6 pieces	1.7	47	33%
sirloin tips/precooked	5 oz	8.2	473	16%
steak				
chopped/precooked	4 oz	16.2	225	65%
	5.3 oz	21.5	296	65%
Kansas city strip/precooked	5 oz	5.7	138	37%
New York strip/pre-cooked	8 oz	10.5	314	30%
	10 oz	14.5	384	34%
porterhouse/precooked	16 oz	30.9	640	43%
rib-eye/precooked	5 oz	12.8	219	53%
	6 oz	14.2	282	45%
sirloin/precooked	7 oz	10.8	241	40%
T-bone/precooked	8 oz	8.5	178	43%
	10 oz	18.4	444	37%
teriyaki/precooked	5 oz	3.0	174	16%

Food and Description	Amount	Fat Grams	Total Calories	% Fat Calories
steak kabobs/precooked/meat only	3 oz	4.8	153	28%
steak sandwich	1 sandwich	11.0	408	24%
swordfish/broiled	1 serving	9.4	271	31%
trout/broiled	1 serving	3.9	228	15%
■ SALAD BAR ITEMS				
apple				
fresh	1 medium	1.0	80	11%
canned	4 oz	–	90	–
apple ring/spiced	4 oz	–	100	–
applesauce	4 oz	–	80	–
banana	1 medium	<1.0	87	2%
banana. chips	2 oz	1.3	25	47%
beets/diced	4 oz	<1.0	55	7%
breadstick				
Italian	1 piece	1.0	100	9%
sesame	2 pieces	–	35	–
broccoli	1 oz	<1.0	9	90%
cabbage				
green	1 oz	–	9	–
red	1 oz	–	1	–
cantaloupe	1 wedge	–	13	–
celery	1 oz	–	4	–
cheese/imitation/shredded	1 oz	7.0	90	70%
cherry peppers	2 pieces	<1.0	7	26%
chicken salad	3.5 oz	15.4	213	65%
chow mein noodles	0.2 oz	1.2	25	43%
coconut/shredded	0.2 oz	1.9	25	68%
cottage cheese	4 oz	5.0	120	38%
crackers/melba snacks	2 pieces	–	18	–
croutons	1 oz	3.7	115	29%
cucumber	1 oz	–	4	–
eggs/hard-cooked/diced	2 oz	6.6	94	63%
fruit cocktail	4 oz	<1.0	97	2%
garbanzo beans	1 oz	–	102	–
gelatin/plain	4 oz	–	71	–
granola	0.2 oz	1.0	24	38%
grapes	10 pieces	<1.0	34	5%
ham/diced	2 oz	10.0	120	75%
honeydew melon	1 wedge	<1.0	25	7%
lettuce	1 oz	–	5	–
macaroni salad	3.5 oz	11.7	335	31%
mushrooms	1 oz	–	8	–
olives				
black	1 olive	<1.0	4	90%
green	1 olive	<1.0	3	90%
onion/red or yellow	1 oz	–	11	–
orange	1 piece	–	45	–
pasta salad/premade	3.5 oz	11.7	269	39%
peaches/canned	4 oz	–	70	–

Food and Description	Amount	Fat Grams	Total Calories	% Fat Calories
peanuts/granulated	0.2 oz	2.3	30	69%
pears/canned	4 oz	<1.0	98	5%
pepper/green	1 oz	–	6	–
pickles				
dill spears	0.14 oz	–	<1	–
sweet chips	0.14 oz	–	4	–
pineapple				
canned/tidbits	4 oz	<1.0	95	2%
fresh/wedges	1 wedge	–	11	–
potato salad	3.5 oz	5.9	126	42%
radish	1 oz	–	4	–
scallion	1 piece	–	7	–
spinach	1 oz	–	7	–
sprouts				
alfalfa	1 oz	–	10	–
bean	1 oz	–	10	–
strawberries	2 oz	<1.0	14	13%
sunflower seeds	0.2 oz	2.8	32	79%
tomato	1 oz	–	6	–
turkey/julienne	1 oz	<11.0	29	19%
turkey-ham salad	3.5 oz	12.8	186	62%
watermelon	1 wedge	<1.0	1ll	7%
yogurt				
fruit	4 oz	1.0	115	8%
vanilla	4 oz	2.0	110	16%
■ SIDE DISHES (*See also* Salad Bar Items in this section)				
baked beans	4 oz	6.0	170	32%
baked potato	1 serving	<1.0	145	3%
carrots	3.5 oz	–	31	–
cauliflower/breaded	4 oz	1.0	115	8%
corn	3.5 oz	<1.0	90	5%
green beans	3.5 oz	–	20	–
macaroni & cheese	1 oz	<1.0	17	26%
mashed potatoes	1 serving	<1.0	62	3%
okra/breaded	4 oz	1.0	124	71%
onion rings/breaded	4 oz	8.8	213	37%
pasta shells	2 oz	<1.0	78	39%
peas	3.5 oz	<1.0	67	4%
potato wedges	1 serving	6.0	130	42%
rice pilaf	1 serving	4.0	160	34%
roll				
dinner	1 roll	3.4	184	17%
sourdough	1 roll	1.0	110	8%
spaghetti				
plain	1 serving	–	80	–
w/sauce	1 serving	4.0	190	19%
stuffing	4 oz	11.0	230	43%
tortilla chips	1 oz	8.0	150	48%
winter mix	3.5 oz	–	25	–
zucchini/breaded	4 oz	<1.0	102	6%

Food and Description	Amount	Fat Grams	Total Calories	% Fat Calories
POPEYE'S CHICKEN & BISCUITS				
■ **CHICKEN & SHRIMP**				
chicken				
mild				
breast	1 serving	30.0	515	52%
leg	1 serving	12.0	200	54%
thigh	1 serving	27.0	386	63%
wing	1 serving	14.0	218	58%
spicy				
breast	1 serving	31.0	529	53%
leg	1 serving	11.0	190	52%
thigh	1 serving	29.0	392	67%
wing	1 serving	15.0	216	63%
■ **DESSERT**				
cinnamon apple pie	1 slice	10.0	250	36%
■ **SIDE ORDERS**				
biscuit	1 biscuit	12.0	227	48%
Cajun rice	1 serving	7.0	181	35%
coleslaw	1 serving	7.0	181	35%
corn on the cob	1 piece	4.0	255	14%
French fries	1 serving	18.0	380	43%
onion rings	1 serving	20.0	379	47%
potatoes/mashed				
w/gravy	1 serving	4.0	121	30%
w/o gravy	1 serving	2.0	96	19%
red beans & rice	1 serving	19.0	338	51%
QUINCY'S				
■ **BREAKFAST**				
bacon	1 serving	3.0	35	77%
corned beef hash	1 serving	15.0	210	64%
country ham	1 serving	6.0	90	60%
escalloped apples	1 serving	2.0	120	15%
oatmeal	1 serving	2.0	175	10%
pancakes	1 serving	3.0	95	28%
sausage gravy	1 serving	6.0	70	77%
sausage links	1 serving	22.0	225	88%
scrambled eggs	1 serving	7.0	95	66%
steak fingers	1 serving	25.0	360	63%
syrup	1 oz	–	75	–
■ **CONDIMENTS**				
margarine	2 Tbs	22.0	200	100%
salad dressing				
blue cheese	1 oz	16.0	155	93%
French				
light	1 oz	4.0	85	42%
regular	1 oz	12.0	125	86%
honey mustard	1 oz	6.0	100	54%
Italian				
creamy/light	1 oz	4.0	65	55%
light	1 oz	2.0	20	90%
regular	1 oz	14.0	135	93%

Food and Description	Amount	Fat Grams	Total Calories	% Fat Calories
Parmesan peppercorn	1 oz	14.0	150	84%
ranch	1 oz	11.0	110	90%
Thousand Island/light	1 oz	4.0	65	55%
■ DESSERT				
banana pudding	1 serving	12.0	240	45%
brownie pudding cake	1 serving	5.0	310	15%
cobbler				
apple	1 serving	8.0	255	28%
cherry	1 serving	8.0	410	18%
peach	1 serving	8.0	305	24%
cookie				
chocolate chip	1 cookie	5.0	60	75%
sugar	1 cookie	3.0	60	45%
topping				
hot caramel	1 oz	1.0	105	9%
hot fudge	1 oz	4.0	105	34%
pineapple	1 oz	–	70	–
yogurt/frozen	1 serving	2.0	135	13%
■ ENTRÉES				
beef stir-fry	16 oz	77.0	950	73%
chicken				
grilled	regular	2.0	125	14%
	large	3.0	250	11%
homestyle/fillet	6 oz	24.0	410	53%
stir-fry	15.75 oz	66.0	780	76%
chopped beef steak	5.75 oz	34.0	470	65%
fillet of beef	5.5 oz	12.0	330	33%
hamburger/quarter pound	1 burger	20.0	410	44%
prime rib	8 oz	46.0	570	73%
	16 oz	93.0	1145	73%
sirloin tips	4 oz	9.0	240	34%
steak				
country style	5 oz	29.0	380	69%
rib-eye	7.25 oz	60.0	670	81%
	9.5 oz	78.0	870	81%
sirloin	petite	37.0	450	74%
	regular	54.0	650	75%
	large	70.0	850	74%
sizzlin strip	9.5 oz	37.0	595	56%
T-bone	14 oz	84.0	1,190	64%
trout/grilled	6 oz	12.0	300	36%
■ SANDWICHES				
country style steak sandwich	1 sandwich	29.0	520	50%
grilled chicken sandwich	1 sandwich	5.0	305	15%
■ SIDE ORDERS				
baked potato/w/o butter	1 serving	–	370	–
black-eyed peas	4 oz	1.0	75	12%
broccoli				
plain	10 oz	1.0	110	8%
w/cheese sauce	12 oz	13.0	250	47%
broccoli & rice casserole	4 oz	5.0	100	45%

Food and Description	Amount	Fat Grams	Total Calories	% Fat Calories
cabbage/steamed	4 oz	4.0	85	42%
carrots/steamed	4 oz	4.0	85	42%
corn				
on the cob	1 piece	1.0	140	6%
whole kernel	4 oz	6.0	110	49%
cornbread	1 piece	5.0	140	32%
green beans	1 serving	1.0	25	36%
hashrounds	1 serving	14.0	230	54%
macaroni & cheese	4 oz	9.0	165	49%
mashed potatoes	4 oz	<1.0	70	6%
mushrooms	1 serving	12.0	115	94%
new potatoes	4 oz	11.0	190	52%
pinto beans	4 oz	–	70	–
refried beans	4 oz	7.0	140	45%
rice pilaf	3.5 oz	2.0	105	17%
squash	4 oz	10.0	110	82%
turnip greens	4 oz	6.0	75	72%
vegetable medley	4 oz	<1.0	35	13%
yams/candied	4 oz	10.0	250	36%
■ SOUP				
chili w/beans	1 serving	11.0	235	42%
clam chowder	1 serving	9.0	180	45%
cream of broccoli	1 serving	10.0	170	53%
vegetable beef	1 serving	2.0	90	20%
RALLY'S				
■ BEVERAGES				
Coca-Cola				
Diet Coke	16 fl oz	–	–	–
	32 fl oz	–	–	–
regular	16 fl oz	–	120	–
	32 fl oz	–	215	–
Dr. Pepper	16 fl oz	–	120	–
	32 fl oz	–	215	–
Fanta				
orange	16 fl oz	–	145	–
	32 fl oz	–	265	–
root beer	16 fl oz	–	130	–
	32 fl oz	–	235	–
iced tea	16 fl oz	–	–	–
	32 fl oz	–	5	–
Ramblin' Root Beer	16 fl oz	–	145	–
	32 fl oz	–	265	–
Shakes				
banana	1 shake	11.0	400	25%
chocolate	1 shake	12.0	410	26%
strawberry	1 shake	11.0	400	25%
vanilla	1 shake	11.0	320	31%
Sprite	16 fl oz	–	120	–
■ BURGERS & SANDWICHES				
Burgers				
Big Buford	1 burger	46.0	745	56%

Food and Description	Amount	Fat Grams	Total Calories	% Fat Calories
cheeseburger				
bacon	2 burgers	40.3	622	58%
super double	1 burger	48.0	762	57%
Rallyburger				
regular	1 burger	22.0	435	46%
w/cheese	1 burger	29.4	485	55%
Sandwiches				
chicken/spicy	1 sandwich	18.0	435	37%
super barbecue bacon	1 sandwich	31.0	595	47%
■ SIDES				
Chili				
w/cheese & onions	7 oz serving	22.0	360	55%
	13 oz serving	41.0	670	55%
French fries	regular	11.0	211	47%
	large	16.0	317	45%
	extra large	21.0	423	45%
RAX				
■ CHOCOLATE SHAKE	11 oz	12.0	445	24%
■ SALADS & DRESSING				
Salad dressings				
blue cheese	2 Tbs	16.0	145	99%
buttermilk ranch	2 Tbs	20.0	175	100%
Catalina/fat-free	2 Tbs	–	50	–
creamy Caesar	2 Tbs	15.0	140	96%
honey French	2 Tbs	5.0	140	32%
Italian/fat-free	2 Tbs	–	15	–
ranch/fat-free	2 Tbs	–	60	–
thousand island	2 Tbs	13.0	130	90%
vinaigrette	2 Tbs	4.0	70	51%
Salads				
Caesar side salad	1 serving	2.0	40	45%
gourmet garden salad	1 serving	9.0	220	37%
grilled chicken Caesar salad	1 serving	5.0	160	28%
side salad	1 serving	4.0	40	90%
■ SANDWICHES				
barbecue beef				
hold the mayo & oil	1 sandwich	10.0	315	29%
regular	1 sandwich	19.5	400	44%
BBQ (beef, bacon, & cheddar)	1 sandwich	51.0	720	64%
cheddar melt				
hold the mayo & oil	1 sandwich	15.6	283	50%
regular	1 sandwich	22.6	346	59%
Deluxe roast beef				
hold the mayo & oil	1 sandwich	13.0	325	36%
regular	1 sandwich	34.6	521	60%
grilled chicken breast				
hold the mayo & oil	1 sandwich	7.0	285	22%
regular	1 sandwich	33.5	526	57%
Jr. deluxe				
hold the mayo & oil	1 sandwich	8.0	215	33%

Food and Description	Amount	Fat Grams	Total Calories	% Fat Calories
regular	1 sandwich	25.0	370	61%
mushroom melt	1 sandwich	37.5	600	56%
Philly, melt	1 sandwich	32.0	540	53%
regular Rax				
hold the mayo & oil	1 sandwich	13.0	305	38%
regular	1 sandwich	22.0	390	51%
turkey				
hold the mayo & oil	1 sandwich	4.0	230	16%
regular	1 sandwich	32.0	485	59%
turkey-bacon club	1 sandwich	46.5	680	62%
■ SIDE ORDERS				
baked potato				
cheese	1 potato	6.0	270	20%
cheese & bacon	1 potato	18.5	336	50%
cheese & broccoli	1 potato	6.0	281	19%
plain	1 potato	–	207	–
w/butter	1 potato	11.3	306	33%
w/sour topping	1 potato	4.0	257	14%
■ SOUP				
chicken noodle	1 serving	1.0	115	8%
chili	1 serving	11.0	235	42%
cream of broccoli	1 serving	10.0	170	53%
RED LOBSTER				
■ APPETIZERS				
Lighthouse selections				
shrimp cocktail				
regular	3 oz	0.5	80	6%
colossal	5.9 oz	1.5	140	10%
regular				
calamari	1 serving	22.0	350	57%
chicken fingers	1 serving	18.0	390	42%
crab add-on	1 serving	1.0	60	15%
crab & shrimp cakes	1 serving	24.0	480	45%
lobster quesadilla	1 serving	47.0	760	56%
mozzarella cheesesticks	1 serving	46.0	730	57%
mushrooms				
fresh/fried	1 serving	51.0	790	58%
lobster-stuffed	1 serving	26.0	400	59%
stuffed	1 serving	27.0	420	58%
Parmesan zucchini	1 serving	40.0	620	58%
shrimp				
chilled/in the shell	6 oz	1.5	110	12%
cocktail/shelled	6 pieces	0.5	50	9%
■ ENTRÉES				
Lighthouse selections				
chicken breast				
garlic herb-seared	13.2 oz	10.0	500	18%
honey BBQ	13.4 oz	11.0	510	19%
spicy grilled	13.2 oz	10.0	500	18%
chicken salad/grilled/	20.3 oz	7.0	270	23%

Food and Description	Amount	Fat Grams	Total Calories	% Fat Calories
w/fat-free ranch dressing				
cod/baked cod	14.2 oz	10.0	450	20%
haddock/baked	14.2 oz	11.0	460	22%
king crab legs	9 oz	3.5	200	16%
mahi mahi/lemon-pepper grilled	14.2 oz	10.0	460	20%
Maine lobster/live	9.2 oz	1.5	190	7%
rock lobster tail/broiled	8 oz	6.0	200	27%
shrimp & scallops/seared	18.6 oz	13.0	610	19%
snow or Dungeness crab legs	7 oz	2.0	140	13%
regular				
Admiral's Feast	1 serving	52.0	1,060	44%
Atlantic cod/haddock/baked	1 serving	6.0	220	25%
broiled fisherman's platter	1 serving	23.0	600	35%
broiled seafarer's platter	1 serving	19.0	450	38%
catfish Santa Fe	1 serving	9.0	340	24%
chicken				
breast				
grilled	1 serving	7.0	230	26%
teriyaki grilled	1 serving	7.0	240	26%
fresco	1 serving	73.0	1,320	50%
smothered	1 serving	31.0	530	53%
chicken salad/grilled/fat-free				
ranch dressing/lunch entrée	20.3 oz	7.0	270	23%
clam strips	1 serving	39.0	720	49%
crab Alfredo	1 serving	66.0	1,170	51%
fish & shrimp combo	1 serving	35.0	730	43%
flounder fillet/baked/lunch entrée	11.6 oz	6.0	350	15%
lobster, shrimp, & scallop scampi	1 serving	33.0	870	34%
mahi mahi/lemon-pepper grilled	1 serving	7.0	240	26%
Maine lobster/live				
steamed	1 serving	1.0	160	6%
stuffed	1 serving	10.0	430	21%
Neptune's Feast	1 serving	62.0	1,210	46%
New York strip steak	1 order	34.0	560	55%
New York strip steak & fried shrimp	1 order	46.0	780	53%
New York strip steak & rock lobster tail	1 order	31.0	570	49%
rock lobster tail/broiled	1 tail	6.0	190	28%
shrimp				
carbonara	1 serving	76.0	1,290	53%
large/fried	1 serving	27.0	500	49%
Milano	1 serving	65.0	1,190	49%
popcorn	1 serving	37.0	580	57%
shrimp & chicken	1 serving	15.0	340	40%
shrimp combo	1 serving	23.0	380	54%
shrimp feast	1 serving	24.0	470	46%
snow crab legs	1 serving	2.0	110	16%
■ SOUP				
bayou style seafood gumbo	6 oz	4.0	120	30%
broccoli cheese soup	1 serving	9.0	160	51%
clam chowder	6 oz	5.0	130	35%

Food and Description	Amount	Fat Grams	Total Calories	% Fat Calories
ROUND TABLE PIZZA				
■ **14" PIZZA**				
Big Vinnie				
Aloha	1 slice	14.0	430	29%
regular	1 slice	19.0	460	37%
Pan Crust				
Bacon Super Deli	1 slice	13.5	260	47%
cheese	1 slice	7.2	210	31%
chicken garlic gourmet	1 slice	8.0	230	31%
classic pesto	1 slice	8.8	230	34%
garden pesto	1 slice	8.6	230	34%
Gourmet Veggie	1 slice	7.4	220	30%
Guinevere's Garden Delight	1 slice	6.2	200	28%
Italian garlic	1 slice	10.5	250	38%
King Arthur's Supreme	1 slice	9.8	240	37%
Maui Zaui	1 slice	10.0	310	29%
pepperoni	1 slice	8.0	220	33%
Salute chicken & garlic	1 slice	5.8	200	26%
Salute veggie	1 slice	5.0	190	24%
Western BBBQ Chicken Supreme	1 slice	6.5	220	27%
Thin Crust				
Bacon Super Deli	1 slice	12.6	200	57%
cheese	1 slice	6.2	160	35%
chicken garlic gourmet	1 slice	7.0	170	37%
classic pesto	1 slice	7.9	170	42%
garden pesto	1 slice	7.7	170	41%
Gourmet Veggie	1 slice	6.5	160	37%
Guinevere's Garden Delight	1 slice	5.6	150	34%
Italian garlic	1 slice	10.4	200	47%
King Arthur's Supreme	1 slice	10.0	200	45%
Maui Zaui	1 slice	6.5	170	34%
pepperoni	1 slice	8.0	170	42%
Salute chicken & garlic	1 slice	5.4	150	32%
Salute veggie	1 slice	4.7	140	30%
Western BBQ Chicken Supreme	1 slice	5.6	170	30%
■ **SANDWICHES, ETC.**				
chicken club	1 sandwich	38.0	800	43%
ham & honey mustard	1 sandwich	33.0	760	39%
garden vegetable	1 sandwich	29.0	670	39%
garlic Parmesan twists	3 twists	15.0	430	31%
turkey pesto	1 sandwich	40.0	830	43%
turkey Santa Fe	1 sandwich	44.0	840	47%
ROY ROGERS				
■ **BREAKFAST ITEMS**				
bagel				
cinnamon raisin	1 bagel	1.0	300	3%
plain	1 bagel	2.0	300	6%
big country breakfast platter				
w/bacon	1 serving	43.0	740	52%

Food and Description	Amount	Fat Grams	Total Calories	% Fat Calories
w/ham	1 serving	39.0	710	49%
w/sausage	1 serving	60.0	920	59%
biscuit				
bacon	1 biscuit	23.0	420	49%
bacon & egg	1 biscuit	26.0	470	50%
cinnamon 'n raisin	1 biscuit	18.0	370	44%
ham & cheese	1 biscuit	24.0	450	48%
ham & egg	1 biscuit	23.0	460	45%
ham, egg, & cheese	1 biscuit	27.0	500	49%
plain	1 biscuit	21.0	390	48%
hashrounds	1 serving	14.0	230	55%
orange juice	11 fl oz	–	140	–
pancakes				
pancakes only	3 pancakes	2.0	280	6%
w/bacon	1 serving	9.0	350	23%
w/sausage	1 serving	16.0	430	33%
sourdough ham, egg, & cheese				
plain	1 serving	21.0	390	48%
regular	1 serving	24.0	480	45%
sausage	1 serving	31.0	510	55%
sausage & egg	1 serving	35.0	560	56%
■ **BURGERS & BEEF**				
cheeseburger				
bacon	1 burger	28.0	490	51%
¼ pound	1 burger	22.0	470	42%
regular	1 burger	13.0	300	39%
sourdough bacon	1 burger	46.0	730	57%
hamburger				
¼ pound	1 burger	18.0	430	38%
regular	1 burger	9.0	260	31%
roast beef sandwich	1 sandwich	4.0	260	14%
■ **CHICKEN & FISH**				
chicken fillet sandwich	1 sandwich	24.0	500	43%
chicken nuggets	6 pieces	18.0	290	56%
	9 pieces	29.0	460	57%
fisherman's fillet	1 sandwich	21.0	490	39%
fried chicken				
breast	1 piece	15.0	370	36%
leg	1 piece	7.0	170	37%
thigh	1 piece	15.0	330	41%
wing	1 piece	8.0	200	36%
grilled chicken sandwich	1 sandwich	11.0	340	29%
Roy's Roaster/ ¼ chicken				
dark meat				
skinless	1 serving	10.0	190	47%
w/skin	1 serving	34.0	490	62%
white meat				
skinless	1 serving	6.0	190	28%
w/skin	1 serving	29.0	500	52%
sourdough grilled chicken sandwich	1 sandwich	21.0	500	38%

Food and Description	Amount	Fat Grams	Total Calories	% Fat Calories
■ DESSERT				
hot fudge sundae	1 sundae	10.0	320	28%
strawberry shortcake	1 piece	21.0	480	39%
strawberry sundae	1 sundae	6.0	260	21%
vanilla frozen yogurt	1 cone	4.0	180	20%
■ SALADS				
garden	1 serving	14.0	190	66%
grilled chicken	1 serving	4.0	120	30%
side	1 serving	–	20	–
■ SIDE DISHES & CONDIMENTS (*See also* Salads in this section)				
baked beans	5 oz	2.0	160	11%
baked potato				
plain	1 potato	1.0	130	9%
w/margarine	1 serving	13.0	240	11%
w/margarine & sour cream	1 serving	19.0	300	57%
coleslaw	5 oz	25.0	295	76%
cornbread	1 piece	17.0	310	49%
French fries	regular	15.0	350	39%
	large	18.0	430	38%
gravy	1.5 oz	–	20	–
mashed potatoes	5 oz	–	92	–
RUBIO'S BAJA GRILL				
■ BAJA BOWLS				
grilled chicken	1 bowl	6.0	260	21%
grilled steak	1 bowl	8.0	270	27%
■ HEALTH-MEX MENU				
Burito				
rice & bean	1 burrito	7.0	340	19%
w/chicken	1 burrito	9.0	380	21%
w/Mahi Mahi	1 burrito	8.0	380	19%
Combo				
regular	1 combo	13.0	690	17%
taco				
w/chicken	1 combo	8.0	480	15%
w/Mahi Mahi	1 combo	7.0	500	13%
w/chicken & Mahi Mahi	1 combo	7.0	490	13%
Taco				
w/chicken	1 taco	3.0	180	15%
w/Mahi Mahi	1 taco	2.0	190	9%
■ KIDS PESKY MEALS				
Add				
beans	1 serving	1.0	80	11%
chips/tortilla	1 serving	18.0	350	21%
"Churro"/mini	1 churro	4.0	65	55%
rice	1 serving	2.0	50	36%
bean/cheese burrito	1 burrito	20.0	480	38%
cheese quesadilla	1 quesadilla	29.0	520	50%
fish taco	1 taco	14.0	280	45%
taquitos	1 serving	17.0	320	48%

Food and Description	Amount	Fat Grams	Total Calories	% Fat Calories
■ LOS OTROS				
beans	1 serving	5.0	200	23%
chips/tortilla	1 order	22.0	420	47%
choco taco	1 taco	10.0	310	29%
churro	1 churro	8.0	130	55%
guacamole	1 serving	34.0	360	85%
nachos grande				
regular	1 serving	91.0	1,400	59%
w/chicken	1 serving	94.0	1,500	56%
w/steak	1 serving	97.0	1,520	57%
rice	1 serving	4.0	100	36%
taquitos	1 serving	12.0	330	33%
■ MAIN MENU				
Burritos				
bean & cheese	1 burrito	20.0	490	37%
carne asada	1 burrito	21.0	470	40%
carnitas	1 burrito	36.0	640	51%
chicken	1 burrito	25.0	540	42%
Especial				
w/carne asada	1 burrito	39.0	690	51%
w/carnitas	1 burrito	51.0	820	56%
w/chicken	1 burrito	36.0	670	48%
fish	1 burrito	30.0	590	46%
Mahi Mahi	1 burrito	31.0	640	44%
shrimp	1 burrito	22.0	480	41%
Combos				
#1-two fish tacos	1 combo	47.0	990	43%
#2-carne asada & carnitas tacos	1 combo	38.0	930	37%
#2-carnitas tacos	1 combo	47.0	1,010	42%
#2-chicken & carne asada tacos	1 combo	31.0	840	33%
#2-chicken carnitas	1 combo	38.0	920	37%
#2-chicken tacos	1 combo	29.0	830	31%
#2-fish & chicken tacos	1 combo	38.0	910	38%
#2-fish & carne asada tacos	1 combo	40.0	920	39%
#2-fish & carnitas tacos	1 combo	47.0	1,000	42%
#2-two carne asada tacos	1 combo	35.0	850	37%
#3-carnitas burrito & fish taco	1 combo	69.0	1,350	46%
#4-grilled chicken	1 combo	58.0	1,250	42%
#5-fish burrito & fish taco	1 combo	63.0	1,300	44%
#6-carne asada burrito & fish taco	1 combo	54.0	1,180	41%
#7-burrito Especial w/carne asada & fish taco	1 combo	72.0	1,400	46%
#7-burrito Especial w/carnitas & fish taco	1 combo	84.0	1,530	49%
#7-burrito Especial w/chicken & fish taco	1 combo	69.0	1,380	45%
Baja Grill	1 combo	45.0	1,100	37%
Cabo	1 combo	55.0	1,190	42%
Pesky's	1 combo	61.0	1,170	47%
Tacos				
carne asada	1 taco	7.0	210	30%

Food and Description	Amount	Fat Grams	Total Calories	% Fat Calories
Carnitas	1 taco	14.0	290	43%
fish				
Especial	1 taco	21.0	370	51%
grilled Mahi Mahi	1 taco	14.0	300	42%
regular	1 taco	14.0	280	45%
grilled				
chicken	1 taco	5.0	200	23%
shrimp	1 taco	13.0	260	45%
■ QUESADILLAS				
carne asada	1	50.0	800	56%
cheese	1	43.0	680	57%
chicken/grilled	1	46.0	780	53%
shrimp	1	43.0	720	54%
SCHLOTSKY'S DELI				
■ BREAD/BUNS				
dark rye	small	1.0	218	4%
	regular	2.0	327	6%
jalapeño cheese	small	3.0	235	11%
	regular	4.0	353	10%
pizza crust	6.7 oz serving	2.0	332	5%
sourdough	small	1.0	225	4%
	regular	2.0	333	5%
	large	4.0	667	5%
wheat	small	2.0	226	8%
	regular	4.0	336	11%
■ CHIPS & PRETZELS				
Potato chips/deli style				
barbeque	1.5 oz	11.0	210	47%
jalapeño	1.5 oz	11.0	210	47%
plain	1.5 oz	11.0	210	47%
salt & vinegar	1.5 oz	11.0	210	47%
sour cream & onion	1.5 oz	11.0	210	47%
Pretzels/sourdough	2.25 oz bag	2.0	240	8%
■ DESSERTS				
Cake/fudge brownie	1 slice	25.0	410	55%
Cheesecake				
cookies & creme	1 slice	18.0	330	49%
New York creamstyle	1 slice	18.0	310	52%
strawberry swirl	1 slice	17.0	300	51%
Cookies				
chocolate chip	1 cookie	7.0	160	39%
chocolate chunk	1 cookie	7.0	160	39%
chocolate pecan chunk	1 cookie	8.0	170	42%
fudge chocolate chunk	1 cookie	8.0	170	42%
oatmeal raisin	1 cookie	1.0	150	6%
peanut butter	1 cookie	8.0	170	42%
peanut butter chocolate chunk	1 cookie	8.0	170	42%
sugar	1 cookie	6.0	160	34%
white chocolate macadamia nut	1 cookie	8.0	170	42%

Food and Description	Amount	Fat Grams	Total Calories	% Fat Calories
■ KIDS DEALS				
Pizza				
cheese	1 serving	14.0	483	26%
pepperoni	1 serving	18.0	530	31%
Sandwich				
cheese	1 sandwich	18.0	426	38%
ham & cheese	1 sandwich	19.0	456	38%
PBJ (peanut butter & jelly)	1 sandwich	16.0	470	31%
■ PIZZAS/8" Sourdough Crust Pizzas				
bacon, tomato, & mushroom	1 pizza	24.0	635	34%
barbeque chicken	1 pizza	20.0	653	28%
chicken & pesto	1 pizza	19.0	649	26%
double cheese	1 pizza	21.0	603	31%
double cheese & pepperoni	1 pizza	16.0	744	19%
fresh tomato & pesto	1 pizza	16.0	539	27%
Mediterranean	1 pizza	19.0	564	30%
New Orleans	1 pizza	20.0	666	27%
smoked turkey & jalapeño	1 pizza	19.0	647	26%
Southwestern	1 pizza	19.0	635	27%
Thai chicken	1 pizza	19.0	681	25%
"The Original" combination	1 pizza	25.0	648	35%
vegetarian special	1 pizza	17.0	551	28%
■ SALADS & SALAD EXTRAS				
Deli Salads/5 oz servings				
cole slaw				
country style	1 serving	16.0	225	64%
shredded	1 serving	16.0	225	64%
macaroni	1 serving	23.0	338	61%
potato				
choice	1 serving	18.0	253	64%
diced w/egg	1 serving	13.0	216	54%
mustard & egg	1 serving	15.0	225	60%
Leaf Salads w/o salad extras				
Caesar	1 salad	8.0	152	47%
chicken Caesar	1 salad	10.0	254	35%
Chinese chicken	1 salad	3.0	150	18%
garden				
regular	1 salad	1.0	61	15%
small	1 sald	1.0	25	36%
Greek	1 salad	12.0	220	49%
ham & turkey Chef's	1 salad	11.0	248	40%
smoked turkey chef's	1 salad	10.0	243	37%
Salad Extras				
Chow mein noodles	1 serving	4.0	74	49%
croutons/garlic cheese	1 serving	2.0	46	39%
dressings				
Greek Balsamic vinaigrette	3 Tbs	17..0	170	90%
Italian/light	3 Tbs	8.0	90	80%
Olde World Caesar	3 Tbs	27.0	260	93%
ranch				
spicy	3 Tbs	25.0	230	98%

Food and Description	Amount	Fat Grams	Total Calories	% Fat Calories
spicy/light	3 Tbs	11.0	140	71%
traditional ranch	3 Tbs	29.0	270	97%
sesame ginger vinaigrette	3 Tbs	15.0	170	79%
thousand island	3 Tbs	21.0	220	86%
■ SANDWICHES				
Light & Flavorful				
Albacore tuna	small	11.0	361	27%
	regular	16.0	533	27%
	large	26.0	1,000	23%
chicken breast	small	7.0	363	17%
	regular	10.0	535	17%
	large	15.0	1,008	13%
Dijon chicken	small	4.0	330	11%
	regular	6.0	497	11%
	large	10.0	972	9%
pesto chicken	small	6.0	346	16%
	regular	9.0	512	16%
	large	15.0	999	14%
Santa Fe chicken	small	13.0	421	28%
	regular	19.0	642	28%
	large	29.0	1,182	22%
smoked turkey breast	small	5.0	335	13%
	regular	7.0	498	13%
	large	13.0	988	12%
Original				
cheese	small	31.0	596	47%
	regular	44.0	854	46%
	large	98.0	1,857	47%
Deluxe	small	65.0	1,044	56%
	regular	75.0	1,296	52%
	large	152.0	2,638	52%
ham & cheese	small	22.0	537	37%
	regular	32.0	789	37%
	large	67.0	1,625	37%
"The Original"	small	41.0	713	52%
	regular	50.0	941	48%
	large	102.0	1,917	48%
turkey	small	41.0	763	48%
	regular	51.0	1,017	45%
	large	104.0	2,083	45%
Specialty Deli				
Albacore tuna melt	small	28.0	562	45%
	regular	40.0	818	44%
	large	77.0	1,631	42%
BLT	small	15.0	379	36%
	regular	24.0	578	37%
	large	46.0	1,141	36%
chicken club	small	15.0	458	29%
	regular	23.0	686	30%
	large	45.0	1,351	30%

Food and Description	Amount	Fat Grams	Total Calories	% Fat Calories
corned beef	small	10.0	388	23%
	regular	15.0	587	22%
	large	25.0	1,134	20%
corned beef Reuben	small	21.0	528	36%
	regular	35.0	833	38%
	large	62.0	1,594	35%
pastrami & swiss	small	24.0	570	38%
	regular	37.0	861	39%
	large	69.0	1,681	37%
pastrami Reuben	small	29.0	619	42%
	regular	43.0	924	42%
	large	77.0	1,777	39%
roast beef	small	11.0	413	24%
	regular	17.0	617	25%
	large	28.0	1,185	21%
roast beef & cheese	small	24.0	580	37%
	regular	34.0	848	36%
	large	70.0	1,749	36%
Schlotzsky's Texas	small	26.0	561	42%
	regular	37.0	816	41%
	large	65.0	1,544	38%
The Philly	small	22.0	559	35%
	regular	32.0	824	35%
	large	66.0	1,709	35%
turkey & bacon club	small	27.0	596	41%
	regular	40.0	874	41%
	large	80.0	1,790	40%
turkey guacamole	small	15.0	449	30%
	regular	24.0	683	32%
	large	42.0	1,317	20%
turkey Reuben	small	26.0	579	40%
	regular	39.0	863	41%
	large	69.0	1,656	38%
vegetable club	small	16.0	393	37%
	regular	25.0	584	39%
	large	41.0	1,112	33%
Western vegetarian	small	23.0	449	46%
	regular	33.0	651	46%
	large	61.0	1,261	44%
■ **SOUPS**				
7 bean medley	1 cup	2.0	145	12%
beef & black bean	1 cup	1.0	150	6%
Boston clam chowder	1 cup	15.0	233	58%
broccoli cheese	1 cup	17.0	252	61%
chick noodle/old fashioned chicken	1 cup	2.0	122	15%
gumbo	1 cup	5.0	110	41%
tortilla	1 cup	3.0	167	16%
w/wild rice	1 cup	28.0	378	67%
corn chowder	1 cup	17.0	284	54%

Food and Description	Amount	Fat Grams	Total Calories	% Fat Calories
minestrone	1 cup	1.0	89	10%
potato/cream of w/bacon	1 cup	13.0	226	52%
ravioli tomato	1 cup	2.0	111	16%
red beans & rice	1 cup	1.0	167	5%
Santa Fe vegetable	1 cup	2.0	120	15%
Schlotzsky's vegetable	1 cup	2.0	220	8%
Timberline chili	1 cup	7.0	210	30%
tomato Milano	1 cup	3.0	89	30%
tortellini	1 cup	3.0	122	22%
Tuscan clam bisque	1 cup	16.0	219	66%
vegetable				
beef barley	1 cup	3.0	100	27%
cheese	1 cup	19.0	289	59%
vegetarian	1 cup	6.0	138	39%
Wisconsin cheese	1 cup	25.0	319	71%

SHONEY'S
■ BREAKFAST

Food and Description	Amount	Fat Grams	Total Calories	% Fat Calories
bacon	3 strips	9.4	109	78%
biscuit	1 biscuit	8.0	170	42%
blueberry muffin	1 serving	7.0	214	29%
country gravy	3 oz	9.8	114	77%
croissant	1 biscuit	16.0	260	55%
egg/fried	1 serving	14.7	159	83%
grits	1 serving	3.2	57	51%
ham/breakfast	2 slices	2.0	59	31%
hash browns	1 serving	3.0	90	30%
home fries	1 serving	3.7	115	29%
honey bun	1 bun	14.0	265	48%
pancake/6" dia	1 serving	<1.0	91	2%
sausage	1 patty	9.6	103	84%
sirloin/charbroiled	6 oz	24.5	357	62%
syrup/low-calorie	2.2 oz	–	98	–
toast w/butter	2 slices	5.2	163	29%

■ BURGERS

Food and Description	Amount	Fat Grams	Total Calories	% Fat Calories
All-American	1 burger	32.6	501	59%
bacon	1 burger	40.0	591	61%
mushroom-Swiss	1 burger	41.7	616	61%
old-fashioned	1 burger	28.2	470	54%
Shoney burger	1 burger	35.7	498	65%

■ CONDIMENTS (*See also* Salads & Dressing in this section)

Food and Description	Amount	Fat Grams	Total Calories	% Fat Calories
BBQ sauce	1 serving	1.0	41	22%
cocktail sauce	1 serving	–	36	–
sweet & sour sauce	1 serving	–	58	–
tartar sauce	1 serving	7.7	84	83%

■ DESSERT

Food and Description	Amount	Fat Grams	Total Calories	% Fat Calories
apple pie à la mode	1 serving	23.0	492	42%
carrot cake	1 serving	26.0	500	47%
hot fudge cake	1 serving	19.7	522	34%
hot fudge sundae	1 serving	22.0	451	44%
strawberry pie	1 serving	16.7	332	45%

Food and Description	Amount	Fat Grams	Total Calories	% Fat Calories
strawberry sundae	1 serving	19.0	380	45%
walnut brownie à la mode	1 serving	33.7	576	53%
■ ENTRÉES				
beef patty/light	1 serving	22.9	289	71%
chicken				
charbroiled	1 serving	7.4	239	28%
Hawaiian	1 serving	7.4	262	25%
chicken tenders	1 serving	20.4	388	47%
country fried steak	1 serving	27.2	449	55%
fish				
baked	1 serving	1.4	170	7%
light fried	1 serving	14.4	297	44%
fish & chips w/fries	1 serving	34.8	639	49%
fish & shrimp	1 serving	25.5	487	47%
Italian feast	1 serving	19.6	500	35%
lasagna	1 serving	9.8	297	30%
liver & onions	1 serving	22.9	411	50%
seafood platter	1 serving	28.0	566	45%
shrimp				
bite-size	1 serving	24.7	387	57%
boiled	1 serving	1.0	93	10%
charbroiled	1 serving	3.0	138	20%
shrimp sampler	1 serving	22.7	412	50%
shrimper's feast	regular	22.2	383	52%
	large	33.3	575	52%
spaghetti	1 serving	16.3	496	30%
steak				
half pound	1 serving	34.4	435	71%
rib-eye	8 oz	50.5	605	75%
sirloin	6 oz	24.5	357	62%
steak 'n shrimp				
w/charbroiled shrimp	1 serving	22.6	361	56%
w/fried shrimp	1 serving	32.7	507	58%
■ SALADS & DRESSING				
ambrosia salad	¼ cup	3.3	75	40%
apple grape surprise salad	¼ cup	–	19	–
beet onion salad	¼ cup	1.3	25	47%
broccoli/cauliflower salad	¼ cup	8.5	98	78%
broccoli/cauliflower/carrot salad	¼ cup	4.4	53	75%
broccoli/cauliflower/ranch salad	¼ cup	6.4	65	89%
carrot apple salad	¼ cup	9.0	99	82%
coleslaw	¼ cup	5.0	69	65%
cucumber salad/lite	¼ cup	–	12	–
Don's pasta salad	¼ cup	4.6	82	50%
fruit delight salad	¼ cup	1.6	54	27%
Italian vegetable salad	¼ cup	–	11	–
kidney bean salad	¼ cup	2.0	55	33%
macaroni salad	¼ cup	13.9	207	60%
mixed fruit salad	¼ cup	–	37	–
mixed squash salad	¼ cup	4.0	49	73%

Food and Description	Amount	Fat Grams	Total Calories	% Fat Calories
oriental salad	¼ cup	2.7	79	31%
pea salad	¼ cup	5.5	73	68%
rotelli pasta salad	¼ cup	4.0	78	46%
salad dressing				
Biscayne/ low-calorie	2 Tbs	1.0	62	15%
blue cheese	2 Tbs	13.0	117	100%
French				
regular	2 Tbs	12.0	124	87%
rue	2 Tbs	10.0	122	74%
honey mustard	2 Tbs	17.0	165	93%
Italian				
creamy	2 Tbs	15.0	135	100%
golden	2 Tbs	15.0	141	96%
ranch	2 Tbs	10.0	95	95%
Thousand Island	2 Tbs	13.0	130	90%
Weight Watchers	2 Tbs	–	10	–
Seigan salad	¼ cup	3.6	72	45%
snow salad	¼ cup	4.0	72	50%
spaghetti salad	¼ cup	4.6	81	51%
spring salad	¼ cup	2.9	38	69%
summer salad	¼ cup	11.6	114	92%
three bean salad	¼ cup	5.0	96	47%
Waldorf salad	¼ cup	5.2	81	58%
■ SANDWICHES				
baked ham	1 sandwich	10.3	290	32%
charbroiled chicken	1 sandwich	17.0	451	34%
chicken fillet	1 sandwich	21.2	464	41%
country fried	1 sandwich	25.8	588	39%
fish	1 sandwich	12.7	323	35%
grilled bacon & cheese	1 sandwich	28.2	440	58%
grilled cheese	1 sandwich	16.9	302	50%
ham club on whole wheat	1 sandwich	35.5	642	50%
patty melt	1 sandwich	41.7	640	59%
Philly steak	1 sandwich	44.0	673	59%
Reuben	1 sandwich	34.7	596	52%
Slim Jim	1 sandwich	23.9	484	44%
turkey club on whole wheat	1 sandwich	32.7	635	46%
■ SIDE DISHES				
baked potato	1 serving	<1.0	264	1%
French fries	3 oz	7.5	189	36%
	4 oz	9.9	252	35%
Grecian bread	1 serving	2.2	80	25%
mushrooms/sautéed	3 oz	6.5	75	78%
onion rings	1 piece	3.0	52	52%
onions/sautéed	2.5 oz	2.0	37	49%
rice	3.5 oz	3.7	137	24%
■ SOUP				
bean	6 oz	1.0	63	14%
beef cabbage	6 oz	3.0	86	31%
broccoli/cauliflower	6 oz	9.2	124	67%

Food and Description	Amount	Fat Grams	Total Calories	% Fat Calories
cheddar chowder	6 oz	2.3	91	23%
cheese Florentine ham	6 oz	7.8	110	64%
chicken gumbo	6 oz	2.0	60	30%
chicken noodle	6 oz	1.4	62	20%
chicken rice	6 oz	<1.0	72	6%
clam chowder	6 oz	5.4	94	52%
corn chowder	6 oz	4.7	148	29%
cream of broccoli	6 oz	4.6	75	55%
cream of chicken	6 oz	8.9	136	59%
cream of chicken vegetable	6 oz	1.3	79	15%
onion	6 oz	2.0	29	62%
potato	6 oz	3.4	102	30%
tomato Florentine	6 oz	1.0	63	14%
tomato vegetable	6 oz	<1.0	46	6%
vegetable beef	6 oz	1.5	82	16%
SIZZLER				
■ **CONDIMENTS**				
buttery dipping sauce	1½ oz	37.0	330	100%
cocktail sauce	1½ oz	–	40	–
guacamole	1 oz	4.0	42	86%
hibachi sauce	1½ oz	–	57	–
Malibu sauce	1½ oz	31.0	283	99%
margarine/whipped	1½ Tbs	12.0	105	100%
marinara sauce	1 oz	–	13	–
nacho cheese sauce	1 oz	10.0	120	75%
salsa	1 oz	–	7	–
sour dressing	2 Tbs	6.0	60	90%
	1½ oz	9.0	89	91%
tartar sauce	1½ oz	17.0	170	90%
■ **DESSERT BAR ITEMS**				
chocolate & vanilla soft-serve				
frozen dessert	4 oz	4.0	136	26%
chocolate syrup	1 oz	–	90	–
strawberry topping	1 oz	–	70	–
whipped topping	1 Tbs	1.0	12	–
■ **ENTRÉES**				
chicken				
breast				
hibachi w/pineapple	5 oz	3.0	193	14%
lemon-herb	5 oz	3.0	140	19%
Santa Fe	5 oz	3.0	150	18%
patty/Malibu	1 patty	19.0	310	55%
hamburger/meat, bun, lettuce, & tomato	1 burger	33.0	626	47%
salmon	8 oz	12.0	247	44%
shrimp				
broiled	5 oz	6.0	150	36%
fried	4 shrimp	2.0	223	81%
mini	4 oz	1.0	152	6%
scampi	5 oz	3.0	143	19%

Food and Description	Amount	Fat Grams	Total Calories	% Fat Calories
steak	6 oz	20.0	316	57%
	8 oz	27.0	421	58%
	9.5 oz	32.0	500	58%
swordfish	8 oz	14.0	315	40%
■ SALADS & SALAD BAR ITEMS				
alfalfa sprouts	¼ cup	–	2	–
avocados	½ avocado	15.0	153	88%
bacon bits	1 Tbs	2.0	27	67%
bean sprouts	¼ cup	–	–	–
beets	¼ cup	–	13	–
bell peppers	2 oz	–	8	–
broccoli	½ cup	–	12	–
cantaloupe	½ cup	–	28	–
carrot & raisin salad	2 oz	10.0	130	69%
carrots	¼ cup	–	12	–
cherry tomatoes	¼ cup	–	12	–
Chinese chicken salad	2 oz	2.0	54	33%
cottage cheese	2 oz	1.0	51	18%
cucumber	2 oz	–	7	–
egg/hard-cooked	1 oz	3.0	44	61%
garbanzo beans	¼ cup	1.0	63	14%
grapes	½ cup	–	29	–
honeydew melon	½ cup	–	30	–
jicama	2 oz	–	13	–
kidney beans	¼ cup	–	52	–
kiwifruit	2 oz	–	35	–
lettuce,				
iceberg	1 cup	–	7	–
romaine	1 cup	–	9	–
Mediterranean minted fruit salad	2 oz	–	29	–
Mexican fiesta salad	2 oz	–	54	–
olives	1 oz	6.0	62	87%
onion/red	2 Tbs	–	8	–
peaches	¼ cup	–	34	–
peas	¼ cup	–	31	–
pineapple	½ cup	–	38	–
potato salad				
old fashioned	2 oz	5.0	84	54%
red herb	2 oz	9.0	121	67%
mushrooms	¼ cup	–	4	–
red cabbage	¼ cup	–	6	–
salad dressing				
blue cheese	1 oz	12.0	1ll	97%
honey mustard	1 oz	16.0	160	90%
Italian				
lite	1 oz	–	14	–
Parmesan	1 oz	10.0	100	90%
Japanese rice vinegar	1 oz	–	10	–
ranch				
reduced calorie	1 oz	8.0	90	80%

Food and Description	Amount	Fat Grams	Total Calories	% Fat Calories
regular	1 oz	12.0	120	90%
Thousand Island	1 oz	15.0	143	94%
seafood Louis pasta salad	2 oz	2.0	64	28%
seafood salad	2 oz	3.0	56	48%
spicy jicama salad	2 oz	–	16	–
spinach	½ cup	–	6	–
strawberries	½ cup	–	22	–
teriyaki beef salad	2 oz	2.0	49	37%
tuna pasta salad	2 oz	10.0	133	68%
turkey ham	1 oz	5.0	62	73%
watermelon	½ cup	–	28	–
zucchini	¼ cup	–	5	–

■ **SIDE ORDERS & APPETIZERS** (*See also* Salads & Salad Bar Items in this section)

baked potato/flesh only	4 oz	–	105	–
cheese toast	1 piece	21.0	273	69%
chicken wings	1 oz	4.0	73	49%
fettuccine	2 oz	1.0	80	11%
focaccia bread	2 pieces	7.0	108	58%
French fries	4 oz	12.0	358	30%
meatballs	4 meatballs	11.0	157	63%
potato skin	2 oz	8.0	160	45%
refried beans	¼ cup	1.0	62	15%
rice pilaf	6 oz	5.0	256	18%
saltine crackers	2 crackers	1.0	25	36%
spaghetti	2 oz	–	80	–
taco filling	2 oz	9.0	103	79%
taco shell	1 shell	2.0	50	36%

■ **SOUP**

broccoli cheese	4 oz	9.0	139	58%
chicken noodle	4 oz	1.0	31	29%
clam chowder	4 oz	6.0	118	46%
minestrone	4 oz	–	36	–
vegetable sirloin	4 oz	2.0	60	30%

SMOOTHIE KING

■ **HIGH CALORIE SMOOTHIES**

The Hulk				
chocolate	20 oz	29.0	846	31%
strawberry	20 oz	29.0	953	27%
vanilla	20 oz	29.0	846	31%
Malts	20 oz	41.4	887	42%
Peanut Power	20 oz	20.8	632	30%
Peanut Power Plus				
w/grape juice	20 oz	20.8	703	27%
w/strawberries	20 oz	20.8	632	30%
Shakes	20 oz	41.4	875	43%

■ **HIGH PROTEIN 40/30/30 SMOOTHIES**

almond mocha	20 oz	12.9	402	29%
banana	20 oz	13.8	412	30%
chocolate	20 oz	12.9	401	29%
lemon	20 oz	12.8	390	29%

Food and Description	Amount	Fat Grams	Total Calories	% Fat Calories
pineapple	20 oz	12.9	380	31%
■ KIDS KUPS				
Berry Interesting	1 kup	–	150	–
Choc-A-Laka	1 kup	2.0	210	9%
Gimme-Grape	1 kup	–	170	–
Sweet Tart	1 kup	–	150	–
■ LOW-FAT FRUIT SMOOTHIES				
Angel Food	20 oz	0.5	330	1%
Blackberry Dream	20 oz	0.3	343	1%
Caribbean Way	20 oz	0.4	392	1%
Celestial Cherry High	20 oz	0.4	285	1%
Cranberry Cooler	20 oz	0.1	538	<1%
Cranberry Supreme	20 oz	0.6	577	1%
GoGuava	20 oz	–	300	–
Grape Expectations	20 oz	0.4	399	1%
Grape Expectations Part II	20 oz	0.4	429	1%
Immune Builder	20 oz	1.0	333	3%
Instant Vigor	20 oz	1.2	359	3%
Island Treat	20 oz	0.8	334	2%
Lemon Twist				
banana	20 oz	0.4	339	1%
strawberry	20 oz	0.3	399	1%
Light & fluffy	20 oz	0.4	389	1%
Mango Fest	20 oz	–	320	–
Muscle Punch	20 oz	1.3	339	3%
Muscle Punch Plus	20 oz	1.2	340	3%
Peach Slice	20 oz	0.2	341	1%
Peach Slice Plus	20 oz	0.2	471	<1%
Pineapple Pleasure	20 oz	0.4	313	1%
Raspberry Sunrise	20 oz	0.7	335	2%
Slim & Trim				
chocolate	20 oz	1.6	270	5%
orange vanilla	20 oz	0.5	199	2%
strawberry	20 oz	1.0	357	3%
vanilla	20 oz	1.0	227	4%
■ SPECIALTY SMOOTHIES				
Coconut Surprise	20 oz	5.9	457	12%
Hawaiian Cafe Au Lait	20 oz	0.3	286	1%
Mo'cuccino	20 oz	12.0	420	26%
Yogurt D-Lite	20 oz	3.9	341	10%
■ WORKOUT SMOOTHIES				
Power Punch	20 oz	1.3	430	3%
Power Punch Plus	20 oz	2.0	499	4%
Super Punch	20 oz	0.4	425	1%
Super Punch Plus	20 oz	0.4	516	1%
The Activator				
banana	20 oz	1.0	429	2%
chocolate	20 oz	1.0	429	2%
strawberry	20 oz	1.0	559	2%
vanilla	20 oz	1.0	429	2%

Food and Description	Amount	Fat Grams	Total Calories	% Fat Calories
SONIC				
■ **BURGERS & HOT DOGS**				
cheese coney				
extra long				
plain	1 coney	39.0	635	55%
w/onions	1 coney	39.0	640	55%
regular				
plain	1 coney	23.0	358	58%
w/onions	1 coney	23.0	361	58%
cheeseburger				
bacon	1 burger	38.6	548	63%
mini	1 burger	14.4	281	46%
chili pie	1 piece	22.6	327	62%
corn dog	1 corn dog	15.0	280	48%
hamburger				
hickory	1 burger	15.7	314	45%
mini	1 burger	11.0	246	24%
#1				
plain	1 burger	26.6	409	59%
w/cheese	1 burger	32.4	479	61%
#2				
plain	1 burger	15.7	323	43%
w/cheese	1 burger	21.5	393	49%
hot dog/regular	1 hot dog	15.0	258	52%
jalapeño burger/double meat & cheese	1 burger	40.6	638	57%
Super Sonic burger/double meat & cheese				
w/mayo	1 burger	51.5	730	63%
w/mustard	1 burger	40.7	644	57%
■ **SANDWICHES**				
BLT	1 sandwich	19.0	325	53%
chicken				
breaded	1 sandwich	24.7	455	49%
grilled	1 sandwich	4.3	215	18%
fish	1 sandwich	7.0	277	23%
grilled cheese	1 sandwich	17.0	288	53%
steak	1 sandwich	41.6	631	59%
■ **SIDE ORDERS**				
French fries				
plain	regular	8.0	233	31%
	large	11.0	315	31%
w/cheese	large	20.7	420	44%
onion rings	regular	26.5	404	59%
	large	37.8	577	59%
Tater Tots				
plain	1 serving	7.0	150	42%
w/cheese	1 serving	13.0	220	53%
SOUP PLANTATION				
■ **CONDIMENTS**				
Croutons/garlic, Parmesan	10 croutons	3.0	40	68%
Salad Dressings				
blue cheese	2 Tbs	14.0	140	90%

Food and Description	Amount	Fat Grams	Total Calories	% Fat Calories
blush vinaigrette	2 Tbs	12.0	120	90%
creamy cucumber	2 Tbs	7.0	80	79%
garden French tomato/low-fat	2 Tbs	1.5	40	34%
honey mustard/fat-free	2 Tbs	13.0	150	78%
Parmesan pepper cream	2 Tbs	17.0	160	96%
ranch house				
fat-free	2 Tbs	–	50	–
regular	2 Tbs	13.0	130	90%
raspberry vinaigrette	2 Tbs	13.0	120	98%
thousand island	2 Tbs	11.0	110	90%
zesty Italian				
fat-free	2 Tbs	–	20	–
regular	2 Tbs	18.0	180	90%
■ DESSERTS				
apple medley	½ cup	–	70	–
banana royale	½ cup	–	80	–
chocolate chip cookie	1 small	3.0	70	39%
muffins				
low-fat/98% fat free	1 muffin	0.5	80	6%
regular				
apple raisin	1 muffin	7.0	150	42%
apricot	1 muffin	7.0	150	42%
banana nut	1 muffin	7.0	150	42%
blueberry/wild				
large	1 muffin	12.0	310	35%
regular	1 muffin	5.0	140	32%
carrot pineapple	1 muffin	6.0	150	36%
cherry nut	1 muffin	7.0	150	42%
Georgia peach poppyseed	1 muffin	6.0	150	36%
lemon	1 muffin	4.0	140	26%
peanut butter				
chocolate chip	1 muffin	9.0	190	43%
nutty	1 muffin	8.0	170	42%
pumpkin raisin	1 muffin	6.0	150	36%
strawberry buttermilk	1 muffin	6.0	140	39%
zucchini nut	1 muffin	7.0	150	42%
pudding				
chocolate	½ cup	4.0	140	26%
rice	½ cup	2.0	110	16%
tapioca	½ cup	3.0	140	19%
vanilla	½ cup	3.0	140	19%
■ PASTAS				
bruschetta				
creamy	1 cup	16.0	360	40%
regular	1 cup	4.0	260	14%
chipotle chicken w/cilantro	1 cup	16.0	390	37%
creamy pesto w/sundried tomatoes	1 cup	21.0	430	44%
fettucine Alfredo	1 cup	18.0	390	42%
garden vegetable				
w/meatballs	1 cup	7.0	270	23%

Food and Description	Amount	Fat Grams	Total Calories	% Fat Calories
w/Italian sausage	1 cup	10.0	300	30%
Italian vegetable beef	1 cup	6.0	270	20%
jalapeño salsa	1 cup	4.0	240	15%
nutty mushroom	1 cup	20.0	390	46%
smoked salmon	1 cup	16.0	360	40%
vegetarian marinara	1 cup	4.0	260	14%
■ SALADS				
Fresh Salads				
antipasto	1 cup	10.0	140	64%
Caribbean Krab	1 cup	7.0	120	53%
classic Caesar	1 cup	14.0	190	66%
Ensalada Azteca	1 cup	9.0	130	62%
Greek	1 cup	9.0	120	68%
mandarin spinach w/walnuts	1 cup	11.0	170	58%
roma tomato, mozzarella, & basil	1 cup	9.0	120	68%
shrimp & krab Louis	1 cup	12.0	180	60%
spinach & pasta w/raspberry vinaigrette	1 cup	6.0	180	30%
won ton chicken	1 cup	8.0	150	48%
Prepared Salads				
artichoke rice	½ cup	8.0	160	45%
Aunt Doris' red pepper slaw	½ cup	–	70	–
Baja bean& cilantro	½ cup	3.0	180	15%
BBQ potato	½ cup	8.0	160	45%
carrot raisin	½ cup	3.0	90	30%
Chinese krab	½ cup	8.0	160	45%
confetti pasta w/cheddar	½ cup	9.0	160	51%
cucumber tomato	½ cup	–	20	–
Dijon potato w/garlic dill vinaigrette	½ cup	7.0	140	45%
German potato	½ cup	3.0	130	21%
Greek couscous	½ cup	9.0	170	48%
mandarin krab	½ cup	3.0	150	18%
mandarin w/broccoli and almonds	½ cup	3.0	120	23%
marinated summer vegetables	½ cup	–	80	–
Mazatian krab & pasta	½ cup	9.0	160	51%
Mediterranean harvest	½ cup	3.0	120	23%
Moroccan marinated vegetables	½ cup	3.0	90	30%
old fashioned macaroni w/ham	½ cup	11.0	180	55%
Oriental ginger slaw w/krab	½ cup	3.0	70	39%
Pesto pasta	½ cup	7.0	160	39%
picnic potato	½ cup	7.0	160	39%
pineapple coconut slaw	½ cup	10.0	150	60%
poppyseed coleslaw	½ cup	9.0	120	68%
roasted potato w/chipotle chile	½ cup	6.0	140	39%
Southern dill potato	½ cup	3.0	120	23%
spicy Southwestern pasta	½ cup	3.0	130	21%
spinach krab	½ cup	12.0	230	47%
summer barley w/black beans	½ cup	3.0	110	25%
Thai noodle w/peanut sauce	½ cup	8.0	170	42%
three bean marinade	½ cup	6.0	170	32%

Food and Description	Amount	Fat Grams	Total Calories	% Fat Calories
tortellini salad	½ cup	10.0	170	53%
tumbleweed tortellini	½ cup	9.0	140	58%
tuna tarragon	½ cup	14.0	240	53%
turkey chutney pasta	½ cup	9.0	230	35%
zesty tortellini	½ cup	15.0	190	71%
■ SOUPS & CHILI				
Chili				
Arizona Red	1 cup	8.0	230	31%
House/low-fat	1 cup	3.0	230	12%
Santa Fe black bean/low-fat	1 cup	3.0	190	14%
Texas Red	1 cup	8.0	230	31%
Yucatan	1 cup	10.0	280	32%
Soups				
Chesapeake corn chowder	1 cup	13.0	310	38%
chicken				
fajitas & black beans	1 cup	7.0	280	23%
jambalaya	1 cup	7.0	160	39%
noodle/low-fat	1 cup	3.0	160	17%
tortilla/low-fat	1 cup	3.0	100	27%
cream of				
broccoli	1 cup	15.0	250	54%
chicken	1 cup	15.0	250	54%
mushroom	1 cup	21.0	290	65%
minestrone w/Italian sausage	1 cup	11.0	210	47%
navy bean w/ham	1 cup	10.0	340	26%
New England clam chowder	1 cup	20.0	330	55%
New Orleans style jambalaya	1 cup	8.0	160	45%
potato				
cheese/chunky	1 cup	10.0	210	43%
Irish leek	1 cup	16.0	260	55%
shrimp bisque	1 cup	19.0	300	57%
split pea w/ham	1 cup	10.0	350	26%
sweet tomato onion/low-fat	1 cup	3.0	110	25%
turkey vegetable	1 cup	12.0	270	40%
vegetarian harvest	1 cup	8.0	190	38%
vegetable medley/low-fat	1 cup	1.0	90	30%
STARBUCKS (*See also* ICE CREAM & FROZEN DESSERTS)				
■ BEVERAGES				
Cocoa-w/whipping cream				
non-fat milk	short	10.0	230	39%
	tall	11.0	300	33%
	grande	12.0	380	28%
	venti	12.0	450	24%
low-fat milk	short	14.0	260	48%
	tall	16.0	350	41%
	grande	18.0	430	38%
	venti	21.0	520	36%
soy milk	short	5.0	140	32%
	tall	8.0	210	34%

Food and Description	Amount	Fat Grams	Total Calories	% Fat Calories
whole milk	grande	10.0	290	31%
	short	17.0	290	53%
	tall	21.0	390	48%
	grande	25.0	490	46%
	venti	29.0	590	44%
Hot Coffee				
Americano	short	–	5	–
	tall	–	10	–
	grande	–	15	–
	venti	–	15	–
cappuccino				
non-fat milk	short	–	60	–
	tall	–	80	–
	grande	–	110	–
	venti	0.5	120	4%
lowfat milk	short	2.5	80	28%
	tall	3.5	110	29%
	grande	5.0	140	32%
	venti	5.0	160	28%
soy milk	short	3.0	60	45%
	tall	4.0	70	51%
	grande	5.0	100	45%
	venti	6.0	110	49%
whole milk	short	5.0	100	45%
	tall	7.0	140	45%
	grande	9.0	180	45%
	venti	10.0	200	45%
caramel macchiato				
non-fat milk	short	0.5	90	5%
	tall	1.0	140	6%
	grande	1.0	190	5%
	venti	1.0	230	4%
low-fat milk	short	2.5	110	20%
	tall	3.5	170	19%
	grande	5.0	225	20%
	venti	6.0	270	20%
whole milk	short	4.5	130	31%
	tall	7.0	190	33%
	grande	9.0	250	32%
	venti	11.0	310	32%
Chai latte				
nonfat milk	short	–	110	–
	tall	–	150	–
	grande	0.5	210	2%
	venti	17.0	400	38%
lowfat milk	short	3.5	130	24%
	tall	5.0	190	24%
	grande	7.0	260	24%
	venti	9.0	330	25%

Food and Description	Amount	Fat Grams	Total Calories	% Fat Calories
soy milk	short	4.0	100	36%
	tall	5.0	140	32%
	grande	8.0	200	36%
	venti	10.0	260	35%
whole milk	short	7.0	160	39%
	tall	9.0	220	37%
	grande	13.0	320	37%
	venti	17.0	400	38%
espresso				
con panna	solo	3.0	35	77%
	doppio	3.0	40	68%
macchiato				
non-fat milk	solo	–	10	–
	dippio	–	15	–
lowfat milk	solo	–	15	–
	dippio	–	20	–
soy milk	solo	–	10	–
	dippio	–	15	–
whole milk	solo	0.5	15	30%
	dippio	0.5	20	23%
plain	solo	–	5	–
	doppio	–	10	–
Frappuccino				
caramel	12 oz	9.0	290	28%
	16 oz	9.0	350	23%
	24 oz	10.0	490	18%
coffee	24 oz	3.5	360	9%
espresso	24 oz	3.5	350	9%
mocha	24 oz	4.5	430	9%
power				
coffee	24 oz	3.5	470	7%
mocha	24 oz	4.5	640	6%
rhumba				
	12 oz	4.0	220	16%
	16 oz	6.0	300	18%
	24 oz	9.0	450	18%
latte				
non-fatmilk	short	–	80	
	tall	0.5	120	4%
	grande	1.0	160	6%
	venti	1.0	200	5%
lowfat milk	short	3.5	110	29%
	tall	6.0	170	32%
	grande	7.0	220	29%
	venti	10.0	280	32%
soy milk	short	4.0	70	51%
	tall	6.0	110	49%
	grande	8.0	150	48%
	venti	10.0	190	47%

Food and Description	Amount	Fat Grams	Total Calories	% Fat Calories
whole milk	short	7.0	140	45%
	tall	11.0	210	47%
	grande	14.0	270	47%
	venti	18.0	350	46%
mocha				
non-fat milk/no whipping cream	short	1.5	120	11%
	tall	2.0	180	10%
	grande	3.0	240	11%
	venti	3.5	300	11%
lowfat milk	short	13.0	230	51%
	tall	15.0	300	45%
	grande	17.0	370	41%
	venti	20.0	450	40%
soy milk/no whipping cream	short	4.5	120	34%
	tall	7.0	180	35%
	grande	9.0	230	35%
	venti	12.0	290	37%
whole milk	short	16.0	250	58%
	tall	20.0	340	53%
	grande	23.0	420	49%
	venti	27.0	510	48%
mocha valencia				
non-fat/no whipping cream	short	1.5	140	10%
	tall	2.0	220	8%
	grande	2.5	290	8%
	venti	3.5	370	9%
lowfat milk	short	12.0	240	45%
	tall	15.0	330	41%
	grande	16.0	420	34%
	venti	19.0	510	34%
soy milk/no whipping cream	short	3.5	140	23%
	tall	6.0	220	25%
	grande	8.0	290	25%
	venti	10.0	360	25%
whole milk	short	14.0	260	48%
	tall	18.0	370	44%
	grande	21.0	460	41%
	venti	25.0	560	40%
Iced Coffee				
Chai latte				
nonfat milk	tall	–	110	–
	grande	–	160	–
	venti	0.5	190	2%
lowfat milk	tall	2.5	130	17%
	grande	4.5	190	21%
	venti	5.0	230	20%
soy milk	tall	3.0	100	27%
	grande	4.5	150	27%
	venti	6.0	190	28%

Food and Description	Amount	Fat Grams	Total Calories	% Fat Calories
whole milk	tall	5.0	150	30%
	grande	8.0	220	33%
	venti	10.0	270	33%
latte				
non-fat milk	short	–	60	–
	tall	–	70	–
	grande	–	100	–
	venti	–	110	–
lowfat milk	short	2.5	80	28%
	tall	3.0	90	30%
	grande	4.5	130	31%
	venti	5.0	140	32%
soy milk	short	3.0	60	60%
	tall	3.5	70	45%
	grande	4.5	90	45%
	venti	5.0	100	45%
whole milk	short	5.0	100	45%
	tall	6.0	120	45%
	grande	8.0	160	45%
	venti	9.0	180	45%
mocha				
w/whipping cream				
non-fat milk	24 oz	3.5	240	13%
1% milk	24 oz	6.0	260	83%
2% milk	24 oz	8.0	270	27%
soy milk	24 oz	7.0	240	26%
whole milk	24 oz	10.0	290	31%
w/o whipping cream				
non-fat milk	short	1.5	100	14%
	tall	2.0	130	14%
	grande	2.5	170	13%
	venti	3.0	210	13%
lowfat milk	short	3.0	110	25%
	tall	4.0	150	24%
	grande	5.0	200	23%
	venti	6.0	230	23%
soy milk	short	3.5	100	32%
	tall	4.0	130	28%
	grande	6.0	170	32%
	venti	6.0	200	27%
whole milk	short	5.0	130	35%
	tall	6.0	160	34%
	grande	8.0	220	33%
	venti	9.0	260	31%
Steamed Milk				
non-fat milk	short	–	90	–
	tall	0.5	130	3%
	grande	1.0	170	5%
	venti	1.0	110	8%

Food and Description	Amount	Fat Grams	Total Calories	% Fat Calories
low-fat milk	short	4.5	120	34%
	tall	6.0	180	30%
	grande	9.0	240	34%
	venti	11.0	290	34%
soy milk	short	4.5	80	51%
	tall	7.0	120	53%
	grande	9.0	160	51%
	venti	12.0	200	54%
whole milk	short	8.0	150	48%
	tall	12.0	220	49%
	grande	16.0	300	48%
	venti	20.0	370	49%
■ EXTRAS				
bar mocha syrup				
short	1 oz	1.0	50	18%
tall	1.5 oz	1.5	70	19%
grande	2 oz	2.0	100	18%
venti	2.5 oz	2.5	120	19%
Frappuccino mocha syrup				
tall	0.375 oz	–	25	–
grande	0.5 oz	–	35	–
venti	0.875 oz	0.5	45	10%
whipped cream topping	0.8 oz	9.0	80	100%
■ FRUIT BEVERAGES				
Tiazzi blended				
berries & cream	tall	13.0	320	37%
	grande	14.0	400	32%
	venti	18.0	530	31%
mango citrus	tall	–	160	–
	grande	–	220	–
	venti	–	290	–
orange & cream	tall	13.0	340	34%
	grande	14.0	420	30%
	venti	18.0	550	29%
peach	tall	–	130	–
	grande	–	180	–
	venti	–	240	–
peaches & cream	tall	13.0	310	38%
	grande	14.0	380	33%
	venti	18.0	500	32%
wild berry	tall	–	150	–
	grande	–	200	–
	venti	–	260	–
■ FROZEN NOVELTIES				
Frappucinno bar				
chocolate covered caramel	1 bar	10.0	190	47%
coffee	1 bar	2.0	110	16%
mocha	1 bar	2.0	120	15%

Food and Description	Amount	Fat Grams	Total Calories	% Fat Calories
STEAK & SHAKE				
■ **BEVERAGES**				
coffee	6 fl oz	–	2	–
Dr. Pepper	10.5 fl oz	–	137	–
hot chocolate	6 fl oz	18.6	686	24%
floats (see DESSERTS in this section)				
Freezes (see DESSERTS in this section)				
tea				
hot	7 fl oz	–	4	–
iced	7.5 fl oz	–	6	–
lemon drink	1 small	–	86	–
milk/whole	8 fl oz	7.9	146	49%
orange drink	1 small	–	83	–
orange juice	7 fl oz	<1.0	105	3%
root beer	10 fl oz	–	115	–
shakes				
chocolate	1 shake	37.8	608	56%
strawberry	1 shake	40.0	648	56%
vanilla	1 shake	38.4	619	56%
■ **BURGERS & CHILI**				
chili & oyster crackers	1 serving	14.0	337	37%
chili mac & 4 saltines	1 serving	12.4	311	36%
chili 3 ways & 4 saltines	1 serving	16.0	402	36%
steakburger				
regular				
plain	1 burger	7.1	277	23%
w/cheese	1 burger	13.3	353	34%
super				
plain	1 burger	12.0	375	29%
w/cheese	1 burger	18.3	451	37%
triple				
regular	1 burger	17.0	474	32%
w/cheese	1 burger	29.5	626	42%
■ **DESSERTS**				
apple Danish	1 Danish	23.8	391	55%
apple pie				
à la mode	1 piece	25.5	549	42%
plain	1 piece	17.65	407	39%
brownie	1 piece	11.5	258	40%
brownie fudge sundae	1 sundae	35.2	645	49%
cheesecake				
plain	1 piece	11.0	368	27%
w/strawberries	1 piece	11.4	386	28%
cherry pie				
à la mode	1 piece	21.6	476	41%
plain	1 piece	13.8	334	37%
Coca-Cola float	1 serving	17.2	514	30%
hot fudge nut sundae	1 sundae	34.4	530	58%
lemon float	1 serving	18.6	555	30%

Food and Description	Amount	Fat Grams	Total Calories	% Fat Calories
lemon freeze	1 serving	24.9	548	41%
orange float	1 serving	16.8	502	30%
orange freeze	1 serving	23.8	516	42%
root beer float	1 serving	16.7	529	28%
strawberry sundae	1 sundae	21.7	330	59%
vanilla ice cream	1½ scoops	11.7	213	49%
■ SALADS				
chef salad	1 serving	17.6	313	51%
lettuce & tomato salad w/1 oz Thousand Island dressing	1 serving	15.3	168	82%
low-calorie platter	1 serving	13.7	293	42%
■ SANDWICHES				
baked ham	1 sandwich	22.0	451	44%
egg	1 sandwich	9.9	275	32%
ham & egg	1 sandwich	17.2	434	36%
toasted cheese	1 sandwich	13.3	250	48%
■ SIDE ORDERS				
baked beans	1 serving	3.7	173	19%
cottage cheese	½ cup	3.6	94	35%
French fries	1 serving	10.2	211	44%
lettuce & tomato	1 serving	–	4	–
SUBWAY				
■ BAKED GOODS				
Bread				
deli style roll	1 roll	2.0	170	11%
Italian bread				
6"	2.5 oz	1.0	190	5%
12"	5 oz	2.0	380	5%
wheat				
6"	2.67 oz	3.0	210	13%
12"	5.35 oz	5.0	420	11%
Cookies				
chocolate chip	1 cookie	10.0	214	42%
chocolate chip M&M	1 cookie	10.0	212	42%
chocolate chunk	1 cookie	10.0	215	42%
double chocolate Brazil nut	1 cookie	10.0	215	42%
macadamia nut	1 cookie	11.0	222	45%
oatmeal raisin				
low-fat	1 cookie	3.0	166	16%
original	1 cookie	8.0	199	36%
peanut butter	1 cookie	12.0	223	48%
sugar	1 cookie	12.0	225	48%
■ BEVERAGES				
Fruisle Smoothies				
Berry Blitz	12 oz	–	129	–
Berry Breeze	12 oz	–	120	–
Berry 'Lishus	12 oz	–	154	–
Island Berry	12 oz	–	120	–
Island Fever	12 oz	–	137	–
Peach Paradise	12 oz	–	119	–

Food and Description	Amount	Fat Grams	Total Calories	% Fat Calories
Peach Pizazz	12 oz	–	126	–
Pineapple Delite	12 oz	–	142	–
Pineapple Passion	12 oz	–	140	–
Sunrise Energizer	12 oz	–	160	–
Tropical Trio	12 oz	–	138	–
Wild Berries	12 oz	–	130	–
■ **FIXINS'**				
Deli Style Sandwiches				
lettuce	1 serving	–	14	–
olives	2 rings	–	2	–
onions	1 serving	–	2	–
peppers	2 strips	–	1	–
pickles	2 chips	–	1	–
tomato	2 slices	–	8	–
Optional				
bacon	2 slices	3.0	42	64%
cheese	2 triangles	3.0	41	66%
mayonnaise dressing				
light	1 tsp	2.0	18	100%
regular	1 tsp	4.0	37	100%
mustard	2 tsp	–	7	–
Standard				
lettuce	1 serving	–	4	–
olives	2 rings	–	2	–
onions	1 serving	–	5	–
peppers	2 strips	–	1	–
pickles	3 chips	–	2	–
tomato	2 large slices	–	6	–
■ **SALAD DRESSINGS & SALADS**				
Salad Dressings				
French				
fat-free	1 pkt	–	18	–
regular	1 pkt	6.0	70	77%
Italian				
creamy	1 pkt	7.0	65	97%
fat-free	1 pkt	–	5	–
ranch				
fat-free	1 pkt	–	15	–
regular	1 pkt	10.0	88	100%
Thousand Island	1 pkt	7.0	65	97%
Salads				
Classic Italian BMT	1 serving	19.0	269	64%
Cold cut Trio	1 serving	12.0	193	56%
ham	1 serving	3.0	112	24%
meatball	1 serving	13.0	232	50%
roast beef	1 serving	3.0	115	23%
roasted chicken breast fillet salad	1 serving	4.0	162	22%
seafood & crab	1 serving	7.0	157	40%
steak & cheese	1 serving	8.0	182	40%
Subway club salad	1 serving	3.0	123	22%

Food and Description	Amount	Fat Grams	Total Calories	% Fat Calories
Subway melt	1 serving	9.0	190	43%
tuna salad-made w/light mayonnaise dressing	1 serving	12.0	198	55%
turkey & ham	1 serving	2.0	107	17%
turkey breast salad	1 serving	2.0	101	18%
veggie delite salad	1 serving	1.0	51	18%
■ **SANDWICHES & SUBS**				
Breakfast				
added cheese	2 triangles	3.0	41	66%
bacon & egg	6" sub	15.0	363	37%
	deli	14.0	323	39%
	wrap	14.0	353	36%
cheese & egg	6" sub	15.0	363	37%
	deli	14.0	323	39%
	wrap	14.0	353	36%
ham & egg	6" sub	13.0	352	33%
	deli	12.0	312	35%
	wrap	12.0	342	32%
western egg	6" sub	12.0	351	31%
	deli	12.0	311	35%
	wrap	12.0	341	32%
Deli-style sandwich				
bologna	1 sandwich	10.0	283	32%
ham	1 sandwich	3.0	224	12%
roast beef	1 sandwich	4.0	236	15%
tuna	1 sandwich	8.0	267	27%
turkey breast	1 sandwich	4.0	227	16%
6" cold sandwiches				
Classic Italian BMT	1 sandwich	21.0	450	42%
Cold cut Trio	1 sandwich	14.0	374	34%
ham	1 sandwich	5.0	293	15%
roast beef	1 sandwich	5.0	296	15%
Seafood & Crab w/cheese & condiments	1 sandwich	9.0	338	24%
Subway Club	1 sandwich	5.0	304	15%
tuna	1 sandwich	14.0	378	33%
turkey breast	1 sandwich	4.0	282	13%
turkey & ham	1 sandwich	4.0	288	13%
Veggie Delite	1 sandwich	3.0	232	12%
6" hot sandwiches				
meatball	1 sandwich	15.0	413	33%
roasted chicken breast fillet	1 sandwich	6.0	342	16%
steak & cheese	1 sandwich	10.0	363	25%
Subway Melt w/cheese & condiments	1 sandwich	11.0	370	27%
6" Super Subs				
Classic Italian BMT	1 sandwich	39.0	668	53%
Cold Cut Trio	1 sandwich	24.0	517	42%
ham	1 sandwich	7.0	354	18%
meatball	1 sandwich	27.0	594	41%
roast beef	1 sandwich	7.0	360	18%
roasted chicken breast	1 sandwich	9.0	453	18%

Food and Description	Amount	Fat Grams	Total Calories	% Fat Calories
Seafood & Crab w/cheese & condiments	1 sandwich	15.0	444	30%
Steak & cheese	1 sandwich	17.0	495	31%
Subway				
Club	1 sandwich	7.0	377	17%
Melt	1 sandwich	19.0	509	34%
turkey breast	1 sandwich	5.0	333	14%
turkey & ham	1 sandwich	6.0	343	16%
tuna w/cheese & condiments	1 sandwich	26.0	525	45%
turkey breast	1 sandwich	4.0	276	13%
turkey breast & ham	1 sandwich	4.0	275	13%
veggie delite	1 sandwich	3.0	223	12%
■ WRAPS				
chicken Parmesan ranch	1 wrap	5.0	333	14%
steak & cheese	1 wrap	4.0	353	10%
turkey bacon deluxe	1 wrap	4.0	355	10%
10.5" wrap only	1 wrap	0.5	200	2%
TACO BELL				
■ BREAKFAST				
Burritos				
Country Breakfast	1 burrito	14.0	270	47%
Double Bacon 7 Egg	1 burrito	27.0	480	51%
Fiesta Breakfast	1 burrito	16.0	280	51%
Grande Breakfast	1 burrito	22.0	420	47%
Hash Brown Nuggets	1 serving	18.0	280	58%
Quesadilla				
Breakfast cheese	1 quesadilla	21.0	380	50%
w/bacon	1 quesadilla	27.0	450	54%
w/sausage	1 quesadilla	25.0	430	52%
■ BURRITOS				
bean	1 burrito	12.0	370	29%
Big Beef				
regular	1 burrito	17.0	400	38%
Supreme	1 burrito	23.0	510	41%
Burrito Supreme	1 burrito	18.0	430	38%
Chicken				
Big Chicken Supreme	1 burrito	17.0	460	33%
grilled	1 burrito	13.0	390	30%
chili cheese	1 burrito	13.0	330	35%
7-layer	1 burrito	22.0	520	38%
■ CHALUPAS				
Baja				
beef	1 chalupa	27.0	420	58%
chicken	1 chalupa	24.0	400	54%
steak	1 chalupa	24.0	400	54%
Santa Fe				
beef	1 chalupa	29.0	440	59%
chicken	1 chalupa	26.0	420	56%
steak	1 chalupa	27.0	430	57%
Supreme				
beef	1 chalupa	23.0	380	54%

Food and Description	Amount	Fat Grams	Total Calories	% Fat Calories
chicken	1 chalupa	20.0	360	50%
steak	1 chalupa	20.0	360	50%
■ GORDITAS				
Baja				
beef	1 gordita	21.0	360	53%
chicken	1 gordita	18.0	340	48%
steak	1 gordita	18.0	340	48%
Santa Fe				
beef	1 gordita	23.0	380	54%
chicken	1 gordita	20.0	370	49%
steak	1 gordita	20.0	370	49%
Supreme				
beef	1 gordita	14.0	300	42%
chicken	1 gordita	13.0	300	39%
steak	1 gordita	14.0	300	42%
■ NACHOS & SIDES				
Choco Taco ice cream dessert	1 ice cream	17.0	310	49%
Cinnamon Twists	1 twist	8.0	180	40%
Mexican rice	1 serving	9.0	190	47%
Nachos				
BellGrande				
chicken	1 serving	36.0	740	44%
regular	1 serving	39.0	760	46%
steak	1 serving	37.0	740	45%
Big Beef Supreme	1 serving	24.0	440	49%
regular	1 serving	18.0	320	51%
pintos'n cheese	1 serving	8.0	180	40%
■ SPECIALTY ITEMS				
Big Beef Meximelt	1 serving	15.0	290	47%
Mexican pizza				
beef	1 pizza	33.0	530	56%
cheese	1 pizza	35.0	540	58%
chicken	1 pizza	32.0	520	55%
quesadilla				
cheese	1 quesadilla	18.0	350	46%
chicken	1 quesadilla	19.0	400	43%
taco salad w/salsa	1 salad	52.0	850	55%
tostada	1 tostada	12.0	250	43%
■ TACOS				
Taco				
chicken/soft	1 taco	7.0	200	32%
Double Decker				
regular	1 taco	15.0	330	41%
Taco Supreme	1 taco	18.0	380	43%
plain				
original				
light	1 taco	5.0	140	32%
regular	1 taco	10.0	170	53%
soft				
light	1 taco	5.0	180	25%

Food and Description	Amount	Fat Grams	Total Calories	% Fat Calories
regular	1 taco	10.0	210	43%
steak, grilled/soft				
regular	1 taco	7.0	200	7%
Taco Supreme	1 taco	11.0	240	41%
Supreme				
original				
light	1 taco	5.0	160	28%
regular	1 taco	14.0	210	60%
soft	1 taco	13.0	260	45%
TACOTIME				
■ **BURRITOS**				
Casita	1 burrito	31.0	647	43%
Crisp				
bean	1 burrito	18.0	427	38%
chicken	1 burrito	25.0	422	53%
meat	1 burrito	30.0	552	49%
Double soft				
bean	1 serving	12.0	506	21%
combination	1 serving	23.0	617	34%
meat	1 serving	33.0	726	41%
Value soft/single				
bean	1 burrito	10.0	380	24%
meat	1 burrito	33.0	726	41%
■ **CONDIMENTS & INDIVIDUAL INGREDIENTS**				
cheese/cheddar	¾ oz	7.0	85	74%
chicken	2.5 oz	6.0	109	50%
chips	2 oz	12.0	266	41%
guacamole	1 oz	2.0	29	62%
taco				
meat	2.5 oz	11.0	208	48%
shell/6" dia	1 shell	6.0	110	49%
tortilla				
flour				
fried				
8" dia	1 tortilla	11.0	205	48%
10" dia	1 tortilla	16.0	318	45%
regular				
7" dia	1 tortilla	1.0	88	10%
8" dia	1 tortilla	3.0	107	25%
12" dia	1 tortilla	4.0	213	17%
wheat/11" dia	1 tortilla	3.0	175	15%
■ **SALADS & DRESSINGS**				
Dressings				
sour cream	3 Tbs	14.0	137	92%
thousand island	2 Tbs	16.0	160	34%
Salads				
chicken taco w/o dressing	1 salad	21.0	370	52%
taco salad w/o dressing	1 salad	28.0	479	53%
■ **SIDE ORDERS**				
Crustos	1 serving	15.0	373	36%

Food and Description	Amount	Fat Grams	Total Calories	% Fat Calories
empañada/cherry	1 empañada	9.0	250	32%
Mexican brown rice	1 serving	2.0	160	11%
Mexi-fries	regular	17.0	266	58%
	large	34.0	532	58%
nachos				
Deluxe	1 serving	57.0	1,048	49%
regular	1 serving	38.0	680	50%
quesadilla/cheese	3.25 oz	11.0	205	48%
refritos w/o cheese	1 serving	10.0	326	28%
■ TACOS				
Crisp	1 taco	17.0	295	52%
Natural Super Taco/meat	1 taco	27.0	627	39%
Soft				
chicken	1 taco	16.0	387	37%
rolled flour/plain	1 taco	23.0	512	40%
Super shredded beef	1 taco	11.0	368	27%
Taco				
cheeseburger w/meat	1 taco	36.0	633	51%
WENDY'S				
■ BEVERAGES				
coffee/regular & decaffeinated	6 fl oz	–	–	–
cola	1 small	–	90	–
diet cola	1 small	–	–	–
hot chocolate	6 fl oz	3.0	80	34%
lemonade	1 small	–	90	–
lemon-lime	1 small	–	90	–
milk/2% reduced fat	8 fl oz	4.0	110	33%
tea/hot or iced	6 fl oz	–	–	–
■ BUNS				
kaiser	1 bun	3.0	190	14%
sandwich	1 bun	2.5	160	14%
■ BURGERS				
Big Bacon Classic on kaiser bun	1 burger	30.0	580	47%
cheeseburger				
bacon/ junior	1 burger	19.0	380	45%
Deluxe	1 burger	17.0	360	43%
kid's meal/2 oz	1 burger	13.0	320	37%
regular				
deluxe junior	1 burger	16.0	360	40%
junior	1 burger	13.0	320	37%
hamburger				
junior	1 burger	10.0	270	33%
kid's meal	1 burger	10.0	270	33%
single				
plain	1 burger	16.0	360	40%
w/everything	1 burger	20.0	420	43%
hamburger patty only				
junior	1 patty	7.0	100	63%
¼ lb	1 patty	14.0	200	63%

Food and Description	Amount	Fat Grams	Total Calories	% Fat Calories
■ **CHICKEN**				
Chicken fillet only				
breaded	1 piece	12.0	230	47%
grilled	1 piece	3.0	110	25%
spicy	1 piece	9.0	110	74%
Chicken Nuggets & sauce				
chicken	5 pieces	14.0	210	60%
	4 pieces/kids	11.0	170	58%
sauce				
barbecue sauce only	1 pkt	–	45	–
honey mustard only	1 pkt	12.0	130	83%
spicy buffalo wingsauce	1 pkt	1.0	25	36%
Chicken Sandwiches				
breaded	1 sandwich	18.0	440	37%
club	1 sandwich	20.0	470	38%
grilled	1 sandwich	8.0	310	23%
spicy	1 sandwich	15.0	410	33%
■ **CHILI, CHEESE, & CRACKERS** (See SIDE ORDERS in this section)				
■ **DESSERT**				
chocolate chip cookie	1 cookie	13.0	270	43%
frosty-dairy	small	8.0	330	22%
	medium	11.0	440	23%
	large	14.0	540	23%
■ **PITAS/STUFFED**				
Pita Dressing				
Caesar vinaigrette	1 Tbs	7.0	70	90%
garden ranch	1 Tbs	4.5	50	81%
Pitas				
Chicken Caesar	1 pita	18.0	490	33%
Classic Greek	1 pita	20.0	440	41%
Garden Ranch Chicken	1 pita	18.0	480	34%
Garden Veggie	1 pita	17.0	400	39%
■ **SALADS & GARDEN SPOT SALAD BAR ITEMS**				
Fresh Salads				
Caesar side	1 salad	4.0	100	36%
Deluxe garden	1 salad	6.0	110	49%
grilled chicken	1 salad	8.0	200	36%
grilled chicken Caesar	1 salad	9.0	260	31%
side	1 salad	3.0	60	45%
taco	1 salad	19.0	380	45%
Garden Spot Salad Bar				
applesauce/chunky	2 Tbs	–	30	–
bacon bits	2 Tbs	2.5	45	50%
banana & strawberry glaze	¼ cup	–	30	–
breadstick/soft	1	3.0	130	21%
broccoli	¼ cup	–	14	–
cantaloupe	1 piece	–	15	–
carrots	¼ cup	–	5	–
cauliflower	¼ cup	–	–	–
cheese/shredded	2 Tbs	4.0	50	72%

Food and Description	Amount	Fat Grams	Total Calories	% Fat Calories
chicken salad	2 Tbs	5.0	70	64%
cottage cheese	2 Tbs	1.5	30	45%
croutons	2 Tbs	1.0	30	30%
cucumber	2 slices	–	–	–
eggs/hard-cooked	2 Tbs	3.0	40	68%
green peas	2 Tbs	–	15	–
green peppers	2 pieces	–	–	–
lettuce				
iceberg	1 cup	–	10	–
romaine	1 cup	–	10	–
mushrooms	¼ cup	–	–	–
orange/sliced	2 slices	–	15	–
Parmesan blend	2 Tbs	4.0	70	51%
pasta salad	2 Tbs	1.5	35	39%
peaches	1 piece	–	15	–
pepperoni/sliced	6 pieces	3.0	30	90%
potato salad	2 Tbs	7.0	80	79%
pudding/chocolate	¼ cup	3.0	70	39%
red onion	3 rings	–	–	–
sunflower seeds & raisins	2 Tbs	5.0	80	56%
taco chips	15 pieces	11.0	210	47%
tomato wedges	1 piece	–	5	–
turkey ham	2 Tbs	4.0	50	72%
watermelon	1 piece	–	20	–
Salad Dressings				
blue cheese	2 Tbs	19.0	180	95%
French				
fat-free	2 Tbs	–	35	–
regular	2 Tbs	10.0	120	75%
Italian				
Caesar	2 Tbs	16.0	150	96%
reduced fat	2 Tbs	3.0	40	68%
ranch/Hidden Valley				
reduced fat & calories	2 Tbs	5.0	60	75%
regular	2 Tbs	10.0	100	90%
salad oil	2 Tbs	14.0	120	100%
Thousand Island	2 Tbs	8.0	90	80%
wine vinegar	1 Tbs	–	–	–
■ SIDE ORDERS				
Baked potato				
bacon & cheese	1 serving	18.0	530	31%
broccoli & cheese	1 serving	14.0	470	27%
cheese	1 serving	23.0	570	36%
chili & cheese	1 serving	24.0	630	34%
plain	1 serving	–	310	–
sour cream & chives	1 serving	6.0	380	14%
sour cream only	1 pkt	6.0	60	90%
whipped margarine only	1 pkt	7.0	60	100%
Chili	small	7.0	210	30%
	large	10.0	310	29%

Food and Description	Amount	Fat Grams	Total Calories	% Fat Calories
cheddar cheese/only	2 Tbs	6.0	70	77%
crackers only	2 crackers	0.5	25	18%
French fries	small	13.0	270	43%
	biggie	23.0	470	44%
	great biggie	27.0	570	43%
WHATABURGER				
■ **BEVERAGES**				
Coca-Cola				
Cherry Coke	medium	–	227	–
classic	medium	–	217	–
Diet Coke	medium	–	1	–
coffee				
black	1 small	–	5	–
w/1 pkt cream	1 small	1.0	15	60%
w/1 pkt sugar	1 small	–	20	–
Dr. Pepper	medium	–	140	–
iced tea	medium	–	5	–
milk/2% reduced fat	1 serving	4.5	115	35%
orange juice	10 fl oz	–	140	–
root beer	medium	–	235	–
Shakes				
Chocolate	junior	9.0	365	22%
strawberry shake	junior	9.0	350	23%
vanilla shake	junior	9.5	325	26%
Sprite	medium	–	210	–
■ **BREAKFAST**				
Biscuit				
bacon	1 biscuit	20.0	359	50%
egg & cheese	1 biscuit	26.5	435	55%
egg, cheese, & bacon	1 biscuit	33.0	515	58%
egg, cheese, & sausage	1 biscuit	42.0	600	63%
gravy	1 biscuit	27.5	480	52%
plain	1 biscuit	13.5	280	43%
sausage	1 biscuit	29.0	450	58%
Breakfast platter				
w/bacon	1 serving	44.0	695	57%
w/sausage	1 serving	53.0	785	61%
Breakfast on a bun				
plain	1 serving	28.0	455	55%
w/bacon	1 serving	19.5	365	48%
Egg omelette sandwich	1 sandwich	13.0	290	40%
Hash browns	1 serving	9.0	150	54%
Mexican breakfast				
taquito				
potato	1 taquito	22.0	450	44%
sausage	1 taquito	26.0	445	53%
w/bacon	1 taquito	16.0	335	43%
Pancakes				
pancakes only	3 pancakes	6.0	260	21%
w/bacon	1 serving	12.4	335	33%

Food and Description	Amount	Fat Grams	Total Calories	% Fat Calories
w/sausage	1 serving	21.0	425	44%
Scrambled eggs	2 eggs	15.0	189	71%
Texas toast	1 slice	4.5	150	27%
■ **BURGERS & FAJITAS**				
Burgers				
Justaburger	1 burger	13.0	297	39%
Whataburger				
double meat	1 burger	42.0	823	46%
junior	1 burger	12.0	300	36%
regular	1 burger	26.0	298	39%
small bun, w/o oil	1 burger	19.0	410	42%
Fajita				
beef	1 fajita	12.0	326	33%
chicken	1 fajita	7.0	275	23%
■ **CHICKEN & FISH**				
chicken strips	2 pieces	20.0	300	60%
grilled chicken sandwich				
regular	1 sandwich	14.0	445	28%
small bun/w/mustard-no oil or dressing	1 sandwich	3.0	300	9%
w/o oil or salad dressing	1 sandwich	5.5	358	14%
w/o salad dressing	1 sandwich	8.5	385	20%
Whatacatch sandwich	1 sandwich	25.0	467	48%
Whatachick'n sandwich	1 sandwich	23.0	500	41%
■ **CONDIMENTS**				
bacon	1 slice	3.5	40	79%
butter	1 serving	4.0	36	100%
cheese slice	1 small	4.0	50	72%
	1 large	7.5	90	75%
grape jelly	1 serving	–	45	–
gravy/peppered chicken	3 oz	4.5	75	54%
honey	1 serving	–	25	–
jalapeño pepper	1 pepper	–	3	–
margarine	1 serving	3.0	25	100%
picante sauce	1 serving	–	5	–
sour cream	2 oz	12.0	125	86%
strawberry jam	1 serving	–	40	–
syrup	1 serving	–	180	–
Texas toast	1 slice	4.5	150	27%
■ **SALADS & RELATED ITEMS**				
club crackers	1 pkg	1.0	30	30%
croutons	1 pkg	1.0	30	30%
garden salad	1 serving	0.5	55	8%
grilled chicken salad	1 serving	1.5	150	9%
salad dressing				
French	1 pkt	21.0	260	73%
ranch	1 pkt	33.0	320	93%
Thousand Island	1 pkt	12.0	160	68%
vinaigrette/lite	1 pkt	2.0	40	45%
■ **SIDE ORDERS**				
baked potato				
plain	1 serving	0.5	310	1%

Food and Description	Amount	Fat Grams	Total Calories	% Fat Calories
w/broccoli & cheese	1 serving	10.0	463	20%
w/cheese	1 serving	16.5	510	29%
French fries	junior	12.0	221	49%
	regular	18.0	332	49%
	large	124.5	445	50%
onion rings	regular	19.0	330	52%
■ SWEETS				
apple turnover/fried	1 turnover	11.0	215	46%
blueberry muffin	1 muffin	8.0	240	30%
cinnamon roll	1 roll	16.0	320	45%
cookies				
chocolate chunk	1 cookie	16.0	250	58%
macadamia nut	1 cookie	16.0	270	53%
pecan Danish	1 Danish	16.0	270	53%
WHITE CASTLE				
■ BEVERAGES				
Coca-Cola				
Classic	20 oz	–	170	–
Diet	20 oz	–	1	–
coffee	small	–	5	–
iced tea	14 oz	–	45	–
shake/chocolate	20 oz	10.0	310	29%
■ BUN				
white bun	1 bun	<1.0	74	6%
■ BURGERS				
Cheeseburger				
bacon	1 burger	13.0	200	59%
double	1 burger	18.0	285	57%
single	1 burger	9.0	160	51%
Hamburger				
double	1 burger	14.0	235	54%
single	1 burger	7.0	135	47%
■ CHICKEN & FISH				
chicken sandwich	1 sandwich	8.0	190	38%
fish sandwich/w/o tartar sauce	1 sandwich	6.0	160	34%
■ CONDIMENTS				
onion chips	3.3 oz	17.0	329	47%
tartar sauce	1 Tbs	8.0	72	100%
■ SIDE ORDERS				
chicken rings	1 serving	21.0	310	61%
French fries	1 serving	6.0	115	47%
onion rings	1 serving	26.0	540	43%

Personal Food Diary

Date	Food	Amount	Fat Grams	Total Calories	% Fat Calories

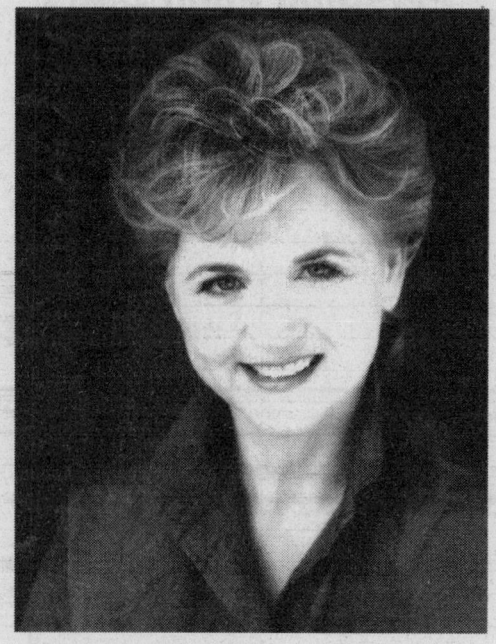

Karen J. Bellerson is the author of *The Shopper's Guide to Fat in Your Food* and *Low-Fat, No-Fat Cookbook*. She has been a nutritional consultant for fifteen years and makes her home in the Southwest.